W9-BAO-791

CONTENTS

Part 1: Introduction to Emerging Infectious Diseases

Part 2: Bacterial Infections

Part 3: Viral Infections

Part 4: Parasitic Infections

Part 5: Infectious Proteins

Part 6: Special Issues in Infectious Diseases

TABLES AND FIGURES

Tables

Figures

This book is dedicated to the health care professionals
at the front line in the battle against infectious diseases
and to the researchers who provide them with information
about the enemies and weapons to defeat them.

HEADLINES AND NEWS REPORTS warn of "Flesh-Eating Bacteria," "Mad Cow Disease," the AIDS pandemic, and flu pandemics. Drug-resistant bacteria are in our hospitals and our locker-rooms, malaria incidence is on the rise, and TB is reemerging. Every year, new infectious threats appear or old diseases spread to new areas or attack with greater viciousness. Some of the new diseases rear their heads and then suddenly vanish, like SARS, while others may be with humanity for the foreseeable future. The media warn and inform of the newly emerging diseases yet also may capitalize on public fears by overstating the real danger or describing the diseases in the most gruesome terms possible before moving on to the next "killer virus" predicted to kill tens of millions of people. Meanwhile, other, less spectacular diseases spread unnoticed through certain segments of the world's population (as babesiosis or cryptosporidiosis in immunosuppressed persons or dengue hemorrhagic fever in many parts of the world). This book attempts to provide a balanced overview of some of the emerging and reemerging diseases of current times. No single text could cover all of these diseases, but a number of illnesses have been selected which are found in different regions of the world. Many of these strike tropical regions or developing countries with particular virulence, others are found in temperate or developed areas, and still other microbes and infections are more indiscriminate. In five or ten years, other diseases may have emerged as major killers of humanity while some of the current threats may have been neutralized by the development of new drugs, vaccines, or other preventive measures. Poverty, civil unrest and war, and lack of access to modern health care supplies and facilities have fueled epidemics of some of the diseases covered in this book. If these underlying causes could be nullified or eliminated, many diseases would be controllable and large numbers of people freed from their crippling effects upon health and prosperity.

Since many of the infectious diseases presented in this book are relatively new or little information is known about the causative agent, much of the material has been derived from recent infectious disease journals or other related articles. Other timely information is derived from the Centers for Disease Control and Prevention, the World Health Organization, or MedLine Plus. The excellent

Emerging Infections series from the American Society for Microbiology have also provided much of the background material for this book.

This text has been written to accommodate several different groups of students, including but not limited to, upper-level undergraduate or graduate students in biology or medically-related professions, public health students, and persons already working in the healthcare arena. Not all of the information may be useful to every audience but the material (especially some of the immunology and microbiology) is presented for use by those who wish to have a greater understanding of how the microbes function and cause disease and how the human body attempts to remove or minimize the damage. This information may be skipped without losing understanding of the disease itself or its prevention and treatment.

The diseases are divided by type of causative agent: bacteria, viruses, protozoa, or infectious protein. Those chapters which deal with diseases induced by infection with a single organism or group of organisms are organized in a similar fashion: introduction, history, the disease(s), the causative agent(s), the immune response, diagnosis, treatment, prevention, and surveillance. The Major Concepts section presents a brief overview of the most important concepts found in the chapter. The Summary is a thumbnail sketch of the basic information about the microbe and the associated disease. Review Questions help students to test their knowledge of the material, while Topics for Further Discussion allow for a wider conversation of the implications of the disease and challenge students to "think outside of the box" to develop new solutions. There are no right answers or solutions to the material found within this section; rather, it is hoped that any students entering into the medical or research fields, as well as those destined to serve in public health, may learn to search for innovative ways of dealing with health-related problems.

The two introductory chapters provide basic information that will be useful for the other chapters, including an introduction to emerging and reemerging infectious diseases, proposed causes for disease emergence, very basic microbiology, and very basic immunology. The latter is included since a discussion of disease needs to include how the host attempts to defend itself as well as what can go wrong with this "protective" response. The last two chapters cover topics of particular interest. Chapter Twenty-Nine discusses emerging diseases in immunocompromised individuals since the numbers of people in this group are increasing rapidly, posing unique challenges to public health. Chapter Thirty describes several of the agents that may be used in acts of bioterrorism. Many of these agents have already been used for this purpose. Hopefully, the spread of knowledge about the threat of bioterrorism will discourage its usage in the future.

New Philadelphia, Ohio   Lisa A. Beltz
February 2011

D R. LISA A. BELTZ is an assistant professor in the Department of Biology at Kent State University at Tuscarawas, in New Philadelphia, Ohio. She has taught a number of medically-related biology courses during her 14 years of teaching at Kent State University and the University of Northern Iowa. Prior to teaching, she studied two of the diseases described in this book. While a graduate student at Michigan State University, she examined the mechanisms by which *Trypanosoma cruzi* inhibits human immune responses, allowing the parasite to kill large numbers of people in Central and South America. Later, at Johns Hopkins University and the University of Pittsburgh, she studied interactions between the simian and human immunodeficiency viruses and bone marrow cells as well as exploring the mechanisms by which HIV kills white blood cells. Dr. Beltz was the co-originator of the course Cancer and Emerging Infectious Diseases during her time in Iowa. The need for a college-level textbook in this field became apparent over her seven years of teaching the course. Dr. Beltz's more recent research has involved studying the impact of nitrate and other environmental contaminants on the human immune system and studying the effects of green tea components upon normal and cancerous white blood cells.

ACKNOWLEDGMENTS

I WOULD LIKE TO THANK the following reviewers for their time and many helpful suggestions: Gokul Das, John E. Gustafson, Kathy Hanley, Carrie Horwich, Frank Jenkins, Stanley Katz, and Terri Rebmann. Mr. Andrew Pasternak and Seth Schwartz of Jossey-Bass played major roles in the writing of this text. Their ideas shaped the book and guided every step of its creation. I am also grateful for the support of the faculty and administration of Kent State University at Tuscarawas and Kent State University at Kent, particularly Dean Gregg Andrews from the Tuscarawas Campus, Dr. James Blank, Chair of the Department of Biology, Dr. Christopher Fenk, and Dr. Donald Gerbig. They provided me with the time and atmosphere in which to develop my ideas into the final product. Finally, I wish to thank my family for their patience and encouragement during the writing process.

—*L.A.B.*

INTRODUCTION TO EMERGING INFECTIOUS DISEASES

CHAPTER 1

INFECTIOUS DISEASES PAST AND PRESENT

LEARNING OBJECTIVES

- Discuss the roles of plague and smallpox in human history

- Discuss the most important infectious diseases in the world today

- Discuss the linkages between infectious diseases, poverty, and civil unrest

- Describe a number of emerging and reemerging infectious diseases found in the Americas, outside of the Americas, and throughout the world

- Discuss a number of factors contributing to the emergence or reemergence of infectious diseases

- Gain a sense of the number of new infectious diseases that have emerged recently and the rapid pace of discovery of the microbes responsible, development of antimicrobial drugs, and evolution of microbial drug resistance

Major Concepts

History

Infectious diseases have had a great impact on human history, killing vast numbers of persons and disabling or disfiguring many others. Some diseases have transformed the social and economic landscape of a region, as when the decline in the peasant population following the Black Death contributed to the end of the feudal system. The fight against smallpox led to the development of vaccination, a weapon in the human arsenal that prevented major loss of life by protecting people from a wide range of diseases. Due to an ever-better understanding of the causative agents of infectious diseases, other tools have been developed to prevent or treat illnesses, including improved sanitation, greater availability of clean drinking water, the increased use of disinfectants, the discovery of antimicrobial compounds, and improvements in the inspection, processing, and preparation of food and drink. The incidence and severity of infectious diseases have fallen in developed nations but are again on the rise worldwide.

Infectious Diseases Today

The leading causes of death due to infectious diseases in the world today are lower respiratory tract infections, diarrheal diseases, HIV/AIDS, tuberculosis, malaria, and dengue hemorrhagic fever and shock syndrome. Many of the victims of these diseases belong to the most vulnerable segments of our population, the very young and the very old, those weakened by other pathological conditions, and those with compromised immune responses. Many other diseases affect smaller segments of humankind. Some of these preferentially strike those living in certain climates or ecosystems, in lower socioeconomic groups, or in regions of civil unrest and war. Other diseases are more prevalent in some racial groups, age ranges, occupations, or one gender. Still other diseases are indiscriminate killers. Incidence of some diseases peaks in certain seasons, while others occur year round.

Emerging and Reemerging Infectious Diseases

Many diseases have either been described for the first time within the past 40 to 50 years or have increased in incidence, severity, or geographical range. This text focuses on a number of such diseases and the associated microbes. Several factors in combination have contributed to the explosion of emerging and reemerging infectious diseases in recent times (as evidenced by the Timeline at the end of this chapter). Our awareness of new infections may be due in part to improved detection and understanding of the underlying causes of illness. Many of the emerging diseases, however, appear to be entirely new to humans, while many reemerging diseases represent increasing threats to humankind. Several of the factors believed to contribute to the emergence or reemergence of infectious diseases include microbial evolution, the trend toward increasing urbanization, population migrations between regions or into formerly uninhabited areas, the ease and speed of long-distance movement of persons and materials, natural disasters, climatic and ecological changes, and decreased vaccination rates in many regions of the world. One of the important factors contributing to the rapid emergence of new infections is the increasingly large numbers of immunocompromised individuals who are vulnerable to the development of severe or life-threatening diseases as a result of infection by organisms formerly viewed as nonpathogenic.

History of Infectious Diseases

Much of the history of humankind has been critically shaped by infectious diseases. Large, widespread outbreaks of bubonic, pneumonic, and septicemic plague, caused by infection with *Yersinia pestis*, have struck repeatedly, including the Plague of Justinian from 542 to 767, which killed 40 million people in Europe and Asia Minor and initiated the Dark Ages, and the Black Death, lasting from the fourteenth to eighteenth centuries. The latter began in Central Asia and subsequently spread to China, India, and Asia Minor, entering Italy in 1347. Twenty-five to fifty percent of the population of Europe succumbed to the plague within the next three years, leading to the death of many peasants and the abandonment of much of the agricultural land. The resulting food shortage and loss of an abundant workforce rendered the existing governments ineffective. These were major factors in the eventual collapse of the feudal system and the rise of middle-class artisans. Improvements in sanitation were also implemented due to lessons learned during the plague years.

Smallpox is another disease that changed the face of human history, quite literally, for over three thousand years, afflicting humans with horrific and disfiguring scars, blindness, and death for most of our known existence. Its eradication has been one of our greatest achievements.

The rich and powerful were not spared the attention of this deadly pestilence. Scars were even found on the mummy of the Egyptian pharaoh Ramses V. Throughout the ages, the fatality rate often approached 30%, with 65% to 80% of the survivors left with pockmarks on their faces as reminders of their ordeal. As late as the 1700s, 10% to 14% of the children in France, Sweden, and Russia died of smallpox. Surviving the disease was almost a rite of passage, and no parent could be totally at ease until his or her children had vanquished that most dreaded foe.

FIGURE 1.1   Child with smallpox

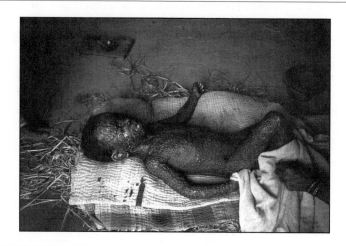

Source: CDC/Jean Roy.

"The smallpox was always present," wrote T. B. Macaulay, "filling the churchyards with corpses, tormenting with constant fears all whom it had stricken, leaving on those whose lives it spared the hideous traces of its power, turning the babe into a changeling at which the mother shuddered, and making the eyes and cheeks of the betrothed maiden objects of horror to the lover."

It was observed in China over a thousand years ago that survivors of smallpox did not contract the disease again, even after extended exposure to infected persons. It was additionally discovered that inoculation of previously unexposed persons with material from dried smallpox scabs derived from persons with mild cases of the disease often safeguarded the inoculated persons against developing severe infection at a later time. This practice was known as **variolation** and occasionally resulted in death. Variolation was brought to Europe in 1721 by Lady Mary Wortley Montagu, the wife of the British ambassador to Turkey. Decades later, Edward Jenner acted on the common observation that milkmaids, who typically developed the mild disease cowpox, did not later suffer from smallpox or develop the hideous scars present on most members of society. In 1796, he modified the practice of variolation by inoculating a young boy, James Phipps, with material from cowpox scabs and subsequently challenging him with smallpox. Fortunately for James (and humanity), the boy was protected.

Thus began the age of **vaccination**, which ultimately led to the eradication of smallpox as a result of the concerted efforts of many dedicated individuals working under difficult conditions throughout the world for a decade. The program featured the quarantine of patients and their contacts as well as vaccination of all

FIGURE 1.2   Sign announcing smallpox vaccination

INOCULATION

Those who are desirous to take the infection of the SMALL - POX, by inoculation, may find themselves accommodated for the purpose, by applying to.

Stephen Samuel Hawley

Fiskdale, in Sturbridge.

February 7, 1801

N. B.   A Pest-House will be opened, and accommodations provided by the first day of March next.

Source: CDC.

potential contacts. Ali Maalin from Somalia is believed to have acquired the last naturally occurring case of smallpox in 1977. Several subsequent cases occurred several years later in England following viral escape from a laboratory.

While smallpox remains the only disease that humans have totally eliminated from nature, the lessons learned during this triumph of humans over one of its most deadly foes have been applied many times in subsequent years. Highly effective vaccines have been developed and brought into widespread use to tame other serious microbial diseases such as polio, whooping cough, German measles, mumps, and tetanus. The science of epidemiology, initiated by John Snow to trace the source of a cholera epidemic in London in the 1850s to a specific water pump, transformed public health. The "germ theory of disease," developed by Louis Pasteur, Robert Koch, John Lister, and others in the 1860s, revolutionized beliefs concerning the origins of diseases. These developments—along with improvements in sanitation, the availability of clean drinking water, practices such as pasteurization and sterilization of beverages and food, increased use of disinfectants, the discovery of antimicrobial compounds such as antibiotics (discussed in Chapter Eleven) and antiviral drugs, improvement in the inspection of meat and processing facilities, more thorough cooking of meat and eggs, and educational programs—eventually served as tipping points for many infectious diseases in the developed areas of the world. The numbers of cases of microbial illnesses dramatically declined: the incidence of tuberculosis, malaria, cholera, and many other diseases fell either regionally or around the world. Many persons in the public health arena in the early 1970s declared an imminent end to threats by infectious diseases.

The victory dance proved premature. A number of factors reversed the gains made in humankind's war against pathogenic microbes. Diseases thought to be on the brink of extinction reemerged with a vengeance, and many new devastating diseases, including AIDS and a variety of hemorrhagic fevers, began to appear at an alarming rate. Rather than an end to the war against microbes, we were surprised to find ourselves facing fresh troops and new enemies. The battle continues as both sides reassess their strategies and struggle to develop new weapons better suited to the continuingly evolving situation.

The Role of Infectious Diseases in the World Today

A number of serious infectious diseases affect humans currently. The type of microbe, the mode of transmission, and the incidence of disease within a population or region varies according to income levels and socioeconomic status, age, gender, type of employment, general health parameters, social customs, housing preferences, climate and ecology of the region (temperature and rainfall; woodland versus prairie versus coastline), and the types and abundance of vector and reservoir species. Many of the diseases strike primarily members of the population with poor immune responses: the very young, the elderly, pregnant women, and immunocompromised individuals. Some infectious diseases, including Lyme disease and hantavirus pulmonary syndrome, preferentially strike men and women between the ages of 20 and 40. Other serious illnesses, such as pandemic influenza, are more indiscriminate with regard to their victims' age. Due to differences in occupational exposure and recreational activity, some infectious diseases, among them the American hemorrhagic fevers and ehrlichiosis, strike men more frequently than women because males are more likely to spend time working in the cornfields and on cattle ranges or hunting and fishing in the wooded areas where the rodent or insect vectors of these diseases are found. Others are more common among women. One such example is the prion disease kuru, which afflicted women exposed to prions while preparing brains for consumption during funeral rites. Persons in poor overall health are more likely to succumb to infectious diseases. Once infected with one microorganism, individuals are more susceptible to other infections due to generalized immunosuppression. Social customs may increase infectious disease incidence as exemplified by funeral rites that exposed women to the Ebola virus. The type of housing common to a given region also affects disease incidence. People living in homes with thatched roofs and no screened windows or doors are exposed to disease vectors, as seen with

Chagas' disease in South America, where the "kissing bug" vector bites humans sleeping in the thatched huts at night. Tropical areas are home to many, but not all, of the emerging infections presented in this book. A hot, humid environment may support large populations of insect vectors year round. Some microbes are unable to survive in colder environments. Vector and reservoir species availability also influences the spread of diseases. Chagas' disease is moving into parts of the southern United States, where the insect vector can survive the winters and where abundant small mammals are present to serve as reservoir hosts.

The population of immunosuppressed individuals in both developed and developing regions is increasing, leading to the emergence or reemergence of many infectious diseases. The AIDS pandemic has been responsible for much of this increase, especially in developing regions. Organisms other than HIV, such as Epstein-Barr virus (causative agent of mononucleosis) and herpesviruses, suppress immune reactivity. The aging of the population in developed regions is also a factor because various immune system components either decrease in mass (thymus), numbers (some populations of T lymphocytes), or effectiveness (T and B lymphocytes, natural killer cells) as persons age. Diabetes and cancer chemotherapy also compromise immune response. The incidence of both diabetes and cancer is increasing in developed nations due to obesity and recent alterations in diet, exercise, lifestyle, and occupation.

Depression also adversely affects various aspects of the immune response because functions of the central nervous system and the immune system are

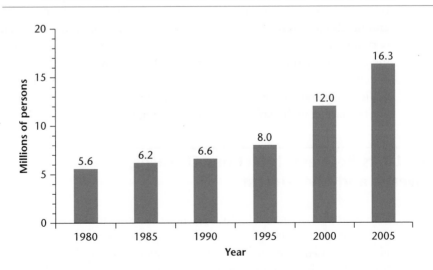

FIGURE 1.3   Incidence of diabetes in the United States

closely linked. Anti-inflammatory medications that are used to treat autoimmune disorders, such as rheumatoid arthritis, Crohn's disease, psoriasis, and systemic lupus erythematosus (such as corticosteroids), suppress lymphocyte responses and increase susceptibility to infectious diseases, such as tuberculosis and staphylococcal infections.

Several infectious diseases cause a great degree of suffering and death in the world today. Lower respiratory tract infections are caused by several bacteria, viruses, and protozoa, including *Streptococcus pneumoniae, Haemophilus influenza,* respiratory syncytia virus, influenza viruses, parainfluenza viruses, and *Pneumocysitis jiroveci* (formerly *P. carinii*). These together constitute the leading cause of death due to infectious disease. Diarrheal diseases are the second leading infectious cause of death throughout the world and are the primary cause of malnutrition. Diarrheal organisms include *Vibrio cholerae, Shigella* spp., *Campylobacter* spp., *Salmonella* spp., rotavirus, *Cryptosporidium* spp., *E. coli,* and *Giardia lamblia.* Children under the age of 2 years are most vulnerable to these infections, and 1.5 million children die annually of diarrheal disease. HIV/AIDS is the single leading infectious cause of death. In 2007, some 33 million persons were living with HIV, and 2.7 million new infections were recorded. Approximately 2 million HIV-related deaths occur each year, and 25 million persons have died from AIDS since the mid-1980s. The tuberculosis bacterium infects about one-third of the world's population and killed almost 1.6 million people in 2007. Many people are coinfected with HIV and *M. tuberculosis:* indeed, tuberculosis is one of the leading causes of death in HIV-positive persons. Malaria caused around 1 million deaths in 2005, and 247 million persons were infected with the parasite responsible. Very young African children are especially vulnerable to infection and death and average 1.6 to 5.4 episodes of malarial fever per year. We are currently in the midst of a pandemic caused by the dengue virus, resulting in the extremely painful dengue fever ("breakbone fever") or the very dangerous dengue hemorrhagic fever, which has a high fatality rate if untreated. Fifty-six million infections occur each year, and the number of cases and disease range are increasing, with explosive outbreaks being reported.

The Links Between Infectious Diseases, Poverty, and Civil Unrest

Infectious diseases continue to be major causes of human death in the world. This is particularly true for areas that are gripped by poverty and the associated ills of decreased access to clean drinking water, malnutrition, overcrowding, substandard housing that does not fully protect against physical or biological threats (temperature extremes, wetness or dryness, insects, and rodents), inadequate health care, and poor educational opportunities. These factors combine to undermine the health of infants, children, and adults in the affected regions, leaving them vulnerable to infectious illnesses. Exposure to insect and rodent vectors in the home increases the spread of pathogenic microbes responsible for diseases such as bubonic plague, malaria, yellow fever, and Lassa fever. Contaminated water supplies transmit diseases such as cholera and schistosomiasis. Overcrowded living conditions, such those found in the slums of major urban centers, homeless shelters, and some prisons, nursing homes, and mental health facilities, permit the rapid spread of infections such as tuberculosis and typhus. Women may be forced into prostitution to obtain money for food for themselves and their children, increasing their risk of acquiring sexually transmitted diseases such as AIDS and syphilis. Children born of infected mothers may become infected in utero, during labor, or via contaminated breast milk. Persons addicted to drugs or alcohol may live in poverty or turn to prostitution in order to obtain funds to feed their habit.

Once individuals in a poverty-stricken region have acquired an infectious disease, they are unlikely to receive adequate treatment due to the inability to pay for services and medications or the lack of health care facilities and practitioners in close proximity to their residence. Many impoverished regions are located in remote areas with few roads. Most of the population may not own a motor vehicle to allow travel to distant sites, and fuel may be either too expensive or too scarce to permit its use by the majority of persons. Roads may be in poor condition or impassable during the wet season. Many governments may be unable or unwilling to provide basic health services or emergency care. Educational programs that could reduce disease incidence or severity are often of limited value because much of the population may not own televisions or radios and may not read newspapers due to illiteracy.

Poverty and disease often form a vicious circle that entraps large regions of the world today. As noted, poverty may set the stage for sickness. Sickness may then deepen the poverty of an area as individuals who could have been vital members of the workforce, producing food and bringing money into the region, are too ill to be fully productive or to work at all. Corporations may be unwilling to bring factories into regions with ill workers. Areas of sub-Saharan Africa suffer from decreased tourism as travelers hesitate to expose themselves to tropical diseases, some of which are difficult to prevent or treat. Ill children may have frequent absences from school. Some infectious diseases impede children's physical and cognitive development, interfering with their ability to learn the information and skills necessary to lead themselves and their societies out of the grip of poverty and increasing the distance between developed and developing regions of the world.

Many regions of the world suffer under the twin burdens of poverty and civil unrest. Civil wars as well as wars between nations force mass population movements. Combatants and refugees carry diseases from an indigenous region to other areas. Agricultural activity and economic development are challenged. Refugee camps may be hotbeds of infectious disease due to overcrowding, inadequate clean water supplies, lack of proper sanitation facilities, and malnutrition. Areas of active combat are barriers to transportation of food, medicine, and vaccines, not only to the involved area but also to areas served by the associated roads or waterways. Civil unrest and wars disrupt the fabric of society and may tear apart the social mores of the culture. This may further the spread of disease as sexual practices change in manners conducive to microbial transmission.

The role of infectious disease in the world today is linked to a region's income level. In the world as a whole, coronary heart disease and stroke and cerebrovascular disease were the leading causes of death, responsible for 12.2% and 9.7% of the deaths, respectively, in 2004, according to the World Health Organization. Four of the remaining ten leading causes of death in the world are due to infectious diseases (lower respiratory tract infections, 7.1%; diarrheal diseases, 3.7%; HIV/AIDS, 3.5%; and tuberculosis, 2.5%; total, 16.8%). Among low-income countries, six of the ten leading causes of death were infectious diseases (lower respiratory tract infections, 11.2%; diarrheal diseases, 6.9%; HIV/AIDS, 5.7%; tuberculosis, 3.5%; neonatal infections, 3.4%; and malaria, 3.3%; total, 34.0%). In middle-income countries, on the other hand, two of the ten major causes of death were of an infectious nature (lower respiratory tract infections, 3.8%, and tuberculosis, 2.2%). Among high-income countries, only one of the ten leading causes of death in 2004 was an infectious disease (lower respiratory tract infections, 3.8%). Less than 25% of the people in low income countries live to the age of 70 years, and more than one-third of the deaths are among individuals under the age of 14 years. In middle-income countries, almost 50% of the population dies after the age of 70, and that figure exceeds 67% in high-income countries. The proportion of deaths among those under the age of 14 years is 10% and 1% in middle- and high-income countries, respectively.

Emerging and Reemerging Infectious Diseases

No one textbook can cover the vast numbers of **emerging and reemerging infectious diseases** that have either been discovered during the past four to five decades or have greatly increased in incidence or virulence regionally or worldwide during that time. A number of these have been selected for inclusion in this book. These include viral, bacterial, and protozoan infections and a number of important diseases found in both tropical and temperate and both developed and developing regions of the world. Some of these are familiar to the general public, while others are virtually unknown even to most members of the medical community in the developed world. The sheer number of new infectious organisms and their spread to novel geographical regions complicates the tasks of physicians, nurses, public health agencies, epidemiologists, and legislators in their roles of safeguarding the general population against infection. This text attempts to draw attention to a subset of these diseases, some of which were once as obscure and remote as slim disease in Africa was to health care personnel before the recognition of the AIDS pandemic. The health and lives of billions of people in the future relies on vigilance of health workers to trends in old diseases and to the emergence of others.

The following diseases are presented in this book:

Diseases Found Primarily in the Americas

- Lyme disease: multisymptom disease transmitted by tick bite; includes rash, arthritis, neurological manifestations

- Ehrlichiosis: potentially serious or fatal bacterial infection of white blood cells; transmitted by tick bite

- Hantavirus pulmonary syndrome: severe to fatal respiratory disease found most commonly in the American Southwest; deer mice serve as disease reservoirs

- West Nile encephalitis in the United States: results in rare but serious neurological disease; transmitted by mosquito bite

- American hemorrhagic fevers: hemorrhagic fevers with high fatality rates found in South and North America; rodents serve as reservoir species

- Chagas' disease in the United States: potentially fatal parasitic infection of the blood that leads to cardiac failure; transmitted by "kissing bugs"

Diseases That Occur Primarily Elsewhere in the World

- Marburg and Ebola hemorrhagic fevers: hemorrhagic fevers with high fatality rates found primarily in Africa

- Lassa fever: a hemorrhagic fever found primarily in western Africa; transmitted by inhalation of contaminated rodent excreta

- Monkeypox: a potentially fatal smallpoxlike disease found primarily in Central Africa; transmitted directly between humans

- Malaria (reemergent and newly drug-resistant): potentially fatal parasitic infection of red blood cells; transmitted by mosquito bites

- Variant Creutzfeldt-Jakob disease and other transmissible spongiform enceph-alopathies: fatal neurological diseases caused by an infectious protein; trans-mitted between humans or by consumption of infected beef

Diseases That Occur Around the World

- Drug-resistant bacteria: includes methicillin- and vancomycin-resistant bac-teria as well as drug-resistant strains of *Pseudomonas aeruginosa* and *Streptococcus pneumoniae*

- Group A streptococci: cause potentially fatal infections such as scarlet fever, necrotizing fasciitis, childbed fever, and toxic shock syndrome

- Legionnaires' disease: a potentially fatal respiratory infection; transmitted by inhalation of bacteria in aerosolized water droplets

- Dengue fever: an extremely painful disease that may progress to the often fatal dengue hemorrhagic fever or dengue shock syndrome

- *Escherichia coli* O157:H7: causes potentially fatal diseases such as hemolytic uremic syndrome and hemorrhagic colitis; transmitted by the oral-fecal route

- *Helicobacter pylori:* causes peptic ulcers and hepatocellular carcinoma

- *Bartonella* species: cause several potentially serious diseases including cat-scratch fever, trench fever, and bacillary angiomatosis

- HIV/AIDS: fatal immunosuppressive disease; transmitted through sexual contact or blood

- Kaposi's sarcoma: cancer caused by human herpesvirus-8 that can be fatal to HIV-positive persons

- Hepatitis C: potentially fatal liver disease caused by a bloodborne virus

- Severe acute respiratory syndrome (SARS): potentially fatal respiratory illness; transmitted via inhalation

- Influenza: pandemic influenza strains result in widespread loss of life; trans-mitted via inhalation

- Tuberculosis: reemergent lung disease that has become resistant to many com-monly used drugs; transmitted by inhalation

- *Cryptosporidium:* causes severe diarrheal disease with a high fatality rate in immunosuppressed persons; transmitted via contaminated water or food

- Babesiosis: potentially fatal parasitic infection of red blood cells; transmitted by tick bite

Other chapters discuss diseases that particularly imperil persons with suppressed immunity (a rapidly growing segment of human societies) and the emerging threat of biological warfare agents.

In addition to the diseases covered in this book, many others are being studied by researchers around the world. For example, in the journal *Emerging Infectious Diseases*, published by the Centers for Disease Control and Prevention, the following microbes or diseases were discussed in the September 2009 issue: avian bornaviruses, *Baylisascaris*, bluetongue virus, bocavirus, *Campylobacter* enteritis, *Candida dubliniensis*, *Chlamydia*, feline infectious peritonitis virus, foot-and-mouth disease, *Gordonia sputa*, hantavirus, Kyasnur Forest disease virus, Merkel cell polyomavirus, rhinovirus C, rotavirus, Saffold cardiovirus, strongyloidiasis, Zika virus, and zygomycosis. The following were covered in the October 2009 issue: acute Q fever, Aichi virus, anthrax, *Borrelia hispanica* relapsing fever, coxsackievirus, human bocavirus 2, Japanese encephalitis virus, leishmaniasis, lymphocytic choriomeningitis virus, melioidosis, nontuberculosis mycoplasma infection, novel arenavirus in southern Africa, plague, *Pneumonocystis jirovecii*, rabies, rickettsia, *Salmonella enterica*, and scrub typhus.

Factors Contributing to the Emergence of New Infectious Diseases and the Spread and Evolution of Older Diseases

A number of factors have led to the recent increase in the emergence and reemergence of infectious diseases. One trivial factor may be increased awareness of a disease or the discovery of an infectious cause for an old affliction. An example of the latter is our relatively recent awareness of the bacterium *H. pylori* as the cause of peptic ulcers and hepatocellular carcinoma. In many cases, however, older diseases have either undergone increases in incidence or virulence regionally or throughout the world or novel diseases have appeared in the human population. Some of these changes result from microbial evolution through mutation of their DNA or RNA or by the acquisition of new genetic material in the form of plasmids or via transformation or transduction by a bacteriophage. Some microbes, such as influenza and HIV, have rapid mutation rates: influenza viruses of pigs, birds, and humans may exchange RNA if they happen to infect the same cell, and HIV uses an error-prone enzyme during replication and lacks a repair mechanism. The pathogenic *E. coli* O157:H7 contains several virulence factors that are borne on either a plasmid or a bacteriophage that has infected the bacterium. These changes in genetic material allow the development of drug-resistant microbes, followed by natural selection processes that are fueled by factors such as medicinal overuse of drugs, agricultural practices, patient noncompliance with correct drug dosage, and failure to complete the course of treatment.

Several additional factors involve the movements of individuals or groups. One such factor is the trend toward increasing **urbanization**, which has moved drawn numbers of people away from their lives in traditional villages to large population centers with different social customs and moral values concerning sexual practices. The rapid increase in city size has not allowed the time and resources necessary for careful planning, resulting in haphazard growth and the appearance of huge slum areas with overcrowded, shoddy housing and very limited access to sanitary waste disposal facilities and clean water for drinking, cooking, bathing, and laundering clothing.

Another factor, noted earlier, is the mass migration of populations (civilians or military personnel) that occurs during war or civil unrest and the result-ing spread of disease to new areas, especially under conditions that also allow movement of disease vectors or reservoir species. Such population movements occurred during the exploration and colonization of the Americas and the importation of slaves followed by the introduction of European and African diseases into New World groups, often with disastrous results for the indigenous peoples. During the Pacific campaign of World War II, North American and European soldiers serving in Asia were heavily afflicted by tropical maladies such as malaria, dysentery, and typhoid fever.

A third factor is the rapid movement of individuals and materials by modern transportation systems. A person may travel around the world by air in several days, carrying pathogenic microbes to a wide range of new hosts. A recent outbreak of mumps was linked to an infected individual flying into and out of a number of American cities within the span of a week. SARS traveled from China to Toronto's Chinatown in a similar manner in 2003. Infected vector spe-cies may also bring diseases into new areas, as occurred with the arrival of West Nile virus via its mosquito vector on a ship that arrived in New York Harbor in the summer of 1999. Reservoir hosts may also travel illicitly aboard ships, as the rats bearing bubonic plague from Asia to California did in the 1800s. Other infected reservoir hosts may be imported as pets (monkeypox-infected African rodents were brought into the United States in 2003) or for medical research purposes (Marburg hemorrhagic fever broke out in Germany and Yugoslavia in 1967 in primate centers housing African green monkeys).

A fourth factor is the settlement and clearing of "virgin" territory for farm-ing in the rain forests of South America, Asia, and Africa. This brought humans into greater contact with new species of animals and disrupted existing ecosys-tems, allowing the emergence of diseases such as Argentine hemorrhagic fever due to shifts in rodent populations inhabiting the newly developed cornfields in the Pampas and the emergence of HIV in humans, believed by many to have entered people when a macaque infected with the simian immunodeficiency virus bit a farmer trying to carve out a living in the rain forests of sub-Saharan Africa.

Natural disasters and climatic factors play roles in disease emergence. A natural disaster triggered a large outbreak of bubonic and pneumonic plague in India in 1994 after a long disease-free period. It was believed to have been initiated by changes resulting from a large earthquake and its aftershocks, followed by mass population movements and rapid expansion of a population of rats that were particularly suited to host and transmit *Yersinia pestis* to humans.

Climatic factors contributed to the recent appearance of a new respiratory disease in the United States. The mild winter and wet spring accompanying El Niño in the southeastern United States in 1993 led to an unusual abundance of pinyon nuts in the Four Corners region of Arizona, New Mexico, Colorado, and Utah. The deer mouse population of that region exploded, leading to crowding among the mice and their increased contact with the Navaho residents of the area. Some members of the mouse population were infected with Sin Nombre virus, which subsequently spread to numerous other mice and then to humans, leading to the first reported outbreak of the often fatal hantavirus pulmonary syndrome. Navaho folklore had previously warned of death stalking the people following a mild winter with many pinyon nuts.

Other factors contributing to the emergence or reemergence of infectious diseases are functions of health care systems. One such factor is the recent decline in quality and availability of local and national health services in many areas of the world, including much of Africa and the former Soviet Union. Changing national alliances at the conclusion of the colonial era decreased the input of European funds for building and maintenance of clinics and hospitals, medical supplies, and personnel. It also set in motion a long series of vicious battles for control of the regions by differing ethnic or religious groups, rival chieftains, and various political factions. Some of the resulting warfare continues to the present. Another factor leading to disease reemergence is decreased vaccination. Many parents in developed countries, including the United States, choose to not vaccinate their children against many potentially serious infectious agents such as the polio virus, the mumps virus, and *Pertussis* (the causative agent of whooping cough). These diseases are no longer common in developed countries, lulling many persons into a false sense of security that is occasionally shattered, as witnessed by the mumps outbreak in Iowa early in this century and the reemergence of measles in children in some parts of the United States. Other parents fear that vaccination may increase the risk for their children to develop autism, a claim based on small bits of unreliable research. Other vaccines, such as that formerly used to protect against smallpox, are no longer widely available. The agent used in the smallpox vaccine, vaccinia virus, may cause serious disease, and the natural transmission cycle of smallpox has been broken for three decades. Despite the inherent risks associated with that particular vaccine, immunization with vaccinia virus during the smallpox eradication program did appear to decrease incidence and severity of monkeypox in humans. Vials of smallpox virus still officially exist in Biosafety Level 4 facilities in the United States and the Russian Federation. A former Soviet bioweapons researcher also claims that very large stocks of the virus are in the hands of terrorist states and could conceivably be used in a bioterrorism attack against the world's almost totally unprotected population.

A major factor influencing the emergence and increased virulence of infectious diseases is the large increase in the numbers of immunosuppressed persons throughout the world today. As noted earlier, a variety of factors lead to decreased competence of the immune system. Immunocompromised individuals, especially HIV-positive persons in late-stage AIDS with extremely low numbers of $CD4^+$ T helper cells, are very vulnerable to infection by a number of microbes, with greater morbidity and higher mortality rates. Many of the diseases covered in this text may be included in this category. These include ehrlichiosis and anaplasmosis; monkeypox; malaria; necrotizing fasciitis following group A streptococcal infection; Legionnaires' disease; life-threatening manifestations of *E. coli* infection; bacillary angiomatosis, bacillary peliosis hepatis, and endocarditis induced by infection by *Bartonella* spp.; infection by human herpesvirus-8 and Kaposi's sarcoma; *Cryptosporidium*-induced diarrheal disease; and babesiosis. Persons with compromised immunity are also vulnerable to potentially fatal manifestations of disease caused by other infectious agents, including gram-positive cocci such as *Enterococcus faecalis* and *E. faecium;* gram-negative bacilli such as *Pseudomonas aeruginosa;* intracellular bacteria such as *Salmonella* and *Listeria monocytogenes;* fungi such as *Candida* spp., *Aspergillus* spp., and *Fusarium* spp., and other organisms such as the *Mycobacterium avium* complex and *Cyclospora*. If the numbers of immunocompromised persons continue to increase, we may expect to see new illnesses arise due to infection of this population by long-established human pathogens.

Timeline

The accompanying timeline traces some of the important events in the history of the emerging infections covered in this book. The incidence of emerging infections has increased in the past several decades, and new organisms have been discovered. The times when antibiotics were first used and resistance to them developed are also listed.

Timeline for Emerging Infectious Diseases

Before 50,000 B.C.	*Helicobacter pylori* (cause of gastric ulcers) believed to have colonized humans in Africa
5000 B.C.	Evidence of tuberculosis found in human bones
1000 B.C.	Hippocrates described disease characterized by lung nodules matching the description of tubercles found in tuberculosis
A.D. 300s	Artemisinin used in China to treat malaria (*Plasmodium* infection)
1600s	Quinine used in South America to treat malaria
1664	Description of scarlet fever (infection with group A streptococci)
1730	Scrapie (prion) discovered in sheep
1736	Major outbreak of severe scarlet fever in the American colonies
Mid-1800s	Beginning of quinine resistance among *Plasmodium*
1800s–1900s	Sanatorium movement for the treatment of tuberculosis in the wealthy
1825–1885	Series of cyclical, highly lethal epidemics of scarlet fever in Paris, London, Dublin, and New York City
1840s	Ignaz Semmelweis suspected an infectious origin for childbed fever (group A streptococcal infection) and initiated handwashing with chlorinated lime solution for people delivering babies, resulting in a rapid decrease in the mortality rate
1871	First description of necrotizing fasciitis (infection by group A streptococci) in the Americas, reported by a Confederate army surgeon during the Civil War
1871	Large outbreak of bartonellosis during the building of the Central Railroad from Lima to Oroya, Peru
1872	Recognition of an unusual pigmented skin cancer (Kaposi's sarcoma caused by human herpesvirus-8) in elderly men in Vienna by Moritz Kaposi
1875	Spiral bacteria found in gastric ulcers and aspirates, postulated to play a causal role in gastric disease
1882	Discovery of *Mycobacterium tuberculosis* by Robert Koch
1885	Discovery of *Escherichia coli* by Theodore von Escherich
1885	Investigation of Oroya fever (caused by *Bartonella*) by Daniel Carrión
1888	First description of *Babesia* species, by Viktor Babe, in cattle erythrocytes
1906–1909	Malaria and yellow fever brought into control in Panama by decreasing numbers of the mosquito vector under the direction of W. C. Gorgas of the U.S. Army Medical Corps
1907	*Cryptosporidium muris* found in asymptomatic mice by Edward Tyzzer
1909	Chagas' disease (caused by *Trypanosoma cruzi*) first described by Carlos das Chagas
1912	Discovery of *Cryptosporidium parvum* by Tyzzer
1915	Large outbreak of trench fever (infection by *Bartonella*) during World War I
1918	"Spanish flu" pandemic (H1N1)
1920s	Discovery of Creutzfeldt-Jakob disease (caused by human prion)
1921	Beginning of widespread use of BCG (bacillus Calmette-Guérin) as a tuberculosis vaccine
1928	Discovery of penicillin by Sir Alexander Fleming
1930s	Benito Mussolini drained swamps near Rome, greatly decreasing the incidence of malaria in Italy
1930s	Recognition of hemorrhagic fever with renal syndrome (infection by hantavirus) among Japanese troops stationed in Manchuria prior to World War II
1930s	Decreased incidence of severe invasive group A streptococcal infections
1933	Isolation of the influenza virus
1936	Scrapie found to be transmissible between sheep
1936	Prontosil, a sulfonamide, used to treat established childbed fever (infection by group A streptococci)
1937	West Nile virus first isolated in the West Nile district of Uganda
1938	Epidemic of bartonellosis in Columbia
1940s	Beginning of widespread use of penicillin, amid reports of drug resistance
1940s–1950s	Major epidemics of rheumatic fever (infection by group A streptococci) in the U.S. military during World War II and the Korean War
1950	Recognition of cat-scratch disease (infection by *Bartonella*)

(Continued)

Timeline for Emerging Infectious Diseases (Continued)

1950s	*Cryptosporidium* linked to diarrheal disease in calves and poultry
1950s	Chloroquine used to treat malaria
1950s–1960s	Malaria Eradication Campaign
1953	Report of sennetsu fever (infection by *Legionella*) in Japan
1955	Description of Argentine hemorrhagic fever
1957	"Asian flu" pandemic (H2N2)
1957	Discovery of kuru (prion disease) in Fore Highlanders of Papua New Guinea
1957	West Nile virus responsible for severe neurological symptoms among residents of Israeli nursing homes
1957	First report of human infection with *Babesia divergens*
1958	Isolation of the Junin virus (cause of a type of American hemorrhagic fever)
1958	Monkeypox virus identified as causative agent of smallpox-type rash in cynomolgus macaques in a primate colony in Denmark
1959	First reported outbreak of Bolivian hemorrhagic fever
Early 1960s	Introduction of methicillin and oxacillin, amid reports of drug resistance
1960s	Appearance of chloroquine-resistant *Plasmodium falciparum*
1961	H5N1 avian influenza first detected in South African terns
1961	Reports of methicillin-resistant strains of *Staphylococcus aureus* (MRSA) in the United Kingdom
1963	Isolation of the Machupo virus (cause of a type of American hemorrhagic fever)
Mid-1960s	First recognition of human babesiosis in the United States, in California
1966	Tikvah Alpers noted that the scrapie agent was extremely resistant to inactivation by ultraviolet light and questioned whether it could replicate without nucleic acids
1967	First report of Marburg hemorrhagic fever; establishment of vaccine production facilities in Marburg and Frankfurt, Germany, and Belgrade, Yugoslavia
1968	"Hong Kong flu" pandemic (H3N2)
1969	First report of Lassa hemorrhagic fever in a missionary hospital in Nigeria
1970	Monkeypox virus first reported in humans in the Democratic Republic of the Congo (DRC)
1970s	Reemergence of malaria
1970s	*Babesia microti* found to cause human illness on Nantucket Island
Mid-1970s	*Pseudomonas aeruginosa* begins to develop resistance to expanded-spectrum cephalosporins, carbapenems, aminoglycosides, and fluoroquin
1976	First reported outbreak of Legionnaires' disease at an American Legion convention in Philadelphia
1976	First report of Lyme disease in Old Lyme, Connecticut
1976	First reported human infection with *Cryptosporidium parvum*
1976	Carleton Gadjusek received the Noble Prize in medicine for his discovery of the transmissibility of Creutzfeldt-Jakob disease and kuru
1976	Isolation of Hantaan virus (causes hemorrhagic fever with renal syndrome)
1976	First report of Ebola hemorrhagic fever in two simultaneous outbreaks in Yambuku and Kinshasa, Zaire (DRC), and Maridi and N'zara, Sudan
1976	"Swine flu" (H1N1); initiation of the National Influenza Immunization Program
1977	Swine flu immunization program halted due to large numbers of vaccine-associated cases of Guillain-Barré syndrome and some deaths
Late 1970s	Slim disease (infection with HIV) appeared in parts of Africa
1977	Emergence of strains of *Streptococcus pneumoniae* resistant to erythromycin, trimethoprim, sulfamethoxazole, vancomycin, tetracycline, chloramphenicol, and ofloxacin
1979–1982	Isolation of *Helicobacter pylori* and its role in gastric diseases postulated by Robin Warren and Barry Marshall
1980	Official elimination of natural transmission of smallpox
1980s	Beginning of resistance to sulfadoxine-pyrimethamine and mefloquine among *Plasmodium*
1980s	Increasing pathology of necrotizing fasciitis and other severe group A streptococcal infections

Timeline for Emerging Infectious Diseases

1981	Unusually aggressive form of Kaposi's sarcoma in young homosexual men in New York and unexpectedly high numbers of cases of *Pneumocysitis carinii* pneumonia in young homosexual men from Los Angeles triggers awareness of the AIDS pandemic; AIDS also found in intravenous drug users
1981	*Borrelia burgdorferi* (cause of Lyme disease) isolated by William Burgdorfer
1982	AIDS found in high numbers in Haitians and hemophiliacs
1982	Prions isolated by Stanley Pruisiner
1982	First reported outbreak of *E. coli* O157:H7 resulting from tainted hamburgers in the U.S. Pacific Northwest and Michigan
1982	Reports of severe diarrheal disease associated with *Cryptosporidium parvum* in persons later found to be HIV-positive
1983	Lymphadenopathy-associated virus (later renamed HIV-1) isolated by Luc Montagnier at the Pasteur Institute
1983	Reports of *E. coli* strains resistant to penicillin
1983	Description of bacillary angiomatosis (infection by *Bartonella*)
1984	Human T lymphotropic virus-III (later renamed HIV-1) isolated by Robert Gallo
Mid-1980s	Appearance of multidrug-resistant tuberculosis
1986	Beginning of the bovine spongiform encephalopathy (BSE) epidemic, in the United Kingdom
1986	Description of human monocytotropic ehrlichiosis (infection by *Ehrlichia chaffeensis*) in Arkansas
1986	Development of zidovudine (AZT) for the treatment of AIDS
1987	Bacillary angiomatosis found as an opportunistic infection in individuals with AIDS
1988	Ban on feeding ruminant-derived protein to other ruminants went into effect
1989	First reported outbreak of Venezuelan hemorrhagic fever
1989	Hepatitis C virus cloned
1989	First reported outbreak of Ebola Reston in nonhuman primates imported from the Philippines to Reston, Virginia
1989–1990	Ban on the use in human or animal foods of brain, spinal cord, tonsil, thymus, spleen, or lower intestine tissue from cattle over the age of 6 months
1990	First reported case of Brazilian hemorrhagic fever
1990	Development of blood test for hepatitis C virus
1990	Isolation of *Ehrlichia chaffeensis* at Fort Chaffee, Arkansas
1990s	Appearance of vancomycin-resistant enterococci
1990s	Increased numbers of tuberculosis and multidrug-resistant tuberculosis in the United States
1990s–2000s	Increasing numbers of severe group A streptococcal infections
1991	*Babesia* isolate type WA-1 discovered to cause an acute malarialike disease in Washington State
1991	*Babesia* isolate type CA-1 identified in California
1992	*Babesia* isolate type MO-1 caused fatal disease in a 73-year-old splenectomized man in Missouri
1992	Global Malaria Control Strategy
1992	Ebola Reston reported in Italy in cynomolgus monkeys imported from the Philippines
1992	Isolation of *Bartonella henselae* and *B. quintana* from bacillary angiomatosis lesions
1993	Large outbreak of waterborne *Cryptosporidium parvum*-associated diarrhea in Milwaukee, Wisconsin
1993	First report of adult respiratory distress syndrome (caused by hantavirus) among Navahos in the American Southwest
1993	Identification of *Bartonella henselae*
1993	*Bartonella elizabethae* isolated from blood of a person with fever and endocarditis
1994	First report of Ebola Ivory Coast in humans and chimpanzees
1994	National Institutes of Health confirm role of *Helicobacter pylori* in gastric ulcers and chronic gastritis
1994	World Health Organization names *Helicobacter pylori* a class I carcinogen

(Continued)

Timeline for Emerging Infectious Diseases (Continued)

1994	Discovery of atypical form of Creutzfeldt-Jakob disease (prion infection), later named variant Creutzfeldt-Jakob disease
1994	Human herpesvirus-8 first identified in Kaposi's sarcoma tissues from an AIDS patient
1994	Recognition of human granulocytic anaplasmosis by Johan Bakken in Minnesota
1995	Large outbreak of Ebola hemorrhagic fever in Kikwit, DRC
1996	Large waterborne outbreak of *Cryptosporidium parvum*–associated diarrhea in Las Vegas, Nevada
1996	Isolation of Whitewater Arroya virus (cause of a type of American hemorrhagic fever) from wood rats
1996	Very large outbreak of *E. coli* O157:H7, from contaminated radish sprouts, in Japan
1996–1997	Large outbreak of Ebola hemorrhagic fever in Gabon
1996–1997	Large outbreak of Lassa hemorrhagic fever in Sierra Leone
1996–2000	Increased numbers of monkeypox outbreaks in DRC
1997	H5N1 influenza A first reported in humans in Hong Kong
1997	Pruisiner receives Noble Prize in medicine for his work on the prion theory
1998	Roll Back Malaria Partnership
1998–2000	Large outbreaks of Marburg hemorrhagic fever among gold miners near Durba, DRC
1999	First reported cases of hemorrhagic fever caused by Whitewater Arroya virus
1999	Description of dog and human disease due to *Ehrlichia ewingii*
1999	First report of West Nile virus in the Western Hemisphere in New York City
2000	Large outbreak of *E. coli* O157:H7 from contaminated municipal water supplies, in Walkerton, Ontario
2000–2001	Increased incidence of extensively drug-resistant tuberculosis
2000–2001	Large outbreak of Ebola hemorrhagic fever in Gulu, Uganda
2001	West Nile disease found south of the United States in the Cayman Islands
2002	West Nile disease reported in humans in Canada
2002	Reports of high-level vancomycin-resistant *Staphylococcus aureus* (VRSA)
2002	Differentiation of *Cryptosporidium parvum* and *C. hominis*
2002–2003	Severe acute respiratory syndrome (SARS) epidemic
2003	Beginning of second wave of H5N1 avian influenza in humans in Southeast Asia
2003	Isolation of SARS-associated coronavirus (SARS-CoV)
2003	First report of monkeypox in the United States, from African rodents imported into Texas
2003	First monkeypox outbreak in the Republic of the Congo
2003–2004	Four mild cases of SARS in China
2004	Avian H7N3 variant causes mild illness in two persons in Canada
2004–2005	Large outbreak of Marburg hemorrhagic fever in the Uige province of Angola
2005	Warren and Marshall receive Nobel Prize in medicine for their work on *Helicobacter*
2005	President's Malaria Initiative
2005–2006	Discovery of natural infection with Marburg virus in a nonprimate species, fruit bats, in Gabon
2006	First reports of human H5N1 influenza outside of Southeast Asia in Turkey, Azerbaijan, Djibouti, Egypt, and Iraq
2007	H7N7 avian virus causes typically mild illness in humans in the Netherlands
2007–2008	Spread of H5N1 influenza to Nigeria and Pakistan
2008	H5N2 avian influenza virus appears as an asymptomatic infection of poultry workers in Japan
2008	First reported cases of hemorrhagic fever caused by Chapare virus
2008	Large outbreak of Marburg hemorrhagic fever in a bat-infested mine in Uganda
2008	First reported case of Marburg hemorrhagic fever in the United States, in a traveler returning from Uganda
2008	First reported cases of hemorrhagic fever caused by a novel Old World arenavirus in Zambia and South Africa
2009	Declaration of "swine flu" pandemic by new strain of H1N1 influenza virus

Summary

Effects of Several Infectious Diseases in History

• Plague resulted in massive population reduction, altered economic and civil structure, and led to reforms in sanitation.   • Smallpox was a major killer of the young and previously unexposed populations and led to the development of vaccination.

Leading Causes of Death Due to Infectious Disease Today

• Lower respiratory tract infections • diarrheal diseases • HIV
• tuberculosis • malaria • dengue hemorrhagic fever and shock syndrome

Poverty-Associated Factors That Increase Infectious Disease Incidence

• Decreased access to clean drinking water • malnutrition
• overcrowding • substandard housing • poor educational opportunities • prostitution as a source of income • inadequate health care due to the inability to pay for services and medications
• lack of local health care facilities and practitioners • lack of roads or their impassability • poor access to motor vehicles or fuel to travel to health care sites

Civil-Unrest-Associated Factors That Increase Infectious Disease Incidence

• Mass population movement due to wars • geographical spread of disease by combatants and refugees • poverty due to loss of crops and economic disruption • amplification of disease in refugee camps • physical inhibition of the transportation of food, medicine, and vaccines by areas of active combat • altered sexual practices due to disruption of social mores

Factors Contributing to the Emergence or Reemergence of Infectious Diseases

• Microbial evolution • urbanization • large population migration
• rapid long-distance transportation of persons and materials • human intrusion into formerly uninhabited territories • natural disasters
• climatic changes • decreased vaccination • increased numbers of immunocompromised individuals

Key Terms

Emerging and reemerging infectious diseases Infectious diseases that have either been discovered during the past 40 to 50 years or greatly increased in incidence or virulence regionally or worldwide

Urbanization Movement of large numbers of people away from traditional villages to large population centers with differing social customs and moral values; may result in overcrowding and decreased sanitation

Vaccination Inoculation with nonpathogenic material derived from infectious agents in order to induce protective immunity against future infection

Variolation Inoculation with material from dried scabs derived from persons with mild cases of smallpox to protect against the future development of severe infection

Review Questions

1. What are variolation and vaccination, and how did each develop?
2. What microbes are responsible for many of the cases of lower respiratory tract infections and diarrheal diseases found in developing nations? Name three of other major microbial diseases leading to death in the world today.
3. How may illness increase the poverty of an area?
4. What are some of the emerging infectious diseases found throughout the world and the organisms that cause them?
5. What are some reasons for the observed decrease in vaccination?

Topics for Further Discussion

1. The Black Death killed a large percentage of the inhabitants of Europe in the fourteenth to eighteenth centuries, leaving a vastly altered society in its wake. In what ways are AIDS and the reemergence of tuberculosis currently inducing societal changes in developed nations?
2. Smallpox was one of the worst scourges of humanity until its eradication in the 1970s, and the practice of vaccination was developed as a result of this disease. Vaccination has gone on to save the lives of untold millions of people infected with other infectious diseases. Research the positive effects that have

come from the AIDS pandemic, including advances in the understanding of the body's defensive systems and treatment of other diseases.

3. Outline several practical ways that might reduce the incidence of lower respiratory tract infections and diarrheal diseases in impoverished regions. Keep in mind limitations (finite financial resources and personnel, educational level of the population, cultural and religious customs, the role of geography and climate, and the ability and willingness of local governments to assist in the effort). Suggest practical ways in which the limitations might be minimized.

4. New diseases have emerged throughout history. Humans have countered with new strategies (sanitation, vaccination, antimicrobial medications) for protection against infection or to decrease the severity of the resulting disease. Discuss possible innovative means by which humans might combat infectious diseases in the future, such as gene therapy or means of eliminating large numbers of closely related microbes from the environment.

Resources

Alibek, K., with Handelman, S. *Biohazard: The Chilling True Story of the Largest Covert Biological Weapons Program in the World—Told from Inside by the Man Who Ran It.* New York: Dell, 1999.

Emerging Infectious Diseases. Monthly journal published by the Centers for Disease Control and Prevention.

Garrett, L. *Betrayal of Trust: The Collapse of Global Public Health.* New York: Hyperion, 2001.

Garrett, L. *The Coming Plague: Newly Emerging Diseases in a World Out of Balance.* New York: Penguin, 1994.

Krause, R. M. (ed.). *Emerging Infections.* New York: Academic Press, 1998.

Macaulay, T. B. *The History of England from the Accession of James II* (Vol. 4). Gloucester, England: Dodo Press, 2009. [Originally published 1855.]

Salyers, A. A., and Whitt, D. D. *Revenge of the Microbes: How Bacterial Resistance Is Undermining the Antibiotic Miracle.* Washington, D.C.: ASM Press, 2005.

Scheld, W. M., Armstrong, D., and Hughes, J. M. *Emerging Infections* (Vol. 1). Washington, D.C.: ASM Press, 1997.

World Health Organization. http://www.who.int/research/en.

CHAPTER 2

OF MICROBES AND MEN

LEARNING OBJECTIVES

- Describe viruses, bacteria, protozoa, and prions and discuss how they differ

- Discuss the differences between prokaryotes and eukaryotes

- Describe the roles of DNA, RNA, proteins, and mutations

- Discuss how bacteria and viruses increase their genetic diversity

- Describe the adaptive and innate immune systems and the functions of the cells found in each

- Describe and differentiate the classes of antibodies and different categories of cytokines

- Describe the different categories of antimicrobial agents and how they act to kill microbes

Major Concepts

Infectious Agents

Several types of infectious agents are described in this chapter. Viruses are obligate intracellular parasites whose small size enables them to pass through most filters. They exist on the border between life and nonlife in that they are not capable of carrying out many of the processes normally associated with living organisms by themselves. Bacteria compose the majority of prokaryotic organisms and are surrounded by cell walls containing peptidoglycan. They are subdivided in several ways, including by shape (round to oval cocci, rod-shaped bacilli, and corkscrew-shaped spirochetes) and staining characteristics (gram-positive, gram-negative, acid-fast). Protozoa are unicellular eukaryotic organisms whose cell wall, if present, does not contain chitin or cellulose. Their ranks include some of the major killers of the residents of tropical regions, including the well-known malaria and the less publicized schistosomiasis. Prions are nonliving, infectious proteinaceous particles. They are misfolded forms of normal cellular proteins that replicate by inducing the normal form of the protein to refold into the prion form. They lack RNA and DNA. All of these infectious agents have developed means of slipping past the skin and mucous membrane barriers of humans to gain entry into their host.

The Production of Protein and Generation of Genetic Diversity

DNA encodes the genetic information of most forms of life. It serves as a template for the production of RNA, which is in turn the code for the production of the proteins that provide much of the structure and direct most activities of organisms. A small group of the viruses that use RNA to store their genetic code must use this RNA as a template for the production of their DNA. HIV is one such virus. This unusual extra step in protein production is the target of some of the drugs used to treat AIDS. Changes in the structure of DNA lead to changes in the structure and functions of proteins, often leading to fundamental changes in the organism. Mutations are one way in which the structure of DNA is altered. Most mutations are detrimental to the organism and may result in decreased chance of survival. In rare instances, however, mutations may lead to a survival advantage. HIV and influenza viruses use a rapid rate of mutation to evade the host immune system as well as drugs and vaccines. Other means of changing the structure of DNA and thus increasing the species' genetic diversity include conjugation, transformation, acquisition of plasmids, and transduction in bacteria. Some viruses have error-prone replication enzymes and fail to correct their mistakes.

The Human Immune System

The human immune system may be divided into adaptive and innate branches. The activity of the adaptive branch is slow to develop but provides a powerful defense targeted very specifically to the present threat. It acts more rapidly and vigorously with repeated exposures to the same microbe. Cell types involved are the B and T lymphocytes, which kill cells infected by microbes and produce five classes of antibodies as well as many of the cytokines that regulate the immune response. The innate branch of the immune system is believed to be more ancient than the adaptive branch. It is faster-acting and nonspecific, each cell responding to a large number of threats. Innate immunity does not improve with subsequent exposures to the threatening agent. Cell types involved include neutrophils, monocytes and macrophages, dendritic cells, natural killer cells, eosinophils, basophils, and mast cells. Some of their actions include ingestion and killing of microbes, killing of infected cells, killing of parasitic worms, and production of allergic reactions. Over the course of history, many microbes have evolved means of evading various components of the immune system. In response, humans have produced additional defensive components such as the adaptive immune system. Throughout time, microbes and humans have continued to evolve new offensive and defensive strategies, each side gaining a temporary advantage but neither achieving total victory.

Antimicrobial Agents

A variety of antimicrobial agents have been developed to protect humans from infection or disease. Some of these are derived from other microbes (fungi or bacteria), some are plant derivatives, and others have been synthesized in the laboratory. Most of the antimicrobial drugs attempt to target differences between the microbe and humans in order to lessen toxicity to the host. Antibiotics kill bacteria or inhibit their growth. They are not active against viruses and may not be able to reach the site of infection. Antiviral drugs attack viruses. Several compounds kill parasitic protozoa and worms. Antifungal drugs kill fungi but may be toxic to human cells. As humans continue to develop newer and more effective drugs, subpopulations of microbes become resistant as the battle between microbes and men continues.

Introduction

Infectious agents range from extremely simple, such as the nonliving prions and the barely living viruses, to the complex (parasitic protozoa and worms). Bacteria are responsible for some of the more common infections and are prokaryotes whose cellular structure differs greatly from that of humans. Many bacteria and protozoa are free-living, some are always parasitic, and others may function in either capacity. Viruses and prions are obligate intracellular parasites that require the machinery of the cells to function and replicate.

Agents that infect humans have forged a complex relationship with us over the course of history. Organisms that have only relatively recently begun to infect humans were originally believed to be more pathogenic than organisms that have interacted with us for long spans of time. This theory, however, has recently been challenged, as it does not explain the serious nature of infections such as malaria, tuberculosis, and smallpox, which have a very long history with humans. Infectious agents must be able to adapt to withstand challenges posed by human defenses, both natural agents (barriers to entry and the immune response) and antimicrobial agents. Over the millennia, humans have also adapted to the changing face of their microbial foes. This process resembles a complex evolutionary waltz in which each partner constantly responds to the actions of the other. The dance continues to the present day.

This chapter describes the various types of infectious agents and how they are able to enter the human body and to adapt rapidly to the changing host environment. Human immune responses are very briefly described next. The chapter concludes with short descriptions of some of the types of antimicrobial agents used in the human battle against infectious invaders.

Infectious Agents: The Enemy Combatants

Microbes: The Good, the Bad, and the Ugly

Microorganisms (microbes) are commonly held in low regard due to the potential of some of their ilk to cause serious, if not fatal, diseases (the bad and the ugly). Microbes, however, serve many beneficial functions and are vital to continuing life on earth (the good). Some of these beneficial activities include the decomposition of wastes and recycling of nutrients (degradation of dead plant and animal matter; components of sewage treatment plants), use by the food and beverage industry (production of sauerkraut, cheese, and alcohol), bioremediation (degradation of oil following oil spills and leaks), pest and pathogen control (killing insects attacking crops; infecting and killing pathogenic bacteria, such as anthrax), use in biotechnology to produce recombinant proteins (insulin or hepatitis B vaccine) within bacteria or fungi and in gene therapy as vehicles to deliver genes to protect against life-threatening human diseases (severe combined immunodeficiency or cystic fibrosis).

Microbes are living organisms too small to be viewed individually without magnification. They include viruses (on the edge of the life-nonlife divide), prokaryotic organisms (bacteria and Archaea), fungi (molds and yeasts), protozoa, and algae. Some of these types of microbes (Archaea, fungi, and algae) will not be extensively covered in this book even though some fungi (*Aspirgillus* and *Candida*) may serve as human pathogens. Although most infectious agents are microbes, not all microbes are infectious agents. Other types of infectious agents include the prions that cause transmissible encephalopathies, such as mad cow disease (discussed in this text), and multicellular parasites, including parasitic helminthes and arthropods (not covered separately in this text). Examples of parasitic worms include *Trichinella spiralis* (the causative agent of trichinosis), *Necator americanus* (the "American killer" species of hookworm), and *Schistosoma* spp. that are responsible for a great deal of suffering and death throughout much of the developing world. Parasitic arthropods include *Ixodes scapularis* (the black-legged tick), *Pulex irritans* (the human flea), and *Pediculus humanus corporis* (the body louse), which transmit viruses and bacteria between animals and humans or from one human to another.

Viruses: Complex Collections of Chemicals or Life Forms?

Viruses (*virus* is Latin for "poison") are tiny agents that pass through most filters. They do not consist of cells but rather are collections of nucleic acid (DNA or RNA) in a core surrounded by a protein coat and sometimes an envelope. Viruses carry out some, but not all, of the normal processes of life. Due to the absence of most metabolic and synthetic enzymes present in living organisms, they are obligate intracellular parasites that must reside within cells in order to reproduce. Although many viruses infect eukaryotic cells, others (**bacteriophages**) inhabit prokaryotic bacteria. In some cases, bacteria are pathogenic to humans only when infected by a certain virus. *Bacillus anthracis*, the causative agent of anthrax, carries several such bacteriophages. A group of viruses, the **retroviruses**, contain an unusual enzyme, reverse transcriptase, which produces DNA using an RNA template (to be discussed shortly). The four well-defined retroviruses of humans (HTLV-1, HTLV-2, HIV-1, and HIV-2) are all serious or deadly pathogens.

Viruses, like bacteria, may act as infectious agents of human disease. Viral diseases include AIDS, yellow fever, hepatitis, hemorrhagic fevers, influenza, polio, and the common cold. Important distinctions exist in the manner by which viruses and bacteria are killed, however. Viruses, unlike bacteria, are not killed by antibiotics but may be killed by interferons (chemical agents produced by host immune cells). A number of antiviral agents have been developed recently, including ribaviran and zidovudine (AZT, used to treat HIV infection).

In addition to causing infectious diseases, viruses may initiate cancer. About 10% of human cancers are of viral origin. Viruses may induce expression of **oncogenes** (genes that cause cancer if mutated, overexpressed, or improperly expressed). Some viruses contain oncogenes within their genetic material, while other viruses "turn on" copies of a human cell's own oncogenes during viral integration into a host cell's chromosome. Some cancer-causing viruses are HTLV-1 (acute T cell leukemia), papillomaviruses (cervical cancer), Epstein-Barr virus (Burkitt's lymphoma), hepatitis B and C (liver carcinoma), and human herpesvirus-8 (Kaposi's sarcoma).

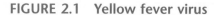

FIGURE 2.1   Yellow fever virus

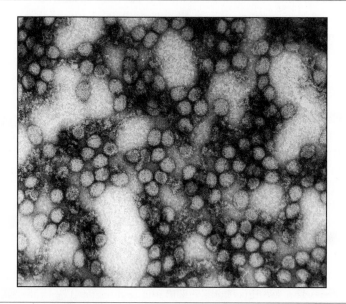

Source: CDC.

Bacteria: Simple Prokaryotic Cells

Bacteria are typically small, unicellular prokaryotes surrounded by cell walls containing peptidoglycan. They take a variety of shapes, including spheroid or ovoid (cocci such as *Streptococcus*), rodlike (bacilli such as *E. coli*), and corkscrew-like (spirochetes such as *Borellia burgdorferi*, the causative agent of Lyme disease). Some bacteria bear projections, such as the long, whiplike flagella of *Helicobacter pylori*, which causes peptic ulcers. Bacteria have differential reactions to various staining procedures. A commonly used stain is the gram stain, which divides bacteria into gram-positive (organisms appear purple) and gram-negative (organisms appear pink). Other bacteria are visualized by special staining techniques; one such bacterium is *Mycobacterium tuberculosis*, which is acid-fast.

Bacteria generally have a single circular chromosome containing DNA for their genetic information in the absence of histone proteins. They usually divide by **binary fission**, an asexual form of clonal reproduction that produces two individuals identical to the parent. This reproductive strategy does not by itself lead to the degree of genetic diversity required to adapt rapidly to environmental changes, such as exposure to antibiotics or the host's immune system. One method of increasing genetic diversity is **conjugation**, a process whereby DNA is exchanged between individuals of opposite mating types. Other means of acquiring different DNA will be discussed later in this chapter.

Bacteria are the most common form of prokaryotic organisms on earth (the other being the nonpathogenic Archaea). Prokaryotic structure differs greatly from that of eukaryotes, and some of these differences have been exploited during drug development. Prokaryotes lack membrane-enclosed organelles found within eukaryotic cells, including the nucleus, endoplasmic reticulum, Golgi apparatus, and lysosomes. Significantly, prokaryotic and eukaryotic ribosomes differ substantially. Prokaryotic ribosomes contain 30S and 50S subunits, while eukaryotic ribosomes contain 40S and 60S subunits, a difference exploited by many antibiotics, which attack components of either the 30S or 50S subunit. Eukaryotic organisms, by contrast, use cell walls (when present) containing cellulose or chitin; contain membrane-enclosed organelles; divide by mitosis; arrange their DNA in multiple, linear chromosomes containing histone proteins; and have carbohydrates and sterols in their plasma membranes. Many eukaryotes multiply sexually, with male and female individuals.

Protozoa: Single-Celled Eukaryotes

Protozoa are unicellular eukaryotic organisms. They may be free-living in soil or water, reside within other organisms parasitically, or have life cycles with both free-living and parasitic components. Some protozoa move using pseudopodia ("false feet"; *Amoeba histolytica*, responsible for severe, bloody diarrhea) or flagella (*Trypanosoma cruzi*, the causative agent of Chagas' disease). Protozoa use linear DNA as their genetic material and may reproduce asexually (amoebas), sexually as males and females, or both asexually and sexually (*Plasmodium* species, which cause malaria). A number of protozoa cause serious human diseases, such as malaria, African sleeping sickness, leishmaniasis, babesiosis, and amoebic meningitis.

Prions: Infectious Proteins?

Prions (infectious proteinaceous particles) are extremely hardy, infectious proteins that lack DNA and RNA but nevertheless divide and infect cells. Although prions are classified as nonliving material, they function as obligate intracellular parasites. They may be acquired in a hereditary fashion, by mutation of a person's DNA, or by infection. Prions are very difficult to inactivate and can withstand almost all types of chemical treatments and normal autoclaving processes that denature virtually all other proteins, due to their ability to fold themselves correctly back to their previous form.

Prions are self-propagating, misfolded proteins closely related to normal proteins encoded by human genes and are found within the cells of normal individuals. They are formed by the interaction between the normal cellular protein (PrP^c) and the protein's prion form (PrP^{sc}). PrP^{sc} induces PrP^c to undergo a change in shape and become a PrP^{sc}. Thus the normal form of the protein and the pathogenic form differ in primarily in shape, the shape of the PrP being its hereditary material rather than DNA or RNA.

Prions are responsible for several universally fatal illnesses that are characterized by spongelike changes to the brain. In humans, these include several forms of Creutzfeldt-Jakob disease (CJD), kuru (once found in members of the formerly cannibalistic Fore Highlander tribe of Papua New Guinea after handling or eating brains of dead relatives), Alpers syndrome (a prion disease of infants), fatal familial insomnia, and variant CJD (a human form of mad cow disease, acquired by eating beef from infected cattle). In addition to infecting cattle, spongiform encephalopathies strike sheep ("scrapie"), deer, elk, and mink.

Modes of Transmission: Penetrating the Human Stronghold

Before microbes can wage war on humans, they must first travel to their next host, breach the external barriers, and gain entry to the correct body region. Some microbes travel between hosts through an airborne route or by respiratory secretions, attached to tiny bits of solid matter (Junin virus, the causative

FIGURE 2.2 Transmission via respiratory secretions

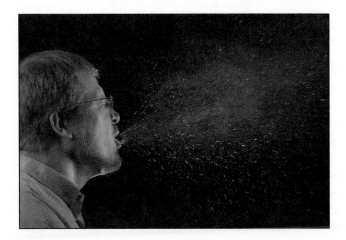

Source: CDC/Brian Judd.

agent of Argentine hemorrhagic fever, and the Sin Nombre virus, responsible for hantavirus pulmonary syndrome, carried by aerosolized rodent excreta) or enclosed within small droplets of liquid (*Legionella pneumophila*, responsible for Legionnaires' disease, via water aerosols). Other microbes gain entry through food (*E. coli* O157:H7 via undercooked hamburgers), drink (major outbreaks of *Cryptosporidium* by ingestion of contaminated water from municipal drinking supplies), or ingestion of recreational water (swimming or diving).

Humans have protective barriers that normally block the entry of foreign life forms: these are primarily the skin and the mucous membranes lining the digestive, respiratory, and urogenital tracts. The latter also contain a specialized type of antibody, IgA, to block microbial entry. Microbes must somehow penetrate these lines of defense in order to infect the interior of the human host. Some organisms enter via breaks in the skin (*Staphylococcus* species causing boils and skin infections; *Trypanosoma cruzi*, the causative agent of Chagas' disease, in the fecal matter of kissing bugs entering through the insects' bite wounds) or mucous membranes (HIV entering through damaged anal membranes following sexual intercourse). Prior infection with other microbes or trauma to these barrier structures aids in microbial entry. Some microbes need a little help from their friends to pass through the skin barrier. Ticks, lice, and mosquitoes serve as vector hosts whose bites transport microbes into humans, as in the cases of *Borrelia burgdorferi* (Lyme disease; *Ixodes* ticks), *Bartonella quintana* (trench fever; *Pediculus* lice), West Nile virus (West Nile encephalitis; *Culex* mosquitoes), and *Plasmodium* spp. (malaria; *Anopheles* mosquitoes). Living conditions that permit interactions between these arthropods and humans facilitate disease transmission. Bites or scratches of animals may also carry microbes past the skin, as exemplified by *Bartonella henselae* (cat-scratch disease) and rabies virus transmission through the bite of infected raccoons or bats. Persons with compromised immunity may have increased susceptibility to infection, especially those with low levels of mucosal IgA antibody.

Other infectious agents may be carried past the skin or into the lungs by medical instruments. For example, HIV may enter by injection with a hypodermic needle, prions may enter via contaminated scalpels during brain surgery, and *Legionella* may be present in the output of nebulizers and ventilators. Hospitals and clinics that use improperly sterilized equipment may thus serve to transmit disease between patients, amplifying a single initial case into a large outbreak, as has occurred several times with Ebola hemorrhagic fever. Transfusions of blood or blood components, organ transplantation, and other human-derived products may also transmit microbes, as occurs with HIV via contaminated blood and platelets and prions during transplantation of infected meninges or growth factor derived from human pituitary glands.

Some microbes exist for part of their life cycle in wild or domestic animals that serve as reservoir hosts until they again infect humans. In some cases, such as monkeypox, the reservoir host (squirrels) may transmit the disease to humans. Other reservoir hosts, like the black rat reservoir of *Yersinia pestis* (plague) and the white-tailed deer reservoir of *Anaplasma phagocytophilum* (human granulocytic anaplasmosis), are themselves hosts to the microbe's arthropod vector. Increases in numbers of the reservoir host or in its contact with humans may lead to increased disease incidence. Such has been the case recently during the population explosion of white-tailed deer and several diseases associated with the arthropods they host, including Lyme disease and ehrlichiosis. Some of the reservoir hosts are human pets, such as prairie dogs, reservoirs for monkeypox. Other reservoir hosts are exotic sources of human food, such as palm civets and raccoon dogs, reservoirs for SARS CoA virus. Still other reservoir hosts are used for medical research, such as the African green monkey hosts of Marburg virus.

Genetic Information and the Making of Proteins: Preparing the Armament

From DNA to RNA to Protein: Making the Weapons of War

One of the most important concepts in the field of biology was the discovery that specific regions of DNA, the genetic material of all living organisms except some viruses, serve as templates for the production of specific, unique messenger

RNA molecules during the process of transcription. These RNA molecules, in turn, serve as keys to produce specific, unique proteins during the process of translation. **DNA** is composed of two long chains of interconnected nucleotides twisted into the form of a double-helix, resembling a spiral staircase. **RNA**, by contrast, consists of much shorter single chains of closely related nucleosides. **Proteins** are long strings of amino acids folded in complex ways. The sequence of amino acids in a protein determines the subsequent folding pattern of that protein. The folding pattern of the protein in turn determines its activity as form dictates function.

Alterations in the sequence of DNA nucleotides (**mutations**) change the sequence of the resulting RNA and the protein. Some proteins determine much of the structural architecture of cells, and other proteins, in the form of enzymes, catalyze the chemical reactions of cells; consequently, changing the structure of proteins fundamentally changes the cell's form and activity. Changing cells' activities may change the processes of the associated tissues and organs and may affect the organism as a whole. Mutations in DNA may thus have large-scale effects on the individual harboring the mutation. Most mutations tend to be deleterious to the individual, inhibiting proper functioning of the resulting protein, and may lead to the death of the individual or impair its ability to compete effectively for resources. Some rare mutations, however, may lead to a more fully functional protein or a protein with new or improved activities. Such mutations benefit the affected individual and may increase its ability to success-fully compete for resources, allow the individual to adapt to changing external conditions, allow it to enter a new ecological niche, or facilitate evasion of the host immune response, drugs, and vaccines. The acquisition of new sequences of DNA by other means may likewise occasionally be beneficial to individual organisms. Species that have the ability to increase their genetic diversity rapidly may also readily adapt to new situations and withstand threats to their survival. Because beneficial mutations are rare and deleterious mutations are common, these species need to reproduce rapidly so that the loss of many individuals due to deleterious mutations is compensated by large numbers of offspring, some of which are better adapted for survival. Microbes multiply very rapidly, producing large numbers of offspring. As will be discussed shortly, they also have means of quickly increasing their genetic diversity.

From RNA to DNA: Unconventional Weaponry

The scheme just described for producing unique proteins from specific regions of DNA containing a unique sequence of nucleotides has subsequently been shown to be a rather simplified description of a far more complex process. For example, a given sequence of DNA may permit the production of more than one sequence of resulting RNA, and a given RNA sequence may be translated into more than one protein. Proteins themselves are often chemically altered after their production, leading to subsequent alterations in their functions. Furthermore, some viruses were found to use RNA as their genetic information, and this RNA may be double-stranded. One group of viruses, the retroviruses, was further found to contain an enzyme that turned the transcription process on its head. The reverse transcriptase enzyme, found in all retroviruses including HIV, uses single-stranded viral genomic RNA as a template to produce first single-stranded and later double-stranded DNA.

The earliest anti-HIV medications, including AZT, targeted reverse transcriptase, believed to be present only in retroviruses. Years later, however, other organisms, including humans, were also found to use reverse transcriptase enzymes. Human telomerase, the enzymatic star of the 2009 Nobel Prize for Medicine or Physiology, is one such enzyme. Lymphocytes and stem cells are some of the few types of differentiated human cells known to use telomerase. Not surprisingly, persons taking AZT often suffer from decreased lymphocyte counts as well as other side-effects.

Increasing Genetic Diversity: Evading the Human Defenses

As discussed earlier, prokaryotes typically reproduce by binary fission, resulting in a clone of progeny that are identical to the original parent bacterium. This does not lead to genetic diversity or allow adaptation to new situations that microbes encounter, such as the adaptive host immune response or antimicrobial agents. Some bacteria partially address this problem by conjugation, an exchange of DNA between bacterial partners of different mating types. Conjugation increases genetic diversity of those species of bacteria.

To further increase diversity, bacteria have developed additional means of acquiring DNA. One such means is **transformation**, a process by which some species of bacteria may under certain conditions acquire pieces of DNA from the external environment. Transformation occurs naturally in *Bacillus* (the causative agent of anthrax), *Haemophilus influenzae* (a causative agent of pneumonia), *Neisseria gonorrhoeae,* and some *Streptococcus* and *Staphylococcus* species.

Another means by which bacteria obtain new DNA is by the acquisition of plasmids. **Plasmids** are small, circular pieces of nonchromosomal DNA that may divide in a somewhat autonomous manner within bacteria. They may travel between bacteria of the same or different species, acting rather like selfish parasitic pieces of DNA that infect bacteria. Plasmids are not typically required for the survival of bacteria under normal circumstances, and bacteria often treat plasmids as junk DNA, expelling them unless the plasmid contains a gene beneficial to the bacteria. Plasmids bearing such "useful" genes are thus more likely to be retained inside their bacterial host and survive. Many plasmids do contain such genes, which allow their host bacteria to compete more successfully by encoding toxins that kill other bacteria or contain antibiotic resistance genes. Plasmid exchange is partially responsible for the rapid spread of antibiotic resistance between bacterial species. For example, in some hospitals, a plasmid containing the vancomycin resistance gene is being passed from some gut bacteria (*Enterococcus faecium*) to *Staphylococcus aureus* present in skin wounds. Some of these staphylococci are already resistant to methicillin and several other antibiotics (MRSA strains) due to their acquisition of a different sort of transmissible DNA, the mobile genetic island staphylococcal cassette chromosome SCC*mec*. Often plasmids accumulate several antibiotic resistance genes, as in the case of the EHEC plasmid found in the virulent O157:H7 strain of *E. coli*. This plasmid carries genes encoding several virulence factors, including the enterohemolysin protein, which lyses red blood cells; espP, an enzyme that cleaves pepsin and human coagulation factor V, inhibiting blood clotting; and catalase peroxidase, which protects the bacteria against toxic reactive oxygen species produced by the host immune system.

Another means by which bacteria increase genetic diversity is **transduction.** In this process, bacteriophages infect different bacteria, transmitting genes between bacteria of the same or different species. *E. coli* O157:H7 are infected by lambdalike bacteriophages that contain genes encoding Shiga toxins, which are very similar to toxins produced by *Shigella dysenteriae* type 1 bacteria. These toxins destroy intestinal blood vessels, resulting in hemorrhagic colitis and leading to the formation of gummy clots that may clog the kidneys and cause the potentially fatal hemolytic uremia syndrome. Some strains of MRSA are infected by bacteriophages encoding the Panton-Valentine leukocidin, which destroys neutrophils, a type of white blood cell, and causes tissue death.

Viruses also have means of increasing genetic diversity. The HIV enzyme reverse transcriptase often makes errors (five to ten per division), and the virus has no enzymes to correct these mistakes, allowing them to become permanent. Hepatitis C virus is another RNA virus whose high mutation rate is combined with the lack of repair mechanisms. Influenza is also an RNA virus, and it uses a different strategy to increase genetic diversity. Influenza A viruses from birds may infect pigs. If the avian influenza virus infects a pig cell containing a swine influenza virus, the two viruses may exchange some of their RNA. This hybrid influenza virus may subsequently infect a human and swap genetic material with a human influenza virus, producing a novel influenza virus. Such viruses are vastly different from typical human influenza A viruses and occasionally cause dangerous pandemics.

The Immune Response: Humans Fight Back, Part One

Humans have developed a dual action defensive system containing a more ancient and rapid response component (innate immunity) and a slow-developing, powerful, more recent component (adaptive immunity). These two components act in an interrelated manner to deal with most of the microbial invaders that threaten human health. Microbes, with their rapid means of increasing genetic diversity, continually evolve new ways to evade the human immune response. Humans respond by increasing and improving their defensive arsenal. Over the course of history, microbes and humans have each evolved means of increasing their own survival at the expense of the other. Both sides have developed elaborate weapons systems, but neither has emerged as the victor in the evolutionary arms escalation race.

Cells of the Immune System: The Members of the Military

The adaptive and innate branches of the immune defensive service each contain their own types of troops, each specializing in a slightly different protective role.

The Adaptive Immune Response By recognizing specific regions of invading microbes and malignant cells (antigens), **adaptive immunity** provides a very powerful, large-scale, extremely precise defense. Individual cells of the adaptive immune system (the lymphocytes) recognize one, and only one, short portion of a protein, usually 8 to 13 amino acids long. The many billions of different lymphocytes present within a given period of time each typically recognize a slightly different antigen. The initial generation of these reactions against a given pathogen (primary immune response) is slow, requiring 10 to 14 days; subsequent exposure to the same pathogen, however, triggers a rapid and overwhelming protective response (secondary response) that is more powerful than the primary response and improves with each subsequent exposure to the same microbe. Vaccination speeds this process by exposing people to antigens from dead or inactivated microbes (**attenuated microbes**), initiating a primary response so that the first exposure of the vaccine recipient to the same live, pathogenic microbe stimulates a secondary immune response that rapidly kills the microbe, often prior to the onset of illness. The precision of this response requires vaccination against each species or strain of pathogen because vaccination protects only against microbes whose antigens were present in the vaccine.

Because adaptive immunity is very precise and specific often to the exact amino acid sequence of the original pathogen, even very minor changes in the

Table 2.1   Immune cells and immune responses

Type of Immune Response	Cell Type	Action
Adaptive	B lymphocyte	Produce antibodies
	T helper lymphocyte	Produce cytokines
	T killer lymphocyte	Kill viruses and cancer cells
Innate	Neutrophil, monocyte, macrophage	Phagocytosis
	NK cell	Kill viruses and cancer cells

antigenic structure of the microbial invader allow it to escape detection by this branch of the immune system. The ability of the HIV virus to generate rapid mutations leading to small changes in its proteins permits it to evade this most powerful arm of the human immune system. The speed and ease of mutation of HIV also complicates the task of producing an effective vaccine, and such a vaccine is not currently available. Influenza strains also mutate rapidly, as noted earlier. They change antigenically from one season to the next, requiring yearly vaccination using antigens from the currently circulating viral strains. Large, unanticipated mutations in these viruses, such as occur during influenza pandemics, render the vaccines ineffective.

Two general classes of lymphocytes generate the adaptive immune response, the closely related B and T lymphocytes. The primary task of B lymphocytes is to produce the five major classes of antibodies (discussed later in this chapter). Antibody responses are most effective against extracellular pathogens such as the majority of bacteria and fungi and extracellular parasites. Antibodies may also block entry of intracellular organisms, such as viruses, into their target cells (neutralizing antibodies) or may inactivate microbial toxins. The tetanus vaccine uses a harmless form of the toxin (tetanus toxoids) to generate antibodies that prevent the pathogenic form of the toxin from killing human cells. B cells also function as "antigen-presenting cells" to aid in activation of $CD4^+$ T helper cells (to be described shortly).

T lymphocytes are subdivided into two major branches: $CD4^+$ T helper cells and $CD8^+$ T cytotoxic (killer) cells. Both cell types require activation following interaction with antigen bound onto surface molecules (major histocompatibility complex molecules—MHC class I and class II) present on other cells from the same individual. $CD8^+$ T killer cells are triggered by contact with antigen bound to MHC class I molecules, which are typically found on most nucleated human cells (but not on red blood cells, sperm, or neurons). T killer cells induce apoptosis (programmed cell death) in atypical cells, such as cells infected by viruses or intracellular bacteria (*Listeria monocytogenes*) and parasites (*Babesia* or *Plasmodium* species), malignant cells, and cells transplanted from another individual. They provide some of the most effective protection against viral infection and cancers. Viruses and cancer cells often attempt to evade killing by these cells by diminishing the expression of MHC class I molecule on cells to decrease the activation of T killer cells.

CD4$^+$ T helper cells act as the officers of the immune system by secreting a large variety of **cytokines** (immune messenger molecules), which direct and control activity of other cells of the immune system or act on microbes directly. HIV specifically infects and kills CD4$^+$ T helper cells, thus throwing the entire immune response into disarray. T helper cells require stimulation by antigen bound to MHC class II molecules on **antigen-presenting cells** (B cells, monocytes and macrophages, and dendritic cells). Several categories of T helper cells exist. Th1 cells compose one such category. These cells secrete Th1 cytokines that primarily induce immune responses against intracellular organisms such as viruses by stimulating activation of CD8$^+$ T killer cells, macrophages, and natural killer cells. Th2 cells fall into another category. They secrete Th2 cytokines, which act mainly on bacterial invaders by stimulating production of specific classes of antibody by B cells. Th2 cells also stimulate production and activation of eosinophils, mast cells, and basophils. Th1 cytokines tend to inhibit activation of Th2 cells, whereas Th2 cytokines tend to inhibit activation of Th1 cells. T regulatory cells (Treg) comprise another category of CD4$^+$ T helper cells. These cells express high levels of the receptor for the cytokine interleukin-2. Treg function to down-regulate activity of Th1 and Th2 cells, acting as a brake on the immune system to avoid consequences of a runaway immune response such as autoimmune diseases and allergies in which members of our body's defense system damage other body cells in a manner resembling immune friendly fire.

The Innate Immune System The components of the **innate immune system** provide immediate, nonspecific protection against microbial and cancerous threats. Individual cells of the innate immune system each recognize multiple antigens present on multiple microbes. Innate immunity, though rapid and versatile, is far less powerful than adaptive immunity and is believed to have evolved far earlier. Its activity level does not improve or react more rapidly after repeated exposures to antigen, as is the case with the adaptive immune system. Components of the innate and adaptive immune systems function interactively, as macrophages and dendritic cells (innate immunity) function as antigen-presenting cells, which activate CD4$^+$ T helper cells (adaptive immunity), whereas cytokines produced by T helper cells stimulate full activation of macrophages and natural killer cells. Antibodies (products of the adaptive immune system) kill bacteria in conjunction with the complement cascade and stimulate release of vasoactive components from basophils and mast cells (components of the innate immune system). Several cell types are involved in the innate immune response.

Polymorphonuclear neutrophils (neutrophils) are phagocytic cells that ingest large particles and microbes, killing them by the combined action of powerful digestive enzymes and reactive oxygen and nitrogen species (ROS and RNS). Neutrophils are the most common of the white blood cells and are vital in the defense against bacterial invaders. These cells may also release enzymes and ROS extracellularly.

Monocytes and macrophages comprise another group of phagocytic cells that kill ingested material in a manner similar to that employed by neutrophils. They, along with dendritic cells, express MHC class II molecules on their surface and function as antigen-presenting cells vital to CD4$^+$ T helper cell activation. Monocytes are immature cells found in the blood. After approximately eight hours, they migrate into the tissues and mature into macrophages. Microglia are brain-dwelling macrophages. Macrophages produce several inflammatory cytokines and may induce either protective or pathological inflammation during diseases such as tuberculosis and rheumatic heart disease following streptococcal infection. These cells, like T helper cells, express CD4 and are infected by HIV.

Natural killer (NK) cells are morphologically similar to lymphocytes and function in a manner reminiscent of the actions of CD8$^+$ T killer cells. NK cells, however, kill virally infected cells and cancerous cells in a nonspecific manner and choose as their targets cells containing few or no MHC class I molecules. As stated previously, some viruses and cancers reduce the expression of MHC class I molecules on cells in order to avoid killing by CD8$^+$ T killer cells; such cells then become better targets for NK cell-mediated killing.

Several other cell types are present at low levels in the blood or tissues. Eosinophils are believed to aid in defense against parasitic worms and protect against severe allergic reactions. Basophils and mast cells are activated by immunoglobulin E (IgE) antibodies to release vasoactive chemicals, such as histamine and the leukotrienes, triggering allergic reactions.

Antibody Classes: The Heavy Artillery

The five classes of antibodies have partially overlapping but also specialized functions. All five are produced by the same adaptive immune cell type, the B lymphocyte. If this cell type is inactivated, all classes of antibody could be lost.

IgG are the most common class of antibodies in the blood. They are able to activate the **complement cascade**, a series of enzymatic reactions that terminates in the formation of large, destructive pores within the plasma membrane of the targeted microbe or cell. Another functions of the complement cascade is to attract other immune cells to the area. IgG adhered to a microbe draws it to the attention of phagocytic cells and NK cells for killing and disposal. These antibodies are able to trigger **agglutination**, the formation of large complexes of antibody and antigen that may be removed from circulation by phagocytic cells. IgG are the only class of antibodies able to cross the placenta in order to protect the fetus.

Immunoglobulin M (IgM) are the largest of the antibodies, over five times as large as IgG. IgM have a superior ability to activate complement and agglutinate antigens. They are the only type of antibody made during a primary immune response and are the first class of antibody made by infants.

Immunoglobulin A (IgA) are more than twice the size of IgG. They are the most abundant of the antibodies in secretions, such as tears, saliva, and mucus, and perform the vital role of blocking microbial entry via the nose, mouth, gastrointestinal tract, and urogenital system. Because IgA are present in breast milk, they help protect newborns against infection.

Immunoglobulin D (IgD) are present almost exclusively on the surface of B lymphocytes. Like the other classes of antibodies, they serve as the B cells' receptor for antigen.

IgE are the least abundant antibody class. These antibodies adhere to receptors on the surface of mast cells and basophils. Upon binding to their antigen, IgE antibodies trigger many of the most common allergic reactions.

Cytokines and Chemokines: Communications Corps and Chemical Weaponry

Cytokines are immune messenger molecules that communicate between cells of the immune system, increasing or decreasing activity of various cells. Some cytokines stimulate hematopoiesis, the formation of all types of blood cells, while others trigger activity of other human cells, such as neurons of the brain or hepatocytes of the liver. Some types of cytokines induce apoptotic death of infected cells or cancerous cells. Still other cytokines directly impair the division of viruses. Cytokines may be divided into several broad categories.

Hematopoietic cytokines stimulate formation of erythrocytes, leukocytes, and platelets by stem cells of the red bone marrow. Erythropoietin (Epo) stimulates production of erythrocytes. Thrombopoietin (Tpo) triggers production of megakaryocytes and, subsequently, platelets. Granulocyte colony-stimulating factor (G-CSF) stimulates the production of neutrophils, eosinophils, and basophils, and macrophage colony-stimulating factor (M-CSF) initiates formation of monocytes and macrophages. Granulocyte-macrophage colony-stimulating factor (GM-CSF) encourages formation of neutrophils, eosinophils, basophils, and monocytes and macrophages.

Th1 cytokines are produced by Th1 cells or other immune cells. They play important roles in the defense against viral infections and cancer by activating macrophages, $CD8^+$ T killer cells, and NK cells. Interleukin-2 (IL-2) serves as a growth factor for T lymphocytes and activates B lymphocytes, NK cells, and macrophages. Interferon-gamma (IFN-γ) inhibits viral growth, activates macrophages and NK cells to kill viruses and cancer cells, and increases the expression of MHC class I and II molecules on cell surfaces. IFN-γ also inhibits release of Th2 cytokines. IL-12 and IL-23, while not Th1 cytokines, stimulate production of the Th1 cytokines and IL-15 functions in a manner similar to that of IL-2.

Th2 cytokines are produced by Th2 cells or other immune cell types. They function primarily in protection against many bacterial, fungal, and parasitic infections by stimulating B lymphocytes, eosinophils, and basophils. IL-10 decreases Th1 cytokine production as well as other functions of the immune system. IL-4 encourages production of IgE antibodies and suppresses production of Th1 cytokines. IL-5 activates eosinophils and stimulates their formation.

Th17 cytokines protect against many bacterial infections. IL-17 is the major representative of this group of inflammatory cytokines. IL-25 is also a member of this group.

Treg cytokines are made by Treg cells. They act to decrease the immune response in order to prevent autoimmune, inflammatory, and allergic reactions. Transforming growth factor-β (TGF-β) and IL-10 are the two primary Treg cytokines.

Proinflammatory cytokines induce **inflammation**, a process characterized by an influx of immune cells, resulting in redness, swelling, pain, heat, and loss of function. IL-1, IL-6, and tumor necrosis factor-α (TNF-α) are members of this group. IL-6 also stimulates acute phase responses by the liver. IL-1 and TNF-α additionally function as endogenous pyrogens ("fire generators") that stimulate the hypothalamus to produce fever that kills many microbes. TNF-α also kills tumor cells and induces wasting (such as occurs during AIDS). Excess levels of this cytokine occurring in diseases such as toxic shock syndrome (massive streptococcal infection) lead to shock and rapid death.

The interferons are so named for their ability to interfere with viral growth. Interferons also have antiproliferative properties and can inhibit cancerous growth. Interferon (IFN)-α and IFN-β are the type I interferons. IFN-γ (immune interferon) is also a Th1 cytokine.

Table 2.2 Actions of selected cytokines

Category	Cytokine	Action
Hematopoietic growth factors	Erythropoietin	↑ erythrocyte production
	Thrombopoietin	↑ platelet production
	G-CSG	↑ production of neutrophils, eosinophils, basophils
	M-CSF	↑ production of monocytes and macrophages
Th1 cytokines	IL-2	Growth factor Activates leukocytes
	IFN-γ	↓ viral growth Activates leukocytes
Th2 cytokines	IL-4	↑ production of IgE
	IL-5	Activates eosinophils
Th17 cytokines	IL-17	Protect against bacterial infections
Treg cytokines	IL-10	↓ autoimmune diseases
	TGF-β	↓ allergies ↓ inflammation
Inflammatory cytokines	IL-6	Induces inflammation
	IL-1	Induces inflammation and fever
	TNF-α	Induces fever

Tumor necrosis factors (TNF) trigger the death of tumor cells. TNF-α is also a proinflammatory cytokine, while TNF-β is a Th1 cytokine.

Chemokines are cytokines with chemotactic activity that attract other cells, primarily those of the immune system, into an area. IL-8 attracts neutrophils. IP-10, I-TAC, and Mig (monocyte induced by IFN-γ), by contrast, attract CD4$^+$ Th1 cells. Migration inhibitory proteins (MIP-1 and MIP-2) decrease migration of macrophages, retaining them in a given area.

Antimicrobial Agents: Humans Fight Back, Part Two

In addition to the body's own natural defensive mechanisms, for several thousand years humans have used medicinal agents derived initially from other organisms, such as plants and fungi, to protect themselves from infectious diseases. More recently, humans have used chemical or molecular biological techniques to design and mass-produce still more effective drugs. Some of the earliest antimicrobial compounds were extracted from medicinal plants by cultures throughout the world, including those of Egypt, the Middle East, India, China, and the Americas, including many plants mentioned in the Bible, such as garlic, white wormwood (used to treat malaria and other infections), aloe, cumin, and chickpea. Traditional healers beginning 2,500 to 3,000 years ago were observant botanists. Today, scientific methods are increasingly being brought to bear in attempts to uncover the mechanisms of action of other plants used in "alternative medicine." A great deal of interest is currently focused on the antibacterial, antiviral, and anticancer activities of plant extracts such as the polyphenols, a large group of antioxidants derived from green tea, acai, soy, and red wine.

Antibiotics are drugs that either kill bacteria or inhibit their growth. Many antibiotics are produced by fungi. Some of the early work on antibacterial agents was performed by René Dubois, who studied the ability of soil extracts to kill *Streptococcus pneumoniae.* He later isolated an antibacterial compound from a soil bacterium, *Bacillus brevis.* Sulfonamides (sulfa drugs) were synthesized after the discovery that a red dye could successfully treat some cases of pneumonia. These drugs, as well as trimethoprim, mimic a precursor of folic acid in such a manner as to inhibit synthesis of this vital compound by bacteria, thus halting their growth. Humans are not affected by sulfa drugs because we do not produce our own folic acid but rather obtain it from dietary sources. Many of the antimicrobial compounds selectively affect microbes by targeting key differences between these organisms and humans. Bacteria are particularly susceptible to antimicrobial drugs because prokaryotes (bacteria) and eukaryotes (humans) differ in several key cellular structures, as described earlier. Some of the bacterial structures and activities targeted by antibiotics include the 30S (neomycin, tetracycline, and aminoglycosides such as streptomycin) and 50S ribosomal subunits (azithromycin, chloramphenicol, clindamycin, erythromycin, linezolid, and quinupristin-dalfopristin), the peptidoglycan layer of the bacterial cell wall (β-lactam antibiotics and glycopeptides and lipoglycopeptides such as teicoplanin, dalbavancin, telavancin, and vancomycin), and the bacterial membrane (daptomycin and polymyxins). Other commonly used antibiotics include the β-lactam compounds such as penicillin, amoxicillin, ampicillin, cephalosporins, and monobactams. The fluoroquinolones act by binding to bacterial DNA gyrase, an enzyme used during DNA replication. Rifampin and mupirocin block synthesis of bacterial RNA.

Antibiotics have limitations. They do not target viruses. Some antibiotics kill bacteria (bacteriocidal compounds), while others block their growth without killing the organisms (bacteriostatic compounds). Antibiotics also have differential abilities to penetrate tissues, enter cells, or pass through the blood-brain barrier. Some antibiotics may be toxic to fetuses. Antibiotics that target the 30S or 50S ribosomal subunits may be toxic to cells because mitochondria, key cellular organelles involved in energy production, contain ribosomes very similar to those found in bacteria.

Relatively few compounds are available that kill viral invaders: acyclovir is the gold standard antiviral agent. Some antiviral compounds inhibit the replication of viral RNA. The benzofuran derivatives, indole-N-acetamine, phenylanlanine, thiophene, etravirine, and efavirenz are non-nucleoside-based RNA replicase inhibitors, while ribavirin, zidovudine (AZT), and stavudine are nucleoside analogs. Some of the former agents may cause rash and liver toxicity, while the latter are toxic to human mitochondria and their use may lead to muscle pain, weakness, fatigue, loss of body fat, and lactic acidosis. Several antiviral agents target serine proteases: these include boceprevir, ciluprevir, and telaprevir. Other drugs target various HIV enzymes, such as protease (indinivar, squinavir, and ritonavir) and integrase (raltegravir). Miraviroc and vicriviroc block the binding of HIV to its CCR5 coreceptor on macrophages. Enfuvirtide blocks HIV fusion with the host cell membrane. Most of these drugs have a number of side effects, some of which are potentially very serious. Highly active antiretroviral therapy (HAART) uses a combination of some of these drugs to inhibit HIV growth. It has greatly extended the life span of many infected persons.

Other agents act against protozoan invaders. Examples of antimalarial compounds include artemisinin and its derivatives, quinine, chloroquine, sulfadoxine-pyrimethamine, and mefloquine. Nifurtimox (lampit) is used to treat infection with *Trypanosoma cruzi*. Nitazoxanide and paromomycin (Humatin) are partially effective against infection with *Cryptosporidium parvum*.

Microbes have developed resistance to many of these agents. The story of drug-resistant microbes is described in the chapters on multidrug-resistant bacteria, drug-resistant malaria, and multidrug-resistant and extensively drug-resistant tuberculosis.

Summary

Types of Infectious Agents
- Viruses • Bacteria • Protozoa • Fungi • Prions

Means of Increasing Genetic Diversity in Bacteria and Viruses
- Bacteria: conjugation, transformation, acquisition of plasmids, and transduction • Viruses: error-prone reproductive enzymes, lack of genomic repair mechanisms, genomic reassortment between similar species

Cells of the Adaptive Immune Response and Their Functions

• B lymphocytes (antibody production, T helper lymphocyte activation via antigen presentation) • T helper lymphocytes (production of many types of cytokines) • T killer lymphocytes (killing of atypical cells, including cells infected by microbes)

Some of the Cells of the Innate Immune Response and Selected Functions

• Neutrophils (phagocytosis, killing of ingested and extracellular microbes) • Monocytes and macrophages (phagocytosis, killing of ingested and extracellular microbes, antigen presentation, production of inflammatory cytokines) • Dendritic cells (antigen presentation) • Natural killer cells (killing of atypical cells, including cells infected by microbes) • Eosinophils (protection against parasites, protection against allergic responses) • Basophils and mast cells (release of vasoactive compounds, production of allergic reactions)

Classes of Antibodies

• IgG • IgM • IgA • IgD • IgE

Major Types of Cytokines

• Hematopoietic • Th1 • Th2 • Th17 • Treg
• Proinflammatory • Interferons • Tumor necrosis factors
• Chemokines

Targets of Antibiotics

• Folic acid synthetic machinery • 30S and 50S ribosomal subunits • Peptidoglycan layer of the bacterial cell wall • Bacterial membrane • DNA gyrase • Bacterial RNA synthetic machinery

Activities of Antiviral Compounds

• Inhibition of RNA replication by non-nucleoside-based RNA replicase inhibitors or nucleoside analogs • Inhibition of enzymatic activity (serine proteases, integrase) • Inhibition of viral binding to receptors • Inhibition of viral fusion with host cell membranes

Key Terms

Adaptive immunity Arm of the immune response that provides very powerful, large-scale, extremely precise defense by recognizing specific regions of proteins

Agglutination Formation of large complexes of antibodies and antigen to be removed from circulation by phagocytic cells

Antigen-presenting cells B cells, monocytes and macrophages, and dendritic cells

Attenuated microbes Weakened, nonpathogenic microbes

Bacteria Prokaryotes surrounded by cell walls containing peptidoglycan

Bacteriophages Viruses that infect bacteria

Binary fission Asexual form of clonal reproduction that produces two individuals identical to the parent

Chemokines Cytokines with chemotactic activity

Complement cascade Series of enzymatic reactions that terminates in the formation of large, destructive pores within the plasma membrane of the targeted microbe or cellular target and also attracts other immune cells to the area

Conjugation Process whereby DNA is exchanged between individuals of opposite mating types

Cytokines Immune messenger molecules

DNA Genetic information composed of two long chains of interconnected nucleotides twisted into the form of a double helix (except in some viruses)

Hematopoietic cytokines Cytokines that stimulate formation of erythrocytes, leukocytes, and platelets by stem cells of the red bone marrow

Inflammation Process characterized by an influx of immune cells and red blood cells followed by redness, swelling, pain, heat, and loss of function

Innate immune system Arm of the immune response that provides immediate, nonspecific protection against microbial and cancerous threats

Mutations Alterations in the sequence of DNA nucleotides

Oncogenes Genes that may cause cancer if mutated, overexpressed, or improperly expressed

Plasmids Small circular pieces of nonchromosomal DNA that may divide in a somewhat autonomous manner in bacteria

Prions Infectious proteinaceous particles; self-replicating, misfolded proteins

Proteins Long strings of amino acids folded into complex patterns; produced from RNA by translation

Protozoa Unicellular eukaryotic organisms whose cell wall, if present, does not contain chitin or cellulose

Retroviruses Viruses that use the enzyme reverse transcriptase to reproduce their genetic material

RNA Single chains of nucleosides (except for some viruses) produced from DNA by transcription

Transduction Transmission of genetic information between bacteria of the same or different species by a bacteriophage

Transformation Process by which some species of bacteria may under special conditions acquire pieces of DNA from the external environment

Viruses Tiny obligate intracellular parasites that pass through most filters

Review Questions

1. How do prokaryotes differ from eukaryotes?
2. How do microbes breach the skin and mucous membranes to gain access to the interior of human hosts?
3. What are four ways in which bacteria increase their genetic diversity? Briefly describe each.
4. How do the adaptive and innate immune systems differ? What cell types function in each?
5. What are some of the limitations of antibiotics?

Topics for Further Discussion

1. The rapid mutation rate of HIV allows it to evade the host immune response and become resistant to antimicrobial agents. Discuss possible reasons why other viruses and bacteria do not mutate as rapidly as HIV.
2. The human immune system contains both innate and adaptive branches. Discuss how these two branches interact and complement each other.
3. The immune system contains cells (basophils and mast cells) and antibodies (IgE) that trigger allergic reactions. Search the Internet for other functions of these cells that may explain why they have been retained as a part of the human defense system.
4. Antimicrobial agents often attack microbial structures or processes that differ from those found in humans. Humans do not use conjugation, transformation, transduction, or acquisition of plasmids in order to increase genetic diversity as bacteria do. Discuss possible ways in which humans may target these processes in order to kill bacteria.

Resources

Centers for Disease Control and Prevention. http://cdc.gov.

Chin, J. *Control of Communicable Diseases Manual* (17th ed.). Washington, D.C.: American Public Health Association, 2000.

Duke, J. A. *Duke's Handbook of Medicinal Plants of the Bible.* Boca Raton, Fla.: CRC Press, 2008.

Goldsby, R. A., Kindt, T. J., and Osborne, B. A. *Kuby Immunology* (4th ed.). New York: Freeman, 2000.

Medline Plus. http://www.nlm.nih.gov/medlineplus.

Ramawat, K. G. (ed.). *Herbal Drugs: Ethnomedicine to Modern Medicine.* New York: Springer, 2009.

Salyers, A. A., and Whitt, D. D. *Revenge of the Microbes: How Bacterial Resistance Is Undermining the Antibiotic Miracle.* Washington, D.C.: ASM Press, 2005.

Tortora, G. J., Funke, B. R., and Case, C. L. *Microbiology: An Introduction* (10th ed.). San Francisco: Benjamin Cummings, 2004.

BACTERIAL INFECTIONS

CHAPTER 3

LYME DISEASE

LEARNING OBJECTIVES

- Define Lyme disease
- Describe the spirochete responsible for causing this illness
- Discuss modes of infection
- Discuss the host's response to infection
- Describe symptomatology and diagnosis
- Discuss methods of treatment
- Discuss methods of prevention

Major Concepts

Outbreak

Lyme disease was first reported in Connecticut in 1976 as an outbreak of arthritis in an unusually large number of children and adults. It was later found to result from infection by a tickborne spirochete bacterium. A spirochete is a spiral-shaped, rodlike bacterium that has caused diseases such as syphilis and relapsing fever. Nymphal and larval forms of the tick transmit the spirochete to humans. Disease incidence is highest during spring and summer when these ticks are seeking new hosts.

Symptoms

The symptoms of Lyme disease include a combination of a tick bite with or without the presence of a tick, an erythema migrans rash, fever, chills, fatigue, weight change, hair loss, swollen glands, sore throat, irritable bowel, chest pain, shortness of breath, heart palpitations, joint pain and stiffness, muscle pain, headache, tingling or numbness, facial paralysis, double vision, buzzing or ringing in the ears, dizziness, poor balance, light-headedness, difficulty walking, tremor, heart murmur, confusion, forgetfulness, poor short-term memory, mood swings, meningitis, sensitivity to light, recurring hepatitis, and adult respiratory distress syndrome. Lack of prompt treatment may lead to persistent fatigue or malaise, migratory musculoskeletal disorders, chronic encephalopathy and encephalomyelitis, peripheral neuropathy, and difficulty with concentration or memory.

Setting

Lyme disease in the United States occurs primarily in the Northeast along the coast from Maine to Maryland, in portions of the Midwest, and in parts of the Far West. It is also found in temperate areas of Canada, Europe, Africa, Asia, and Australia. Incidence of Lyme disease has been on the rise due to increased habitats for the tick vectors and the mice and deer on which they feed. The rising incidence is also influenced by greater use of tick habitat by humans and an increase in the construction of human residences in these regions. Southern-tick-associated rash illness (STARI) is a similar disease found in the American Southeast. It results from infection with *Borrelia lonestari*, transmitted by the bite of the lone star tick.

Infection

Lyme disease is the result of infection by genospecies of *Borrelia burgdorferi* sensu lato. These are gram-negative, flagellated spirochetes, similar to the causative agent of syphilis. Over 300 strains of these bacteria are found worldwide. In Europe and Africa, *B. afzelii* and *B. garinii* may also cause Lyme disease, while *B. japonica* and *B. miyamoto* cause the disease in Japan. Borrelia species have a small linear chromosome and up to 9 circular and 12 linear plasmids. These plasmids are involved in the infection of mammals and ticks and in drug resistance. The spirochetes contain very limited numbers of biosynthetic proteins, relying instead on the host for most of their nutritional needs (importantly, *B. burgdorferi* does not require iron for survival, permitting it to avoid host defense mechanisms that limit microbial access to iron). Following a localized skin infection, bacteria enter the blood and cerebrospinal fluid and may migrate to the myocardium of the heart, retina, muscle, bone, spleen, liver, meninges, and brain. As systemic infection declines, some organisms persist for years in areas such as the joints, nervous system, and skin.

Immune Response

The reaction of the immune system to *B. burgdorferi* is complex, involving complement-mediated lysis, antibody production by B lymphocytes, Th1 cytokine secretion by T helper lymphocytes, activation of macrophages, and phagocytosis by neutrophils. These cells, acting together, kill bacteria and limit their dissemination. The immune response may, however, also induce pathology. Persons suffering from moderate to severe arthritis often have very high levels of antibody in their blood and joints, which may contribute to arthritis. The bacteria trigger macrophages to produce proinflammatory cytokines such as IL-1 β, TNF-α, and IL-6, worsening joint damage. *Borrelia* also have mechanisms to evade the immune system, such as complement regulatory factors, rapid antigenic variation to avoid recognition by T cells, and triggering apoptotic death pathways in macrophages.

Medicinal Therapy

Various bacteriostatic or bacteriocidal drugs are available to treat Lyme disease, including the tetracyclines, doxycycline, minocycline, penicillins (amoxicillin but not penicillin G), macrolides, and cephalosporins. These vary widely in their ability to penetrate tissues and enter the central nervous system. Antibiotic use may result in the Jarish-Herxheimer reaction, a temporary increase in discomfort due to shedding toxins released by dead spirochetes stimulating an intense immune response.

Prevention

Ticks are found mainly in leaf litter and low-lying vegetation. Prevention of Lyme disease involves avoiding tick habitat; wearing light-colored, protective clothing that covers the arms and legs; wearing closed shoes; and using tick repellents containing DEET (an oily, colorless chemical that is the active ingredient in the most widely used insect repellents that may be safely applied to the skin) on clothing and exposed skin. The removal of leaf litter, tall grass, woodpiles, and brush from residential areas may reduce vector and reservoir habitat. Following visits to tick-inhabited areas, it is essential to inspect the skin and hair, and promptly remove ticks using methods that completely eliminate all tick parts.

Introduction

Lyme disease, spread by the bite of deer ticks, is the most prevalent arthropod-borne illness in temperate climates due to reforestation, decreased hunting, increased human habitation near woodlands, and the subsequent increases in deer numbers and in human-deer interactions. First reported in Connecticut, this disease has been found in all states in the United States. It is concentrated in three regions: the Northeast coast from Maine to Maryland, the Midwestern states of Wisconsin and Minnesota, and parts of the Far West. It is endemic in New York, New Jersey, Connecticut, Pennsylvania, Massachusetts, Rhode Island, Delaware, Maryland, Wisconsin, Minnesota, California, and Oregon. While the absolute number of cases in the United States are highest in New York and Pennsylvania, the incidence is highest in Delaware (77 per 100,000 population) and Connecticut (51 per 100,000). Numbers of cases in other coastal or midwestern states are increasing as the causative bacterium, **Borrelia burgdorferi**, spreads to new areas. It is estimated that only 10% of the true number of cases are accurately diagnosed and reported to the Centers for Disease Control and Prevention. Lyme disease also occurs in Canada, much of Europe, the former Soviet Union, northern China, Japan, North Africa, and eastern Australia. The areas of Europe with highest incidence of disease are Germany, Austria, Slovenia, and Sweden, in which the infection rate approaches that of Connecticut.

In the United States, Lyme disease most commonly strikes individuals between the ages of 5 and 14. Incidence decreases between the ages of 15 and 30 and then slowly increases until 70 years, followed by declining numbers in older persons. Males are infected at a higher rate than females, perhaps due to a greater exposure to ticks.

Table 3.1 Incidence of Lyme disease by state

State	2004	2005	2006	2007	2008
Alabama	0.1	0.1	0.2	0.3	0.1
Alaska	0.5	0.6	0.4	1.5	0.9
Arizona	0.2	0.2	0.2	0.0	0.0
Arkansas	0.0	0.0	0.0	0.0	0.0
California	0.1	0.3	0.2	0.2	0.2
Colorado	0.0	0.0	0.0	0.0	0.0
Connecticut	38.5	51.7	51.0	87.3	78.2
Delaware	40.8	76.7	56.5	82.7	88.4
District of Columbia	2.9	1.7	10.7	19.7	12.0
Florida	0.3	0.3	0.2	0.2	0.4
Georgia	0.1	0.1	0.1	0.1	0.4
Hawaii	0.0	0.0	0.0	0.0	0.0
Idaho	0.4	0.1	0.5	0.6	0.3
Illinois	0.7	1.0	0.9	1.2	0.8
Indiana	0.5	0.5	0.4	0.9	0.7
Iowa	1.7	3.0	3.3	4.1	2.8
Kansas	0.1	0.1	0.1	0.3	0.6
Kentucky	0.4	0.1	0.2	0.1	0.1
Louisiana	0.0	0.1	0.0	0.0	0.1
Maine	17.1	18.7	25.6	40.2	59.2
Maryland	16.0	22.1	22.2	45.8	31.0
Massachusetts	23.9	36.3	22.2	46.3	60.9
Michigan	0.3	0.6	0.5	0.5	0.8
Minnesota	20.1	17.9	17.7	23.8	20.0
Mississippi	0.0	0.0	0.1	0.0	0.0
Missouri	0.4	0.3	0.1	0.2	0.1
Montana	0.0	0.0	0.1	0.4	0.6
Nebraska	0.1	0.1	0.6	0.4	0.4
Nevada	0.0	0.1	0.2	0.6	0.3
New Hampshire	17.4	20.3	46.9	68.1	92.0
New Jersey	31.0	38.6	27.9	36.1	37.0
New Mexico	0.1	0.2	0.2	0.3	0.2
New York	26.5	28.8	23.1	21.6	29.5
North Carolina	1.4	0.6	0.4	0.6	0.2
North Dakota	0.0	0.5	1.1	1.9	1.2
Ohio	0.4	0.5	0.4	0.3	0.3
Oklahoma	0.1	0.0	0.0	0.0	0.0
Oregon	0.3	0.1	0.2	0.2	0.5
Pennsylvania	32.1	34.6	26.1	32.1	30.7
Rhode Island	23.0	3.6	28.8	16.7	17.7
South Carolina	0.5	0.4	0.5	0.7	0.3
South Dakota	0.1	0.3	0.1	0.0	0.4
Tennessee	0.3	0.1	0.2	0.5	0.1
Texas	0.4	0.3	0.1	0.4	0.4

(Continued)

Table 3.1   Incidence of Lyme disease by state (Continued)

State	2004	2005	2006	2007	2008
Utah	0.0	0.1	0.2	0.3	0.1
Vermont	8.0	8.7	16.8	22.2	53.1
Virginia	2.9	3.6	4.7	12.4	11.4
Washington	0.2	0.2	0.1	0.2	0.3
West Virginia	2.1	3.4	1.5	4.6	6.6
Wisconsin	20.8	26.4	26.4	32.4	26.5
Wyoming	0.8	0.6	0.2	0.6	0.2

Note: Confirmed cases per 100,000 persons, calculated using July 1 population estimates for each year.
Source: CDC.

FIGURE 3.1   Annual incidence of reported cases of Lyme disease in the United States, by age group and sex, 1992–2004

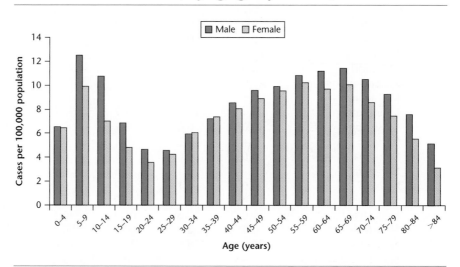

Note: Age- and sex-specific incidence was calculated using Census Bureau population estimates for July 1, 2000.
Source: CDC.

History

Lyme disease was named after the town of Old Lyme, Connecticut, where it was reported in 1976 to cause an unusually large number of arthritis cases in children (39 cases in children and 12 in adults). The arthritis presented as intermittent episodes

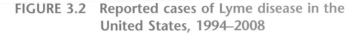

FIGURE 3.2   Reported cases of Lyme disease in the United States, 1994–2008

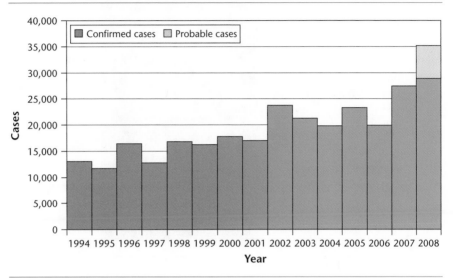

Source: CDC.

of asymmetric pain and swelling, particularly in large joints such as the knees. A search of historical records indicates that a similar condition was reported in 1883 in Breslau, Germany, by Alfred Buchwald, who described a degenerative skin condition, acrodermatitis chronica atrophicans. In the early 1900s, Arvid Afzelius observed a ringlike lesion that he believed resulted from the bite of an *Ixodes* tick.

In the Americas, Lyme disease was present in Cape Cod during the 1960s. DNA from the causative organism, however, was detected by polymerase chain reaction (PCR) in museum specimens of ticks and mice from Long Island dating from the late nineteenth and early twentieth centuries. After European colonization, much of the habitat required for Lyme disease transmission was removed as wooded areas were cleared for farmland. During the twentieth century, however, much of the area was returned to forests, and the deer, rodent, and tick populations grew, as did the incidence of Lyme disease. This disease now affects suburban locations in some of the most heavily populated regions of the country, including Boston, New York, Philadelphia, and Baltimore.

The Disease

The initial symptoms are known as early localized Lyme borreliosis and include a rash, **erythema migrans** (EM), in 60% to 80% of infected individuals. This rash appears between 2 and 30 days after the bite of an infected tick and often

FIGURE 3.3 Erythema migrans

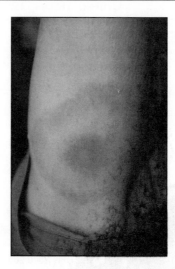

Source: CDC/James Gathany.

has a bull's-eye appearance that may be circular or oval. The rash may be quite large, up to 30 inches in diameter. It is often accompanied by a nonspecific fever.

Although up to 10% of infections may be asymptomatic, Lyme disease is usually associated with a variety of symptoms that allow it to be confused with other diseases. It presents as a combination of several of the following symptoms: tick bite, erythema migrans rash at the tick bite site or other areas, fever, chills, sweats, fatigue, weight change, hair loss, swollen glands, sore throat, irritable bowel, chest pain or rib soreness, shortness of breath, heart palpitations, joint pain or swelling, stiffness of joints, neck, or back, muscle pain, headache, tingling or numbness, facial paralysis (such as Bell's palsy), double or blurry vision, buzzing or ringing in the ears, dizziness or poor balance, light-headedness or difficulty walking, tremor, heart murmur, confusion, difficulty thinking, forgetfulness, poor short-term memory, disorientation, mood swings, meningitis, sensitivity to light in the eyes, mild transient or recurring hepatitis, or adult respiratory distress syndrome. Patients do not manifest all of the listed symptoms. If the infection is not promptly treated in a manner leading to its elimination, several manifestations may occur several years later, including persistent fatigue and malaise, together with migratory musculoskeletal disorders, such as Lyme arthritis, chronic encephalopathy and encephalomyelitis, peripheral neuropathy, and difficulty with concentration and memory. These symptoms are believed by some to result from persistent infection. Host immunogenetic background may influence disease course, with individuals with major histocompatibility complex class II HLA-DRB1*0401 and 0101 alleles at increased risk for chronic joint inflammation or nonresponsiveness to antibiotic therapy. Coinfection with the protozoan parasite *Babesia microti* or the bacterial causative agent of human granulocytic ehrlichiosis, both transmitted by deer ticks and endemic to regions with high incidence of Lyme disease, may lead to acute flulike symptoms.

A disease similar to Lyme disease, **southern-tick-associated rash illness (STARI)**, is present in the American Southeast and is transmitted by the bite of the lone star tick, *Amblyomma americanum*. This tick carries a newly described spirochete, ***Borrelia lonestari***. This spirochete may be widespread in the southeastern United States.

The Causative Agent

Borrelia burgdorferi was isolated by William Burgdorfer at the Rocky Mountain Laboratory in 1981. Lyme disease results from infection with genospecies of *B. burgdorferi* sensu lato, gram-negative, flagellated spirochetes. These highly motile, tightly-coiled spiral bacteria are similar to the causative agent of syphilis. Over 300 strains of these bacteria are found worldwide. The causative genospecies in the United States is *B. burgdorferi* sensu stricto. The A, B, I, and K clones, distinguished by their outer surface protein C (OspC), are often associated with disseminated Lyme disease. The A clone is prevalent in both the Americas and Europe and its OspC gene is fairly uniform in both locations, suggesting recent migration. The B clone, by contrast, has greater variability between the continents, indicative of a longer period of geographical isolation. In Europe, additional species of *Borrelia* also cause Lyme disease, including ***B. afzelii*** and ***B. garinii***. The latter two strains also occur in Africa; ***B. japonica*** and ***B. miyamoto*** are found in Japan.

The spirochetes' cell wall consists of a cytoplasmic membrane surrounded by peptidoglycan with internal flagella and a loosely associated outer membrane. It was one of the first microbes to be fully sequenced and has a segmented genome with a small, 900-kilobase linear chromosome and up to 9 circular and 12 linear plasmids. The plasmids have roles in infectivity and drug resistance. One of these, the 36-kilobase linear plasmid lp36, is important in allowing infectivity of mammalian cells. The responsible region is the bbk17 (adeC) gene, encoding an adenine deaminase that allows production of hypoxanthine through the de novo pathway of nucleotide and nucleoside synthesis. Another linear plasmid, lp25, and its gene encoding nicotinamidase are vital to infectivity of ticks and mice. Another lp25 gene encodes a lipoprotein involved in persistence in ticks.

FIGURE 3.4   Spirochete

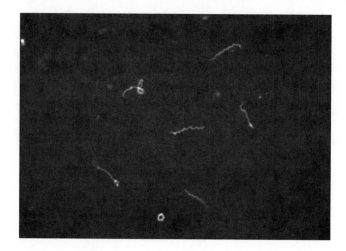

Source: CDC/W. F. Schwartz.

B. burgdorferi uses a large number of lipoproteins, including the outer surface proteins that have been used in vaccine development. The surface-exposed lipoprotein, VlsE, undergoes extensive antigenic variation and may aid the spirochete in avoiding the host adaptive immune response. These bacteria contain few biosynthetic proteins and must therefore rely on the host to supply many of their nutritional needs. *B. burgdorferi* is unusual in that it does not require iron for survival, at least in vitro. This allows it to avoid host defense mechanisms that limit microbes' supply of iron. The spirochete also does not produce toxins.

The Lyme disease agent is transmitted from host to host by hard ticks in temperate zones of the Northern Hemisphere. In the United States, these are most commonly the deer tick (*Ixodes scapularis*, formerly *I. dammini*) or the western black-legged tick (*I. pacificus*). The preferred host of the former tick is the white-footed mouse. In the northeastern United States, 10% to 50% of the deer ticks are infected with the spirochete. In Europe, Lyme disease occurs throughout the range of the sheep tick, *I. ricinus*, and in Asia, the vector is the taiga tick, *I. persulcatus*. The natural life cycle of *B. burgdorferi* involves transfer between the hard ticks and small mammals. The major reservoirs of *B. burgdorferi* in the eastern United States are white-footed mice and eastern chipmunks. In Europe, other vertebrate species also host the spirochete, including birds, reptiles, and many small to medium-sized mammals. In Asia, the immature ticks feed on voles, shrews, and birds, and the adult form feeds on most larger animals, including hares, deer, and cattle. Humans are accidental hosts and are infected by the bite of either the larval or the nymphal stage of the ticks. During these stages, the ticks are very small, approximately the size of the period at the end of this sentence, and are difficult to detect, particularly because they prefer hairy areas (armpits, groin, scalp). Early removal of the ticks is important to prevent Lyme disease because transmission of the spirochete takes at least 36 hours, the time needed for the spirochete to migrate from the tick's midgut to its salivary glands. Transmission of spirochetes to humans on the West Coast involves two

FIGURE 3.5   Nymphal *Amblyomma americanum* (lone star tick) (above) and engorged tick (below)

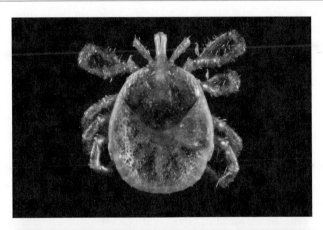

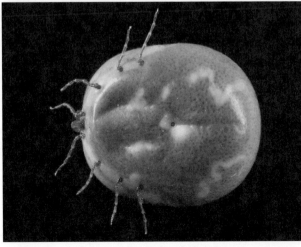

Source: CDC/Amanda Loftis, William Nicholson, Will Reeves, and Chris Paddock.

intersecting cycles. The first of these involves dusky-footed wood rats and *Ixodes spinipalpis*, which do not bite humans but maintain the cycle in nature. The second cycle involves wood rats and *I. pacificus* ticks, which do bite humans but are less commonly infected. Nymphs of *I. scapularis* in the southeastern United States feed mainly on lizards. Lizards are not infected by *B. burgdorferi* due to their innate ability to kill the bacteria using the complement cascade of the innate immune system; consequently, Lyme disease is not common in that region.

The transmission season peaks between April and July when the nymphs are seeking hosts. Ticks are found mainly in leaf litter and low-lying vegetation. Unlike many other arthropod disease vectors, such as mosquitoes, ticks take a large blood meal only once per life cycle stage, ingesting 10 to 100 times their body weight. Larvae and nymphs feed on a range of hosts, while the adults require large animals, such as deer, cattle, sheep, or horses. *B. burgdorferi* also infects and causes disease in dogs, cats, cattle, and horses. In a nymphal tick host, the spirochete remains dormant in the midgut from fall until late spring; OspA is the primary antigen expressed. As the nymph feeds, OspA expression decreases and that of OspC increases. The latter is needed for infection of mammals, and it is predominantly expressed when the spirochete moves to the salivary glands.

In the mammalian host, localized skin infection occurs. Within weeks, the bacteria begin to disseminate by binding to integrins, proteoglycans, and glycoproteins on cells or in tissues. These include heparin sulfate and dermatan sulfate on epithelial cells and neurons, and decorin, which associates with collagen and may allow its association with the extracellular matrix of the heart, nervous system, and joints. The spirochetes also bind the receptors for fibronectin and vitronectin. They move into the blood and cerebrospinal fluid, and small numbers may be found in the myocardium, retina, muscle, bone, spleen, liver, meninges, and brain. Later, systemic infection declines, with the organisms persisting for years in the joints, nervous system, or skin. The different *Borrelia* species vary in ability to persist and cause pathology in the different sites. *B. burgdorferi* appears to favor the joints and is the most capable of inducing arthritis. *B. afzelii*, however, may remain in the skin for decades and cause acrodermatitis chronica atrophicans, mainly on sun-exposed surfaces of the distal extremities in elderly women. *B. garinii* is the most neurotropic, resulting in many types of neurologic abnormalities, including borrelial encephalomyelitis, which is similar to multiple sclerosis.

The Immune Response

Soon after the appearance of the EM rash, complement begins to lyse the spirochetes. Several of the *Borrelia* species produce complement regulatory factors that result in cleavage of C3b, vital to host complement-mediated microbial killing. A humoral immune response then occurs, with the production of antibody, mostly IgM reactive to OspC, and later IgG. In individuals with moderate to severe arthritis, very high levels of antibody may be found in the blood and in the joints. This antibody may contribute to the arthritic manifestations of the disease. Cell-mediated immunity is also present, as T lymphocytes respond to bacterial antigens, secreting interferon-γ and activating macrophages. The VslE lipoprotein, previously mentioned, undergoes antigenic variation to escape recognition by these cells.

Bacterial lipoproteins stimulate the innate immune system by binding to several microbial recognition receptors on macrophages, including CD14 and the Toll-like receptor 2 (TLR2)/TLR1 heterodimer. These cells, together with neutrophils, phagocytize and destroy bacteria in the lesions and limit their dissemination. *B. burgdorferi* also kill macrophages by triggering cytoplasmic signals that induce cytokine production and activation of caspase-1, resulting in apoptotic death of the immune cell. The syphilis spirochete fails to kill the macrophages in this manner, while dendritic cells are spared by *Borrelia*. In Lyme disease, ingestion of spirochetes also induces macrophages to produce transcripts for the proinflammatory cytokines pro-IL-1β (IL-1β), TNF-α, and IL-6, which may worsen joint damage. Caspase-1 must be active to process and secrete IL-1β. The immune response thus functions to both contain the spirochetes and cause much of the pathology.

Diagnosis

Lyme disease has been called the "great pretender" due to its similarity to several other disease conditions, including multiple sclerosis, systemic lupus erythematosus, amyotrophic lateral sclerosis (Lou Gehrig's disease), fibromyalgia, chronic fatigue syndrome, and Alzheimer's disease. Isolation and culture of *B. burgdorferi* from infected individuals is considered the gold standard for diagnosis, and most commonly uses material from skin biopsies or cutaneous lavage from EM lesions or blood from patients with early disseminated disease.

Many of the common diagnostic tests for Lyme disease detect antibodies, such as the enzyme-linked immunosorbent assay (ELISA) and the indirect fluorescent-antibody assay (IFA). These tests are not highly sensitive or specific, for an infected individual may test negative for antispirochete antibodies and still have the disease if infected with a different strain of *B. burgdorferi* than was used in the diagnostic test. An infected person may also test negative for antibodies in the blood but still have them in the spinal fluids. An antibody-based test might alternatively suggest that a person who is not infected indeed has the disease. This is particularly true for individuals with syphilis, which is caused by another bacterial spirochete, *Treponema pallidum*, as antibodies developed against this bacterium may cross-react with *B. burgdorferi*. Occasional false-positive tests also occur in individuals with infectious mononucleosis, systemic lupus erythematosus, or rheumatoid arthritis. A second test, such as Western blot, is needed to confirm the diagnosis. This test directly detects the antibodies to the correct spirochete antigens. A positive result is indicated by positive reactions against any two of the following antigen bands: 20, 23, 35, 39, 41, or 88 kilodaltons (kD). PCR may also be used to detect *B. burgdorferi* DNA in synovial fluid samples of individuals with arthritis or skin biopsy samples from those with EM.

The Lyme urine antigen test (LUAT) identifies spirochete antigens shed in the urine. This test has greater reactivity after the spirochetes begin to die, as occurs following antibiotic treatment, and is not as useful as serological or other molecular techniques. Other tests may search for the presence of antibodies in the cerebrospinal fluid.

Treatment

In its early stages, Lyme disease almost always responds to antibiotic treatment. If untreated, however, it can progress to late Lyme disease, with arthritic, neurological, and cardiac manifestations. These require more intensive therapy and may be permanent. A number of antibiotics may be used; these are administered either orally or intravenously, and each has its positive characteristics. Tetracyclines are bacteriostatic, halting the growth of bacteria without killing them. These drugs are taken into infected cells to fight intracellular bacteria. Doxycycline and minocycline are able to penetrate the spinal fluid and the brain. The penicillins, for their part, are bacteriocidal, killing bacteria, but are not effective against intracellular organisms. Among this group, amoxicillin is effective for the treatment of Lyme disease and is safe for pregnant women, whereas penicillin G is ineffective. The macrolides are bacteriostatic but kill the bacteria when used at high concentrations. They have good tissue penetration and attack intracellular bacteria. The cephalosporins are bacteriocidal. They penetrate tissues, as well as the spinal fluid and the brain. An earlier treatment option was the use of colloidal silver, which may be effective as a drug supplement. An unfortunate side effect of this treatment is the tendency of one's skin to turn gray. The Food and Drug Administration does not recommend the use of the injectable compound bismacine (chromacine), prescribed by some alternative medicine practitioners. This drug contains high levels of bismuth and is not approved for use in an injectable form or as a treatment option for Lyme disease. Its use may lead to bismuth poisoning, resulting in heart or kidney failure.

Antibiotic therapy may also lead to short-term problems. The prolonged use of antibiotics may kill beneficial bacteria inhabiting the digestive system, leading to an overgrowth of yeast and possibly causing thrush. Eating yogurt with live cultures or taking acidophilus tablets restores the bacterial flora. The **Jarish-Herxheimer reaction** is a temporary increase of patient discomfort after antibiotic treatment. This reaction was first described in syphilis and occurs when the spirochetes die, shedding toxins that induce an intense immune response. This results in headache, chills, fever, neck pain, rashes, and fatigue.

Antibiotic-resistant strains of *B. burgdorferi* have arisen. Some isolates of strain B31 are resistant to macrolide, lincosamide, or streptogramin A antibiotics. This resistance was not due to inactivation of the antibiotics or to their removal by efflux pumps but resulted from modification of the bacterial ribosomes to decrease their binding to these antibiotics. Resistance could be transferred by conjugation to other bacterial species, such as the gram-positive *Bacillus subtilis* and *Enterococcus faecalis*. Several plasmids have been postulated to be involved in the transfer of resistance. A recent report suggests the role of an outer membrane protein, BesC, in a tripartite multidrug drug export system of the resistance nodulation division type that may be at least partially responsible for the natural ability of *B. burgdorferi* to resist antibiotics. This protein is homologous to the TolC protein in *Escherichia coli* and forms membrane channels in planar lipid bilayers. Its removal prevents successful bacterial infection of mice.

Prevention

The best way to prevent acquiring Lyme disease is to prevent the transmission of the spirochetes from ticks to humans. Risk of infection is highest when the nymphal forms are most actively feeding, during the late spring and early summer. Many people are exposed during recreational activities, such as hiking, camping, and fishing. Others are at risk due to jobs that result in exposure, such as construction, farming, landscaping, forestry, brush clearing, surveying, park or wildlife management, and railroad, oil field, or utility line work.

Several guidelines to prevent tick attachment and subsequent transmission of bacteria are as follows: (1) wear light-colored clothing to readily permit viewing of ticks before their attachment; (2) wear a long-sleeved shirt, long pants, and closed shoes with socks, and tuck the shirt into the pants and the pants into the socks; (3) use tick repellant containing N,N-diethyl-m-toluamide (**DEET**) on the skin (must be reapplied after several hours; check for adverse reactions in children) or permethrin for longer protection (several days) on clothing and boots; and (4) carefully check skin and hair for ticks soon after leaving their

RECENT DEVELOPMENTS

Antibodies may be protective against the development of Lyme disease. In animal models, immune serum (containing antibodies against *B. burgdorferi*) prevents infection of naive animals upon challenge. In dogs, a vaccine (Bacterin) exists that uses whole, killed organisms. In humans, much of the vaccine work has focused on the use of recombinant outer surface proteins (Osp). Recombinant OspA vaccines were developed in the 1990s. One such vaccine, licensed in the United States, was withdrawn by 2002 due to limited public acceptance resulting from the low risk of Lyme disease in many regions, the need for booster shots every year or two, and the relatively high cost compared with antibiotic treatment for early infection.

habitat. DEET should not be applied to the hands or face or to irritated skin. The CDC provides detailed instructions on tick removal at http://www.cdc.gov/ ticks/removing_a_tick.html. Folk remedies such as hot matches and petroleum jelly are not advised. Take care to not touch the tick with bare hands.

Risk of infection may also be decreased by removing tick, rodent, and deer habitat. This may be accomplished by application of chemicals to kill ticks and mites (acaricides) and removing leaf litter, tall grass, woodpiles, and brush at one's residence. Other methods include chemical treatment of deer and rodents by means of deer feeding stations and bait tubes and biological control with fungi

FIGURE 3.6   Approved method of tick removal

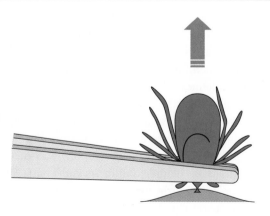

Source: CDC/DVBID

or parasitic worms or wasps. If one does visit areas inhabited by ticks, carefully inspect skin and hair soon after leaving the area, promptly removing any ticks detected using approved methods that completely remove all tick parts.

Surveillance

Recent technological advances like remote sensing methods, including satellite-determined environmental variables such as temperature, humidity, elevation, and land cover type, together with information about vector density, have been used to identify and characterize tick habitats. This information is then analyzed with georeferenced epidemiological data to yield a comprehensive picture and to produce risk maps and to suggest how alterations in environmental factors might influence disease occurrence and severity. Such studies have been performed in Baltimore County, Maryland, and in Wisconsin.

Summary

Disease
- Lyme disease

Causative Agents
- *Borrelia burgdorferi* • *B. afzelii* • *B. garinii* • *B. japonica*
- *B. miyamoto*

Agent Type
- Gram-negative, flagellated spirochete

Genome
- DNA

Vectors
- Deer tick (*Ixodes scapularis*) • Western black-legged tick (*I. pacificus*)
- Sheep tick (*I. ricinus*) • Taiga tick (*I. persulcatus*)

Common Reservoirs
- Mammals (white-footed mouse, eastern chipmunks, voles, shrews, hares, dusky-footed wood rat, dogs, cats, cattle, and horses) • Birds • Reptiles

Mode of Transmission
- Tick bite

Geographical Distribution

- Temperate areas throughout the world

Year of Emergence

- 1976

Key Terms

Borrelia afzelii Agent of Lyme disease in Africa

Borrelia burgdorferi Spirochete agent of Lyme disease

Borrelia garinii Agent of Lyme disease in Africa

Borrelia japonica Agent of Lyme disease in Japan

Borrelia lonestari Spirochete agent of southern-tick-associated rash illness

Borrelia miyamoto Agent of Lyme disease in Japan

DEET A tick repellent that is safe to apply to intact skin

Erythema migrans Large circular or oval rash with a bull's-eye appearance; often associated with Lyme disease

Jarish-Herxheimer reaction Augmentation of symptoms (headache, chills, fever, neck pain, rashes, and fatigue) following antibiotic therapy of spirochete-associated diseases; due to an excessive immune response triggered by antigens released by dying bacteria

Lyme disease Most prevalent arthropod-borne illness in temperate climates; characterized by a wide range of symptoms, including erythema migrans, migratory arthritis, fever and chills, and neurological symptoms following a tick bite

Southern-tick-associated rash illness (STARI) Disease similar to Lyme disease that is found in the southeastern United States; transmitted by *Borrelia lonestari*

Review Questions

1. What areas of the United States and the world have the highest incidence of Lyme disease?
2. What symptoms are typically associated with disseminated Lyme disease?
3. What compounds are used to treat Lyme disease?
4. What bacteria cause Lyme disease in the United States, Africa, Europe, and Asia? What are the vector and reservoir species for each of these?
5. *Treponema pallidum* is caused by a similar bacterium. What disease does this organism cause, and how does infection with *T. pallidum* complicate diagnosis of Lyme disease?

Topics for Further Discussion

1. Other than the methods listed in this chapter, what other means might be devised to reduce human exposure to ticks or to interrupt the *Borrelia* life cycle?
2. Because the genome of *B. burgdorferi* encodes few biosynthetic proteins, the spirochete depends on its host to supply many of its nutrients. How might this characteristic be used to protect infected humans?
3. What other diseases are caused by spirochetes, and how are they similar to Lyme disease? What other diseases are transmitted by *Ixodes* ticks?
4. Describe how various *Borrelia* genes protect the bacteria against antibiotics or the host immune response. Many of these are encoded by plasmids. How might this location influence drug resistance?

Resources

Bunikis, I., and others. "An RND-Type Efflux System in *Borrelia burgdorferi* Is Involved in Virulence and Resistance to Antimicrobial Compounds." *PLOS Pathogens*, 2008, *4*, 1–11.

Burkot, T. R., and others. "*Borrelia lonestari* DNA in Adult *Amblyomma americanum* Ticks, Alabama." *Emerging Infectious Diseases*, 2001, *7*, 471–473.

Cruz, A. R., and others. "Phagocytosis of *Borrelia burgdorferi*, the Lyme Disease Spirochete, Potentiates Innate Immune Activation and Induces Apoptosis in Human Monocytes." *Infection and Immunity*, 2008, *76*, 56–70.

Jackson, C. J., Boylan, J., and Frye, J. G. "Evidence of a Conjugal Erythromycin Resistance Element in the Lyme Disease Spirochete *Borrelia burgdorferi*." *International Journal of Antimicrobial Agents*, 2007, *30*, 496–504.

Jewett, M. W., Lawrence, K., and Bestor, A. C. "The Critical Role of the Linear Plasmid lp36 in the Infectious Cycle of *Borrelia burgdorferi*." *Molecular Microbiology*, 2007, *64*, 1358–1374.

Kalluri, S., Gilruth, P., Rogers, D., and Szczur, M. "Surveillance of Arthropod Vector–Borne Infectious Diseases Using Remote Sensing Techniques: A Review." *PLOS Pathogens*, 2007, *3*, 1361–1371.

Persing, D. H. "A Convergence of Tick-Transmitted Diseases Within the Lyme Disease Transmission Cycle." In W. M. Scheld, D. Armstrong, and J. M. Hughes (eds.), *Emerging Infections* (Vol. 1). Washington, D.C.: ASM Press, 1998.

Qiu, W.-G., and others. "Wide Distribution of a High-Virulence *Borrelia burgdorferi* Clone in Europe and North America." *Emerging Infectious Diseases*, 2008, *14*, 1097–1104.

Reed, K. D. "Laboratory Testing for Lyme Disease: Possibilities and Practicalities." *Journal of Clinical Microbiology*, 2002, *40*, 319–324.

Steere, A. C., Coburn, J., and Glickstein, L. "The Emergence of Lyme Disease." *Journal of Clinical Investigation*, 2004, *113*, 1093–1101.

Stites, D. P., Terr, A. I., and Parslow, T. G. *Basic and Clinical Immunology* (8th ed.). Norwalk, Conn.: Appleton & Lange, 1994.

CHAPTER 4

HUMAN EHRLICHIOSIS

LEARNING OBJECTIVES

- Define and contrast ehrlichiosis, anaplasmosis, and related diseases

- Describe the *Ehrlichieae* bacteria responsible for causing these illnesses

- Discuss modes of infection

- Discuss the host's response to infection

- Discuss methods of treatment

- Describe symptomatology and diagnosis

- Discuss methods of prevention

Major Concepts

Diseases

Bacteria of the *Ehrlichieae* group cause several tickborne infections of humans and animals which include human monocytotropic ehrlichiosis (HME; caused by *Ehrlichia chaffeensis*), human granulocytic anaplasmosis (HGA; caused by *Anaplasma phagocytophilum*), human disease due to *Ehrlichia ewingii*, and sennetsu fever (caused by *Neorickettsia sennetsu*). Tickborne fever of sheep, cattle, and goats and pasture fever of sheep, cattle, bison, deer, and rodents, as well as serious disease in horses, dogs, and cats, may resulting from infection with *A. phagocytophilum* as well.

Symptoms

Although many ehrlichial infections remain asymptomatic, severe illness may occur, with up to half of infected individuals hospitalized. Early symptoms include fever, malaise, muscle and bone aches, headache, and gastrointestinal abnormalities with or without rash. Blood cell numbers are decreased. Serious disease manifestations include prolonged fever, kidney failure, disseminated intravascular coagulation, meningoencephalitis, seizures, coma, and adult respiratory distress syndrome. Death occurs in 2% to 5% of the cases for HME and 7% to 10% of cases of HGA. The latter is associated with fungal or viral infection, possibly indicating an immunosuppressive effect of the bacteria. Immunosuppressed persons, especially those who are HIV-positive, are more likely to develop severe disease: the fatality rate in this group is 25%. Alveolar damage and interstitial pneumonia; lymphohistiocytic infiltrates; focal necrosis of the spleen, liver, and lymph nodes; and diffuse hemorrhaging may occur during cases of lethal infection. *E. ewingii* also causes serious disease in immunosuppressed persons. Sennetsu fever is a rare and mild disease.

Infection

The ehrlichial bacteria are small, obligate, intracellular, gram-negative cocci residing within phagocytic white blood cells, such as monocytes and macrophages or neutrophils, in which they may form microcolonies called morulae. *E. chaffeensis* is transmitted primarily by adult lone star ticks. High rates of infection occur in Arkansas, North Carolina, Missouri, Oklahoma, New Jersey, and Tennessee. Because these diseases are tickborne, the majority of cases occur in rural settings or, less commonly, in suburban locations. The median age of infected individuals is 44 years, and males are more commonly infected than females. Persons spending large amounts of time in wooded areas (foresters, rangers) have an increased risk of infection. *A. phagocytophilum* is spread by nymphal and larval stages of the blacklegged and western blacklegged ticks in the United States and is found in Connecticut, Minnesota, Rhode Island, New York, Wisconsin, and California. HGA is also found in a number of European countries, including Slovenia, the Netherlands, Spain, Sweden, Norway, Croatia, Poland, Italy, Austria, and France. A number of animal species serve as reservoir hosts for these bacteria, including white-tailed deer, dogs, wolves, coyotes, sheep, cattle, goats, horses, and some rodents.

Immune Response

Protective immunity against ehrlichiosis and anaplasmosis is provided by $CD4^+$ T helper cells and $CD8^+$ T killer cells, the cytokines interferon-γ and tumor necrosis factor-α, and antibodies produced by B lymphocytes. *Ehrlichia* bacteria evade the immune response by (1) not expressing lipopolysaccharide and peptidoglycan typically used by immune cells to recognize bacteria, (2) preventing lysosomes from fusing with endosomes containing bacteria, (3) failing to activate enzymes within the host cells that generate bacteriotoxic reactive oxygen species, and (4) blocking apoptotic self-destruction by infected cells.

Treatment and Prevention

HME and HGA may be successfully treated by antibiotics such as doxycycline, another tetracycline, or rifampin. Preventive measures include avoiding exposure to or attachment of ticks, their prompt removal, and elimination of tick habitat.

Introduction

Some 1,200 cases of human ehrlichiosis and anaplasmosis were reported to the CDC between 1986 and 1997. *Ehrlichia* species are found globally, mainly in temperate regions of the world. Individuals with antibody reactivity to ***Ehrlichia chaffeensis*** have been seen in countries as diverse as Argentina, Belgium, Israel, Italy, Mali, Mexico, Portugal, Thailand, and the United States. Human infection with ***Anaplasma phagocytophilum*** has been reported in Belgium, Denmark, Hungary, Slovenia, and Sweden, and antibody reactivity to the granulocytic form has been found in Germany, Israel, Italy, Norway, Switzerland, and the United States.

Ehrlichiosis and anaplasmosis are tickborne zoonoses and are transmitted by some of the same vector species as *Borrelia burgdorferi*, resulting in the possibility of coinfection. Most infections occur during the spring and summer (55% to 70% between May and July), reflecting times of greatest exposure to the appropriate life stage of the tick vectors. Infection rates are higher among older adults (usually over the age of 40), with the highest rates found in adults aged 70 to 79. The resulting diseases, when present, range in severity from mild to very severe, especially in immunosuppressed persons. In addition to humans, infection is found in many common domestic and wild animal populations.

History

The first human disease found to result from infection with an *Ehrlichia*-like species was **sennetsu fever**, caused by ***Neorickettsia*** (formerly *Ehrlichia*) ***sennetsu***, in Japan in 1953. This is a mononucleosis-like illness with fever and swollen lymph nodes. It is very rare, with most of the cases occurring in western Japan and Malaysia. There have been no reported deaths.

FIGURE 4.1   Range of one of the principal tick vectors in the United States

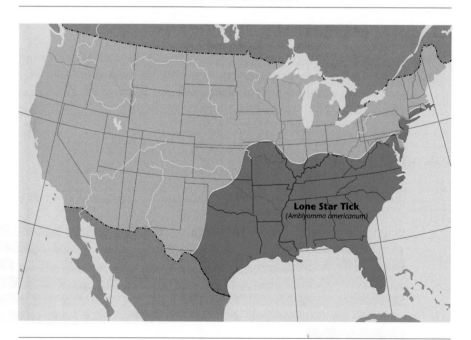

Lone Star Tick
(Amblyomma americanum)

Human monocytotropic ehrlichiosis (HME) was described in 1986 in Arkansas and is found mainly in the southern and southeastern parts of the United States. The causative bacterium was isolated in 1990 from Fort Chaffee, Arkansas. **Human granulocytic anaplasmosis (HGA**; formerly human granulocytic ehrlichiosis) was first recognized by Johan Bakken in 1994 after the discovery of microcolonies of an *Ehrlichia*-like species in a patient's neutrophils.

One of the important factors in the recent increase of HGA is the explosive rise in the population of white-tailed deer, which increased an estimated 50-fold during the twentieth century. The deer is the primary host for all stages of the tick vector. Populations of other hosts for this tick, including the wild turkey and the coyote, have grown as well. There has also been an increase in the number of humans particularly vulnerable to severe disease manifestations, including individuals who are older, have cancer, or are immunosuppressed.

The Diseases

Infected individuals may remain asymptomatic. In those in whom disease does develop, symptomatic illness follows an incubation period of five to ten days. Initial signs include fever, malaise, muscle and bone aches, headache, and gastrointestinal abnormalities. Rash may or may not be present, in contrast to Rocky Mountain spotted fever, a similar condition in which rash is typically found. Individuals may become severely ill, and up to half of them require hospitalization. Severe reactions occurring in these illnesses include prolonged fever, kidney failure, disseminated intravascular coagulation, meningoencephalitis, seizures, coma, or adult respiratory distress syndrome. Death occurs in 2% to 3% of the cases, with HME being more pathogenic, while HGA infection may lead to serious secondary infections due to *A. phagocytophilum*–induced loss of neutrophil competence. Individuals with prior immunosuppression are at the highest risk for severe disease manifestations.

Human Monocytotropic Ehrlichiosis (HME)

HME is a moderate to severe disease whose symptoms include fever (occurring in more than 95% of cases), headache (60% to 75%), myalgia (40% to 60%), nausea (40% to 50%) and vomiting (36%), joint pain (30% to 35%), rash

(35%, mostly pediatric cases or HIV-positive adults), cough (25%), sore throat, diarrhea, swollen lymph nodes, abdominal pain, and neurological symptoms (meningitis- or encephalitis-like illness, cognitive impairment) (10% to 40%). Adult respiratory distress syndrome may also occur. Laboratory reports often indicate a decrease in the numbers of red blood cells (50% of cases), white blood cells (60% to 70%), and platelets (70% to 90%), accompanied by increased lymphocyte counts (45% to 85% of the white blood cells). Elevated levels of liver enzymes (transaminase—80% to 90%; alkaline phosphatase and bilirubin—25% to 60%) occur. Hyponatremia (decreased urination) is seen in up to 50% of infected adults and 70% of infected children. Serum sodium levels may be under 130 milliequivalents per liter. Some 41% to 63% of patients are hospitalized (median duration of seven days). HME closely resembles the granulocytic forms of the disease, but rash, central nervous system involvement, and gastrointestinal disturbances are more common.

Asymptomatic cases have also been reported but not conclusively documented. Disease is particularly severe in the immunosuppressed and may involve acute kidney or respiratory failure, metabolic acidosis, a profound decrease in blood pressure, widespread blood clotting within vessels (disseminated intravascular coagulopathy), liver failure, adrenal insufficiency, and myocardial dysfunction. One study indicated a 25% mortality rate in immunosuppressed patients; 67% of the fatalities were HIV-positive. Respiratory symptoms in patients with severe disease may include interstitial pneumonitis, pulmonary edema, pleural effusions, and acute respiratory distress syndrome. Other hematological manifestations include pulmonary or conjunctival hemorrhage, gastrointestinal bleeding, subdural hematoma, and bloody urine (hematuria). Secondary infections with cytomegalovirus, *Candida,* and *Aspergillus* suggest that immunosuppression may be occurring. The overall mortality rate is 2% to 5%. In immunosuppressed patients with fatal outcome, alveolar damage and interstitial pneumonia; lymphohistiocytic infiltrates; focal necrosis of the spleen, liver, and lymph nodes; and diffuse hemorrhaging have been seen. In a retrospective study of 133 HIV-positive individuals in Nashville, Tennessee, in 1999, two cases of HME were detected by indirect immunofluorescence, for a seroincidence rate (percentage of persons with antibodies to the microbe) of 6.7% among symptomatic individuals and an overall rate of 1.6%. One of the two patients required hospitalization. False negative readings by serology are possible due to the suppressed immunity found in this population.

Both cell-mediated and humoral immunity appear to play important roles in defense against attack by *E. chaffeensis.* Major histocompatibility complex class II antigens, TLR4, and production of IL-6 by macrophages have been implicated in efficient clearance of bacteria. SCID mice, which lack mature T and B lymphocytes, do not survive infection. In the absence of anti-ehrlichial antibodies, infected monocytes produce the cytokines IL-1β, IL-8, and IL-10, while in the presence of hyperimmune serum, IL-6 and tumor necrosis factor-α are also made. Several of these cytokines are proinflammatory or induce fever. Lymphocytosis (elevated lymphocyte count) is a common finding, with unusually high numbers of rare $CD3^+CD4^-CD8^-$ γ~GD T cells. This T cell subset is also elevated during infection with other intracellular pathogens, such as *Listeria, Mycobacterium,* and *Leishmania* species.

HME is spread primarily by nymphal or adult lone star ticks, *Amblyomma americanum,* but bacteria have been found by PCR in the dog tick (*Dermacentor variabilis*) and the western black-legged tick (*Ixodes pacificus*) as well. Both male and female ticks feed on humans, but the females are believed to be primarily involved in disease transmission. All stages of the tick life cycle bite humans, and prevalence ranges from 5% to 15%. Adult ticks may acquire their infections by transstadial transmission from the nymphal stage or directly by feeding on an infected vertebrate host. Transovarial infection of eggs or unfed larvae has not been documented. White-tailed deer (definitive host), dogs, wolves, goats, coyotes, and red foxes are naturally infected with *E. chaffeensis* and may serve as disease reservoirs. This tick may be found in meadows, woodlands,

FIGURE 4.2 Lone star tick

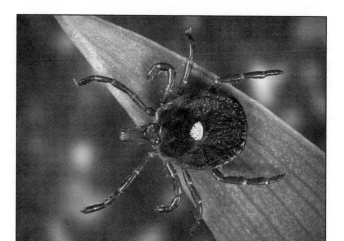

Source: CDC/Amanda Loftis, William Nicholson, Will Reeves, and Chris Paddock.

FIGURE 4.3 Number of ehrlichiosis cases in the United States, 1999–2006

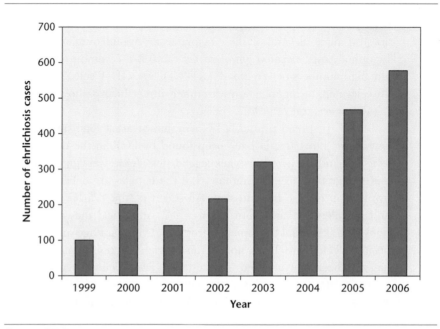

Source: CDC.

and hardwood forests. No incidence has been reported in rodents. From 1997 to 2001, there were 503 cases reported in the United States; 338 of these were confirmed, occurring in 23 states, particularly in Arkansas, North Carolina, Missouri, Oklahoma, New Jersey, and Tennessee. The incidence rate is 7 to 57 per 1,000,000 population. Severe HME has been found to be more common in Georgia and North Carolina than Rocky Mountain spotted fever, a tickborne disease that it resembles.

Most of the cases occur in rural locations and the remainder primarily in suburban locales. The majority of cases are found in males (more than twice as often as in females), and the median age of patients is 44 years.

Human Granulocytotropic Anaplamosis (HGA)

This form of the disease was first detected in the United States in Minnesota in 1994 and in Europe, in Slovenia, in 1997. In the majority of cases, HGA is a mild and self-limiting infection that resolves in about a month, but it

FIGURE 4.4   Ehrlichiosis by state, 2001–2002

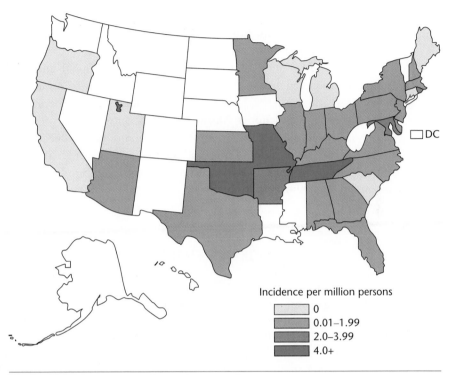

Incidence per million persons

- 0
- 0.01–1.99
- 2.0–3.99
- 4.0+

□DC

Note: Nonreporting states do not have a value.
Source: CDC.

may become a severe illness. Its symptoms include undifferentiated high fever occurring in the spring or summer (98% of cases), severe headache (77%), myalgia (81%), rigors, nausea, anorexia, and vomiting (25%), nonproductive cough (20%), confusion (14%), and rash (8% to 10%). Laboratory findings show a high number of patients with a decrease in platelet numbers, and many also have a lowered white blood cell count. Lymphocytosis with atypical cells may be found after the second week of illness. Anemia is less frequent. As in HME, liver enzymes are elevated. About half of patients (48% to 53%) are hospitalized. Symptoms may be particularly severe in the elderly, the immunosuppressed (including HIV-positive persons and those with monoclonal gammapathy, sickle β-thalassemia, and Down syndrome and persons without a spleen), and patients with cancer or chronic inflammation. Sulfa drugs may exacerbate HME. In people with severe disease manifestations, morulae

(Ehrlichia colonies) may be readily observed in peripheral blood. Disease is generally less severe in Europe than in the United States, and morulae are less frequently noted. The mortality rate is 7% to 10% and is often associated with infection by opportunistic fungi or viruses due to the ability of *A. phagocytophilum* to inhibit neutrophil functions.

In the United States, HGA is spread by the nymphal and larval stages of the black-legged and western black-legged ticks (*Ixodes scapularis* and *Ixodes pacificus*), which are active in the spring and summer. The former is found in the northeastern and upper Midwest and the latter in northern California. Hosts of the immature ticks include small mammals (especially the white-footed mouse), reptiles, and birds, and the adults have a high affinity for biting humans. Many of the cases occur in regions with high levels of Lyme disease and babesiosis, the causative agents of which the tick may be coinfected.

RECENT DEVELOPMENTS

Anaplasma phagocytophilum decreases neutrophil functions such as adherence to endothelial cells, transmigration, phagocytosis, and production of reactive oxygen species via the oxidative burst. The mechanisms by which the bacterium blocks protective neutrophil activities are being uncovered. Bacterial infection increases the binding of a repressor protein, the CCAAT displacement protein (CDP), to the promoter region of the DNA of several genes, inhibiting their transcription. The suppressed genes include gp91phox, involved in the oxidative burst; human neutrophil peptide 1 (HNP-1); CCAAT enhancer binding protein epsilon (C/EBPε), and neutrophil gelatinase, involved in neutrophil migration. HNP-1 is a transcription factor critical for myeloid differentiation and for the expression of genes that produce secondary granule proteins, such as lactoferrin, gelatinase, and collagenase, important for the activity of mature neutrophils. People with granule disorder have a greater tendency for recurrent bacterial infections. Mice without functional C/EBPε have impaired defense mechanisms because their neutrophils have defective uptake and killing of bacteria: these mice often die of secondary infections. *A. phagocytophilum* also increases the activity of the cathepsin L enzyme, a protease that cleaves CDP into a form that has enhanced ability to bind to DNA. Higher activity of cathepsin A thus leads to increased cleavage of CDP during HGA. When cathepsin L activity was inhibited chemically or by the use of small interfering RNA (siRNA), the extent of neutrophil infection by *A. phagocytophilum* was decreased. Drugs that block the actions of *A. phagocytophilum* on cathepsin L may thus reduce the numbers of lethal opportunistic infections arising during HGA.

FIGURE 4.5   Black-legged tick

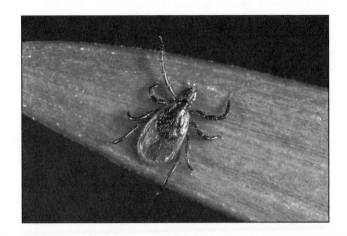

Source: CDC/Michael L. Levin.

FIGURE 4.6   Anaplasmosis cases in the United States, 1999–2006

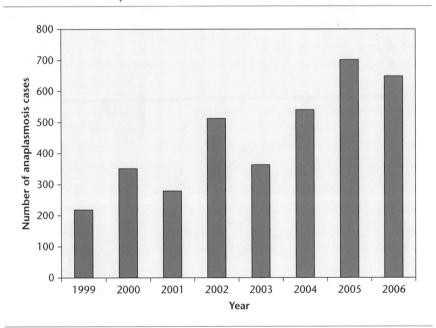

Source: CDC.

These regions include Connecticut, Minnesota, Rhode Island, New York, and Wisconsin. The illness has also been reported in eastern states and California. In Georgia, a study conducted in 1987 and 1988 found an incidence rate of 53 cases per 1,000,000 per year for HGA. From 1997 to 2001, 654 confirmed and 434 probable cases were reported from 21 states. In European countries ranging from the west to Central Asia, *Ixodes ricinus* is the disease vector. It is maintained in nature in sheep, goats, cattle, horses, dogs, cats, deer, elk, mice, shrews, and voles. In 2005, just 20 cases were reported throughout the continent, in Slovenia, the Netherlands, Spain, Sweden, Norway, Croatia, Poland, Italy, Austria, and France. Seroprevalance rates in northern and central Europe ranged from 0% to 2.9% in blood donors and from 1.5% to 21% in individuals exposed to ticks.

FIGURE 4.7   Anaplasmosis by state, 2001–2002

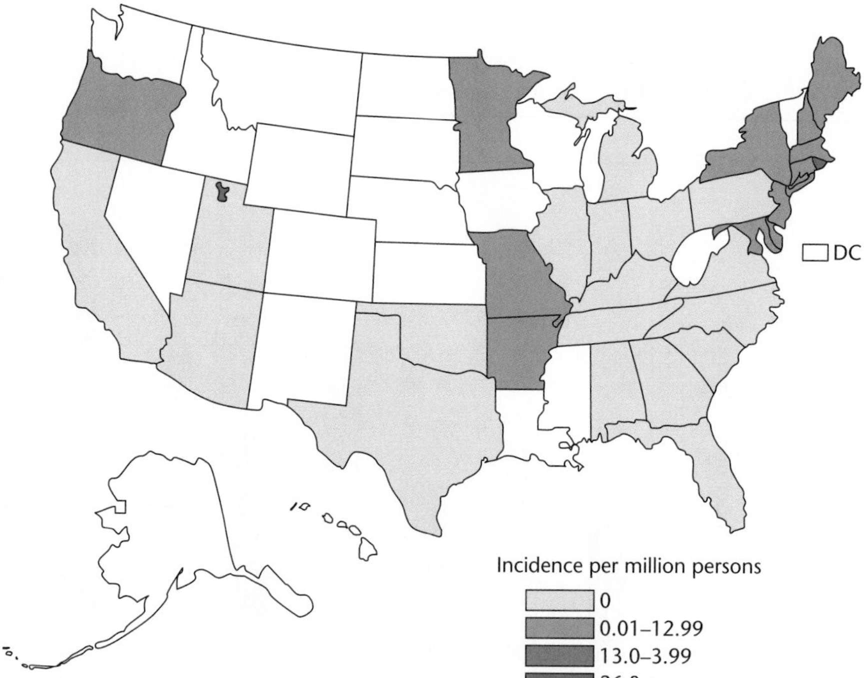

Incidence per million persons

- 0
- 0.01–12.99
- 13.0–3.99
- 26.0.+

Note: Nonreporting states do not have a value.
Source: CDC.

Tickborne fever is found in sheep, cattle, and goats in northern and central Europe. This illness is characterized by a high fever and a decrease in milk production and may be accompanied by a loss of appetite, depression, cough and a nasal discharge, diarrhea, abortion, and mastitis. In horses in the United States and Europe, symptoms include fever, depression, loss of appetite, edema in the lower limbs, petechiae, and reluctance to move. In infected dogs, fever and lethargy are noted. Similar findings have been reported in cats with feline granulocytic ehrlichiosis, with loss of appetite and rapid breathing, as well as increased numbers of neutrophils and a drop in lymphocyte numbers. Other potential reservoir hosts include the white-footed mouse, rabbits, wild boar, foxes, and birds in the United States and Europe.

HGA is found mainly in males (79%), and the median age of infection is 58 years. Its occurrence peaks between May and October and corresponds to times of human exposure to ticks. Sitting on logs, gathering wood, and sitting against trees are particularly risky activities, along with disturbing leaf litter.

Dog and Human Disease Due to *Ehrlichia ewingii*

The human disease was first recognized in 1999, and its symptoms include fever (100%), headache (63%), muscle aches (37%), nausea and vomiting (25%), lowered platelet numbers with or without a corresponding decrease in red or white blood cell counts, elevated transaminase levels, and hyponatremia. Hospitalization is required in 75% of patients. This disease has been reported in only a few people in Missouri, Oklahoma, and Tennessee, with no deaths. It occurs primarily in people with compromised immune systems, including those with HIV infection. The lone star tick is believed to be the vector for **Ehrlichia ewingii**, and dogs and white-tailed deer may serve as reservoir hosts. Disease in canines includes fever, lameness, polyarthritis, and reluctance to move and has been reported in the south central and southern states, including Arkansas, Georgia, Mississippi, Missouri, Tennessee, North Carolina, Oklahoma, and Virginia. The rate of infection of dogs in the last three states has been reported as ranging from 6% to 16%.

Sennetsu Fever

Sennetsu fever was the first human disease known to result from infection with an erhichlial-type bacterium. It is caused by *Neorickettsia sennetsu* and is a mononucleosis-like disease. It is hypothesized to be contracted by eating fish infected with the worm vector.

The Causative Agents

The Bacteria

Ehrlichiosis and related diseases are caused by bacteria of the tribe *Ehrlichieae* of the *Anaplasmataceae* family, and similar agents include the causative agents of Rocky Mountain spotted fever and typhus. They are small (1 to 3 micrometers), obligate, intracellular, gram-negative cocci that live within phagocytic white blood cells—monocytes or macrophages (which are different stages of maturation of the same cell type) for HME or neutrophils for HGA. A microcolony of these bacteria is called a **morula**, after the Latin word for "mulberry." Infected cells usually contain only one or two morulae, although up to 15 have been seen in a single cell. The cell wall of *Ehrlichia* species is unusual in that it lacks lipopolysaccharide and peptidoglycan but does contain glycoproteins and members of a 28-kilodalton gene family. The latter contains three hypervariable domains (which vary greatly between individuals) that are exposed to the surface.

Ehrlichia chaffeensis, isolated in 1991, is the causative agent for HME and has thus far been isolated only in the United States. It resides primarily in monocytes, macrophages, and endothelial cells but may sometimes be found in lymphocytes and neutrophils as well. *E. ewingii* uses granulocytes as host cells and also occurs in the United States. Similar bacteria, *Ehrlichia* (formerly *Cowdria*) *ruminantium*, are known to cause heartwater in cattle and other ruminants. These bacteria and their close relatives *Ehrlichia canis* and *Ehrlichia muris* have a genome of 1,250 kilobases, have 97.7% or more 16S rRNA similarity, and cause disease in their host species.

Ehrlichia may be adapted for growth in tissue culture, growing in cell lines such as human microvascular endothelial cells, Vero cells from African green monkeys, HeLa human cervical epithelioid carcinoma cells, THP-1 human monocytic leukemia cells, embryonic mouse cells, murine fibroblasts, and buffalo green monkey cells. One strain of *E. chaffeensis* is able to survive for 11 days in human blood and for 21 days in tissue culture at 4°C to 6°C.

A number of genes from *E. chaffeensis* have been characterized, including the variable-length PCR target; 120-, 106-, and 37-kilodalton protein genes; the *groESL* heat-shock operon, the quinolate synthetase A gene, and the *p28* multigene family. The former two genes contain repeated elements and display interstrain variability. Members of the *p28* multigene family include at least 16 transcribed alleles and encode the outer membrane proteins whose variability may be a means of immune evasion. The genome encodes at least eight major immunoreactive proteins.

Two *Ehrlichia* cell types may be observed by electron microscopy: reticulate cells containing coccoid and coccobacillary forms with uniformly distributed ribosomes and nucleoid DNA fibrils and dense-cored cells containing predominantly the coccoid form with its ribosomes and nucleoid DNA centrally condensed. Both reproduce by binary fission and have been found in samples of patients' blood. All members of the genus contain insignificant amounts of peptidoglycan. The morulae are 1 to 6 micrometers wide and contain from a single bacterium to more than 40. They sometimes contain a fine, striated fibrillar matrix and tubules originating from the reticular cells. The mitochondria of the host cells are often seen next to the borders of the morulae.

Anaplasma phagocytophilum infects neutrophils and sometimes macrophages and endothelial cells to cause HGA. Seven-eighths of the cases occur in people with compromised immunity. This disease is found in the United States and Europe. *A. phagocytophilum* causes tickborne fever and pasture fever in sheep, cattle, bison, deer, and rodents. It is found in Europe. *A. equi* causes disease in horses, but also occurs in llamas and rodents. It resides in the U.S. and Europe. *Ehrlichia ewingii* is transmitted by *A. americanum* and has the same geographical range as *E. chaffeensis*. *Neorickettsia sennetsu* lives within helminthes (worms) and may be found in Japan and Malaysia.

The Life Cycle of *E. chaffeensis* in Macrophages

The 120-kilodalton outer membrane protein of *E. chaffeensis* may function in adhesion to and internalization by macrophages. The bacteria are covered by host cell membrane within a cytoplasmic vesicle resembling an early endosome. This does not fuse with a lysosome. Iron is required for the growth of *Ehrlichia*-like species. Transferrin and its receptor are host proteins used to bring iron into the cell. They progressively accumulate within the endosome. Furthermore, infection of the macrophage induces production of iron-response protein 1 by the host cell. This protein raises transferrin receptor mRNA levels. The host cytokine interferon-γ (IFN-γ) kills *E. chaffeensis* by lowering the numbers of transferrin receptors; the bacteria can prevent interferon activity by blocking Jak-STAT signaling and by increasing activity of the host's own immunosuppressant, protein kinase A. Another protein that may aid in iron acquisition by these bacteria is a 37-kilodalton protein similar to iron-binding proteins of other gram-negative bacteria.

The Immune Response

In mouse models of infection with *E. chaffeensis*, both CD4$^+$ and CD8$^+$ T lymphocytes were needed for survival, although a stronger role was postulated for the latter cell type. IFN-γ and TNF-α appear to act together, since inactivation of both genes resulted in a 75% fatality rate, while the depletion of either cytokine alone was far less severe. Humoral immunity also plays an important role in controlling *E. chaffeensis*–related disease. Antibodies can protect SCID mice from lethal infections. IgG2a directed against the outer membrane proteins, working together with Fc receptors, clear bacteria from tissue as early as 24 hours after infection. No protective role was assigned to neutrophils, natural killer cells, complement, or reactive nitrogen species. Cell-free plasma was surprisingly found to contain infective bacteria (10% of *Ehrlichia* in the blood). When incubated at either 25°C or 37°C in plasma, these cell-free bacteria replicated, as determined by PCR, ^{3}H-thymidine incorporation, or microscopic counts.

Ehrlichial species use several methods to evade the host defense system. First, in addition to lacking lipopolysaccharide and peptidoglycan, which are commonly used by hosts to recognize bacterial invaders, *E. chaffeensis* and *A. phagocytophilum* acquire cholesterol from their hosts, which may aid in membrane stabilization. Second, upon entry into their host phagocytic cells, the bacteria alter trafficking of vesicles to prevent lysosomal fusion. Third, since a major mechanism by which both monocytes and neutrophils kill internalized microbes relies on reactive oxygen species and these bacteria lack several key detoxifying enzymes, they avoid killing by failing to activate NADPH oxidase. Fourth, *E. chaffeensis* transiently activates nuclear factor κ of B lymphocytes (NF-κB) and the p38 mitogen-activated protein kinase, causing the monocyte hosts to become less receptive to external stimulation. Finally, infected host cells may limit disease by self-destruction by the process of apoptosis. *A. phagocytophilum* circumvents this process by preventing the decrease in a bcl-2 family member, bfl-1, that occurs normally in neutrophils.

Diagnosis

In the case of HME, usually too few morulae are present in the blood, buffy coats, or bone marrow aspirates to be diagnostically useful by viewing with conventional light microscopy (20% to 30% sensitivity). By contrast, other cellular inclusions and familial conditions have resulted in false positives. Moreover, isolation of these bacteria from blood, bone marrow aspirates, or cerebrospinal fluid has proved to be very insensitive. Antibody tests for IgM or IgG (fourfold rise in indirect immunofluorescence titer to *E. chaffeensis* in paired serum samples taken over a three- to six-week interval or a single titer of >256) may be used diagnostically. However, one may not always have HGE even if one makes an antibody response, for *E. chaffeensis* shows antigenic cross-reactivity with the other species. In a prospective study conducted in Cape Girardeau, Missouri, from 1997 to 1999, 90% of the identified cases were antibody-positive and 31% had cross-reactivity to *A. phagocytophilum* (end point titer ≤160). A 21-kilodalton protein has been used in ELISAs with a sensitivity of 95% and a specificity of 100%. Western blotting to the 120-kilodalton protein or detection of the 16S rRNA or the *groESL* gene by PCR may be used to confirm the diagnosis. In the Cape Girardeau study, sensitivity using PCR was 52% to 56%, with a specificity of 100%.

With HGA, morulae containing hundreds to thousands of bacteria are often visible within neutrophils in Wright- or Giemsa-stained smears of buffy coats or peripheral blood, but this may not be the case in mild disease. At least 800 to 1,000 granulocytes should be examined at 50x to 100x magnification before reporting a negative finding. The bacteria may be cultured in HL-60 promyelocytic leukemia cells to amplify bacterial numbers. EDTA-treated blood is added to HL-60 cells, and the cultures followed for up to two weeks. However, culture isolation may not be clinically useful. Antibody tests (fourfold rise in titer in paired acute and convalescent samples) are more sensitive, with greater than 95% of patients developing antibodies during the course of illness. This technique has limitations, however, since 11% to 15% of people living in endemic areas are seropositive, and higher rates are seen in those testing positive for the Lyme disease agent. Confirmation is by detection of a 44-kilodalton protein by Western blot. PCR is a sensitive technique for detecting infections, with a sensitivity of 80% to 87% and 100% specificity. Targets for amplification include gene encoding the 16S rRNA, *groESL*, *epank1*, and a 44-kilodalton antigen.

Treatment

Antibiotic therapy should be started immediately if HME or HGA is strongly suspected. The drug of choice is doxycycline or another tetracycline antibiotic. Failure to respond rapidly to this drug suggests that the patient does not have one of these diseases. Treatment is usually continued for three to five days after fever reduction in adults, with a longer course required for more severe disease. A shorter treatment is recommended for children under the age of 8 years due to the possibility of dental staining in younger children. A seven- to ten-day treatment with rifampin may be used alternatively for HGA, especially for milder cases and those occurring during pregnancy. Although this drug is bactericidal in vitro, no clinical data support its usage in the case of HME. Aminoglycosides, macrolides and ketolides, sulfa drugs (cotrimoxazole), penicillin, cephalosporin, fluroquinolones, and chloramphenicol have not proved to be effective. With treatment, the fever usually is reduced in one to three days.

Prevention

One of the most important means of avoiding ehrlichiosis and related diseases is to limit one's exposure to the tick vectors. Because several hours may occur between tick attachment and the actual transmission of bacteria to the human host, inspection for and removal of ticks after exposure to their habitat is vital. Several methods of reducing rodent, deer, and tick habitat and for decreasing tick attachment and transmission of the bacteria are described in Chapter Three.

Surveillance

Surveillance data have been available for about 15 years from a number of states but not on a national level. Based on 1995 census data from across the United States, HME was more commonly found in the Southeast and South-Central region and HGA was more often detected in the Northeast and Upper Midwest. The highest incidence of HGA occurred in Connecticut, Wisconsin, Minnesota, and New York, and the incidence of HME was greatest in Arkansas, North Carolina, Missouri, Oklahoma, and New Jersey. Because the southern portions of Iowa border states with high rates of HME, surveillance of white-tailed deer has been conducted to ascertain the rate of infection of this common reservoir host. In a study of 2,277 deer, antibodies against *Ehrlichia chaffeensis* were found in 12.5% of the animals in 1994 and 13.9% in 1996. Although a high incidence of human HME is not reported in this state, the causative agent is thus present in many members of one reservoir host.

Ehrlichiosis became a reportable disease in Connecticut in 1995 and in New York in 1996. The state laboratories assayed serum specimens for bacteria-specific antibodies by indirect fluorescent antibody assays and tested either whole blood or serum for bacterial DNA by polymerase chain reaction. In Connecticut, 90% of the reported cases were HGA and 5% were HME; 5% of specimens had antibodies against both *E. chaffeensis* and *A. phagocytophilum*. Ehrlichial cases were reported in all months except January, and the majority (77%) occurred during May through September. Illness occurred equally in males and females. Mean patient age was 53 years: the 11% of patients who were hospitalized were older than the other patients (mean of 62 versus 45 years). In New York, 88% were HGA and the remainder HME. Cases occurred during all months, with 81% being reported May through September. More than half (55%) of the cases occurred in males. Mean patient age was 50.1 years. More than one-third of the patients were hospitalized.

HGA is present in parts of Europe. In 1995 and 1996, a retrospective serologic study collected serum samples from 554 residents of the wooded areas of the northeastern Alpine region of Italy believed to be at high risk because they spent large amounts of time outdoors. *A. phagocytophilum* antibodies were detected in 8.6% of the foresters, 5.5% of the hunters, and 1.5% of other area residents. *Borrelia* antibodies were found in 14.6% of these people. Other studies have reported antibodies against *A. phagocytophilum* in forestry workers in Switzerland (17.1%), the United Kingdom (5.0%), Italy (6.3%), and Sweden (11.4%).

Summary

Diseases
• Human monocytotropic ehrlichiosis • Human granulocytotropic anaplamosis • Dog and human disease due to *Ehrlichia ewingii* • Sennetsu fever

Causative Agents
• *Ehrlichia chaffeensis* • *Anaplasma phagocytophilum* • *Ehrlichia ewingii*
• *Neorickettsia sennetsu*

Agent Types
• Gram-negative cocci of the tribe *Ehrlichieae* of the *Anaplasmataceae* family

Genome
• DNA

Vectors
• Lone star tick, dog tick, western black-legged tick • Black-legged and western black-legged ticks, *Ixodes ricinus* • Lone star tick • Worms

Common Reservoirs
• White-tailed deer, dogs, wolves, goats, coyotes, and red foxes • Sheep, goats, cattle, horses, dogs, cats, deer, elk, mice, shrews, and voles • Dogs and white-tailed deer • None

Modes of Transmission
• Tick bite for all except sennetsu fever • Eating fish infected by the worm vector

Geographical Distribution

- United States • United States and Europe • United States • Japan and Malaysia

Year of Emergence

- 1986 • 1994 • 1999 • 1953

Key Terms

Anaplasma phagocytophilum Gram-negative cocci that cause human granulocytic anaplasmosis

Ehrlichia chaffeensis Gram-negative cocci that cause human monocytotropic ehrlichiosis

Ehrlichia ewingii Gram-negative cocci that cause a rare febrile disease, symptoms of which may include headache, muscle aches, nausea and vomiting, and lowered platelet numbers, that occurs primarily in immunocompromised persons

Human granulocytic anaplasmosis (HGA) Mild, self-limiting infection of neutrophils involving high fever, severe headache, myalgia, rigors, nausea, anorexia, vomiting, nonproductive cough, and confusion

Human monocytotropic ehrlichiosis (HME) Moderate to severe febrile infections of monocytes that may include headache, myalgia, nausea and vomiting, joint pain, rash, cough, swollen lymph nodes, abdominal pain, and neurological symptoms

Morula Microcolony of *Ehrlichieae* bacteria

Neorickettsia sennetsu Gram-negative cocci that cause sennetsu fever

Sennetsu fever Mononucleosis-like disease caused by *Neorickettsia sennetsu*

Tickborne fever Infection of sheep, cattle, and goats characterized by high fever and decreased milk production

Review Questions

1. What are the four species of bacteria of the tribe *Ehrlichieae* of the *Anaplasmataceae* family that cause disease in humans? With which disease is each associated?

2. What are the symptoms of the two major human diseases caused by *Ehrlichia*-type bacteria?

3. How do *Ehrlichia*-type bacteria evade the host's defense system?
4. What are the vectors for *Ehrlichia chaffeensis*? What animal species serve as its common reservoirs?
5. How may infection with *Ehrlichia*-type bacteria be avoided?

Topics for Further Discussion

1. Several diseases are transmitted by the same species of ticks. Make a list of all of the important pathogens of humans and their pets that are transmitted by the lone star tick and the dog tick in the United States.
2. Ehrlichiosis and anaplasmosis are not commonly recognized by the general population or health care providers in many parts of the United States. Discuss the potential for these diseases to be overlooked or misdiagnosed in states such as Nebraska and Kansas. What measures might be implemented to prevent this from occurring?
3. The white-tailed deer is the definitive host for several of the tick species that transmit *E. chaffeensis*. How might the rate of bacterial infection be decreased in the deer population? How might tick populations in areas with high numbers of deer be decreased?
4. Immunosuppressed persons are more likely to develop severe HGA. What measures might be taken to boost the appropriate types of protective immunity in these populations?

Resources

Aguero-Rosenfeld, M. E. "Laboratory Aspects of Tick-Borne Diseases: Lyme, Human Granulocytic Ehrlichiosis and Babesiosis." *Mount Sinai Journal of Medicine*, 2003, *70*, 197–206.

Bakken, J. S., and others "Human Granulocytic Ehrlichiosis in the Upper Midwest: A New Species Emerging?" *Journal of the American Medical Association*, 1994, *272*, 212–218.

Blanco, J. R., and Oteo, J. A. "Human Granulocytic Ehrlichiosis in Europe." *Clinical and Microbiological Infections*, 2002, *8*, 763–772.

Dawson, J. E., and others. "Isolation and Characterization of an *Ehrlichia* sp. from a Patient Diagnosed with Human Ehrlichiosis." *Journal of Clinical Microbiology*, 1991, *29*, 2741–2745.

Li, J. S., and Winslow, G. M. "Survival, Replication, and Antibody Susceptibility of *Ehrlichia chaffeensis* Outside of Host Cells." *Infection and Immunity*, 2003, *71*, 4229–4237.

Olaono, J. P., Masters, E., Hogrefe, W., and Walker, D. H. "Human Monocytotropic Ehrlichiosis, Missouri." *Emerging Infectious Diseases*, 2003, *9*, 1579–1586.

Paddock, C. D., and Childs, J. E. "*Ehrlichia chaffeensis:* A Prototypical Emerging Pathogen." *Clinical Microbiology Reviews*, 2003, *16*, 37–64.

Parola, P. "Tick-Borne Rickettsial Diseases: Emerging Risks in Europe." *Comparative Immunology, Microbiology, and Infectious Diseases*, 2004, *27*, 297–304.

Parola, P., Davoust, B., and Raoult, D. "Tick- and Flea-Borne Rickettsial Emerging Zoonoses." *Veterinarian Research*, 2005, *36*, 469–492.

Rikihisa, Y. "*Ehrlichia* Subversion of Host Innate Responses." *Current Opinions in Microbiology*, 2006, *9*, 95–101.

Safdar, N., Love, R. B., and Maki, D. G. "Severe *Ehrlichia chaffeensis* Infection in a Lung Transplant Recipient: A Review of Ehrlichiosis in the Immunocompromised Patient." *Emerging Infectious Diseases*, 2002, *8*, 320–323.

Talbot, T. R., Comer, J. A., and Bloch, K. C. "*Ehrlichia chaffeensis* Infections Among HIV-Infected Patients in a Human Monocytic Ehrlichiosis–Endemic Area." *Emerging Infectious Diseases*, 2003, *9*, 1123–1127.

Thomas, V., Samanta, S., and Fikrig, E. "*Anaplasma phagocytophilum* Increases Cathepsin l Activity, Thereby Globally Influencing Neutrophil Function." *Infection and Immunity*, 2008, *76*, 4905–4912.

Walker, D. H., and others. "*Ehrlichia chaffeensis:* A Prevalent, Life-Threatening, Emerging Pathogen." *Transactions of the American Clinical Climatological Association*, 2004, *115*, 375–384.

Wormser, G. P., and others. "The Clinical Assessment, Treatment, and Prevention of Lyme Disease, Human Granulocytic Anaplasmosis, and Babesiosis: Clinical Practice Guidelines by the Infectious Diseases Society of America." *Clinical and Infectious Diseases*, 2006, *43*, 1089–1134.

CHAPTER 5

BARTONELLA INFECTIONS

LEARNING OBJECTIVES

- Define bartonellosis, cat-scratch disease, trench fever, bacillary angiomatosis, bacillary peliosis hepatis, and endocarditis

- Describe the bacilli responsible for causing these illnesses

- Discuss modes of infection

- Discuss the host's response to infection

- Describe symptomatology and diagnosis

- Discuss potential methods of treatment

- Discuss methods of prevention

Major Concepts

Diseases

Four *Bartonella* species cause human disease. These are *B. bacilliformis*, *B. henselae*, *B. quintana*, and *B. elizabethae*. These small gram-negative bacilli belong to the α-2 subgroup of *Proteobacteria*. They produce bartonellosis (Oroya fever and verruga peruana), cat-scratch disease, and trench fever in immunocompetent persons and cause bacillary angiomatosis, bacillary peliosis hepatis, and endocarditis in immunocompromised individuals, especially those who are HIV-positive. Several of these conditions induce fever; others cause skin lesions or vascular endothelial proliferation. Oroya fever, with its severe hemolytic anemia, has a high mortality rate if untreated, and the accompanying endocarditis often necessitates heart valve replacement.

Transmission

Arthropods play important roles in the transmission to humans of several *Bartonella* species. The vectors for *B. bacilliformis* are members of a group of sand flies with a very restricted geographical range. The human body louse is the vector for *B. quintana*. The cat flea transmits *B. henselae* between cats; the cats subsequently infect humans by scratching, biting, or licking. Surveillance studies show that high numbers of cats either are currently infected or have previously been infected with *B. henselae*. Some areas of the world also have significant proportions of the arthropod vector population infected with *Bartonella* bacteria. Methods that decrease human exposure to the arthropod vectors help control diseases associated by *Bartonella* and other bacterial species.

Immune Response

The immune system plays an important protective role in host defense against *Bartonella*-induced diseases, involving both humoral (IgG_1 and IgA) and cell-mediated (Th1 T helper cells and interferon-γ) immunity. Immunosuppressed individuals develop more severe pathology than those with intact defense mechanisms, particularly HIV-positive persons who have defective $CD4^+$ T helper cell responses.

Protection

The mild or self-limiting illnesses produced by *Bartonella* infection, such as cat-scratch disease, are often not treated with drugs. Other diseases, such as Oroya fever, bacillary angiomatosis, and bacillary peliosis hepatis, are treated with antibiotics, which also kill microbes that cause problematic secondary infections. Other treatment options, such as blood transfusion, draining or excising lesions, or replacing damaged heart valves, may also be employed.

Introduction

A wide spectrum of diseases results from infection with the four *Bartonella* bacterial species that infect humans. Although some of these diseases have been known since the early 1900s, they are increasing in incidence and expanding their range in human hosts. The most recently described illnesses associated with *Bartonella* infection were identified in 1987 and 1993. They may lead to serious illness in immunocompromised persons, especially those who are HIV-positive. The AIDS pandemic has contributed to the impact of these bacteria on the human race. *Bartonella* infection results in bartonellosis, cat-scratch disease, trench fever, bacillary angiomatosis, bacillary peliosis hepatis, and endocarditis.

Bartonellosis is a potentially severe disease resulting from infection with a small bacterium from the *Bartonella* genus that is transmitted by sand flies. These insect vectors have a very restricted range in the Andes mountain region; accordingly, bartonellosis is confined to a small area. The disease consists of two stages that were originally believed to be distinct illnesses. The first stage is characterized by fever and hemolytic anemia, which may be fatal. The second stage is a mild cutaneous infection. Cat-scratch disease results from infection by another *Bartonella* species. It is widespread and affects over 22,000 persons annually, costing over $12 million in the United States alone. It is a mild infection that causes enlarged lymph nodes that exude pus. Trench fever is also caused by a *Bartonella* bacterium. It is found among individuals living in crowded conditions with poor hygiene. This illness is characterized by fever, headache, and soreness and is usually not fatal but may be more serious among people with AIDS, the homeless, and alcoholics. Bacillary angiomatosis may develop following *Bartonella* infection of immunocompromised individuals, especially those who are HIV-positive.

History

Bartonellosis (also known as **Carrión's disease**) was so designated in honor of Daniel Carrión, a Peruvian medical student in 1885 who investigated the initial stages of a cutaneous disease known as **verruga peruana** (Peruvian warts) by injecting himself with material taken from skin infected with *Bartonella bacilliformis*. Unfortunately, his experiment proved deadly, for he developed **Oroya fever**, a severe and often lethal hemolytic infection that was not then known to be the first stage of infection with *Bartonella*. Under appropriate conditions, epidemics of bartonellosis may occur within its narrow geographical confines. The building of the Central Railroad from Lima to Oroya in 1871 occasioned such an outbreak. Some 10,000 Chileans and Chinese with no prior immunity to *Bartonella* infection were brought into an endemic area of the Peruvian Andes. Approximately 7,000 workers were infected, and the mortality rate approached 40%. Another outbreak occurred in 1938 when *B. bacilliformis* spread into an adjacent region of Columbia where the population's immunity to the bacterium was lower; 4,000 persons died in that epidemic. Archaeological evidence of verruga peruana suggests that it has afflicted persons in the Andes of Peru since pre-Columbian days.

The disease that was later designated **cat-scratch disease** was first recognized in the United States in the 1950 by Lee Foshay while he was studying tularemia. At approximately the same time, Robert Debré linked the occurrence of suppurative (pus-exuding) adenitis in children with multiple scratches from cats. He then studied ill persons who produced positive skin tests (Type IV hypersensitivity reaction) to Foshay's antigen, leading to the clinical description of the illness. The causative agent was first visualized in lymph node samples in 1983 and identified in 1993.

Trench fever caused epidemics involving tens of thousands of troops and prisoners of war in Europe during World War I and again during World War II as a result of crowded, unsanitary living conditions that favor human infestation by lice, the disease vectors. Though not fatal, trench fever nevertheless led to prolonged periods of disability resulting from relapsing episodes of high fever and severe back and shin pain. Decreased use of trench warfare and improving hygienic conditions greatly reduced disease incidence in later wars. During the 1990s, a form of trench fever appeared among alcoholic, homeless individuals in Seattle, Washington, and also in France.

Bacillary angiomatosis was discovered in 1983, and in 1987 was found to be an opportunistic infection in individuals with AIDS. The lesions closely resembled those occurring during verruga peruana and those seen in Kaposi's sarcoma (a skin cancer often found in AIDS patients; described in Chapter Seventeen). Kaposi's sarcoma is caused by a viral infection, whereas the bacillary angiomatosis lesions contain bacilli and respond to antibiotics. The two *Bartonella* species that induce this condition were isolated from bacillary angiomatosis lesions beginning in 1992. One of these, *Bartonella henselae*, is also linked to cat-scratch disease; the link between the two diseases was suggested by the finding that individuals who developed bacillary angiomatosis had often done so following contact with cats. When serum samples were analyzed by the CDC, antibodies to *B. henselae* were found in patients with both conditions. Moreover, when the cats of several persons with bacillary angiomatosis were tested, the animals were found to be bacteremic for *B. henselae*.

The Diseases

Bartonellosis (Carrión's Disease)

Bartonellosis is restricted to humans and other primates and shows no preference based on age, gender, or race. It manifests initially as a severe acute febrile illness (characterized by fever) with hemolytic anemia that is often fatal (Oroya fever). This stage usually persists for two to three months but may last as long as four months. Some persons may develop flulike prodromal symptoms, such as fever, muscle and joint aches (myalgia and arthralgia), and bone pain. These may be the only evidence of disease in persons with low-level infection. People with a higher level of infection rapidly progress to a toxic state characterized by high fever, chills, headache, and delirium. This is followed by **hemolytic anemia** resulting from destruction of large numbers of erythrocytes infected by the bacteria. This form of anemia (low number of erythrocytes in the blood) is due to the destruction of red blood cells rather than their loss by hemorrhage or decreased production. The hemolytic anemia induced by *Bartonella bacilliformis* is extremely rapid, second only to malaria in the rate of drop in hematocrit. Blood smears of infected persons contain large numbers of **reticulocytes** (immature red blood cells) that are rapidly produced by the bone marrow in an attempt to replace the mature erythrocytes that have been lost. The reticulocytes are **polychromatic** (stained blue-pink) and are slightly larger than mature cells. Erythrocyte inclusions, such as **Howell-Jolly bodies** (round remnants of the nucleus), Cabot rings, and **basophilic stippling** (punctuate, bluish inclusions composed of aggregated ribosomes) may also be present. The anemia leads to the development of jaundice, pallor (pale color), and apathy. Thrombocytopenia (low numbers of platelets) may occur. Nontender lymphadenopathy (swelling of the lymph nodes) and hepatomegaly (enlargement of the liver) may occur, as well as petechiae in some persons. Those who present meningeal symptoms or coma often die. Untreated, the mortality rate for Oroya fever averages 40% (range from 10% to 90%), and many of the fatal cases may be associated with malaria or secondary infection with *Salmonella*, *Mycobacterium*, or protozoa species due to immunosuppression following this stage of infection. If treated with antibiotics, mortality drops to 8%.

Table 5.1   Human diseases caused by *Bartonella* species

Disease	Causative Agent	Symptoms
Bartonellosis (Carrión's disease)	*B. bacilliformis*	High fever, chills, headache, jaundice, apathy, delirium, hemolytic anemia, lymphadenopathy, hepatomegaly, petechiae, meningeal symptoms, coma
Cat-scratch disease	*B. henselae*	Lesions with hyperplasia, granuloma, suppuration with central liquification necrosis, microabscesses, macroabscesses
Trench fever	*B. quintana*	High fever, headache, malaise, severe pain of the back and shins, splenomegaly
Bacillary angiomatosis and bacillary peliosis hepatis	*B. henselae, B. quintana*	Chronic, multifocal vascular cutaneous lesions; erosive vascular proliferative lesions in bone, brain parenchyma, lymph nodes, gastrointestinal, or respiratory systems
Endocarditis	*B. henselae, B. quintana, B. elizabethae*	Inflammation of the heart or the aortic valves, high fever, heart murmur, acute cardiac failure, dyspnea, echocardiographic vegetations, bibasilar lung rales

If the infected individual survives this stage of the disease, a second, benign cutaneous stage may develop (verruga peruana), preceded by a shifting pain, sometimes severe, in the muscles, bones, and joints that lasts from minutes to several days. The dermal stage is characterized by widely disseminated, hemangiomatous (blood-filled) lesions with diameters of several millimeters or larger and deeper nodular lesions several centimeters in diameter that are found most commonly on the extensor surface of the extremities. The nodules over the joints may become tumorlike with ulcerated surfaces. Histiocytes within the lesions contain *Bartonella* bacilli. Angioblastic changes (increased growth of blood vessels) are seen upon microscopic examination of the dermis as the endothelial cells divide. Lymphocytes, plasma cells, and neutrophils also infiltrate the area. Other symptoms that may be present during this stage of infection include fever, malaise, and anemia, which are less severe than those occurring in Oroya fever. Verruga peruana may reflect the development of an immune response to the bacteria that prevents their continued infection of the bloodstream. This stage of infection is rarely fatal.

Cat-Scratch Disease

Cat-scratch disease (CSD) or cat-scratch fever (benign lymphoreticulosis; non-bacterial regional lymphadenitis) is seen throughout the world in immunocompetent persons, primarily in children or young adults, and may affect more than one member of a family. Regional outbreaks have also been reported. Humans are the only species known to develop this disease, which typically manifests as a slowly progressive or chronic enlargement of either a single or regional lymph nodes, accompanied by malaise and possibly fever. It may rarely affect other organs as well.

In CSD, lesions develop in one or more lymph nodes, beginning with a primary lesion in the vicinity of the scratch or injury. The lesions are characterized by hyperplasia (increased cell number), formation of a granuloma, and suppuration with a central liquification necrosis (pus-exuding lesion with a dead liquefied center). The nodes become moderately tender. Their pathology is divided into early, intermediate, and late stages. The initial primary lesion may present as a small red papule, vesicle, or pustule occurring approximately 13 days after infection. Few changes are seen in node architecture in the early stage of CSD and include enlargement of the lymphoid follicles and their germinal centers. The follicles are areas of the lymph node rich in lymphocytes of the adaptive

FIGURE 5.1   Small, localized lesion of cat-scratch disease

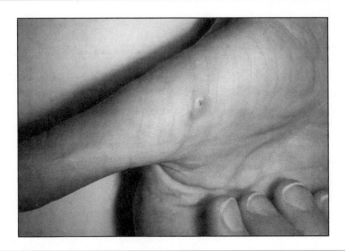

Source: CDC/Thomas F. Sellers, Emory University.

immune system, and the germinal centers contain activated B lymphoblasts that secrete antibodies. Regional lymphadenopathy is seen after 3 to 50 days but rarely becomes generalized or involves nodes of other regions.

The lesion may regress or may progress to the intermediate stage, in which tuberculoid foci appear but multinucleated giant cells (resulting from cell fusion) are rare. Node architecture is noticeably distorted, and the surrounding capsule is often broken. During the late stage, microabscesses and macroabscesses develop, usually within a region of epithelioid cells in a palisade arrangement. The lesions may persist for months.

CSD is usually self-limiting, and lymphadenopathy is the sole symptom in about one-third of affected persons. Fewer than half of those with CSD develop mild fever and malaise. Chills, generalized aching, and nausea are uncommon. Occasionally, infected persons have conjunctivitis (inflammation of the mucous membrane lining the underside of the eyelid) with preauricular, tender lymphadenopathy (oculoglandular syndrome of Parinaud). Less frequently, CSD includes encephalitis or meningitis, pneumonitis (inflammatory lesion of the alveoli of the lungs and interstitial spaces), erythema nodosum (painful, nodular inflammatory lesions of dermal and subcutaneous tissue), thrombocytopenia (low numbers of platelets), osteolytic lesions (lytic bone lesions), optic neuritis (inflammation of the optic nerve), or necrotizing hepatic or splenic granulomata (aggregates of macrophages, lymphocytes, or fibroblasts in the liver or spleen).

Trench Fever

Trench fever (also known as **quintana fever**, shin fever, and Wolhynia fever) is a febrile illness with either a sudden or slow onset following an incubation period of 7 to 30 days. It is characterized by high fever, headache, malaise, and severe pain, particularly affecting the back and shins. The fever may occur in a single episode lasting several days or may be relapsing and typhoidlike. Splenomegaly (enlargement of the spleen) is commonly seen. A transient, macular rash may also be present. Infectious bacteria may persist in the blood for months to years, and subclinical symptoms may recur for several years after the initial infection. Immunocompromised individuals, particularly those who are HIV-positive, may develop bacteremia (bacterial growth in the blood) or osteomyelitis (inflammation of the bone marrow) and may also develop bacillary angiomatosis. Endocarditis (inflammation of the heart lining) may occur in homeless alcoholics and others with poor nutritional and health status.

Bacillary Angiomatosis and Bacillary Peliosis Hepatis

Bacillary angiomatosis (BA) is characterized by chronic, benign tumors consisting of blood vessels and are induced by two *Bartonella* species infecting humans, *Bartonella henselae* and *Bartonella quintana*. It occurs almost solely in immunosuppressed persons and is one of the manifestations of late-stage AIDS; it typically occurs when the $CD4^+$ T helper cell count falls below $100/mm^3$. Other individuals who are at increased risk for BA include those receiving chemotherapy for cancer or immunosuppressive drugs to prevent rejection after organ transplantation. BA is manifested as multifocal vascular cutaneous lesions or by vascular proliferative lesions in other tissues, such as bone, brain parenchyma, lymph nodes, or the gastrointestinal or respiratory systems. These lesions may be erosive in tissues, including the epidermis, bone, and the intestines. Because BA lesions are highly vascular, they may be misdiagnosed as cancer, such as Kaposi's sarcoma or lymphoma, in HIV-positive persons.

Bacillary peliosis hepatis (BP) is another pathological condition characterized by vascular proliferation. It primarily affects the liver and spleen but may also occur in the lymph nodes. It is associated with *Bartonella* infection in HIV-positive individuals. Affected persons may have decreased numbers of platelets or blood cells and elevated liver enzyme levels, particularly alkaline phosphatase.

BA or BP in immunocompromised individuals may be accompanied by prolonged bacteremia. It may also be seen in immunocompetent persons with complicated CSD. Relapses often occur in both populations even after antibiotic therapy.

Endocarditis

Endocarditis may result from infection of either immunosuppressed or immunocompetent individuals with several *Bartonella* species. A person may be symptomatic for months before diagnosis, and the disease course is often subacute. Replacement of the infected heart valve and antibiotic therapy are necessary in 80% of the cases, but people typically recover afterward; the mortality rate is 20%, primarily in patients with delayed diagnosis. Interestingly, endocarditis associated with *B. henselae*, but not *B. quintana*, is often linked to prior heart valve injury. The latter type of endocarditis is found mainly in alcoholic homeless persons. The median age of those affected is 48 years, and 85% of these people are male.

Individuals typically present with acute cardiac failure and often have a fever exceeding 38°C (100.4°F). Frequent symptoms include cardiac murmur, dyspnea (difficulty breathing) on exertion, echocardiographic vegetations, and bibasilar lung rales. Aortic valves are the most often affected and suffer destructive damage. Emboli are found in approximately 40% of the individuals.

The Causative Agents

Bartonella bacilliformis

Bartonellosis is caused by a small (0.2–0.5 μm wide by 0.3–1.5 μm long) bacillus, **Bartonella bacilliformis,** which was described in 1909 by Alberto Barton and isolated in 1926. The gram-negative rods are motile by the actions of a brush of at least ten unipolar flagella. These bacteria are obligate aerobes (absolutely require oxygen) and may be cultured at 28°C (85.6°F) under the surface of a semisolid agar containing 10% rabbit serum plus 0.5% rabbit hemoglobin. Growth is apparent after seven to ten days. *Bartonella* species belong to the α-2 subgroup of *Proteobacteria.*

Humans become infected with *B. bacilliformis* via the bite of infected members of the nocturnal *Lutzomyia* genera of sand flies. These species reside in valleys of the Andes mountain range in Peru, Ecuador, and Columbia between 600 and 2,800 meters (2,000–9,200 feet) above sea level, where the bacteria are highly endemic and may cause epidemics. No reservoirs for *B. bacilliformis* exist other than humans, in whom the bacteria persist for prolonged periods of time during which infection may be propagated by blood transfusion. After the bacteria are introduced into a human host, they enter into endothelial cells lining blood vessels, where they divide in the cytoplasm for two to three weeks. Bacteria then pass into the blood to infect erythrocytes. Up to 90% of a person's erythrocytes may be infected by the bacteria, which subsequently destroy them, causing hemolytic anemia that may be severe. After Giemsa staining, multiple bacilli are seen on the erythrocyte surfaces. The bacteria are also present in cells of the innate immune system in the lymph nodes, liver, and spleen.

Table 5.2 *Bartonella* species that infect humans

Bacteria	Vector
B. bacilliformis	*Lutzomyia* sand flies
B. henselae	cats
B. quintana	human body lice
B. elizabethae	rat fleas

Bartonella henselae

Bartonella henselae infection may induce illness with different presentations, depending on the immune status of the human host. It is responsible for most cases of CSD in persons with intact immune responsiveness and for many cases of bacillary angiomatosis and bacillary peliosis hepatis in immunocompromised persons. Infection of humans with *B. henselae* (formerly known as *Rochalimaea henselae*) is accomplished by scratches, licks, or bites from infected cats or exposure to their excreta or saliva; greater than 95% of individuals with CSD report contact with a cat. Young cats are the most common sources of human infection and do not themselves suffer illness. Transmission may also occur from scratches or bites of dogs or monkeys or from inanimate objects. Cat fleas (*Ctenocephalides felis*) can host viable bacilli and may aid in transmission of *B. henselae* between cats but do not appear to infect humans with these bacteria. CSD incidence is highest in the late fall through early spring.

RECENT DEVELOPMENTS

During both CSD and BA, *B. henselae* bacteria target and infect endothelial cells, resulting in the formation of a host cellular structure called the invasome. After entry into the endothelial cells, the bacteria then divide repeatedly in the cytoplasm in the vicinity of the nucleus. CSD and BA are also characterized by an inflammatory influx of white blood cells into the area, including neutrophils of the innate immune system. In one study, when bacteria derived from a BA lesion were added to cultures of human umbilical cord vein endothelial cells in vitro, they potently stimulated these cells by a pathway involving activation of the transcription factor, NF-κB. The magnitude of the endothelial cell stimulation was on the order of that induced by tumor necrosis factor-α, a powerful inflammatory cytokine. NF-κB binds to the promoters of cellular adhesion molecules, particularly E-selectin and ICAM-1, enhancing their expression. The adhesion molecules increase the numbers of neutrophils rolling on and adhering to infected endothelial cells. Antibodies against E-selectin significantly reduced neutrophils' interaction with these cells. The strain of *B. henselae* used in this study had been growing in culture for just a short period of time. Other isolates that had been maintained longer in the laboratory had a lesser ability to induce neutrophils' rolling and adhesion. Neither live bacteria nor their lipopolysaccharides were required to up-regulate adhesion molecules and this effect could be reproduced using bacterial outer membrane proteins.

Bartonella quintana

Bartonella quintana (formerly *Rickettsia quintana* and *Rochalimaea quintana*) is the bacterium responsible for trench fever and endocarditis and also causes bacillary angiomatosis and bacillary peliosis hepatis in immunocompromised persons. It was first grown in culture in 1961. These bacteria are associated with crowded and unhygienic conditions in which the human body louse vector (*Pediculus humanus corporis*) thrives and which allow ease of transit between its hosts. The bacteria multiply extracellularly in the lumen of the louse's gut throughout its five-week life span. *B. quintana* are passed in the louse's feces and enter humans through skin breaks, including the louse bite site. New lice are then infected by feeding on the blood of infected humans. Bacteria-laden feces are produced by the lice 5 to 12 days after their infection. Disease spreads from person to person as the lice leave abnormally hot (feverish) or cold (dead) humans and infest a new host that has a normal body temperature. Direct human-to-human transmission of *B. quintana* does not occur, but due to the long time bacteria remain in the blood (over a year in some cases), individuals who have developed trench fever are permanently prohibited from donating blood.

In addition to epidemic outbreaks during disruptive conditions such as war and movement of civilians into refugee camps, endemic foci of trench fever are found in Poland, countries of the former Soviet Union, Burundi, Ethiopia, northern Africa, Mexico, and Bolivia. Trench fever is also found in

FIGURE 5.2 Human body louse

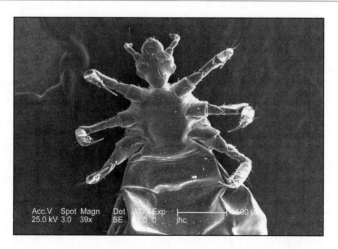

Source: CDC/Joseph Strycharz, Kyong Sup Yoon, and Frank Collins.

some segments of the U.S. population, particularly as an opportunistic disease of AIDS patients and a febrile illness sometimes associated with endocarditis in homeless or alcoholic persons ("urban trench fever").

Bartonella elizabethae

Bartonella elizabethae (formerly *Rochalimaea elizabethae*) was isolated in 1993 from the blood of a person with a fever and endocarditis. This is the only known case of human disease due to it. These bacteria may infect rat fleas (*Xenopsylla cheopis*).

Other *Bartonella* Species in Domestic Animals

Bartonella vinsonii subspecies *berkhoffi* and *B. clarridgeiae* have been isolated from domestic dogs and cats, respectively. The former also infects wild members of the canine family. Neither bacterial species has been found in humans.

The Immune Response

Several aspects of the immune response play an important role in controlling *Bartonella* infections and decreasing pathology. This protection may be long-term, as those who recover from untreated Oroya fever usually develop a state of lifelong immunity, whereas verruga peruana may recur. The importance of a functional immune response is demonstrated by *B. henselae* infection, which results in BA or BP in immunocompromised persons but the milder, self-resolving CSD in those with intact immunity.

Both aspects of the adoptive immune system are activated during infection. A B lymphocyte-mediated humoral (antibody) response to *Bartonella* may be important to the control of the infections. Serum from the blood of a number of patients with CSD contains antibodies that recognize a conserved 83 kilodalton kD molecular weight protein from *B. henselae* that is not recognized by sera from patients infected with other bacteria, including *Rickettsia rickettsii*, *Chlamydia*, *Treponema pallidum*, *Fransciscella tularensis*, *Ehrlichia chaffeensis*, *Mycoplasma pneumoniae*, and *Escherichia coli*. This bacterial molecule does react with antibodies in sera from *B. quintana*–infected patients, however, demonstrating partial cross-reactivity between the two *Bartonella* species. The antibodies are of the IgG (IgG$_1$) and IgA classes. The fact that the IgG antibodies are predominantly of the IgG$_1$ subclass suggests that the antibodies were directed against protein antigens and that their production was dependent on T lymphocyte activity. During *Bartonella* infections, this subclass appears to function by stimulating opsonization, a process that enhances uptake of the bacteria by phagocytic cells prior to their destruction. A cell-mediated immune response due to the action of T lymphocytes is also prominent, with delayed-type hypersensitivity being produced in 95% to 98% of infected individuals. The CD4$^+$ T helper cell response is generally protective and is of the Th1 type, with lymphocytes producing the cytokine interferon-γ but not interleukin-4. HIV infection diminishes Th1 responses, which may partially account for the severity of *Bartonella* infections in the HIV-infected segment of the population.

Diagnosis

Bartonellosis may be suspected in persons from the limited endemic areas who present with fever, headache, and progressive hemolytic anemia. Diagnosis may be confirmed by finding bacteria on the surface of erythrocytes, in sections of cutaneous lesions, or in cultures from blood or affected skin. As many as 90% of the host's erythrocytes may be parasitized. Polymerase chain reaction (PCR) may also be employed.

CSD should be considered in persons presenting with regional or local lymphadenitis, especially those who report having contact with or being scratched by a cat. Infection with *B. henselae* may be determined by lymph node histology and a positive skin test (Type IV hypersensitivity reaction to bacterial antigen) after 36 to 48 hours, similar to that used to detect infection with *Mycobacterium tuberculosis* (causative agent of TB, discussed in Chapter Ten). Other diseases with similar pathology include infection with atypical mycobacteria, tularemia, toxoplasmosis, infectious mononucleosis, lymphogranuloma venereum, brucellosis, plague, and coccidioidomycosis. A titer greater than or equal to 1:64 by indirect fluorescent-antibody assay (IFA) is also considered to be a positive reaction.

Trench fever is diagnosed by the culture of *B. quintana* from the blood on chocolate or blood agar in the presence of 5% CO_2. Microcolonies are visible after 8 to 21 days. IFA may detect the presence of genus-specific antibodies.

Diagnosis of BA and BP is difficult, and these conditions are often not recognized or misdiagnosed as other HIV-associated cancers. Immunological detection by skin test or IFA may not be useful because of the patients' deficient immune responses. The bacteria are difficult to culture but may be visualized in biopsy material treated with hematoxylin and eosin followed by Warthin-Starry silver stain. The tissue contains dividing endothelial cells with new, small-diameter blood vessels and is typically infiltrated by lymphocytes and neutrophils and clusters of granular material, which are bacterial clumps. PCR amplification may be necessary for detection.

Treatment

Salmonellosis is a common and serious complication of the Oroya fever stage of bartonellosis; consequently, infection with *B. bacilliformis* is often treated with chloramphenicol or ampicillin, antibiotics to which both diseases respond. Penicillin, streptomycin, and tetracyclines are also effective against *B. bacilliformis* and in reducing the fever. If the anemia is severe, blood transfusion may be necessary. Because large skin lesions of verruga peruana may be easily abraded and become susceptible to secondary infections, they may be excised. No specific treatment is usually administered for this cutaneous manifestation; however, tetracycline may aid the healing process.

No specific treatment is usually used for cases of CSD, but large and tender lymph nodes may be surgically removed if good cosmetic results are obtainable. Pus may be removed from the nodes by needle aspiration.

Tetracyclines, such as doxycycline, are used to treat trench fever. Special care must be taken in monitoring patients with endocarditis. Relapse may occur after treatment, regardless of the immune competence of the person.

Immunocompromised persons, especially those who are HIV-positive, may be treated with several antibiotics, such as rifampin, erythromycin, and doxycycline, in cases of *Bartonella* infections such as BA or BP. Treatment should be continued for three to four months for these individuals in order to prevent relapse. Unlike CSD, antibiotic therapy for these conditions is often quite effective.

Prevention

Because bartonellosis is transmitted by sand flies, prevention efforts focus on decreasing human contact with these insects. Some of these measures include

Table 5.3   Treatment for diseases associated with *Bartonella* infection

Disease	Treatment Option
Carrión's disease	Chloramphenicol, ampicillin, penicillin, streptomycin, tetracyclines Blood transfusion Excision of skin lesions
Cat-scratch disease	Removal of large lymph nodes Needle aspiration of pus
Trench fever	Tetracyclines
BA and BP	Rifampin, erythromycin, doxycycline

avoiding areas infested by these nocturnal vectors after sundown, applying insecticides to one's clothing and exposed skin, wearing clothing that covers the legs and arms, using fine mesh bed netting, and the spraying of insecticides such as DDT. DDT has greatly reduced the incidence of bartonellosis and prevented large outbreaks during the past 20 years. Blood donated from individuals living in endemic areas should be tested before use. The fact that the pertinent vector species have a very restricted geographical range should be kept in mind.

In the case of CSD, given the mild and self-limiting nature of the infection, avoidance of cats in general is not recommended. Care should be taken to avoid being scratched, and scratches and bites that do occur should be thoroughly cleaned. Removal of cat fleas from pets may decrease transmission between animals.

Because human body lice are the vectors for trench fever, delousing procedures decrease transmission. These may include dusting clothing and bodies of louse-infested persons with insecticides. During epidemics, systemic application of insecticides to members of the affected population is recommended. Ideally, people should avoid living conditions in which louse infestation may occur. This may not be practical, however, for troops during combat or for persons living in refugee camps or in areas experiencing disruptions and massive displacement of populations, as during civil wars or following natural disasters such as earthquakes, hurricanes, and floods. Persons living in crowded, unsanitary conditions—particularly the homeless, impoverished residents of urban slums, and institutionalized persons (in prisons, mental hospitals, and nursing homes)—are also at higher risk and may lack the financial means or be otherwise unable to improve their environment. Local or regional governmental or health agencies may also not have the funding or the personnel to increase the hygiene for these persons. Louse control, whenever possible, also decreases the incidence of other more serious louseborne diseases, such as epidemic typhus (caused by *Rickettsia prowazekii*) and relapsing fever (caused by *Borrelia recurrentis*).

Surveillance

Because epidemics of Oroya fever may result in great loss of life, intensive case-finding efforts should be employed during those times to identify affected areas for systematic spraying of homes with residual insecticides, particularly DDT.

Surveillance of impounded cat and pet cat populations in the San Francisco Bay area of California found that 40% and 41% were bacteremic for *B. henselae*, respectively. Kittens were most likely to have these bacteria in their blood. Other studies examined the proportion of cats with antibodies to this microbe, which would indicate past or current infection; 81% were seropositive in San Francisco, 15% in Baltimore and Japan, and 33% in Austria. The areas of the United States with the highest percentage of seropositive cats were the areas with high numbers of cat fleas, reflecting the roles of these insects in transmission between cats.

Surveillance efforts have included surveys of the arthropod vectors for *Bartonella* species. In a multicountry study of human body lice, more than 10% of the lice from Burundi, France, the Netherlands, Russia, and Zimbabwe were PCR-positive for *B. quintana*. Fewer than 3% of the body lice were infected in Algeria, Australia, Congo Republic, Peru, Rwanda, and Tunisia. The highest percentages of infected lice were found in refugee camps. *B. quintana* were not detected in any of the tested head lice. Several species of *Bartonella*, including *B. quintana* and *B. henselae*, were found in 19% of the *Ixodes pacificus* ticks from California. *B. henselae* were detected in less than 2% of the *I. ricinus* ticks from persons in Italy. Over 60% of rat fleas were also found to be infected with *Bartonella*, including *B. elizabethae*.

Summary

Diseases

- Bartonellosis (Carrión's disease and Oroya fever)
- Cat-scratch fever • Trench fever (quintana fever)
- Bacillary angiomatosis and bacillary peliosis hepatis • Endocarditis

Causative Agents

- *Bartonella bacilliformis* • *B. henselae* • *B. quintana*
- *B. henselae and B. quintana* • *B. henselae, B. quintana, and B. elizabethae*

Agent Type

- Gram-negative bacillus of the genus *Bartonella*, α-2 subgroup of *Proteobacteria*

Genome

- DNA

Vectors

- *Lutzomyia* sand flies • None • Human body louse • Unknown

Common Reservoirs

- Humans • Cats • Humans • Unknown

Modes of Transmission

- Sand fly bite • Cat scratch • Louse feces rubbed into skin wound
- Unknown

Geographical Distribution

- Valleys in the Andes Mountains of Peru, Ecuador, and Columbia
- Worldwide • Epidemic in areas experiencing crowded and unsanitary conditions and endemic in parts of Poland, the former Soviet Union, Burundi, Ethiopia, northern Africa, Mexico, Bolivia, and the United States • Unknown

Year of Emergence

- 1871 • 1950 • 1915 • 1983 • 1993

Key Terms

Bacillary angiomatosis Chronic, benign tumors due to proliferation of blood vessels that are induced by *Bartonella henselae* and *B. quintana* and typically affect immunosuppressed persons

Bacillary peliosis hepatis Vascular proliferative disease of the liver and spleen due to infection of immunosuppressed persons by *Bartonella*

Bartonella bacilliformis Gram-negative bacilli that cause bartonellosis

Bartonella elizabethae Gram-negative bacilli that cause endocarditis

Bartonella henselae Gram-negative bacilli that cause cat-scratch disease

Bartonella quintana Gram-negative bacilli that cause trench fever

Bartonellosis Disease caused by *Bartonella bacilliformis,* consisting of an initial acute febrile stage with potentially lethal hemolytic anemia and a later cutaneous stage

Basophilic stippling Punctuate, bluish erythrocyte inclusions; aggregated ribosomes

Carrión's disease Bartonellosis

Cat-scratch disease Mild, self-limiting swelling of pus-exuding lymph nodes caused by *B. henselae*

Hemolytic anemia Low number of erythrocytes in the blood as a result of their destruction

Howell-Jolly bodies Erythrocyte inclusions; round nuclear remnants

Oroya fever Initial, acute stage of bartonellosis; a severe acute febrile illness with hemolytic anemia; often fatal

Polychromatic Bluish pink, the color of reticulocytes after Giemsa staining

Quintana fever Trench fever

Reticulocytes Immature red blood cells

Trench fever Febrile disease associated with living conditions that favor human body lice

Verruga peruana Second, cutaneous stage of bartonellosis

Review Questions

1. Which *Bartonella* species cause disease in humans? With which diseases are each of these bacterial species associated? Which diseases are most often found in immunosuppressed persons?
2. What are the vectors and reservoir hosts for the pathogenic *Bartonella* species that infect humans? Where are these bacteria concentrated geographically?
3. What are the symptoms of the four diseases caused by *B. henselae*?
4. Why can skin tests and IFA be used in the diagnosis of CSD but not BA or BP?
5. What measures may be employed to decrease the incidence of trench fever during warfare? What measures might decrease the incidence of Oroya fever?

Topics for Further Discussion

1. Impoverished or homeless persons, alcoholics, and HIV-positive persons are at highest risk for either acquiring infection or suffering severe disease manifestations due to *Bartonella* species. Unhygienic living conditions that encourage louse infestation and reduce immune responsiveness put these individuals at risk. Discuss means by which disease incidence or severity might be decreased among these people in a manner that is economically and socially feasible.
2. How might the limited geographical distribution and vector preference of Oroya fever and verruga peruana be exploited to reduce or eliminate these diseases?
3. How might the association between young cats and CSD and many cases of BA and BP in immunocompromised persons be exploited to reduce or eliminate these diseases?
4. Discuss the effects of louseborne illnesses in human history.

Resources

Arvand, M., and others. "*Bartonella henselae*–Specific Cell-Mediated Immune Responses Display a Predominantly Th1 Phenotype in Experimentally Infected C57BL/6 Mice." *Infection and Immunity*, 2001, *69*, 6427–6433.

Brouqui, P., and Raoult, D. "Endocarditis Due to Rare and Fastidious Bacteria." *Clinical Microbiology Reviews*, 2001, *14*, 177–207.

Chin, J. *Control of Communicable Diseases Manual* (17th ed.). Washington, D.C.: American Public Health Association, 2000.

Cramblett, H. G. "Cat-Scratch Fever." In P. D. Hoeprich (ed.), *Infectious Diseases*. New York: Harper & Row, 1977.

Fournier, P.-E., and others. "Human Pathogens in Body and Head Lice." *Emerging Infectious Diseases*, 2002, *8*, 1515–1518.

Fuhrmann, O., and others. "*Bartonella henselae* Induces NF-κB-dependent Upregulation of Adhesion Molecules in Cultured Human Endothelial Cells: Possible Role of Outer Membrane Proteins as Pathogenic Factors." *Infection and Immunity*, 2001, *69*, 5088–5097.

Goldstein, E. "Bartonellosis." In P. D. Hoeprich (ed.), *Infectious Diseases*. New York: Harper & Row, 1977.

Koehler, J. E. "*Bartonella:* An Emerging Human Pathogen." In W. M. Scheld, D. Armstrong, and J. M. Hughes (eds.), *Emerging Infections* (Vol. 1). Washington, D.C.: ASM Press, 1998.

McGill, S. L., Regnery, R. L., and Karem, K. L. "Characterization of Human Immunoglobulin (Ig) Isotype and IgG Subclass Response to *Bartonella henselae* Infection." *Infection and Immunity*, 1998, *66*, 5915–5920.

Sanogo, Y. O., and others. "*Bartonella henselae* in *Ixodes ricinus* Ticks (Acari: Ixodida) Removed from Humans, Belluno Province, Italy." *Emerging Infectious Diseases*, 2003, *9*, 329–332.

CHAPTER 6

GROUP A STREPTOCOCCI

LEARNING OBJECTIVES

- Define and compare the variety of diseases caused by group A streptococci

- Describe the cocci responsible for causing these illnesses

- Discuss modes of infection

- Discuss the host's response to infection

- Discuss potential methods of treatment

- Describe symptomatology and diagnosis

Major Concepts

Diseases

Infections caused by group A streptococcus (GAS) bacteria are common throughout the world and result in a wide variety of illnesses, ranging from mild to debilitating or lethal. The rate of incidence of the more severe, invasive GAS infections, such as necrotizing fasciitis and streptococcal toxic shock syndrome (STSS), peaks and ebbs over time and has increased significantly in developed countries since the 1980s. Other potentially severe manifestations of GAS infection include erysipelas, scarlet fever, meningitis, rheumatic fever, acute glomerulonephritis, and childbed fever.

Infection

GAS (*Streptococcus pyogenes*) bacteria are gram-positive cocci that characteristically lead to β-hemolysis on sheep blood agar. They are common residents of the skin and throat and may enter the body through skin breaks or respiratory secretions or via contaminated food or drink. Different strains of these bacteria possess different virulence factors, a number of which are controlled by the *mga* gene, which up-regulates their expression. A particularly important virulence factor is the M protein which is required for adherence to target cells, such as skin keratinocytes, and resistance to phagocytosis. GAS also encode several exotoxins, which contribute to the disease process by inducing pathogenic overstimulation of the immune system or disrupting the extracellular matrix, resulting in damage to soft tissues.

Immune Response

GAS have several means of avoiding destruction by the innate and adaptive arms of the immune system, including phagocytosis, the complement cascade, and neutralizing antibodies. They also cause harmful immune responses, such as the overproduction of inflammatory cytokines during STSS, and autoimmune reactions during rheumatic fever and acute glomerulonephritis. Care must be taken during vaccine development to avoid the induction of such pathogenic immunity.

Treatment

Early treatment with antibiotics, particularly penicillin, is often effective in eliminating most strains of GAS and decreasing the risk for serious disease manifestations. Individuals who are allergic to penicillin may be treated with erythromycin, cephalexin or cephradine, or macrolides. Drug resistance, however, is becoming increasingly common; a sizable number of GAS strains are resistant to tetracycline, and resistance to erythromycin and macrolides is increasing. Newer drugs, such as telithromycin, are effective against some of these strains. Other treatment options include administration of massive amounts of intravenous fluids for individuals with severe hypotension, extensive debridement for those with necrotizing fasciitis, and absolute bed rest and anti-inflammatory drugs for those with rheumatic fever.

Prevention

Preventive measures include basic hygienic practices, such as hand-washing after coughing or sneezing and before eating to prevent infection by respiratory secretions or contaminated food. Pasteurization of milk and the exclusion of persons with skin lesions from food preparation are also effective means of decreasing GAS infection. Objects used in such medical procedures as liposuction, hysterectomy, childbirth, and bone pinning need to be disinfected to avoid noscomial transmission.

Introduction

Some 10,000 to 15,000 cases of invasive **group A streptococcus (GAS)** infections occur in the United States each year, resulting in 2,000 deaths. GAS causes a variety of diseases, ranging in severity from mild to life-threatening. These conditions include streptococcal septic sore throat (strep throat); pharyngitis; tonsillitis; impetigo; erysipelas; scarlet fever; meningitis; necrotizing fasciitis, myositis, and myonecrosis; rheumatic fever, myocarditis, and valvulitis; acute glomerulonephritis; childbed fever; streptococcal toxic shock syndrome (STSS); otitis media; pneumonia; and septicemia. GAS infections result in 500 to 1,500 cases of necrotizing fasciitis in the United States yearly. Increased morbidity and mortality in recent decades have resulted in the classification of GAS infections as reemerging diseases. Annual costs in the United States due to strep throat alone approach $1 billion. Antibiotics have greatly reduced the incidence of rheumatic fever, an autoimmune complication of GAS infection, in the developed world, but it remains a major health factor in underdeveloped nations. Although some of the illnesses associated with GAS infections are mild, the consequences of invasive GAS may be very serious, and the overall mortality rate is 21%, complicated by the development of drug resistance in children and adults. The incidence of invasive GAS among individuals who inject illegal drugs is increasing.

History

Some of the diseases associated with GAS infections have been known since antiquity and periodically shift their severity. In 1664, Thomas Sydenham described "febris scarlatina." A major epidemic of this condition, scarlet fever, occurred in 1736 in the American colonies, ultimately claiming the lives of 4,000 people. For centuries prior to this time, scarlet fever had existed either endemically or as relatively mild epidemics separated by long periods of time. Between the years 1825 and 1885, however, a series of cyclical and frequently highly lethal epidemics began in various urban centers, including Paris, London, Dublin, and New York City. The mortality rate in some of these outbreaks approached 30%. After that, the severity of scarlet fever decreased in developed regions.

The Greek physician Hippocrates recorded a disease that meets the clinical description of necrotizing fasciitis. This condition was first described in the United States by a Confederate Army surgeon during the American Civil War. It was determined to be of bacterial origin in 1918 and received its current name in 1952. During the 1800s and 1900s, necrotizing fasciitis occurred only sporadically, primarily in military hospitals during conflicts. It increased in virulence in the United States during the 1980s due to the emergence of toxin-producing strains, and by 1999, approximately 600 cases of this serious condition had been reported in the United States.

A decreased incidence of severe invasive GAS infections occurred in the United States during the 1930s, when mortality rates fell from 72% to between 7% and 27% even prior to the introduction to antibiotics. This was not accompanied by a decline in mild disease manifestations or in the prevalence of GAS colonization and infection. Developing regions of the world continued to suffer from highly pathogenic infections. The more lethal expressions of GAS inexplicably rebounded in developed nations throughout the world in the 1980s (with mortality rates ranging from 35% to 48%) as these bacteria reemerged as modern killers. Jim Henson, the creator of the Muppets, died of STSS. Other conditions caused by GAS bacteria have been known for millennia but have reemerged in recent decades. One such condition is necrotizing fasciitis, an extremely rapid pathogenic destruction of connective tissue and fat that may be lethal if not treated promptly. It is caused by the so-called flesh-eating bacteria. This condition was described by Hippocrates in ancient Greece, but the numbers of cases have greatly increased recently and periodically receive much attention in the popular press.

Major epidemics of rheumatic fever struck the U.S. military during World War II and the Korean War. Large numbers of cases also occurred in Utah between 1985 and 1998.

The Diseases

GAS infection results in a wide variety of conditions, some of which are minor (sore throat, tonsillitis, and impetigo), while others (rheumatic fever, necrotizing fasciitis, and streptococcal toxic shock syndrome) may result in long-term disability or death. People are more likely to develop serious illnesses caused by invasive GAS infection if they have skin lesions (including chickenpox or cuts), cancer, diabetes, or a skin ulcer or if they abuse drugs or are using steroids. The elderly are also at increased risk. GAS infections occur year round, but incidence peaks in late winter and early spring.

Entry into the respiratory tract is followed by a 36- to 72-hour latent period. As the bacteria grow, they induce a sore throat, inflammation of the pharynx

Table 6.1   Diseases associated with GAS infection

Disease	Symptoms	Persons Affected
Impetigo	Reddened skin, fluid-filled blisters	Children
Scarlet fever	Sore throat, fever, and rash; "scarlet tongue"; nausea and vomiting	Children
Erysipelas	Acute cellulitis: fever; chills; leukocytosis; lymphadenopathy; painful, fiery red skin lesion	Infants and persons over the age of 20 years
Necrotizing fasciitis	Fever, severe pain, swelling, extreme thirst, diarrhea, nausea, confusion, dizziness, gangrene with extensive necrosis of tissues over large areas of skin, septic shock	Young, healthy adults
Rheumatic fever	Fever, inflammation of joints and heart valves, myocarditis, erythema marginatum, Sydenham's chorea	Persons aged 3–15 years
Acute glomerulonephritis	Inflammation of glomeruli (filtering tubules of the kidneys)	All
Childbed fever	Fever	Women following childbirth
Streptococcal toxic shock syndrome (STSS)	Fever, chills, myalgia, dizziness, confusion, severe abdominal pain, vomiting, diarrhea, hypotension, shock, generalized erythematous macular rash; acute respiratory distress syndrome, renal failure, disseminated intravascular coagulation	All

and tonsils (pharyngitis and tonsillitis) with or without exudate, fever, and leuko-cytosis (increased white blood cell count). Severe, uncomplicated streptococcal pharyngitis typically diminishes after five to seven days. Before the development of penicillin, the death rate from this disease manifestation was 1% to 3%.

Impetigo

Impetigo is a superficial skin infection occurring primarily in children, usually in the late summer or fall in hot climates. This condition is characterized by reddened skin and fluid-filled blisters, mainly on the legs and arms and around the nose and mouth. These blisters later burst, releasing a thin, yellowish fluid. Fever is usually absent. Following antibiotic therapy, the prognosis is excellent. Several million cases occur each year in the United States.

Scarlet Fever

Scarlet fever usually occurs in children and is most commonly found in temperate zones and slightly less frequently in subtropical regions. It typically manifests as sore throat, fever, and rash in response to a pyrogenic exotoxin. The rash begins as a mass of tiny red spots on the neck and upper trunk and then spreads to other parts of the body, including the inner surfaces of the thighs and

FIGURE 6.1   Skin lesions due to impetigo

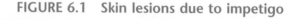

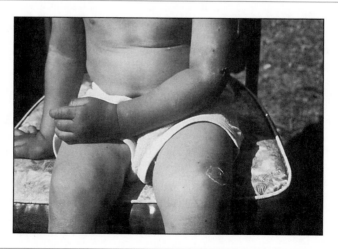

Source: CDC.

FIGURE 6.2   "Strawberry tongue"

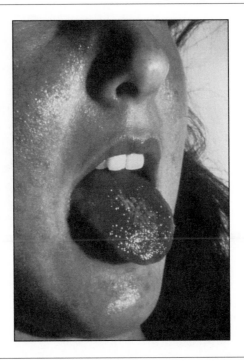

Source: CDC.

the folds of the axillae (armpits), elbows, and groin. The tongue may be covered with a white coating containing red spots; the coating later peels away to give a bright-red appearance (strawberry tongue). A peeling of skin, particularly the tips of the fingers and toes, may occur during convalescence. Severe infections may be accompanied by high fever, nausea, and vomiting. Scarlet fever may be a very severe condition, resulting in large and lethal epidemics. Highly virulent strains of GAS resulted in mortality rates of 25% to 35% among children during the 1880s, but current rates are much lower.

Erysipelas

Erysipelas is a recurrent form of acute cellulitis commonly located on the legs or the face. The symptoms are fever and chills, blisters, leukocytosis (elevated white blood cell count), lymphadenopathy (swollen lymph nodes), and a painful, fiery red, spreading skin lesion with a raised border. Bacteremia may be

FIGURE 6.3   Erysipelas

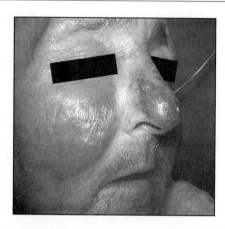

Source: CDC/Thomas F. Sellers, Emory University.

present. Although the prognosis is generally good following antibiotic therapy, erysipelas may be severe or fatal in individuals who are debilitated. It develops most commonly in infants and persons over the age of 20 years.

Necrotizing Fasciitis

Necrotizing fasciitis has also been known as malignant ulcer, putrid ulcer, gangrenous ulcer, and hospital gangrene. It is the rapid, extremely dangerous destruction of fascia (connective tissue) and other soft tissue following infection by **"flesh-eating bacteria"**—often GAS but sometimes *Clostridium perfringes* or other bacteria. Infection with these bacteria often occurs at the site of an insignificant trauma during common activities, such as a scratch from a rose thorn during gardening. The destruction of fascia and fat (adipose tissue) begin within hours of infection by GAS. Early symptoms include fever, severe pain, swelling, redness at the wound site, extreme thirst, diarrhea, nausea, confusion, and dizziness. Over next two days, the wound becomes a purplish or bluish color with blisters containing a clear yellow fluid. Two or three days after that, gangrene develops, with extensive necrosis of the underlying tissues occurring in the next week over large areas of skin. Potent toxins render the patients unresponsive or delirious. Afflicted persons may lose consciousness and develop septic shock due to severe decreases in blood pressure. Some 500 to 1,500 cases of this condition are reported in the United States each year. Even after extensive debridement and irrigation of the wound (removal of dead material and washing), the fatality rate is 20%.

This disease manifestation most often occurs in young, strong persons following minor skin trauma rather than in older people with multiple medical problems. It is rare in children. The increased incidence of this disease may reflect the appearance of more virulent GAS strains. The development of necrotizing fasciitis is associated with immunosuppression in 91% of the cases, especially among persons with diabetes, alcoholism, end-stage renal disease, cancer, and malnutrition; persons using immunosuppressants; and women during the peripartum period occurring around the time of childbirth.

Current cases of necrotizing fasciitis are more likely to display systemic manifestations (shock or organ failure) associated with STSS than previously, even after antibiotic therapy. Another worrisome finding has been the increase in reports of myositis or myonecrosis in conjunction with GAS infections. These manifestations, with destructive damage to muscles and tendons, occur either alone or accompanying necrotizing fasciitis.

Rheumatic Fever

Rheumatic fever usually affects children between the ages of 3 and 15 years; however, large outbreaks have also occurred among adults, particularly those in military service. This condition involves fever of 38.3°C to 40°C (101°F to 104°F) and inflammation of tissues throughout body. The joints are usually involved in this extremely painful reaction, particularly the knees, ankles, elbows, and wrists, and it tends to migrate between joints. In 40% to 50% of the affected children, this condition progresses to myocarditis or valvulitis and causes damage to the heart that may be permanent. The valves undergo thickening and scarring, which is detectable as a heart murmur due to mitral regurgitation (backflow of blood through the damaged valve from the left ventricle into the left atrium). Enlargement of the heart occurs in 50% of patients with rheumatic fever, and congestive heart failure is seen in 5% to 10%. Rapidly progressive carditis results in death in less than 1% of the affected persons. Those with severe carditis may develop subcutaneous nodules over the extensor aspects of their joints. Other complications of rheumatic fever include erythema marginatum (pinkish-red macular lesions with a central area of clearing) in 10% to 15% of children and Sydenham's chorea (spasmatic muscular movements and incoordination) in 5% to 15% of patients. Differential diagnosis of rheumatic fever includes conditions such as rheumatoid arthritis, septic arthritis, systemic lupus erythematosus, serum sickness, sickle cell hemoglobinopathies, infective bacterial endocarditis, and early-stage leukemia.

Rheumatic fever develops between several days and five weeks after symptomatic GAS infection and is believed to be an autoimmune response to infection arising by molecular mimicry. Immunoglobulin (IgG) antibodies formed against bacterial protein M cross-react with similar antigens that are components of the heart, resulting in permanent damage to cardiac tissues and mucopolysaccharides of the valves. M protein types 1, 3, and 18 are most likely to induce these autoreactive antibodies. Persons developing carditis are more prone to having higher levels of antibodies to group A carbohydrates persisting longer than those without this manifestation. The risk of developing rheumatic fever is 0.5% to 3%. It usually is associated with infection via the respiratory tract.

Streptococcal Acute Glomerulonephritis

This form of glomerulonephritis (inflammation of the glomeruli, the filtering tubules of the kidneys), known as **streptococcal acute glomerulonephritis**, is believed to arise as an autoimmune complication, appearing one to five weeks after GAS infection. In this case, antibodies to bacterial antigens form large immune complexes that deposit in the small glomeruli filtering tubules. Once lodged there, they activate the complement cascade to produce a pathogenic inflammatory reaction in the kidneys as a Type III hypersensitivity reaction. Acute glomerulonephritis may arise following infection via the skin or the respiratory tract and is more common in individuals with a M12 type of M protein, although types 1, 3, 4, and 25 are also associated with the development of this condition.

Childbed Fever (Streptococcal Puerperal Fever)

Childbed fever (also known as **streptococcal puerperal fever**) was once one of the major causes of death among women immediately after giving birth. It has also been known to occur following an induced abortion. The streptococci enter the woman through the endometrium and infect the genital tract and occasionally the bloodstream. This acute illness usually induces a fever; mortality rates are currently low in most developed countries thanks to hygienic practices and antibiotic treatment.

The cause of this illness was unknown in the past and was attributed to such conditions as "miasma" or a disturbed state of mind occurring during labor. British physicians began to suspect that childbed fever resulted from a contagious infection in the late eighteenth century, but the concept was largely ignored. In 1844, a physician named Ignaz Semmelweis noted that the mortality rate in the First Obstetric Division of the Vienna Lying-In Hospital, responsible for training medical students, was 16% between 1841 and 1843, while it was only 2% in the Second Division, which used midwives or midwifery students. He learned that the medical students, but not the midwives, spent mornings doing autopsies before performing deliveries. Semmelweis later linked the mothers' deaths with an infectious agent that occasionally killed attending physicians. In 1847, he initiated a hand-washing routine using chlorinated lime solution for everyone working in the First Division. The mortality rate subsequently dropped to 3% within six months. In 1936, prontosil, a sulfonamide, was found to be very effective in treating childbed fever. This drug was later replaced by penicillin.

Streptococcal Toxic Shock Syndrome (STSS)

Streptococcal toxic shock syndrome (STSS) is an extremely dangerous or lethal manifestation of GAS infection found primarily in the United States and Europe. Its early symptoms include fever, chills, myalgia (muscle ache), dizziness, confusion, severe pain of the abdominal or other area, vomiting and diarrhea, and thrombocytopenia (low numbers of platelets). This rapid infection may subsequently lead to hypotension (low blood pressure) and shock as a result of the release of excessive levels of TNF-α and other inflammatory cytokines by overstimulated $CD4^+$ Th1 helper lymphocytes. This may cause severe damage to internal organs, including the kidneys, liver, and lungs. The syndrome may be associated with bacteremia (bacteria growing in the bloodstream) and aggressive soft tissue invasion, leading to necrotizing fasciitis. Other symptoms of STSS include elevated levels of bilirubin; generalized erythematous macular rash; acute respiratory distress syndrome, requiring oxygen and mechanical ventilation; renal failure, requiring dialysis; and disseminated intravascular coagulation. STSS affects people of all age groups. Some 2,000 to 3,000 cases are reported in the United States each year, with a fatality rate of 30% to 70%.

The Causative Agents

Streptococcus pyogenes is a gram-positive streptococcal group A bacterium that measures 0.5 to 0.75 micrometers in diameter and occurs in pairs or chains. The bacteria appear as small, unpigmented colonies on sheep blood agar and cause β-hemolysis (clear ring around bacterial colonies due to lysis of the red blood cells). They commonly inhabit the skin and throat. Infection of a human host usually occurs through a skin break or via the respiratory tract but may also result from contaminated food (milk products) or objects or following medical procedures, especially surgery. Roughly half of persons infected with GAS develop

FIGURE 6.4   Group A streptococci growing in chains

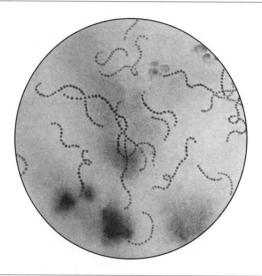

Source: CDC.

symptomatic infection. The bacteria may persist in the remaining individuals for prolonged periods of time, particularly if the organisms are present in the throat. Persons with acute respiratory infections are more contagious than chronic carriers. Infection through a skin break or the endometrium requires smaller inocula than are necessary for respiratory tract infection. Viable bacteria remain in the environment for extended periods.

After binding to host cells, the bacteria may remain at the site of colonization in the throat or on the skin or, less commonly, spread to and destroy other tissues or become widely disseminated by the blood. Some strains of GAS are more likely than others to cause severe disease. Tissue destruction by the more aggressive strains may be rapid and extensive and may result in near total destruction of the extracellular matrix, as in the case of necrotizing fasciitis. Such destruction may also occur at remote sites in the absence of any viable bacteria.

GAS bacteria contain a number of virulence factors that aid in their transmission between hosts, multiplication within a host, and infection of host cells or that protect them from the host's immune response. Organisms with the greatest genetic variability have the best chance of evolving novel virulence factors and thus becoming more pathogenic for their hosts. Genetic variability among GAS strains arises by both intragenic and intergenic recombination. The *emm* gene, in particular, may be transferred between group A and group G streptococci.

Table 6.2 Actions of streptococcal virulence factors

Protein	Action
M protein	Adhesion; ↓ phagocytosis; ↓ activity of complement system
ScpA	↓ activity of complement system
SIC extracellular protein	↓ activity of complement system
Mga	Changes in pH, temperature, partial CO_2 pressure, and iron levels
Exotoxin A	Fever; superantigen (↑ production of inflammatory cytokines)
Exotoxin B	Fever; ↓ monocyte movement; superantigen
Streptokinase	Activates plasmin, ↑ invasion of tissue
Streptolysin O	Lyses blood cells
Hyaluronic acid	↑ survival in upper respiratory tract
Opacity factor	Adhesion and infection of respiratory epithelial cells

The *mga* regulatory gene encodes a molecule that up-regulates the expression of bacterial virulence factors, including the M protein, which is found on the bacterial surface and is encoded by the *emm* gene. The M protein is required for the bacteria's adherence to their target cells and resistance to phagocytosis by cells of the host's innate immune system, such as neutrophils and macrophages. The M protein binds to a membrane cofactor protein on keratinocytes (cells that produce the tough, protective keratin protein in the skin), allowing the bacteria to penetrate the epidermis. More than 80 types of the M protein have been reported. Patients developing invasive diseases are most commonly infected by bacteria expressing M protein types 1 or 3. The M protein additionally binds to several proteins, including kininogen, plasmin, and albumin, a common component of serum. Activation of kininogen by GAS bacteria is followed by the release of kinins, such as bradykinin. These are powerful proinflammatory peptides whose release may result in fever, vasodilation, and increased vascular permeability. The latter two activities decrease blood pressure and, in excess, may induce shock. The *emm* gene belongs to a larger family that includes the *enn* and *mrp* genes in the *vir* chromosomal region. This region is flanked by the *mga* and *spc* genes. The ScpA protein is discussed later in connection with the immune response. The *mga* gene is responsive to variations in pH, temperature, partial CO_2 pressure, and iron concentration.

Invasive GAS strains also express one or both of the *speA* and *speB* (streptococcal pyrogenic exotoxin) genes, which produce the pyrogenic (fever-inducing) exotoxins A and B. These exotoxins may be transmitted to other bacterial strains by bacteriophages (viruses that infect bacteria) or by recombination of genes between bacteria. SPE A, along with several other GAS proteins, acts as a **superantigen**. Superantigens are proteins that cause massive, pathogenic activation of the immune system. While individual lymphocytes typically respond to a specific antigen, producing a moderate and limited immune response involving about one lymphocyte in a million, superantigens are polyclonal activators that nonspecifically stimulate the activity of large numbers of $CD4^+$ T helper cells (as many as 30% to 40% of the T lymphocytes). This massive induction of T lymphocyte activation induces overproduction of the inflammatory cytokines, TNF-α and IL-1, by the host immune system. Both of these cytokines stimulate the brain to raise body temperature in an attempt to kill the bacteria. When levels of these cytokines become too high, the result is high fever, shock, and possibly death. SPE B is the precursor to an extracellular cysteine protease that acts on the precursor to IL-1 and fibronectin and vitronectin (to be described shortly). Degradation of the latter two extracellular matrix proteins may contribute to the soft tissue destruction occurring during necrotizing fasciitis. SPE B also removes the urokinase plasminogen activator receptor from monocytes. This receptor allows cellular migration; thus its removal may inhibit the movement of these phagocytic cells to the infected area.

The increase in GAS virulence observed in European countries was paralleled by an increase in the M1/T1 strain, which uses the M1 type of the M protein virulence factor. M1/T1 strains had a case fatality rate of 33%, while that of other strains was 15%. In North America, strains with M protein type 1, 3, or 18 were the most virulent. M1 strains comprised 35% of the isolates in Canada, and M3 strains accounted for another 25%. Between 1992 and 1995, the proportion of M3 strains almost tripled. Among M1 strains, the M1inv$^+$ clone was most likely to be highly pathogenic. This clone contains the *speA* gene and carries the T12 bacteriophage.

Streptokinase is an enzymatic protein produced by all GAS bacteria that converts the host molecule plasminogen into plasmin. The latter is a serine protease enzyme that degrades extracellular matrix components, such as the fibrin component of clots that walls in bacteria, controlling their spread out of the immediate area; it may thus be hijacked by the bacteria to increase GAS tissue invasion. Plasmin is usually inactivated by the host protein α_2-antiplasmin, but in the presence of bacteria, fibrinogen bound to the bacterial surface provide binding sites for a complex of streptokinase and plasminogen that is not inactivated by α_2-antiplasmin, thus allowing unrestricted enzymatic tissue degradation. Plasmin may also bind directly to the M protein to stabilize its fibrin-degrading activity.

Other bacterial virulence factors include the cytolysins (molecules that lyse cells by damaging their membranes), hyaluronic acid, and serum opacity factor.

Streptolysin O is a cholesterol-binding toxin produced by all GAS bacteria that kills white blood cells, red blood cells, and myocardial cells of the heart. Streptolysin S lyses red and white blood cells and platelets and is responsible for hemolysis seen in blood agar cultures. Because GAS bacteria are unable to acquire the iron required for growth from transferrin or lactoferrin, the lysis of red blood cells by streptolysins releases iron-rich proteins, such as heme and hemoglobin, that may provide them with this vital metal. Expression of streptolysin S is regulated by the Mga protein. The hyaluronic acid capsule aids in GAS survival in the upper respiratory tract. Opacity factor, as well as several other bacterial molecules, acts as an adhesin by binding to fibronectin, a component of the extracellular matrix that may be associated with cell surfaces. Binding to fibronectin allows GAS to adhere to and infect respiratory epithelial cells. Opacity factor also cleaves serum high-density lipoproteins. It is not expressed by all GAS strains and strains lacking this protein are more likely to cause invasive disease. Bacterial lipoteichoic acid may also aid in adherence to epithelial cells.

The Immune Response

GAS uses several mechanisms to avoid the host immune response. The bacterial M protein and the hyaluronic acid capsule both have antiphagocytic properties that decrease bacterial engulfment and destruction by cells of the innate immune system, such as macrophages and neutrophils. The M protein may act by binding to host IgG antibody in a manner that does not trigger immunity but rather prevents this antibody from binding to its receptor on phagocytic cells, aiding in phagocytic ingestion of the bacteria. This antibody-binding activity is important in the establishment of invasive skin infections. Neutralizing antibodies against the M protein, by contrast, block bacterial attachment to the cells of the upper respiratory tract and are thus protective to the human host.

Another important part of innate immunity is the complement cascade. This complex system has several functions, including induction of large pores in microbial membranes, the coating of microbes with protein fragments that increase their attractiveness to ingestion by phagocytic cells, and the attraction of additional white blood cells. The bacterial protein ScpA cleaves and inactivates C5a, a complement fragment that is important for microbial phagocytosis by neutrophils and for attracting more immune cells to the area. The M protein binds to several complement regulatory factors, such as factor H and the C4b-binding protein. Factor H acts together with Factor I to degrade C3b, a critical component of the C3 and C5 convertases, which are necessary for most

Table 6.3 GAS and the human immune response

Effect on Host Immune Response	Consequence
↓ phagocytosis by neutrophils and macrophages	↓ ingestion and killing of bacteria
Degradation of complement components C4b, C3b, C5a	↓ bacterial phagocytosis and lysis; ↓ recruitment of leukocytes
↑ production of IL-1, TNF-α, IL-6, IFN-γ	↑ inflammation

of the functions of complement. The C4b-binding protein also acts with Factor I to degrade C4b, an early component of the classical pathway of complement activation. The SIC extracellular protein also inhibits bacterial lysis by the complement system. The expression of all three of these proteins is regulated by bacterial Mga.

During GAS infections, overstimulation of the immune system, particularly the inflammatory cytokines, may be extremely pathogenic or lethal to the host. One of the key inflammatory cytokines is IL-1, a fever-inducing molecule. SPE B is a major secretory molecule of GAS and may compromise 95% of the protein secreted by some bacterial strains. It is a cysteine protease that cleaves the inactive host IL-1B precursor to produce the active form of IL-1β. SPE A, B, C, and F, streptococcal superantigen, and *S. pyogenes* mitogen all act as superantigens, inducing the overproduction of the inflammatory IL-1 and TNF-α cytokines as described earlier, as well as IL-6 and IFN-γ.

Diagnosis

The "rapid strep test" may be used to quickly detect the presence of GAS in the throat. This test has high specificity but low sensitivity; hence many infections may be overlooked. If the rapid strep test is negative, a throat culture may be performed. GAS infections may also be diagnosed by colony morphology and the patterns of β-hemolytic growth on agar containing 5% sheep red blood cells. Incorporation of neomycin sulfate into the cultures suppresses the growth of staphylococci and other hemolytic bacteria. GAS growth on blood agar is inhibited by the presence of the antibiotic bacitracin. The direct fluorescence antibody test may also be used to identify GAS from throat swabs or spinal fluid. Past infections may be confirmed by detecting the presence of antibodies to streptolysin O, hyluronidase, or bacterial DNase-B.

FIGURE 6.5 Beta-hemolytic growth: ring of clearing around colonies grown on agar containing sheep red blood cells

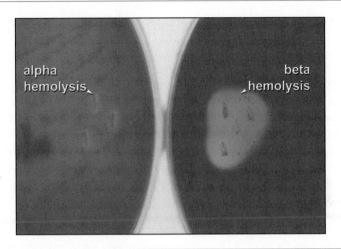

Source: CDC/Richard R. Facklam.

Treatment

Early treatment is important to decrease the death rate among individuals with invasive GAS infections. Antibiotics, particularly penicillin, are effective against many, but not all, GAS bacterial strains. Antibiotics used to treat GAS infections in persons with allergies to penicillin include erythromycin and cephalexin or cephradine. Drug resistance is becoming problematic: a substantial proportion of GAS strains are resistant to tetracycline, and erythromycin-resistant clones are also increasing in number. Clindamycin is not recommended due to the potential for the development of enterocolitis.

In patients experiencing severe hypotension, massive amounts of intravenous fluids may need to be administered to prevent shock. Extensive debridement is necessary for those with necrotizing fasciitis. In addition to antibiotic therapy, those with rheumatic fever need to receive anti-inflammatory drugs. These may include salicylates alone for those without carditis and in combination with corticosteriods, such as prednisone, for those who develop carditis. Absolute bed rest is recommended until resolution of clinical symptoms for those with rheumatic fever, with activity restricted for greater periods of time for those who experienced enlargement of the heart.

RECENT DEVELOPMENTS

Drug resistance is becoming increasingly common among GAS isolates found in Europe and North America. In Canada, rates of erythromycin resistance rose from 2% to 14% over a four-year period. Cross-resistance to clindamycin is also increasing. Several mechanisms are involved. One of these is drug efflux, encoded by the *mefA* gene, which causes a low degree of resistance to erythromycin but not clindamycin. Another method the bacteria employ is methylation of the ribosomal binding site of the drug by products of the *ermB* and *ermTR* genes, whose expression may be either constitutive or inducible. These genes convey resistance to a wider range of therapeutic agents, such as the macrolides, lincosamides, and streptogramin group B. In a study of the mechanisms of drug resistance in Ottawa, 8% of the clinical isolates were resistant to erythromycin and 1% to clindamycin. Resistance to the former was due to *mefA* (67% of the isolates) or inducible (18%) or constitutive (10%) *erm* expression, primarily *ermTR*. In a study of clinical isolates from London between July and October 2003, 7% of the isolates were resistant to erythromycin, 20% were resistant to tetracycline, and a small number were resistant to both drugs. Increases in the rates of erythromycin resistance may be driven in part by clinical use of this agent, and there is concern that resistance genes may be transmitted between GAS strains by bacteriophages, as has been the case for other virulence factors.

Macrolides, especially azithromycin, are being used increasingly to treat strep throat, and resistance to these drugs is also being found. A new agent, telithromycin, is highly effective against all macrolide-susceptible strains and about 75% of macrolide-resistant strains. Telithromycin resistance was found in less than 5% of GAS isolates with the inducible *erm* genes and almost half of those with the constitutive genes.

Prevention

GAS organisms are transmitted by contact with nose or throat secretions or by an airborne route. Exudate material from skin sores is also infectious. Various medical procedures, such as liposuction, hysterectomy, childbirth, and bone pinning, have resulted in noscomial transmission. Dishes, toys, and other inanimate objects usually do not spread these diseases. Milk should be pasteurized, and individuals with skin lesions should be excluded from food preparation. Hand-washing is recommended after coughing or sneezing and before eating to prevent infection. Spread of GAS from person to person is facilitated by close contact between susceptible persons, such as occurs among elementary school children, military recruits, and indigent populations. Special attention needs to be given to educating these populations in good hygienic practices.

No vaccine is currently available for the prevention of GAS infection; however, research is under way. Care must be taken when selecting the antigenic component to be used because some of the bacteria's antigens (such as the superantigens) induce a pathogenic autoimmune response that may lead to rheumatic fever or acute glomerulonephritis. Another obstacle is the large number of serotypes of M protein; immunity is generally serotype-specific. Work is proceeding with a conserved M protein epitope, J14, which is found in approximately 70% of the isolates. Other vaccine candidates include the ScpA peptidase, the fibronectin-binding protein I, and toxoids (inactivated toxins) prepared from the SPE A or SPE C exotoxins.

Persons with rheumatic fever need to receive prophylactic treatment with penicillin or oral sulfonamides for five years afterward to prevent recurrence. Regular administration of these drugs is necessary to maintain their effectiveness.

Surveillance

The results of studies of the incidence of severe manifestations of GAS infections in recent years have been alarming. Between 1992 and 1995, the annual incidence of necrotizing fasciitis rose from 0.85 per million persons to 3.5 per million. A separate survey of the prevalence of all forms of invasive GAS occurring in Montreal between 1995 and 2001 revealed a yearly incidence of 24 infections per million people, with a 14% death rate. Streptococcal pneumonia increased 8.3-fold during that period. The death rate was 38% for persons with pneumonia, 35% for those with STSS, and 16% those with necrotizing fasciitis. Among individuals who had prior infection with varicella (chickenpox), the risk of soft-tissue infection rose sixfold and the risk of death fivefold.

In a 2006 survey of the incidence of severe GAS infections in ten U.S. states involving over 30 million people, 33% of these infections resulted in primary bacteremia, 32% in cellulitis, 15% in pneumonia, 7% in necrotizing fasciitis, and 5% in STSS. The age groups most affected were the very young (9.2% of the infected were aged 1 year or less) and the elderly (10.1% were 65 years or older).

Summary

Diseases

- Strep throat • impetigo • scarlet fever • necrotizing fasciitis
- rheumatic fever • carditis • acute glomerulonephritis
- childbed fever • streptococcal toxic shock syndrome

Causative Agent

- Group A (β-hemolytic) streptococci (*Streptococcus pyogenes*)

Agent Type

- Gram-positive streptococcus

Genome

- DNA

Vector

- None

Common Reservoir

- Humans

Modes of Transmission

- Contact with nose or throat secretions or material from skin sores
- Airborne route, through contaminated food, or contamination during medical procedures

Geographical Distribution

- Worldwide

Year of Emergence or Reemergence

- 1980s in developed areas

Key Terms

Childbed fever (streptococcal puerperal fever) Acute febrile condition arising from group A streptococcal infection of the genital tract following childbirth or abortion

Erysipelas Acute cellulitis due to infection with group A streptococci

"Flesh-eating bacteria" Bacteria that induce necrotizing fasciitis, such as group A streptococci

Group A streptococci β-hemolytic (*Streptococcus pyogenes*) streptococci

Impetigo Infection of the skin around the nose and mouth by group A streptococci, which causes reddening of the area and fluid-filled blisters

Necrotizing fasciitis Rapid, dangerous destruction of fascia and fat caused by "flesh-eating bacteria" such as group A streptococci or other bacteria

Rheumatic fever Autoimmune disorder that damages heart valves following infection by group A streptococci

Scarlet fever Infection with group A streptococci that causes sore throat, fever, and rash beginning with tiny red spots on the neck and upper trunk; the tongue is covered by a white coating with red spots that later peels away, yielding a bright-red appearance

Streptococcal acute glomerulonephritis Inflammatory autoimmune consequence of infection by group A streptococci

Streptococcal toxic shock syndrome (STSS) Severe febrile manifestation of infection by group A streptococci characterized by extremely low blood pressure and shock due to overproduction of TNF-α

Streptokinase Enzyme produced by group A streptococci that converts plasminogen into plasmin, permitting bacterial invasion of tissues

Superantigens Proteins that overstimulate the immune system, resulting in pathological reactions, including shock or death

Review Questions

1. What specific type of bacteria causes scarlet fever and impetigo? Briefly describe the properties of these bacteria and their location in the human body.
2. What are the symptoms of streptococcal toxic shock syndrome (STSS) and necrotizing fasciitis?
3. How do GAS bacteria cause rheumatic fever and acute glomerulonephritis?
4. How do people become infected with GAS? How might infection be prevented?
5. What means are used to diagnose infection with GAS?

Topics for Further Discussion

1. Many of the early proponents of an infectious cause of diseases, such as child-bed fever, who suggested that physicians may be transmitting illness to their patients were ostracized. Discuss the history of the "germ theory" of disease and how it resulted in the hygienic practices currently used in developed regions.
2. The incidence of invasive GAS infections decreased in developed nations in the early twentieth century but remained high in less developed countries. Discuss the factors that may have accounted for the differences in these areas.
3. Describe some of the possible reasons for the resurgence of invasive GAS in the developed world during the past three decades. How might modern medical technology be used to combat the increase in severe disease?
4. Discuss the protective and pathogenic roles of the immune response during GAS infections and how researchers might manipulate the immune system to accentuate the former while reducing the latter.

Resources

Centers for Disease Control and Prevention. *Active Bacterial Core Surveillance Report, Emerging Infections Program Network, Group A Streptococcus, 2006.* Atlanta, Ga.: Centers for Disease Control and Prevention, 2007.

Chin, J. *Control of Communicable Diseases Manual* (17th ed.). Washington, D.C.: American Public Health Association, 2000.

Desjardins, M., and others. "Prevalence and Mechanisms of Erythromycin Resistance in Group A and Group B Streptococcus: Implications for Reporting Susceptibility Results." *Journal of Clinical Microbiology,* 2004, *42,* 5620–5623.

Green, M., and others. "In Vitro Activity of Telithromycin Against Macrolide-Susceptible and Macrolide-Resistant Pharyngeal Isolates of Group A Streptococci in the United States." *Antimicrobial Agents and Chemotherapy,* 2005, *49,* 2487–2489.

Low, D. E., Schwartz, B., and McGeer, A. "The Reemergence of Severe Group A Streptococcal Disease: An Evolutionary Perspective." In W. M. Scheld, D. Armstrong, and J. M. Hughes (eds.), *Emerging Infections* (Vol. 1). Washington, D.C.: ASM Press, 1998.

McGregor, K. F., and Spratt, B. G. "Identity and Prevalence of Multilocus Sequence Typing–Defined Clones of Group A Streptococci Within a Hospital Setting." *Journal of Clinical Microbiology,* 2005, *43,* 1963–1967.

Taviloglu, K., and Yanar, H. "Necrotizing Fasciitis: Strategies for Diagnosis and Management." *World Journal of Emergency Surgery,* 2007, *2,* 19.

Vosti, K. L. "Streptococcal Diseases." In P. D. Hoeprich (ed.), *Infectious Diseases.* New York: Harper & Row, 1977.

CHAPTER 7

ESCHERICHIA COLI 0157:H7

LEARNING OBJECTIVES

- Define hemolytic colitis, hemorrhagic uremic syndrome, and thrombotic thrombocytopenic purpura

- Describe the cocci responsible for causing these illnesses

- Discuss modes of infection

- Discuss the host's response to infection

- Describe symptomatology and diagnosis

- Discuss potential methods of treatment

- Discuss methods of prevention

Major Concepts

Disease

Infection with the enterohemorrhagic O157:H7 strain of *Escherichia coli* may lead to mild, self-resolving intestinal illness (in the majority of cases) or life-threatening conditions such as hemorrhagic colitis, hemolytic uremic syndrome (HUS), and thrombotic thrombocytopenic purpura. HUS is most common in infants, the elderly, and immunosuppressed persons, and antibiotic use appears to increase the risk of developing this disease manifestation. The first reported outbreaks with O157:H7 occurred in 1982 in the American Pacific Northwest and later in Michigan. Large and small outbreaks have been reported in many other areas of the world since that time. Disease severity, as assessed by frequency of hospitalizations and HUS incidence, is increasing as infection with the more pathogenic clade 8 becomes more prevalent.

Infection

O157:H7 is a pathogenic strain of *E. coli*, a species of gram-negative cocci. The bacteria contain genes for several virulence factors that increase their ability to survive and disseminate under the diverse conditions to which they are exposed as they pass through the guts of mammals and into the external environment. These virulence factors include the Shiga toxins, proteins encoded by the LEE genes, enterohemolysin, EspP, catalase peroxidase, and an iron-transporting protein. These are found on the bacterial chromosome, a plasmid, and a bacteriophage.

Transmission

The O157:H7 strain is carried in the digestive tract of normal healthy ruminants, such as cattle and sheep, and is shed into the external environment during defecation. Animals from different feedlot pens may have very different prevalences of infection, as reflected in the wide-ranging percentages of infectious feces and contaminated hides found in the different pens. Both materials contribute to infection of meat during processing. If the external surface of the meat becomes infected and the meat is subsequently ground, bacteria are spread to the internal portions. Ground meat therefore needs to be prepared in a manner that thoroughly cooks all regions. Refrigeration, freezing, and conditions of low pH will not kill the majority of these bacteria. In addition to the infected meat itself, materials and surfaces coming into contact with uncooked meat may spread the bacteria onto other food items, some of which are consumed raw. Raw milk, tap water, vegetables, fruits, and fruit juices may also become infected by contact with manure used in fertilization or water contaminated with manure. Human-to-human transmission may occur when fecal material from an ill person comes into contact with food or with objects in day care centers or in health care settings. Infections may also result from swimming in contaminated, unchlorinated water.

Protection

Treatment for *E. coli* O157:H7 infections is typically supportive and involves balancing fluid and electrolyte levels, and for more severe cases, blood transfusions, renal dialysis, or both. Antibiotic use is not recommended, as killing the bacteria releases toxins and increases the risk of developing HUS. Several vaccine candidates have been tested in cattle, with poor results.

Introduction

Escherichia coli is a common commensal bacterium found in the guts of humans and some other mammals, including cattle and sheep. Though normally beneficial for their human hosts, some strains of *E. coli* cause serious disease. Pathogenic groups of *E. coli* include enterohemorrhagic strains, such as **O157:H7**. Presently as many as 30 outbreaks with that strain alone occur in the United States each year, during which about 20,000 people become ill and approximately 250 die. Transmission often occurs by eating or drinking food or liquid tainted with fecal material. The sources of contamination range widely and include hamburgers, alfalfa sprouts, yogurt, fruit juices, and tap water. Humans are infected by other materials as well. Day care centers may allow transmission of *E. coli* between young children as toys and other objects come into contact with fecal material and the bacteria are transferred to fingers and then to food items or directly to the mouth. People have also been infected in public pools from ill infants placed into the water without proper swimming diapers.

Although the general public is aware of the dangers of eating undercooked hamburgers and of the importance of properly washing one's hands after using the restroom or changing diapers, particularly for those employed in the food industry or in the care of children or patients, compliance is not complete. Due to greater public awareness and governmental regulation of restaurants, the overall numbers of infections with O157:H7 strains have been decreasing; however, several disturbing trends have also been noted. First, bacterial transmission is continuing to occur through contaminated fruits and unpasteurized fruit juices and vegetables, particularly those consumed raw in salads, such as lettuce, spinach, and tomatoes. Second, the bacterial population appears to be shifting in favor of more pathogenic strains of O157:H7 clade 8, which have increased expression of toxin genes. Progress has been made, however, in detecting conditions that may lead to bacterial survival and transmission in cattle and sheep and may decrease the rate of infection and production of infectious feces by these hosts. Similarly, factors are being identified that increase bacterial persistence on lettuce and other produce.

History

E. coli was discovered by Theodore von Escherich in 1885. Outbreaks of **enterohemorrhagic *E. coli* (EHEC)**, especially the O157:H7 strain, often occur through contamination of food or water supplies. These outbreaks have occasionally been quite large and have infected large numbers of people before the source of infection was discovered. In the first such reported outbreak, transmission was found to have occurred through hamburgers served by the popular Jack-in-the-Box fast-food restaurant chain in the Pacific Northwest in 1982. During this outbreak, four children died and 732 people became ill. Another outbreak occurred that year from tainted hamburgers in Michigan. A high proportion of infected individuals were hospitalized (70%), but none of them developed one of the most dangerous manifestations of *E. coli* infection, **hemolytic uremic syndrome (HUS)**. An *E. coli* outbreak in Alpine, Wyoming, resulted from the presence of the O157:H7 strain in area tap water. The water did not taste or smell any differently from uncontaminated water but caused a sometimes serious infection. A very large outbreak due to contaminated food occurred in Japan in August 1996. During that outbreak, 6,309 children and 92 staff members from 62 municipal schools were infected with O157:H7 obtained from radish sprouts. Hundreds of persons were hospitalized, and approximately 100 developed HUS. Canada was struck by a large outbreak involving contaminated municipal water supplies in Walkerton, Ontario, in May 2000. Seven people died and another 2,500 became ill, making this episode one of Canada's worst public health emergencies. In the United States between 1982 and 2002, some 350 outbreaks of O157:H7 infection occurred, resulting in illness in more than 8,500 persons, 17% of whom were hospitalized and 4% of whom developed HUS. Two U.S. outbreaks in 2006 resulted from consumption of contaminated spinach or lettuce; 275 persons were infected, 51% to 75% required hospitalization, and 11% to 15% developed HUS. A trend toward higher incidence of HUS appears to be developing. This trend may be due to a shift in bacterial populations in favor of more virulent subpopulations.

Infection may also occur between infants, through feces in diapers coming into contact with objects that other infants place in their mouths and may be transferred to their fingers and then contaminate food. In one day care center in Washington, seven children became ill playing with sand, soil, modeling clay, and toys that were soiled with infected feces. Infection may also occur in public pools if ill infants are placed into the water without proper swimming diapers.

The Diseases

Hemorrhagic Colitis

Infection with as few as 10 viable organisms of EHEC strains may result in a variety of symptoms ranging from asymptomatic or mild (primarily diarrhea) to severe and life-threatening. The incubation period is one to six days. Disease manifestations include vomiting and nausea, abdominal tenderness and severe cramps, and diarrhea, which in 35% to 90% of infected individuals becomes bloody after two to three days (the syndrome is known as **hemorrhagic colitis**). Another symptom of hemorrhagic colitis is the marked edema of portions of the colon in the absence of other stool pathogens. Symptoms do not improve if one does not eat. If a fever is present, it is low-grade. The lack of significant fever together with abdominal tenderness may suggest a variety of noninfectious causes, including inflammatory bowel disease, appendicitis, ischemic or ulcerative colitis, diverticulitis, and Crohn's disease. Neurological symptoms, including seizures and blindness, may also be present. Symptoms may also be confused with those caused by other infectious microorganisms, such as *Campylobacter, Clostridium difficile, Entamoeba histolytica, Salmonella, Shigella,* and *Yersinia enterocolitica.* Some of the virulence genes from O157:H7 bear a great degree of homology with those found in several of these other bacteria and may in fact have been acquired from them via motile genetic elements, such as plasmids and bacteriophages. Symptoms usually resolve within a week; however, some individuals develop more serious or life-threatening infections. The chance for developing severe disease is greatest in children under the age of 5 years and the elderly.

Hemolytic Uremic Syndrome (HUS)

In addition to hemorrhagic colitis, the young and the elderly also have an increased susceptibility to HUS. Early symptoms of HUS include irritability, fever, lethargy, weakness, vomiting and diarrhea, and bloody stools. Later signs may include bruising; paleness due to extensive lysis of red blood cells (hemolytic anemia);

petechial rash; decreased platelet numbers (thrombocytopenia); decreased levels of consciousness, seizures, or other central nervous symptoms; jaundice; and lowered urine output with or without kidney failure (in 2% to 7% of cases). Over 85% of the cases of postdiarrheal HUS are believed to be due to infection with O157:H7, and the majority of the remaining cases are attributed to infection with other *E. coli* strains that produce Shiga toxins (described later in this chapter). The overall mortality rate is 1% to 5%, and deaths occur primarily in children, the elderly, and immunosuppressed individuals. The fatality rate for this syndrome among children is 3% to 5%. Those who survive have an increased incidence of high blood pressure or kidney impairment (or both) later in life.

Thrombotic Thrombocytopenic Purpura (TTP)

Another serious result of O157:H7 infection is **thrombotic thrombocyto-penic purpura** (TTP). It includes many of the symptoms listed for HUS, but with less prominent neurological manifestations and diminished renal damage. It additionally includes bleeding under the skin, resulting in the formation of purple-colored spots (purpura), fatigue, headache, tachycardia (elevated heart rate),

Table 7.1   Diseases associated with *E. coli* O157:H7 infection

Disease	Symptoms	Groups Affected	Mortality Rate
Hemorrhagic colitis	Abdominal tenderness with severe cramps, severe bloody diarrhea, marked edema of the colon, seizures, blindness	Children under 5 years old, the elderly	Usually resolves
Hemolytic uremic syndrome (HUS)	Irritability, fever, lethargy, weakness, vomiting, diarrhea with bloody stools, bruising; paleness, hemolytic anemia, petechial rash; thrombocytopenia, decreased levels of consciousness, seizures, jaundice; lowered urine output, kidney failure	Children, the elderly, immuno-suppressed individuals	1%–5%
Thrombotic thrombocytopenic purpura (TTP)	Similar to HUS plus purpura, fatigue, headache, tachycardia, shortness of breath, speech changes	Adults	1.2%

shortness of breath, and speech changes. TTP is also more often reported in adults and is usually not preceded by diarrhea. In some of the early outbreaks in the United States, the hospitalization rate was 23%, HUS or TTP developed in 6%, and death occurred in 1.2% of the cases; not all of the fatalities were related to either HUS or TTP.

The Causative Agents

General Characteristics of *E. coli* O157:H7

E. coli bacteria are typically harmless commensal gram-negative rods that reside in two very different types of environments: (1) in the rumen or the large or small intestine of humans and some other mammals and (2) in the external environment, with its limited nutrients and variable temperature and water availability. They are usually beneficial to their mammalian hosts and help metabolize food in the digestive tract. Several strains of *E. coli*, however, cause disease in humans. Some strains of these bacteria, such as the EHEC group, are pathogenic; one such strain is O157:H7, which may cause severe or fatal illness. Infection with other EHEC strains, including O26:H11, O111:H8, and members of the O103 and O118 serogroups, are

FIGURE 7.1   Scanning electron micrograph of *E. coli* O157:H7

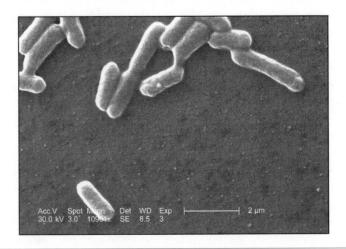

Source: CDC/National Escherichia, Shigella, Vibrio Reference Unit.

becoming emerging problems and appear to be more common than O157 strains in some regions. "Montezuma's revenge," a bane of travelers, is due to infection with EHEC strains. Other major groups of pathogenic *E. coli* strains are the enteroaggressive strains (which cause persistent diarrhea in very young children from developing countries), enteropathogenic (EPEC) strains (infantile diarrhea), enteroinvasive strains (watery diarrhea), entero-toxogenic strains (traveler's diarrhea), and diffuse adherent strains (diarrhea in preschool-aged children).

Phylogenetic analysis of over 500 clinical isolates of the O157:H7 strain have allowed it to be divided into nine distinct clades. Of these, infection with clade 8 bacteria is associated with the highest risk of developing HUS. This clade has become increasingly prevalent since 2003, and a particularly virulent sub-population of this clade is evolving. Changing O157:H7 population dynamics may thus be at least partly responsible for the recent increased pathology in infected humans. O157:H7 strains differ from commensal *E. coli* strains in their ability to ferment sorbitol and dulcitol and to oxidize other carbon sources. They contain over 1,600 genes that are not found in commensal strains; the vast major-ity of these are not virulence factors but may allow the bacteria to outcompete other strains for limiting nutrients.

E. coli, like other gram-negative bacteria, contain lipopolysaccharide (LPS) in their cell walls. Strains of these bacteria are defined by their somatic (O) and flagellar (H) antigens. Differences in the LPS O-antigen have been found in different diseases of humans and animals. The O157 antigen may be involved in virulence (discussed later in this chapter). H7 specifies the type of flagellin protein and is encoded by the *fliC* gene. It has been hypothesized that O157:H7 may be derived from the EPEC strain O55:H7, which is able to adhere tightly to epithelium in the gut. This strain is believed to have acquired the *fliC* gene for H7 flagellin, followed by the Stx2 toxin and EHEC plasmid (to be discussed shortly). The gene for the Stx1 toxin was a later addition, and the ability to ferment sorbitol and β-glucuronidase activity was lost during evolution of the EHEC O157:H7 strain that is commonly found throughout North America and Europe. It is closely related to the O157:H- strain, which causes hemolytic uremic syndrome in Bavaria in Germany. That strain lacks the H7 flagellin and Stx1 but has β-glucuronidase activity and can ferment sorbitol.

O157:H7 bacteria prefer to grow at human body temperature, 37°C (98.6°F), but may grow at a wide range of temperatures from 10°C to 50°C, allowing them to withstand many conditions that they may encounter in the external environment before infecting a suitable host. The O157:H7 strain is also better able to survive and reproduce in acidic conditions than nonpathogic strains of *E. coli*, including food with a pH as low as 4.4. This acid resistance allows the majority of these bacteria to survive passage through the stomach. Acid tolerance is increased at low temperatures, as in refrigerated salad dressing or apple juice.

Bacterial Reservoirs and Transmission

E. coli normally resides, in addition to humans, in the rumen and terminal colons of both ill and healthy cattle and sheep, which serve as disease reservoirs. Examination of healthy cattle in the United Kingdom found that the O157:H7 strain could be isolated in 0.9% to 15.7% of the animals. Calves are more commonly infected than adult cattle and appear more susceptible to developing disease. Raw milk from infected dairy cows may transmit disease. Transmission through the fecal route may be seasonal, as infected sheep from Idaho did not

RECENT DEVELOPMENTS

Bacteria are able to grow on crops such as lettuce and spinach after harvesting or during processing, particularly if the leaves have been damaged physically or due to disease. *E. coli* preferentially attach to areas of lettuce leaf injury or openings, such as at the cut ends of the stem or in cuts in the cuticle. Once attached, the bacteria grow at these sites on the harvested leaves for long periods of time at temperatures between 10°C and 15°C (50°F to 59°F), especially after pretreatment with chlorinated water. The warm temperatures and high humidity found in the temporary storage containers where lettuce leaves are placed in the fields immediately after harvest may also provide ideal conditions for bacterial growth. In one study, as little as four hours after inoculation onto intact harvested romaine lettuce leaves, the *E. coli* O157:H7 population doubled. When the leaves were cut into large pieces, the population increased 4.5-fold, and when the leaves were shredded, the population grew 11-fold. Twenty-two hours after inoculation onto the ends of stems, the population had risen over 20,000-fold. Infection of leaves with other bacteria also affected the growth of *E. coli*: on young leaves (inner leaves) damaged by soft rot resulting from infection with *Erwinia chrysanthemi*, the *E. coli* population was 27 times greater than on healthy middle-aged leaves (middle of lettuce head). Soft rot also encourages growth of other human pathogens on vegetables, including *Salmonella* and *Listeria monocytogenes*. Healthy young leaves are also able to support a 10-fold higher level of bacteria than middle-aged leaves due to the greater availability of nitrogen in these leaves. Areas of leaf tip burn lesions also harbored high levels of bacteria.

shed virus via defecation in November, but many (approximately 30%) did so in the warmer month of June.

Transmission may occur through a variety of routes. The most common of these is consumption of undercooked food contaminated from a fecal source. Ground beef appears to be the most prevalent source of infection. During the slaughter of cattle and processing of beef, meat may come into contact with feces or with bacteria found on the animals' hides. Only the outer portions of many types of beef (steaks, roasts) are contaminated, and bacteria on the surfaces of these cuts of meat are killed during cooking. When beef is ground , however, meat from the outer, contaminated regions is mixed throughout the product; therefore, the entire portion must be cooked thoroughly in order to kill bacteria at the center of the meat. During food preparation, bacteria from infected meat may be transferred to other foods that are consumed raw, including salad greens and other vegetables, by using the same cutting boards and utensils for meat and then other food without cleansing them between uses. In areas where cattle manure is used as a fertilizer for vegetables and fruit crops or where manure may enter irrigation water, food may be exposed to the bacteria during growing or by falling into the manure on the soil surrounding crops. In the case of apples, fallen fruit may be used to produce contaminated cider if the beverage is not pasteurized. Unpasteurized milk may also be a vehicle for bacterial transmission. Food may also be infected if the individuals preparing it do not properly wash their hands after using the restroom.

Drinking-water sources may also be contaminated by mixing of the water supply with unsanitary sewer water, from inadequate sewage treatment, or by agricultural run-off into rivers, lakes, or other sources of drinking water. Chlorination of water reduces the bacterial load, as does boiling, although the latter also concentrates any toxic chemicals that may also be present, including nitrate, pesticides, arsenic, and other metals. Infected babies may contaminate swimming pools if placed into the water without properly fitting swimming diapers. Other persons using public pools have acquired the infection in this manner.

Table 7.2   Routes of transmission of *E. coli* O157:H7

Food and drinks	Undercooked ground meat
	Fecally contaminated fruits and vegetables
	Drinking water
	Unpasteurized milk or fruit juices
Other routes	Fecally contaminated swimming pools
	Oral-fecal route in day care centers
	Contact with animals in petting zoos

Although human-to-human transmission is uncommon, young children may pass bacteria among themselves in day care centers. Children's hands may come into contact with fecal matter that is then transferred to other objects such as toys and from there to hands or food. Very young children may place contaminated objects or hands into their mouths. Adults changing babies' diapers may not wash or otherwise cleanse their hands before interacting with another child. Children may also acquire infection from animals in petting zoos.

E. coli O157:H7 Virulence Factors

Pathogenic strains of *E. coli* have evolved mechanisms that increase bacterial survival or dissemination via a number of virulence factors that often result in increased harm to the host. Some of these factors are encoded by the bacterial chromosome, while others have been introduced to the bacteria by **bacteriophages** or **plasmids**. Bacteriophages are viruses that infect bacteria, and plasmids are small, circular regions of nonchromosomal DNA. Plasmids may be either accepted or rejected by bacteria and are under selective pressure to carry genes encoding virulence factors that enhance bacterial survival under adverse conditions, thus encouraging acceptance by their bacterial hosts. These mobile genetic elements may be transmitted between individual bacteria of the same or different species, aiding in the intra- and interbacterial dissemination of virulence factors. Disease outbreaks have differing clinical features due to the presence of different bacterial clades with differing kinds of virulence factors. O157:H7 outbreaks have become more pathogenic recently and able to spread by a greater number of routes due to evolution of the bacterial populations.

O157:H7 produce **Shiga toxins** (Stx; formerly known as Vero cytotoxins) with a great degree of similarity to a cellular toxin produced by the *Shigella dysenteriae* type 1 bacteria. These toxins are encoded by lambdalike bacteriophages rather than by the bacterial chromosome. Other pathogenic strains of *E. coli* and other bacterial species have also acquired these bacteriophages. Many of the genetic variations between different O157:H7 isolates appear to have resulted from bacteriophages creating insertions, deletions, or duplications of DNA fragments. Shiga toxins destroy blood vessels in the intestines, leading to hemorrhagic colitis, and also damage other blood vessels throughout the body. This leads to the production of gummy clots that may clog the kidneys (which function as filters), resulting in hemolytic uremia syndrome, or harm the heart, lungs, other organs, and the central nervous system. Stx may also increase bacterial survival in the ruminant hosts. These grazing mammals contain in their lower colon several species of protozoa that ingest bacteria. *E. coli* strains that bear Stx are better able to survive in food vacuoles of protozoa such as *Tetrahymena* and may thus escape predation in the bovine digestive tract.

O157:H7 may produce several distinct types of Shiga toxins (Stx1 in 64.9% of isolates, Stx2 in 98.5%, and Stx2c in 28.3%), which may be transmitted by different bacteriophages and share approximately 60% sequence homology. These toxins consist of one A and five B subunits that are encoded by two different genes. The B units bind to a cell membrane glycolipid that is present on both intestinal cells and kidney cells. The toxin is then internalized into cells by endocytosis. Once taken into the cells, the A subunit cleaves an N-glycoside bond, removing an adenine from the 28S ribosomal RNA in the 60S ribosomal subunit. This prevents elongation-factor-1 from binding aminoacyl-tRNAs to the ribosome during the translation process, thus blocking protein synthesis and leading to cell death. Infection of kidney cells leads to damage to the blood vessels, perhaps as a result of production of the proinflammatory cytokine TNF-α by macrophages. In several instances, bloody diarrhea and renal disease are caused by *E. coli* strains other than O157:H7 that also produce Stx; however these strains have not led to large outbreaks.

Another virulence factor shared with the EPEC strains is the **locus of enterocyte effacement (LEE) genes**, which have been inserted into the selenocysteine tRNA gene. The LEE gene *eaeA* encodes the intimin protein, which disrupts the intestinal epithelium by attaching to it and destroying its microvilli by the formation of **attaching and effacing lesions**. Microvilli play an essential role in the human digestive system by increasing the intestinal surface area that absorbs nutrients from food. Intimin binds to the bacterial protein Tir that is translocated onto the surface of gut cells by a secretion system that is a part of the LEE complex. It also binds to host β-integrins. Intimin is homologous to proteins found in other species of bacteria, including *Yersinia pseudotuberculosis* and *Yersinia enterocolitica*. Another protein encoded by LEE genes is **EspB**, a secreted protein that induces signal transduction involving the addition of a phosphate group to the amino acid tyrosine in host cell proteins. EspB is exported from cells by the action of proteins encoded by the LEE *sepB* gene.

E. coli O157:H7 and several other EHEC strains have acquired the 90-kilobase EHEC plasmid, carrying genes for several virulence factors, including the **enterohemolysin** protein, encoded by the RTX gene. Possession of this gene correlates with the ability to induce hemorrhagic colitis because enterohemolysin causes the lysis of red blood cells. This plasmid also encodes **espP** and catalase peroxidase. EspP is a secreted serine protease that cleaves pepsin and human coagulation factor V. Elimination of the latter human protein inhibits blood clotting, enabling mucosal hemorrhaging to occur in the gut and possibly aiding in microbial dissemination. This enzyme is similar to proteases

Table 7.3   *E. coli* O157:H7 virulence genes

Virulence Factor	Gene Location	Action
Shiga toxin	Lambdalike bacteriophage	Destroys blood vessels, forms bloody clots
Intimin protein	LEE gene locus	Attaches to and destroys intestinal epithelium
EspB	LEE gene locus	↑ signal transduction
Enterohemolysin	EHEC plasmid	Lyses red blood cells
EspP	EHEC plasmid	Cleaves plasmin and coagulation factor V
Catalase peroxidase	EHEC plasmid	Protects bacteria from killing by host innate immune response
LPS O-antigen	*rfdE* gene region	↑ adherence to intestinal epithelium

found in the pathogenic *Haemophilus influenzae* and *Neisseria* species. Catalase peroxidase is used to protect the bacteria against toxic reactive oxygen species produced by the host immune system, thus aiding in bacterial survival.

The O157:H7 gene *chuA* encodes a gene that transports iron, a limiting resource for *E. coli* growth, allowing its utilization from heme, the iron-binding portion of the human hemoglobin molecule found in erythrocytes. *ChuA* is similar to the heme utilization locus gene *shuA* of *Shigella dysentariae:* these genes are not found in other *Shigella* species or nonpathogenic *E. coli* strains.

The O157 O-antigen of LPS may be involved in virulence by affecting bacterial adherence to epithelial cells, such as those that line the human intestines. This antigen is encoded by the *rfbE* gene region, which has similarities to the gene from *Vibrio cholerae* (the causative agent of cholera). The O55:H7 strain is very closely related to O157:H7 and is suggested to have evolved from a common ancestor. This EPEC strain was isolated from a child with infantile diarrhea and lacks *rfbE, stx1,* and *stx2* but does contain the *eaeA* and *chuA* genes.

The Immune Response

Because cattle are a major reservoir for *E. coli* O157:H7 and transmit the bacteria to humans via their manure, a vaccine that prevented infection of these animals should decrease the infection rate in humans. A recent vaccine was developed that contained two *E. coli* O157:H7 virulence factors encoded by the LEE genes. This vaccine was administered to cattle by the intramuscular route and boosted intranasally. It successfully induced production of IgG1 and IgA antibodies yet did not lower the levels of bacteria excreted in feces or reduce bacterial colonization of the cattle's intestines. Similarly, a vaccine preparation using formalin-killed EHEC O157:H7 was able to induce a specific IgG1 antibody response but did not prevent infection. Also, prior infection of calves with pathogenic *E. coli* strains does not protect against reinfection, and the immune response against the LEE-encoded proteins is weak or absent in naturally infected animals. Taken together, this information suggests that either the LEE virulence factors may be an inappropriate choice as vaccine antigens or perhaps that an IgG1 and IgA antibody immune response alone is not protective and that other components of the immune system also need to be stimulated.

O157:H7 infection may be immunosuppressive. Exposure of T lymphocytes from blood or intraepithelial T lymphocytes to purified Stx1 or Stx2 decreased their ability to divide in response to *E. coli* antigens. Because T lymphocytes regulate many of the other components of the immune response, suppression of T lymphocyte activity may allow the bacteria to successfully evade the host's immune response. Interestingly, immunization of calves with O157:H7 lacking Stx2 generated a T lymphocyte response that also responded to O157:H7 containing Stx2, a finding that may have relevance in vaccine design.

Diagnosis

Diagnosis with *E. coli* O157:H7 or other pathogenic bacterial strains may involve isolating the bacteria in a person's stool if this test is performed within the first several days of infection. O157:H7 bacteria do not ferment sorbitol, unlike the vast majority of other *E. coli* strains. For diagnostic purposes, stool samples should be inoculated onto sorbitol-MacConkey agar, on which the bacteria grow as colorless colonies. O157:H7 also do not have β-glucuronidase activity and test negative in the fluorogenic 4-methylumbelliferyl β-D-glucuonide assay. Several immunological test kits are also available that use antibodies to detect the presence of various strains of *E. coli*, allowing the determination of the correct causative agent.

The association of some O157:H7 clades with greater pathology in humans led to the suggestion that phylogenetic testing to identify single-nucleotide polymorphism (SNP) loci may allow determination of the specific clade type that is infecting a given individual. These molecular tests are rapid and inexpensive and may have prognostic value, suggesting which persons are at highest risk for developing HUS and guiding treatment options. Such testing may also be useful in predicting the potential severity during outbreaks, particularly those involving children, as in infections acquired from contaminated water or food in school systems or in day care centers.

**FIGURE 7.2   Inoculation of bacteria from a fecal sample onto
an agar plate for isolation**

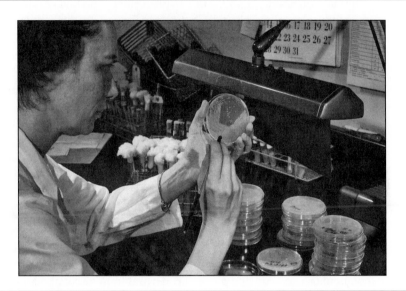

Source: CDC/Dr. Kokko.

Treatment

Most individuals infected with EHEC survive if they are able to remain hydrated. Treatment for those with watery diarrhea includes maintenance of fluid and electrolyte balance. Antibiotics such as TMP-SMX fluoroquinolones are not beneficial and may be detrimental in that they kill the bacteria, releasing more Shiga toxin and increasing the risk of serious renal complications. Antidiarrheal drugs should also be avoided. HUS is treated by blood transfusions and kidney dialysis in an intensive care unit. In most people, however, illness usually resolves in five to ten days.

Prevention

O157:H7 is very acid-resistant; 95% of the bacteria survive for one hour in synthetic gastric fluid (pH 1.5). The bacteria also survive refrigeration and freezing of contaminated food and drink but may be killed by proper cooking. Several simple means of preventing disease have been suggested. One important method is to cook meat properly, especially ground meat such as hamburger, so that the internal temperature is 68°C (155°F) (the center is no longer pink and the juices are clear). Care should be taken when purchasing hamburgers from restaurants to ensure that the meat has been sufficiently cooked. All cutting boards, bowls, and utensils that have come in contact with raw meat should be cleansed with detergent. Wooden instruments and cutting boards are hard to disinfect properly because they may sequester bacteria away from cleaning agents. Fruits and vegetables need to be washed with soap. Irradiating food may decrease disease incidence without compromising taste or nutritional value. To reduce the transmission of fecal material to food, one should always wash one's hands prior to meal preparation and after using the restroom. Infected persons should not be employed to handle food or care for children or patients until at least two negative fecal samples have been collected.

Unpasteurized milk or fruit juices may transmit pathogenic *E. coli* strains. Pasteurization may alter juice taste or affect its vitamin content. Recent work has attempted to find other ways to decrease bacterial survival in juices that avoid these undesirable effects. The addition of the natural antimicrobial phenolic compounds carvacrol and *p*-cymene, derived from essential oils of oregano and thyme, decreased survival of O157:H7 in chilled unpasteurized apple juice from 19 days to undetectable levels within one to two days. These and other phenolic compounds are already in use as flavoring agents in baked goods, beverages, and chewing gum.

To avoid acquiring pathogenic *E. coli* from water, one should avoid drinking or swimming in unchlorinated water. Babies should not be allowed to enter swimming pools unless they are wearing properly fitting swimming diapers.

Another method for preventing human infection with EHEC strains is to decrease bacterial growth in the cattle or sheep hosts or their fecal matter. Fiber content of feed may affect the rate of passage and clearance of *E. coli* through the ruminants' digestive tract. Growth of *E. coli* O157:H7 in rumen fluid of sheep was decreased when the fluid was derived from sheep that were fed a diet containing some grains (50% wheat and 50% hay) in comparison with rumen fluid from sheep receiving a diet of 100% hay. In fecal suspensions, bacterial growth was blocked by the presence of a probiotic strain of *Lactobacillus acidophilus*. Administration of other probiotic bacteria reduced fecal shedding and contamination of the hides of naturally or experimentally infected cattle and lambs, both of which may lead to contamination of meat during processing. Treatment with probiotic bacteria also boosted the average daily weight gain and gain-to-feed ratio of lambs, indicating that animal health was not adversely affected by the treatment. Dietary alterations and supplementation with lactic acid bacteria

PREVENTION OF *E. COLI* INFECTION

Food Preparation

- Cook meat to an internal temperature of 155°.
- Clean surfaces and utensils in contact with raw meat.
- Clean fruits and vegetables with soap.
- Irradiate food.
- Pasteurize milk and juice.
- Add natural phenolic compounds to juices.

Other Means of Decreasing Infection in Humans

- Wash hands prior to food preparation and after using the restroom.
- Don't drink or swim in unchlorinated water.

Decreasing Infection in Cattle and Sheep

- Increase fiber content in feed.
- Administer probiotics.

may thus reduce the numbers of pathogenic *E. coli* organisms to which humans are exposed and improve herd health.

Surveillance

Surveillance efforts have revealed a steady decrease in the number of cases of human infections with O157:H7 in the United States since 2002. One recent study found that the frequency of the more highly pathogenic clade 8 strains, however, greatly increased from 10% in 2002 to 46% in 2006. Continuing surveillance efforts may need not only to determine the *E. coli* strain but also to identify the clade.

Surveillance studies also track O157:H7 numbers in domestic animals. A large study of over 27,000 cattle in feedlot pens in Canada between 2003 and

2004 used sampling devices prepared from manila ropes. These devices revealed that 48% of the pens were contaminated and that pens varied greatly in the prevalence of contaminated fecal matter (0% to 80%) and animal hides (0% to 30%). Such information could be useful in reducing contamination of meat during processing if animals from pens determined to contain a high prevalence of infection were to be processed after animals from low-prevalence pens, followed by thorough cleansing of the equipment. These studies are also being conducted to determine what pen conditions lead to high prevalence of infection, including temperature, dry versus muddy floors and bedding, humidity, number of animals per pen, and water cleanliness.

New methods are needed to detect the presence of pathogenic *E. coli* in tap water, river water, and irrigation water in order to more accurately determine contamination of drinking water and to survey environmental infection. One problem is the difficulty of assessing numbers of bacteria that are viable but not able to be cultured (VBNC). In one recently described method, bacteria were captured on a membrane, followed by extraction and purification of RNA and reverse transcription-PCR plus detection of O157:H7 *rfbE* and *fliC* genes by electronic microarray. This method was able to detect as few as three to four colony-forming units (CFU) per liter in tap water, 7 CFU per liter in river water, and 50 VBNC per liter of river water without detecting nonviable, nonpathogenic bacteria. This represents the best level of detection for VBNC bacteria in environmental water and is important because these organisms can still produce Stx and may be reactivated under certain circumstances.

Summary

Diseases

- Hemorrhagic colitis   •   Hemolytic uremic syndrome
- Thrombotic thrombocytopenic purpura

Causative Agent

- Enterohemorrhagic *E. coli* O157:H7 strain

Agent Type

- Gram-negative coccoid bacterium

Genome

- Circular, double-stranded DNA

Vector

- None

Common Reservoirs

- Cattle, sheep, humans

Modes of Transmission

- Orally via fecal-contaminated food, drink, objects, or water ingested during swimming

Geographical Distribution

- Worldwide

Year of Emergence

- 1982

Key Terms

O157:H7 Enterohemorrhagic strain of *E. coli* that may cause hemorrhagic colitis and hemolytic uremic syndrome

Attaching and effacing lesions Digestive tract lesions induced by the *E. coli* O157:H7 intimin protein, which disrupts intestinal epithelium by attaching to it and destroying microvilli

Bacteriophages Viruses that infect bacteria

Enterohemolysin *E. coli* O157:H7 plasmid-encoded protein that lyses erythrocytes, leading to hemorrhagic colitis

Enterohemorrhagic *E. coli* (EHEC) Pathogenic strains of *E. coli* that produce Shiga toxin and carry a plasmid encoding several virulence factors; includes the O157:H7 strain

Escherichia coli A common commensal bacterium found in the guts of humans and some other mammals

EspB Secreted *E. coli* O157:H7 protein that induces transduction in the host cell via protein tyrosine phosphorylation

EspP Serine protease that cleaves human coagulation factor V; found in *E. coli* O157:H7

Hemolytic uremic syndrome (HUS) Disorder resulting from a digestive system infection that produces toxins that destroy red blood cells and damage the kidneys; may be caused by enterohemorrhagic *E. coli*, *Shigella*, or *Salmonella* infection

Hemorrhagic colitis Severe cramping abdominal pain, grossly bloody diarrhea with little to no fever, and marked edema of portions of the colon

Locus of enterocyte effacement (LEE) genes Group of genes from some types of pathological *E. coli* that encode virulence factors associated with establishing infection in the digestive tract

Plasmid Circular DNA found in some bacteria that are not part of a bacterial chromosome

Shiga toxins Also known as *Vero cytotoxins;* toxins in several pathological strains of *E. coli* that are homologous to a cellular toxin from *S. dysenteriae* type 1 bacteria

Thrombotic thrombocytopenic purpura (TTP) Blood disorder in which blood clots form in small blood vessels throughout the body, leading to a reduction in platelet numbers, bleeding beneath the skin, and purple-colored spots (purpura)

Review Questions

1. Briefly describe hemorrhagic colitis and hemolytic uremic syndrome.
2. What are the functions of the Shiga toxins and the LEE genes?
3. What are two ways in which the transmission of O157:H7 to humans from meat may be decreased? What are two ways to decrease transmission to humans from vegetables or fruit juices?
4. Why are antibiotics not commonly used to treat O157:H7 infection?
5. Other than bacterial chromosomal DNA, what are two other kinds of DNA that carry virulence factors in *E. coli* O157:H7?

Topics for Further Discussion

1. Probiotic ("good") bacteria that inhibit the growth of potentially pathogenic bacteria and fungi are widely available in drugstores for consumption by the general public. These probiotics decrease survival of *E. coli* O157:H7 in calf and lamb feces. Research the use of probiotic bacteria to prevent human infection by pathogenic *E. coli*. What are the potential drawbacks to this preventive approach?
2. Stx-containing strains of O157:H7 are able to decrease the ability of cattle T lymphocytes to grow in culture. Vaccination with various *E. coli* proteins produces a vigorous IgG1 antibody response but this antibody provides little

to no protection against infection of cattle or shedding of infectious bacteria in their feces. What implications might this suggest for the development of human vaccines against this strain?

3. Outline strategies to decrease human disease associated with O157:H7 that involve (a) bacterial survival in cattle and sheep, (b) transmission to humans by contaminated feces or animal hides, (c) transmission to humans through the use of cattle manure as a fertilizer or its introduction into irrigation water, and (d) bacterial ability to colonize and survive in the human digestive tract.

4. Vaccines not only kill pathogenic microorganisms but also inactivate their toxins (as is the case with vaccines that produce antibodies to tetanus toxin or diphtheria toxin). Discuss how a similar vaccine might be developed to induce antibodies to Stx or other virulence factors of *E. coli* O157:H7 and how such antibodies might also protect against diseases caused by other gut bacteria that produce similar sorts of toxins.

Resources

Brandl, M. T. "Plant Lesions Promote the Rapid Multiplication of *Escherichia coli* O157:H7 on Postharvest Lettuce." *Applied and Environmental Microbiology*, 2008, *74*, 5285–5289.

Brandl, M. T., and Amundson, R. "Leaf Age as a Risk Factor in Contamination of Lettuce with *Escherichia coli* O157:H7 and *Salmonella enteric.*" *Applied and Environmental Microbiology*, 2008, *74*, 2298–2306.

Chaucheyras-Durand, F., Madic, J., Doudin, F., and Martin. C. "Biotic and Abiotic Factors Influencing In Vitro Growth of *Escherichia coli* O157:H7 in Ruminant Digestive Contents." *Applied and Environmental Microbiology*, 2006, *72*, 4136–4142.

Griffin, P. M., and Boyce, T. G. "*Escherichia coli* O157:H7." In W. M. Scheld, D. Armstrong, and J. M. Hughes (eds.), *Emerging Infections* (Vol. 1). Washington, D.C.: ASM Press, 1998.

Hoffman, M. A., and others. "Bovine Immune Response to Shiga-Toxigenic *Escherichia coli* O157:H7." *Clinical and Vaccine Immunology*, 2006, *13*, 1322–1327.

Kiskó, G., and Roller, S. "Carvacrol and *p*-Cymene Inactivate *Escherichia coli* O157:H7 in Apple Juice." *BMC Microbiology*, 2005, *5*, 36–44.

Liu, Y., Gilchrist, A., Zhang, J., and Li, X.-F. "Detection of Viable but Nonculturable *Escherichia coli* O157:H7 Bacteria in Drinking Water and River Water." *Applied and Environmental Microbiology*, 2008, *74*, 1502–1507.

Manning, S. D., and others. "Variation in Virulence Among Clades of *Escherichia coli* O157:H7 Associated with Disease Outbreaks." *Proceedings of the National Academy of Sciences*, 2008, *105*, 4868–4873.

Renter, D. G., and others. "Detection and Determinants of *Escherichia coli* O157:H7 in Alberta Feedlot Pens Immediately Prior to Slaughter." *Canadian Journal of Veterinary Research*, 2008, *72*, 217–227.

Steinberg, K. M., and Levin, B. R. "Grazing Protozoa and the Evolution of the *Escherichia coli* O157:H7 Shiga Toxin–Encoding Prophage." *Proceedings of the Royal Society, B,* 2007, *274,* 1921–1929.

van Diemen, P. M., and others. "Subunit Vaccines Based on Intimin and Efa-1 Polypeptides Induce Humoral Immunity in Cattle but Do Not Protect Against Intestinal Colonisation by Enterohaemorrhagic *Escherichia coli* O157:H7 or O26:H-." *Veterinary Immunology and Immunopathology,* 2007, *116,* 47–58.

Whittam, T. S., McGraw, E. A., and Reid, S. D. "Pathogenic *Escherichia coli* O157:H7: A Model for Emerging Infectious Diseases." In R. M. Krause (ed.), *Emerging Infections.* San Diego, Calif.: Academic Press, 1998.

CHAPTER 8

HELICOBACTER PYLORI, ULCERS, AND CANCER

LEARNING OBJECTIVES

- Define peptic ulcers, chronic gastritis, intestinal metaplasia, and gastric adenocarcinoma
- Describe the bacilli responsible for causing these illnesses
- Discuss modes of infection
- Discuss the host's response to infection
- Describe symptomatology and diagnosis
- Discuss potential methods of treatment
- Discuss methods of prevention

Major Concepts

Infection

Helicobacter pylori is a spiral-shaped, mobile, gram-negative bacillus with two to seven flagella. These bacteria inhabit the human gastric mucosa, like the *Campylobacter* species they resemble. The bacteria produce a powerful urease enzyme that increases stomach pH by degrading urea into ammonia and carbonic acid, as well as several virulence factors. Other *Helicobacter* species also inhabit humans. These include *H. cinaedi* and *H. fennelliae* from the intestines or blood of homosexual men with proctitis, colitis, or HIV infection; infections with these bacteria result in bacteremia, fever, leukopenia and thrombocytopenia. *H. westmeadii* is also found in the blood of HIV-positive individuals. *H. pullorum*, *H. canis,* and *H. rappini* from chickens, cats, dogs, sheep, and mice cause diarrhea in humans as well.

Diseases

Infection with *H. pylori* is associated with several gastrointestinal (GI) tract diseases. Most persons with gastric or duodenal ulcers, chronic gastritis, intestinal metaplasia, gastric adenocarcinoma of the distal stomach, and gastric MALT lymphoma are infected with these bacteria. Treatments that eradicate the organisms decrease gastritis and ulcers and lower the risk of developing gastric malignancies. In contrast, due to *H. pylori*'s ability to increase gastric pH, infection appears to lower the chances of developing GERD, Barrett esophagus, and the highly pathogenic adenocarcinoma of the lower esophagus.

Immune Response

H. pylori infection promotes transit of neutrophils and lymphocytes into the gastric mucosa, where they produce several immune mediators, including Th1-related cytokines, chemokines, inflammatory cytokines, and regulatory cytokines. Regulatory cytokines may decrease protective immunity to the extent that the host is unable to completely eliminate the bacteria, resulting in lifelong infection. Vaccine attempts have been largely unsuccessful when tested in phase I clinical trails, but some promising work has been reported in the mouse model of infection. Protection in these animals is associated with the induction of Th1 immunity.

Setting

H. pylori is one of the most common bacterial species that infects humans, and it has done so for over 50,000 years. Developing areas of the world have high rates of infection, and colonization usually occurs during childhood. Persons from developed nations have much lower rates of infection that increase with age. Persons colonized early in life are more likely to develop gastric symptoms, while those infected later in life are more likely to present with duodenal ulcers instead. Infection rates and gastric diseases are decreasing in developed areas but not in developing regions. Socioeconomic factors such as crowding, proper hygiene, and access to treatment help determine prevalence in a given population. Within a given geographical area, the incidence of infection may differ greatly; this is true for the Native Alaskans and Canadian First Nation communities in comparison with the Caucasian population of the regions.

Protection

Bacteria are usually eradicated by a combination of agents that suppress acidity, a bismuth compound, and several antibiotics. While highly effective, the cost of such treatment may be not be affordable by many persons in developing regions. Research is being conducted to determine the utility of less costly and more readily available alternatives in the form of neutraceuticals.

Introduction

Helicobacter pylori bacteria have inhabited the stomach mucosa of men, women, and children throughout the world since before the emergence of the human species from Africa. They are currently one of the most prevalent micro-organisms of humans and are responsible for the majority of peptic ulcers and gastric cancer, yet they were not isolated until 1982 and their role in disease was not acknowledged until 12 years later after much dissention from the medical and scientific communities. In developing nations, most people are colonized with these bacteria before the age of 10 years, and 70% to 90% of the people are eventually infected. In developed countries, the rate of infection is much lower (20% to 50%) and increases with age. Colonization of children in developed countries (currently approximately 10%) is believed to have been more common several decades ago (40% to 60%) because infection rate has been linked to socioeconomic conditions—infection is higher among individuals living in larger families or crowded conditions, those raised in poorer or less hygienic conditions, smokers, and those who consume less fruit, and such conditions are less common in developed areas now than in the past. In developed nations, however, groups with higher incidence of infection persist, including Native Alaskans in the United States. Once infected, people usually remain infected throughout their lives unless treated or unless severe chronic gastritis occurs, killing the bacteria. *H. pylori* infection is classified as emerging not because of its actual entry into the human population but rather due to our relatively recent discovery of the link between these bacteria and a variety of gastroduodenal diseases.

History

In 1875 and 1889, spiral bacteria were discovered in gastric ulcers and gastric aspirations and a potential role in causing peptic ulcers was first postulated. These and other findings of similar bacteria in gastric mucosa of dogs, cats, and monkeys were largely ignored, however, until 1979 and 1982 when two Australian researchers began the lengthy process of altering long-held views concerning gastric disease. At that time, infection with the spiralbacteria was suggested to lead to gastric disorders by Robin Warren, and following up on this hypothesis, the bacteria were successfully cultured and isolated by Barry Marshall. The bacteria were initially named *Campylobacter pyloridis* but were reclassified as *Helicobacter pylori* in 1989. Although Marshall and Warren's work presented strong evidence that the bacterial infection caused conditions such as chronic gastritis and peptic ulcers, the scientific community preemptively rejected their findings because they contradicted conventional knowledge that taught that ulcers were due to stress and dietary factors and urged bed rest and bland food for ulcer sufferers, treatment modalities that did nothing to prevent ulcer recurrence. The validity of their claims was eventually proved by human volunteers ingesting the spiral bacteria and subsequently contracting peptic ulcers that were later cured by the eradication of the bacteria. In 1994, Marshall and Warren's claims were substantiated by the National Institutes of Health, and persons throughout the world suffering from peptic ulcers and chronic gastritis were able to be cured by a relatively quick and simple treatment regimen. The dedication of these scientists in the face of firm opposition by most physicians and researchers has improved the quality of many persons' lives. In recognition of their efforts, Warren and Marshall received the Nobel Prize in Medicine or Physiology in 2005. Recently, additional members of the *Helicobacter* genus have been discovered in domestic animals. Several of these species also infect humans' stomach, intestines, gallbladder, and blood and are associated with gastrointestinal diseases, leading to the suggestion that infection of animals may lead to zoonotic transmission to humans.

H. pylori infection was also found to cause cancers, such as distal gastric adenocarcinomas and gastric MALT lymphomas. Eradication of *H. pylori* in Alzheimer's disease patients was also found in one study to lead to increased cognitive and functional status two years later. Infection has been suggested to play a causal role in a subset of individuals with autoimmune thrombocytopenic purpura as well because antibodies against the bacteria's urease B protein are cross-reactive with a glycoprotein found on human platelets and inhibited the aggregation of these cells. Interestingly, the bacteria have also been postulated to play a protective role against the development of gastroesophageal reflux disease, Barrett esophagus, and adenocarcinoma of the lower esophagus.

The Diseases

Almost all persons infected by *H. pylori* develop chronic gastric inflammation; however, many never develop any corresponding symptoms. Other infected persons do suffer from one or more upper abdominal disorders.

Peptic Ulcer Disease

The origin of **peptic ulcer disease** has long been a matter of contention. Certain peptic ulcers are known to be caused by aspirin and other nonsteroidal anti-inflammatory drugs, excessive alcohol use, or other illnesses such as Crohn's disease or Zollinger-Ellison syndrome. But the cause of approximately 80% of ulcers was unknown until it was discovered that *H. pylori* bacteria were almost always present in such ulcers. Eradication of the bacteria dramatically decreased the rate of ulcer recurrence, which had been greater than 30% in the first year in patients continuing acid-suppressive therapy without killing the bacteria.

Most people who are infected with *H. pylori* (90% of those in developed regions) do not develop peptic ulcers. Ulcers occur more readily in individuals infected by *cagA*$^+$ strains of *H. pylori* and strains that produce more vacuolating cytotoxin (described in the discussion of the causative agent). Environmental and genetic factors also affect the chances that an infected person will develop an ulcer. These factors include cigarette smoking, having blood type O, and certain major histocompatibility class II antigens. Ulcer location may be a function of age of infection, for people living in developing regions where colonization generally occurs during childhood tend to produce gastric ulcers, whereas people living in developed regions where colonization occurs later in life have a higher prevalence of duodenal ulcers. Alterations in gastric acid production may lead to the production of duodenal gastric metaplasia, in which the duodenal epithelium cells assume a more gastriclike morphology, enhancing the ability of *H. pylori* to colonize this region. The presence of duodenal gastric metaplasia and infection with *H. pylori* is associated with increased risk of developing duodenal ulcers.

Gastric Cancer

Chronic inflammatory responses directed against *H. pylori* lead to long-term destruction of the normal gastric mucosal architecture (**chronic gastritis**) as the gastric glands that secrete "gastric juice" are lost and replaced by fibrotic and intestinal metaplastic cells differing in histological type (**intestinal metaplasia**). The gastric glands are responsible for the secretion of the digestive enzyme pepsin, hydrochloric acid, intrinsic factor (required for vitamin B_{12} absorption and red blood cell production), and the mucus that protects the mucosal cells lining the stomach from acid-related damage. Chronic gastritis and intestinal metaplasia increase the risk for **gastric cancer** by 5- to 90-fold, depending on their severity and the type of metaplasia. Individuals whose metaplastic cells are similar to colon epithelium have a higher risk than those whose cells are similar to small intestinal epithelium. People infected with *H. pylori* are most likely to develop the inflammatory conditions that cause gastric cancer, and infection with these bacteria is linked to cancer of the distal stomach. Because of the link between *H. pylori* infection and gastric cancer, the World Health Organization's International Agency for Research on Cancer classified these bacteria as a class I carcinogen

FIGURE 8.1   Gastric cancer

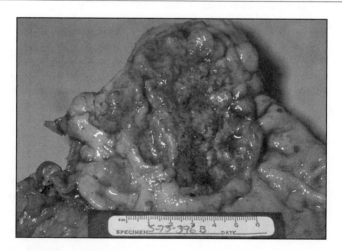

Source: CDC/Edwin P. Ewing.

in 1994. As socioeconomic conditions have improved over the past six decades in developed countries, the rate of infection with *H. pylori* and the prevalence of gastric cancer have decreased from 30 cases per 100,000 persons per year to 5 cases per 100,000. Perhaps the decreasing incidence of *H. pylori* infection in developing countries will have a similarly positive effect on gastric cancer occurrence. As with peptic ulcers, *cagA*$^+$ strains of bacteria cause more severe inflammation and are associated with a higher risk for developing gastric cancer.

Stomach acidity may play a role in the development of gastric cancer. *H. pylori* typically inhabits and causes cancer in the distal portions of the stomach where the pH is in the range 5–6 because this region of the stomach is away from the acid-producing parietal cells. If acid production is decreased by either the use of acid-suppressive medications or destruction of parietal cells by atrophic gastritis, the higher pH may allow *H. pylori* to inhabit more proximal portions of the stomach or penetrate more deeply into gastric pits. Persons with gastric ulcers have lower levels of acid production than those with duodenal ulcers and have a fourfold higher risk of developing gastric cancer.

Gastric MALT Lymphoma

Gastric MALT lymphoma is the result of large numbers of lymphocytes entering into the stomach and forming a solid mass. (MALT refers to mucosal-associated lymphoid tissue—collections of immune cells in mucous-producing regions, such as the Peyer's patches of the intestine.) Lymphocytes are not typically found in the stomach mucosa in the absence of infection by bacteria such as *H. pylori*. When these bacteria do infect the stomach, lymphocytes, usually B cells, enter the gastric epithelium and form lymphoid follicles. This may form the basis of the finding that almost all individuals with gastric lymphomas are also infected by *H. pylori* and that a one-week course of bacterial eradication leads to a 70% rate of complete remission of the lymphoma.

Association with Other Diseases

Hypertrophic Protein-Losing Gastritis **Hypertrophic protein-losing gastritis** is characterized by chronic gastritis with giant folds in the stomach wall, protein loss in the stomach, and hypoalbuminemia (low levels of albumin, the most prevalent blood protein). Although the cause of this condition remains unknown, treatment that eradicates *H. pylori* leads to significant improvement.

Gastroesophageal Reflux Disease (GERD), Barrett Esophagus, and Adenocarcinoma of the Lower Esophagus Recent evidence suggests that the incidence of

gastroesophageal reflux disease (GERD) and its complications of **Barrett esophagus** and **adenocarcinomas of the lower esophagus** may be decreased by *H. pylori* infection. During GERD, the acidified food or liquid contents of the stomach travel backward into the lower esophagus, possibly leading to irritation. Approximately 40% of the population of the Western world experiences symptoms of GERD (heartburn, belching, nausea, vomiting, sore throat, difficulty swallowing) in a given month. Barrett esophagus is a metaplastic alteration of the esophageal epithelium that occurs in 10% to 20% of individuals with GERD and is about twice as common in males as in females. Barrett esophagus results from attempts to repair acid-induced damage to the lower esophagus in which the normal esophageal lining of stratified squamous epithelium is replaced by the more acid-resistant columnar epithelium, which has a greater tendency to undergo malignant transformation. It is a predisposing factor for adenocarcinoma of the lower esophagus, a particularly pathogenic malignancy whose incidence is rapidly increasing in the United States. This cancer has a poor prognosis, with a three-year survival rate of 20%. The recent decrease in rates of *H. pylori* infection in developed countries has been paralleled by an increase in the prevalence of adenocarcinomas of the lower esophagus. Eradication of these bacteria also increases the incidence of GERD. The ability of *H. pylori* to raise stomach pH by decreasing acid production together with the activity of its urease enzyme (discussed further later in this chapter) may help protect the host against GERD and its complications. $CagA^+$ strains appear to be most protective in decreasing incidence of Barrett esophagus and adenocarcinoma of the esophagus.

The Causative Agent

Helicobacter pylori bacteria are highly mobile spiral or slightly curved gram-negative rod-shaped bacilli that may round up into a more coccoidal form after prolonged growth in culture or after antibiotic treatment. The coccoidal form is not able to be cultured but is believed by some scientists to remain viable. This form has been detected in water but not in food. *H. pylori* bear two to seven unipolar flagella to propel them through the thick gastric mucus in which they reside. They were originally grouped with the *Campylobacter* genus based on their location in the gastrointestinal tract and their shape, motility, and ability to grow under microaerobic conditions. Differences in rRNA sequences led to the creation of the genus *Helicobacter,* which now contains at least 20 species derived from the GI tract or the liver of humans, other mammals, or birds. *H. cinaedi* and *H. fennelliae* (originally also designated as *Campylobacter* species) have been isolated from the intestines of homosexual men with proctitis, colitis, or HIV infection. Both of these bacteria may also be present in blood, and *H. cinaedi* may inhabit joints and soft tissues. *H. cinaedi* also infects chronic alcoholics and immunocompetent men, women, and children and may lead to bacteremia, fever, leukopenia, and thrombocytopenia. A new species, *H. westmeadii*, was cultured from the blood of two HIV-positive individuals. Other *Helicobacter* species found in chickens, cats, dogs, sheep, and mice—*H. pullorum, H. canis,* and *H. rappini (Felxispira rappini)*—cause diarrhea in humans as well. *H. rappini* was isolated from several persons with cellulitis, one of whom had developed this condition following a cat scratch. *H. bilis,* from the intestines of rodents, cats, and dogs, as well as *H. pullorum* and *H. rappini,* may reside in the human gallbladder. In contrast, *H. pylori* usually infects only primates, although infection is seen in domestic cats on occasion. *H. hepaticus* infection in mice is associated with hepatic adenomas and hepatic adenocarcinoma.

H. pylori is rarely detected outside of the stomach mucosal layer except in metaplastic gastric lesions in the esophagus, duodenum, jejunum, or much farther down the GI tract in the rectum. These bacteria are able to survive in the harsh, highly acidic pH of the stomach interior thanks to the production of a very potent urease enzyme. Urease breaks down the waste product urea into ammonia and carbonic acid. Ammonia, which is itself a very weak acid, nevertheless is much more basic than the gastric environment and thus increases the pH while serving as a nitrogen source for bacterial growth. Other *Helicobacter* species infecting the intestines of humans may lack this enzyme. Two other species, *H. felis* and *H. heilmannii (Gastrospirillum hominis)*, have been detected in human gastric tissues. These organisms also have urease activity. Infection with the latter bacterium is associated with gastritis, gastric ulcers, and gastric lymphoma.

Table 8.1 *Helicobacter* species associated with human disease

Bacterial Species	Location	Disease or Symptoms
H. pylori	Stomach	Peptic ulcers, gastric cancer, gastric MALT lymphoma
H. cinaedi	Blood, joints, soft tissues	Proctitis, colitis
H. fennelliae	Blood	Proctitis, colitis
H. pullorum	Gallbladder	Diarrhea
H. canis	Unknown	Diarrhea
H. rappini	Gallbladder	Diarrhea, cellulitis
H. heilmannii	Stomach	Gastritis, gastric ulcers, gastric lymphoma

Different strains of *H. pylori* show a large range of genetic diversity because some of the conserved genes (genes found in most species) have a high rate of point mutations, while other genes appear to be mosaics produced by the combination of genes from several bacterial strains. Other factors that contribute to genetic diversity include chromosomal rearrangements and insertions and plasmids (extrachromosomal DNA). *H. pylori* bacteria are competent; that is, they are able to take up DNA from other bacteria from their external environment. Some bacterial strains also contain nonconserved DNA fragments, such as the *cag* pathogenicity island, a 35-kilobase segment with around 20 genes, including the *cagA* and *picB* genes. *PicB* encodes a type III secretion protein that induces gastric cells to secrete the chemokine interleukin-8. The *cagA* gene is the cytotoxin-associated gene, a potent virulence factor. Infection with *cagA*$^+$ strains increases the risk for developing severe chronic gastritis, gastric cancer, and peptic ulcers. These strains compose 40% to 60% of the U.S. and European isolates but may account for greater than 80% of the strains in developing nations. *VacA* is also found in only some *H. pylori* strains and contains both conserved and diverse regions, leading to mosaic structures that differ greatly in the levels of production of the *vacA* vacuolating cytotoxin. *VacA* induces vacuolization of the hosts' cells, and the amount of toxin corresponds to the severity of gastritis or risk of peptic ulcer disease. Another gene that has variant forms is the *iceA* gene, and infection with an *iceA1* strain is associated with a greater risk for developing a duodenal ulcer. Lipopolysaccharides of the bacterial outer membrane contain Lewis antigens, which are identical to those found on human red blood cells and epithelial cells. *CagA*$^+$ strains generally express higher levels of Lewis antigens than *cagA*$^-$ strains. Studies that correlate genetic variation occurring among bacterial strains with strain distribution suggest that humans were infected with *H. pylori* prior to their emergence from East Africa between 50,000 and 70,000 years ago.

The exact modes of bacterial transmission are unclear because colonization is usually not detected during the acute stage but rather later in the course of infection. Transmission has been reported by contact with vomit during mouth-to-mouth resuscitation and ingestion in a laboratory setting. Infection rates are higher among gastroenterologists and nursing personnel and patients in institutions that care for the mentally disabled. One potential route of transmission is oral to oral, as may occur when mothers chew food for their infants. Although the bacteria may occasionally be found in saliva and dental plaque, dentists are not at high risk of infection. Because *H. pylori* have been found in contaminated water and in the feces of children with diarrhea, a second potential route is oral-fecal transmission via water or vegetables treated with infected "night soil." Transmission has also been shown to occur iatrogenically, through the use of contaminated endoscopes or pH electrodes.

The Immune Response

In response to the presence of bacterial antigens in the distal regions of the stomach, phagocytic cells—neutrophils and monocytes—accumulate in the gastric mucosa during the acute phase of infection. This enhances epithelial permeability, leading to acute damage to this layer. Blood monocytes are better able to kill *H. pylori* than the tissue macrophages are. The inflammatory reaction continues later during the course of infection as lymphocytes enter the area. Th1 responses predominate, with increasing production of interferon-γ and IL-12 but no change occurs in the levels of the Th2 cytokines IL-4 and IL-5. IFN-γ serves as a growth factor for gastric epithelial cells, which express a receptor for this cytokine. IL-12 serves to drive Th1 types of immune responses. Bacterial neutrophil-activating protein appears to be responsible for driving Th1-mediated inflammation and inhibiting Th2 responses both in vitro and in vivo. Levels of IL-8, a chemokine that serves to attract neutrophils, is also elevated in the gastric mucosa, as are the inflammatory cytokines IL-1β, IL-6, and TNF-α, and the protective regulatory cytokine TGF-γ. Inflammation due to cytokines and infiltration of neutrophils and Th1 helper lymphocytes appears to play a major causal role in the subsequent gastric pathology. The bacteria additionally trigger a vigorous antibody response.

The immune response triggered by the bacteria in the gastric mucosa does not appear to confer long-term protection against natural infection, as the risk of colonization is similar among persons who were never infected and those who were cured of a previous infection. CD4$^+$ T helper cells are an important component of protective host immunity. Gastric epithelial cells constitutively produce the chemokines IP-10, Mig and I-TAC, which attract CD4$^+$ Th1 cells into the infected area. IFN-γ together with TNF-α induce secretion of these chemokines. Fragments of *H. pylori* are able to significantly reduce the production of IP-10 and Mig in response to IFN-γ and TNF-α. Decreased trafficking of Th1 cells to the gastric mucosa may partially explain the lack of elimination of these bacteria by the host immune response but may also serve in a beneficial capacity to limit the severity of the gastritis, in that activated Th1 lymphocytes acting together with neutrophils are postulated to play a key role in triggering this condition.

The situation in the duodenal epithelium may differ from that occurring in the stomach. Cytokine analysis reveals that persons developing duodenal ulcers have lower levels of IFN-γ, TGF-β, and IL-8 in their normal duodenal epithelial cells than asymptomatic persons infected by *H. pylori*. Furthermore, those with ulcers have a higher bacterial load. In the duodenal lamina propria, however, *H. pylori*–infected persons have increased numbers of immune cells producing

Table 8.2   *H. pylori*–induced changes in production
of cytokines and chemokines

Type of Immune Molecule	Cytokine or Chemokine	Change in Production
Th1-like cytokine	IFN-γ, IL-12	↑
Inflammatory cytokine	IL-1β, IL-6, TNF-α	↑
Regulatory cytokine	TGF-β	↑
Chemokine	IL-8	↑
	IP-10, Mig	↓

these cytokines and IL-6 in comparison with uninfected control persons. Those with duodenal ulcers appear to have higher levels of TGF-β production than the asymptomatic infected persons. The regulatory action of TGF-β often leads to decreased production of other cytokines. This suggests that in individuals who develop duodenal ulcers, cytokine down-regulation in the gut epithelium occurred, permitting increased numbers of bacteria to survive and cause pathology. Persons developing duodenal ulcers are reported to have higher levels of Treg cells, which may lead to the decreased cytokine responses to *H. pylori* via increased their secretion of TGF-β. Further evidence for the importance of this regulatory cytokine in gastric disease is provided by findings that specific genetic variants of the TGF-β gene are associated with precancerous gastric lesions induced by *H. pylori*.

Diagnosis

Screening for infection with *H. pylori* may be accomplished by invasive procedures such as endoscopy or noninvasive methods. During the invasive procedures, a sample of the gastric lining is obtained for morphological examination, detection of urease activity using commercially available kits, or for in vitro culture of the bacteria. *H. pylori* may be cultured in either specific solid or liquid media, such as brain-heart infusion agar plus horse blood, and may also require micro-aerobic conditions with approximately 5% O_2. These bacteria obtain maximal growth at human body temperature (37°C, 98.6°F) and neutral pH unless urea is provided. They show strong urease, catalase, and oxidase activities, which aid in their identification. The sugars glucose, pyruvate, succinate, and citrate are not required for *H. pylori* growth, but certain amino acids (arginine, histidine, isoleucine, leucine, methionine, phenylalanine, and valine) are necessary.

The bacteria are typically resistant to the antibiotic agents trimethoprim, nalidixic acid, sulfonamides, and vancomycin, and sensitivity tests performed during culture may establish whether a given isolate has developed any resistance to additional antibiotics.

Noninvasive tests include assays for the presence of antibacterial antibodies by ELISA, by urease breath testing, or by the stool antigen test. IgG ELISA results range in sensitivity and specificity from 80% to 95%. In urease breath testing, ^{13}C- or ^{14}C-labeled urea is ingested and the person's breath is then tested for the presence of radioactive CO_2 produced by the action of bacterial urease. Sensitivity and specificity for the urease breath test are 94% to 98%. The breath test is, however, costly and may yield false-negative results if the individual is using a proton pump inhibitor. The stool antigen test is a useful alternative, and its results show a 94.7% concordance with those of the urease breath test. This test is less expensive, is simpler to perform, and does not require overnight fasting.

In culture samples, *Helicobacter* may be mistaken for *Campylobacter* species. These bacterial genera also share some immunological features, and antibodies specific for *H. pylori* may cross-react with *Campylobacter jejuni*.

Treatment

Single-drug therapy is not useful in vivo, despite its efficacy in vitro. Treatment regimens typically involve a combination of several drugs, including a means of suppressing acidic conditions such as a proton pump inhibitor (omeprazole or Prilosec) or a histamine H2 receptor blocker; a bismuth subsalicylate compound, such as Pepto-Bismol; and one or more antibiotics, such as metronidazole, amoxicillin, or tetracycline. The related species of *Helicobacter* that infect humans, *H. cinaedi* and *H. fennelliae,* are susceptible to tetracycline, for the former, and ciprofloxacin, doxycycline, gentamycin, rifampin, and sulfamethoxazole, for the latter. The combination treatment is administered for two to four weeks and has a 90% success rate in the eradication of *H. pylori*. Socioeconomic conditions and presence of resistance to some antibiotics may affect the ability of a given population to use some otherwise beneficial regimens. In Brazil, triple therapy using a proton pump inhibitor together with the antibiotics amoxicillin and clarithromycin for seven days has proved to be very efficacious in eradicating bacteria, has high compliance rates, and has few problems with bacterial resistance. Its cost (approximately $75), however, may restrict its usefulness in that nation because it is not affordable by the majority of individuals or the public health system.

Given the difficulty of paying for effective antibiotic therapy regimens in parts of the developing world, a great degree of attention has focused in recent years

Table 8.3   Agents used in combination for the treatment of *H. pylori* infection

Type of Agent	Agents
Agents that ↓ stomach acidity	Proton pump inhibitor
	Histamine H2 receptor blocker
Antibiotics	Metronidazole
	Amoxicillin
	Clarithromycin
	Tetracycline
Plant-derived antioxidants	Tea polyphenols
	Apple peel polyphenols

on potential beneficial roles of neutraceuticals derived from inexpensive, readily available foods and beverages. A 2009 study found that high levels of extracts of the tea plant, *Camellia sinensis,* which contains many biologically active antioxidative polyphenols, are able to kill *H. pylori* in vitro and that lower amounts prevent production of the urease enzyme necessary for bacterial survival in the harsh gastric environment. Green tea extracts were more active than those of black tea. Another 2009 study reported that high-molecular-weight polyphenols from Granny Smith apple peels also inhibit *H. pylori* urease activity. Many other fruits and plant extracts contain high levels of these potent traditional medicine compounds.

Prevention

Because the exact route of bacterial transmission is uncertain, precise preventive measures are difficult to implement; however, some practices appear to have reduced the infection rate among children in some areas of the world. Given the link between low socioeconomic status and infection at an early age, efforts should be made to increase sanitary conditions and reduce crowding. In the latter part of the twentieth century, such improvements in general hygiene occurred in developed nations, which also reported a corresponding decrease in *H. pylori* infection during childhood and subsequent development of *H. pylori*–related disorders, such as gastric cancer. To prevent iatrogenic transmission, all endoscopes, pH electrodes, and other medical devices entering the stomach need to be thoroughly decontaminated.

Several attempts to produce useful vaccines have been disappointing in phase I clinical trials, partially due to the need to establish strong mucosal protection, which often requires vaccine administration via a mucosal route. The use of a recombinant urease vaccine incorporated into an attenuated *Salmonella* vector did not provide strong immune reactivity when given by the oral route. Several other potential vaccines, such as an oral whole-cell vaccine, were not further pursued due to excessive side effects. A recombinant vaccine containing the bacterial proteins VacA, CagA and NAP in alum is more promising, however, and has proved safe and strongly immunogenic. Protective immunity appears to be produced by vaccine protocols that induce Th1 rather than Th2 responses. Accordingly, protective vaccines in the mouse model appear to function via increased production of the cytokine IL-17 or IL-12 or the presence of antibacterial IgG1 or IgG2a antibodies in the blood. Mice that were not protected, however, had greater amounts of IgA in the blood and in Peyer's patches of the intestine. IL-12 and IgG antibodies are associated with a Th1 immune response, while IgA is associated with Th2 responses. Interestingly, protection in these systems was obtained by vaccination via either the oral and intramuscular routes or via the intramuscular route alone.

Whereas on the one hand, prevention of bacterial colonization or eradication of the bacteria from an infected person may reduce the risk of developing peptic ulcer disease, gastric cancer, and gastric lymphoma, infection with *H. pylori* with its ability to raise gastric pH appears, on the other hand, to play a protective role against the likelihood of developing GERD or its serious complications, such as Barrett esophagus and cancer of the lower esophagus. The potential consequences of routine eradication of *H. pylori* should therefore be carefully weighed before action is undertaken.

Surveillance

Incidence of *H. pylori* infection and gastric cancer is higher in developing areas of the world. In Georgia, a developing nation with a postcommunist economy in transition, more than 70% of the adults are infected and the rate of gastric cancer is 18 cases per 100,000 population, six to nine times higher than the rate in the United States. In a study of persons undergoing upper endoscopy in Georgia in 2003 to 2005, *H. pylori* was found in 78% of those with gastritis, 58% of those with peptic ulcer, and 58% of those with dysplasia or gastric cancer. Previous infection with *H. pylori* may have been even higher because the bacterium requires gastric mucus to grow, and mucus produced by metaplastic and neoplastic cells has been suggested to lack the ability to sustain bacterial growth.

In Canada, the overall rate of *H. pylori* infection in asymptomatic persons is similar to that of other comparable developed nations. In a 2000 study conducted in Nova Scotia, seroprevalance for *H. pylori* (percentage of the population with antibacterial antibodies) was 21% for persons in their thirties and 50% for those in their eighties. In a 2007 study, women under the age of 60 years are significantly less likely to be infected than men (17.3% versus 29.4%, respectively), while among persons over the age of 70 years, the infection rate is very similar (36.0% versus 38.7%). Certain population groups in Canada, however, have much higher infection rates. For example, 95% of a Manitoba First Nations community was infected, including 67% of the children who were under the age of 2 years. Infection rates were also higher among individuals with lower levels of education and income. Interestingly, infection rate dropped as moderate levels of alcohol consumption increased and rose as antacid consumption increased. This may be due to the antibacterial effects of moderate levels of alcohol and to increased stomach pH providing more favorable growth conditions for the bacteria, respectively.

RECENT DEVELOPMENTS

High rates of iron deficiency anemia were found to occur among Native Alaskans in the 1950s, despite the availability of adequate iron in the diet. This anemia was later determined to result from the presence of blood in the stool. This blood loss was linked in 1997 to chronic gastritis resulting from infection by *H. pylori* (99% of this population with iron deficiency anemia had gastritis due to bacterial infection). Rates of infection among Native Alaskans range from 32% in children under the age of 4 years to 86% among adults over the age of 20. Rates were higher among rural inhabitants than among people residing in urban areas and in those with young children in the household. The infection rate among nonnative Alaskans, by contrast, was 23%, similar to that found in other areas of North America. Many of the bacterial isolates taken from Native Alaskans were found to have antibiotic resistance—33% were resistant to clarithromycin and 48% to metronidazole. This correlated with high rates of disease recurrence among Native Alaskans following standard regimens for the elimination of *H. pylori*. Studies of the prevalence of ulcers and gastric cancer among Native and nonnative Alaskans are being planned.

HIV-positive persons in China have a rate of *H. pylori* infection far lower than that of the general population (16.5% versus 47.1%). Different rates of infection were also found during different stages of HIV disease progression, with higher rates occurring in asymptomatic persons than in symptomatic persons and those with AIDS. The presence of severe immunosuppression in the gastric mucosa during advanced stages of HIV infection was postulated to be responsible for decreased bacterial infection.

Summary

Diseases
- Chronic gastritis • Peptic ulcers • Distal gastric adenocarcinomas
- Gastric MALT lymphomas

Causative Agent
- *Helicobacter pylori*

Agent Type
- Spiral, gram-negative bacillus

Genome
- DNA

Vector
- None

Common Reservoir
- Human stomach

Mode of Transmission
- Unclear; may occur during mouth-to-mouth resuscitation and via contaminated endoscopes or pH electrodes

Geographical Distribution
- Worldwide

Year of Emergence
- Bacteria discovered in 1982 and postulated to play a causal role in peptic ulcer formation; causal role accepted in 1994

Key Terms

Adenocarcinoma of the lower esophagus Cancer of the esophagus with poor prognosis; often associated with prior GERD and Barrett esophagus

Barrett esophagus Metaplastic alteration of the esophageal epithelium, which is a predisposing factor for adenocarcinomas of the esophagus

Chronic gastritis Prolonged inflammation of the mucosal lining of the stomach; often due to infection with *H. pylori*

Gastric cancer Malignancy of the stomach lining; most frequently, adeno-carcinoma; incidence is linked to infection with *H. pylori*

Gastric MALT lymphoma Cancerous growth of lymphoid cells in the stomach; may be due to infection with *H. pylori*

Gastroesophageal reflux disease (GERD) Condition in which acidified stomach contents travel backward into the lower esophagus

Helicobacter pylori Gram-negative, spiral, rod-shaped bacterium that colonizes the gastric mucosal layer and is responsible for chronic active gastritis, peptic ulcers, distal gastric adenocarcinomas, and gastric lymphomas

Hypertrophic protein-losing gastritis Disorder characterized by chronic gastritis with giant folds in the stomach wall, gastric protein loss, and hypoalbuminemia

Intestinal metaplasia Replacement of cells of the stomach or esophagus (stratified squamous epithelium) with cells resembling histological types usually found in the intestine (simple columnar epithelium)

Peptic ulcer disease Erosion of the lining of the stomach or the duodenum, usually attributable to infection with *H. pylori*

Review Questions

1. Other than *H. pylori*, what species of *Helicobacter* infect humans, what part of the human body do they inhabit, and with which diseases are they associated?
2. How does *H. pylori* infection differ between developing and developed regions of the world? Why does this occur, and what effect does this have on disease?
3. What type of bacterium is *H. pylori*?
4. How are *H. pylori* bacteria transmitted?
5. How is *H. pylori* infection treated?

Topics for Further Discussion

1. Th1 but not Th2 immune responses are induced by infection with *H. pylori* and appear to be needed for protection after successful vaccination of mice. Discuss why the immune response in most persons appears to be largely inef-fective, leading to lifelong infection of the host. Play particular attention to the role of Treg cells and TGF-β.
2. Infection with *H. pylori* is often pathogenic but has been associated with posi-tive effects on human health as well, such as decreasing the risk of developing

GERD, Barrett esophagus, and adenocarcinoma of the lower esophagus. Other, more contested findings suggest that *H. pylori* may decrease asthma. Discuss ways in which live or dead bacteria or isolated bacterial components might be used to aid human health without the risk of pathogenic side effects.

3. Combination therapy that uses several antibiotics is efficacious in eliminating *H. pylori* from human gastric mucosa but is often too costly to be beneficial to the individuals in developing regions among whom the infection rate is highest. Tea extracts, which contain many potent bioactive polyphenols such as epigallocatechin gallate (EGCG), and apple peel polyphenols were shown to have antibacterial activity against *H. pylori* as well as other bacteria and some viruses, including HIV-1. Search for other polyphenolic compounds from foods or beverages that kill microbes. Explore the mechanisms by which they kill the bacteria or viruses.

4. In the United States and Canada, Native Alaskans and First Nations communities have a higher rate of infection with *H. pylori* than surrounding population groups. What might explain this discrepancy? Suggest other ethnic or geographical populations in North America that may also have higher incidence of infection. Search the scientific literature to determine whether studies have been conducted on these groups and the findings of such studies.

Resources

Chin, J. *Control of Communicable Diseases Manual* (17th ed.). Washington, D.C.: American Public Health Association, 2000.

Fox, J. G. "*Helicobacter* Species Other Than *Helicobacter pylori:* Emerging Pathogens in Humans and Animals." In W. M. Scheld, W. A. Craig, and J. M. Hughes (eds.), *Emerging Infections* (Vol. 4). Washington, D.C.: ASM Press, 2000.

Hassani, A. R., and others. "In Vitro Inhibition of *Helicobacter pylori* Urease with Non- and Semifermented *Camellia sinensis*." *Indian Journal of Medical Microbiology*, 2009, *27*, 30–34.

Kountouras, J., and others. "Eradication of *Helicobacter pylori* May Be Beneficial in the Management of Alzheimer's Disease." *Journal of Neurology*, 2009, *256*, 758–767.

Kraft, M., and others. "IFN-γ Synergizes with TNF-α but Not with Viable *H. pylori* in Up-Regulating CXC Chemokine Secretion in Gastric Epithelial Cells." *Clinical and Experimental Immunology*, 2001, *126*, 474–481.

Kuipers, E. J., and Blaser, M. J. "*Helicobacter pylori* and Gastroduodenal Disorders." In W. M. Scheld, D. Armstrong, and J. M. Hughes (eds.), *Emerging Infections* (Vol. 1). Washington, D.C.: ASM Press, 1998.

Modiano, N., and Gerson, L. B. "Barrett's Esophagus: Incidence, Etiology, Pathophysiology, Prevention and Treatment." *Therapeutics and Clinical Risk Management*, 2007, *3*, 1035–1045.

Naja, F., Kreiger, N., and Sullivan, T. "*Helicobacter pylori* Infection in Ontario: Prevalence and Risk Factors." *Canadian Journal of Gastroenterology,* 2007, *21,* 501–506.

Silva, F. M., and others. "Short-Term Triple Therapy with Azithromycin for *Helicobacter pylori* Eradication: Low Cost, High Compliance, but Low Efficacy." *BMC Gastroenterology,* 2008, *8,* 20–25.

Strömberg, E., Edebo, A., Svennerholm, A.-M., and Lindholm, C. "Decreased Epithelial Cytokine Responses in the Duodenal Mucosa of *Helicobacter pylori*–Infected Duodenal Ulcer Patients." *Clinical and Diagnostic Laboratory Immunology,* 2003, *10,* 116–124.

Tarkhashvili, N., and others. "*Helicobacter pylori* Infection in Patients Undergoing Upper Endoscopy, Republic of Georgia." *Emerging Infectious Diseases,* 2009, *15,* 504–505.

CHAPTER 9

LEGIONNAIRES' DISEASE AND PONTIAC FEVER

LEARNING OBJECTIVES

- Define Legionnaire's disease and compare and contrast it with other severe respiratory illnesses

- Describe the bacteria responsible for causing the illness

- Discuss modes of infection

- Discuss the host's response to infection

- Describe symptomatology and diagnosis

- Discuss potential methods of treatment

- Discuss methods of prevention

Major Concepts

Symptoms

In 1976, a frightening new severe respiratory illness emerged during a meeting of the American Legion in Philadelphia, Pennsylvania, that was later named Legionnaires' disease and was found to result from a bacterial infection. In its early stages, Legionnaires' disease is characterized by low-grade fever, headache, decreased energy, myalgia, and loss of appetite. Later symptoms include high fever, chills, cough, difficulty breathing, chest pain, vomiting and diarrhea, abdominal pain, rigor, and delirium. Infection often leads to a form of pneumonia that may be responsible for 15% to 30% of the cases of pneumonia treated in intensive care units. The causative bacteria may cause wound infections, pericarditis, endocarditis, and kidney impairment. A much milder, self-limiting form of infection is Pontiac disease, a flulike disease with fever, chills, headache, fatigue, myalgia, nausea, and a dry cough. This disorder is believed to be the consequence of an allergic response to dead bacteria.

Infection

Legionnaires' disease is caused by infection with bacteria of the genus *Legionella* of the γ-2 subdivision of the family *Proteobacteria*, most commonly *L. pneumophila* and less often *L. longbeachae*. The bacteria are non-spore-forming, gram-negative rods with flagella. Forty-eight species of *Legionella* are known, and at least 20 of these are human pathogens. The bacteria have a complex life cycle that involves infection of freshwater protozoa and human monocytes and macrophages. They may also exist in biofilms. *L. pneumophila* inhabit natural and artificial water sources, including lakes, rivers, air-conditioning cooling towers, water-heating units, showerheads, grocery store misting machines, humidifiers, hot tubs, whirlpools, ventilators, and nebulizers. Infection results from inhalation of aerosols and sprays generated by these sources. Smokers and persons with respiratory illness are at higher risk for developing disease because they are less able to prevent aspiration of infectious droplets. Infants using respiratory equipment are also vulnerable. *L. longbeachae* may be acquired via cutaneous exposure to contaminated potting soil.

Immune Response

The innate and adaptive immune responses act in a cooperative manner to defend against infection with *Legionella*. The bacteria infect predominantly macrophages, triggering the toll-like receptors, which in turn stimulate the cells to produce the cytokine IL-12. IL-12 induces production of IFN-γ by Th1 helper cells. IFN-γ activates macrophages to generate reactive oxygen species that kill intracellular bacteria. The bacteria attempt to evade death by decreasing host production of IFN-γ.

Protection

Legionnaires' disease is typically treated by either erythromycin or an azithromycin type of drug. Tigecycline is also protective in animal models. Treatment is usually effective if begun promptly. Preventive measures include stopping the smoking of cigarettes, wearing a HEPA-filtered mask when cleaning or collecting water samples from cooling towers, rinsing respiratory equipment with sterile rather than distilled water, and raising water temperature at the fixtures. Water sources containing the bacteria are often difficult to decontaminate but may be subjected to heat-and-flush treatment; chlorine, monochloramine, or ozone treatment; UV radiation, or copper-silver electrode ionization.

Introduction

In 1976, a mysterious and sometimes lethal respiratory disease struck the city of Philadelphia, generating fears of widespread infection of unknown cause. That same year saw the reappearance of a strain of H1N1 influenza virus, antigenically similar to the virus responsible for the Spanish influenza epidemic of 1918, which left tens of millions of people dead throughout the world. The year also witnessed the appearance of another frightening and often fatal viral disease, Ebola hemorrhagic fever, in two unrelated outbreaks in Zaire (today's Democratic Republic of Congo) and Sudan. The Philadelphia respiratory outbreak was later named Legionnaires' disease and was found to result from exposure to *Legionella* species bacteria. These bacteria are also responsible for the mild, self-limiting Pontiac fever. Approximately 90% of *Legionella* exposures in the United States appear to involve ***Legionella pneumophila***; this may be an overestimation because most diagnostic tests are specific to that particular species. In some outbreaks, a portion of infected individuals develop Legionnaires' disease and the remainder experience Pontiac fever. In the United States alone, more than 25,000 cases of Legionnaires' disease occur annually, resulting in 8,000 to 18,000 hospitalizations and more than 4,000 deaths. Although large outbreaks do occur (approximately 11% of cases), most incidences of this disease involve only a person or two. A preponderance of cases of the disease (90% to 98%), however, are believed to remain undetected. Since 1980, an annual average of around 350 cases have been reported to the CDC.

History

The first reported occurrence of Legionnaires' disease was July 21–24, 1976, in the Bellevue Stratford Hotel in Philadelphia. At that time, the hotel was hosting a meeting of the Pennsylvania branch of the American Legion. A total of 221 people became ill with bacterial pneumonia, two-thirds were hospitalized, and 34 (15%) died. The incidence of disease correlated with the amount of time spent in the hotel lobby.

Serological data available from a 1966 outbreak of acute pneumonia in a psychiatric hospital in Washington, D.C., were later found to record antibodies to the bacteria linked to Legionnaires' disease. That outbreak involved 94 cases with 16 deaths, for a fatality rate of 17%. Even earlier, a "rickettsia-like agent," isolated in 1947, was later shown to be the Legionnaires' disease bacterium.

More recently, a series of outbreaks occurred between July and October 1993 in Massachusetts (11 persons, 3 deaths), a state prison in Michigan (17 persons, 1 death), and Rhode Island (17 persons, 2 deaths), all of which were associated with cooling towers from which *L. pneumophila* serogroup 1 was cultured. This serogroup is the one most commonly recovered from the environment. Overall, *Legionella* bacteria may be cultured in up to 40% of cooling towers. In July and August 1994, the New Jersey State Department of Health informed the CDC of 14 cases of Legionnaires' disease (and another possible 28 cases) in persons who had recently sailed to Bermuda on the cruise ship *Horizon*. This was the first report of Legionnaires' disease from a cruise ship docking in a U.S. port. Whirlpool usage correlated with the development of illness, and *Legionella* was cultured from a sand filter used for recirculation of whirlpool water.

Many cases of Legionnaires' disease are acquired by nosocomial transmission. Two hospitals (in Arizona and Ohio) were found in 1996 to have sustained transmission of this pneumonia for an extended period of time. In the Arizona hospital, 16 definite cases of Legionnaires' disease (resulting after ten days of continuous hospitalization for a nonpneumonia illness) and 9 possible cases occurred between 1987 and 1996. Most of the patients had received either a heart-lung or bone marrow transplant (76%), and the others were either immunocompromised or had a chronic illness; 48% died during their hospitalization. *L. pneumophila* serogroup 6 was cultured from taps and showers in the patients' rooms, from droplets small enough to be inhaled from air samples of the showers, from a carpet-cleaning unit from the transplant unit, and from the hospital's hot-water distribution system and water softeners. In the Ohio hospital, 9 definite cases and 29 possible cases of Legionnaires' disease were identified between 1989 and 1996. Of these, 39% had a chronic medical condition and another 34% were immunocompromised; 16% were inpatients on the psychiatric ward, and 29% died during their hospital stay. Nonpsychiatric cases were more likely to have received medication by nebulizer; however, only 40% were medicated by this route. This equipment was at times rinsed with tap water between doses. *L. pneumophila* serogroup 1 was cultured from both the psychiatric and nonpsychiatric buildings' hot-water distribution systems, including potable water samples. Several rounds of decontamination were required to stop the nosocomial transmission at both hospitals.

The Diseases

Legionnaires' Disease (Legionellosis)

Many persons with confirmed exposure to *Legionella* species seroconvert but nevertheless remain asymptomatic. Other persons develop **Legionnaires' disease**, a severe multisystem disorder, an important feature of which is pneumonia. Approximately 2% to 5% of people exposed to the responsible *Legionella* species subsequently develop this disease manifestation. It is not uncommon, however, being found in 15% to 30% of pneumonia cases in intensive care units. After infection, an incubation period of two to ten days ensues. Early symptoms include low-grade fever, headache, decreased energy, myalgia, and loss of appetite. Subsequently, a high fever of 38.9°C to 40°C (102°F to 104°F), chills, productive or nonproductive cough, difficulty in breathing, chest pain, vomiting and diarrhea, abdominal pain, and rigor occur. Other manifestations include confusion, delirium, and dyspenia. In many cases, pneumonia results. *Legionella*-induced pneumonia is clinically indistinguishable from forms of pneumonia arising from other sources. Chest X-rays are inconclusive as well; however, alveolar infiltrates occur at higher frequencies in individuals with Legionnaires' disease. *L. pneumophila* has also been associated with wound infections, pericarditis, endocarditis, and kidney impairment.

Fatality rates typically range from 5% to 30% in this form of *Legionella* infection. While even healthy people may present with this disease manifestation, the populations at greatest risk are smokers, heavy drinkers, the elderly and the immunosuppressed (including transplant recipients and individuals with cancer, diabetes, and kidney disease), and patients with chronic obstructive pulmonary diseases. In nosocomial infections (about 23% of the total number of cases), fatality rates approach 40%. Procedures associated with *Legionella* infection include heart-lung or bone marrow transplants and rinsing respiratory equipment, such as nebulizers, with tap water.

FIGURE 9.1   Bilateral pulmonary infiltrates during Legionnaires' disease

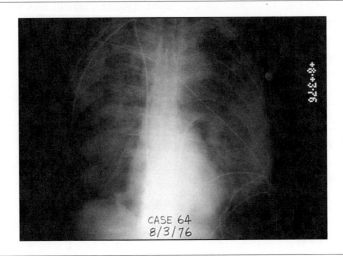

Source: CDC.

Pontiac Fever

Most people (90% to 95%) exposed to *L. pneumophila* develop **Pontiac fever** rather than Legionnaires' disease. Pontiac fever is a mild, self-limiting illness without symptoms of pneumonia. The incubation period ranges from hours to three days. Spontaneous recovery occurs after two to five days. No deaths have been reported from this form of the disease.

Pontiac fever manifests as a flulike illness in normally healthy people. Its symptoms include fever, chills, headache, fatigue, myalgia, nausea, and a dry cough. Pontiac fever is associated with exposure to dead Legionella bacteria and may result from allergic responses to them.

The Causative Agent

The Bacteria

Legionnaires' disease is caused by live bacteria of the genus *Legionella* of the γ-2 subdivision of the family *Proteobacteria*. The bacteria are non-spore-forming, gram-negative motile rods with lateral or polar flagella. Some 48 species encompassing 70 serogroups of *Legionella* are currently recognized; 20 species

FIGURE 9.2 *Legionella pneumophila* bacilli

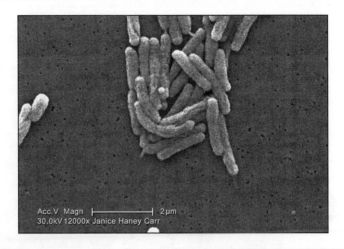

Source: CDC/Margaret Williams, Claressa Lucas, and Tatiana Travis.

(39 serogroups) are known human pathogens. Most cases of Legionnaires' disease, however, result from infection with *L. pneumophila* serotype 1, isolated in 1977. As early as 1943, Hugh Tatlock isolated strains of *Legionella,* using procedures designed for *Rickettsia.* In 1954, Wincenty Drozanski isolated a *Legionella* species from free-living soil bacteria. The organism most closely related to *Legionella* is *Coxiella burnettii,* another bacterial pathogen that causes Q fever.

Legionella bacteria are intracellular parasites of freshwater protozoa (14 amoeba species, 2 species of ciliated protozoa, 1 species of slime mold) that live in artificial or natural warm-water systems with temperatures of 25°C to 42.2°C (77°F to 108°F). They grow best at 35°C to 45°C (95°F to 113°F). The bacteria were detected by polymerase chain reaction (PCR) in 80% or more of the tested freshwater sites. In aquatic systems where the water temperature is artificially elevated, the balance between protozoa and bacteria is altered, with ensuing rapid bacterial growth. Increasing numbers of such systems over the past half century have made *Legionella*-induced illness, once extremely rare, much more common. Construction projects have also been sites of disease outbreaks as changes in water pressure led to descalement of plumbing systems. The bacteria similarly multiply within mammalian phagocytic cells, although such hosts are opportunistic. Most *Legionella* species survive within **biofilms**. One such biofilm contains *Pseudomonas aeruginosa, Klebsiella pnuemoniae, Flavobacterium,* and the amoeba *Hartmannella vermiformis.* The presence of the amoeba appears to be required for *Legionella* growth in this system.

FIGURE 9.3   Scanning electron micrograph demonstrating the association of *Hartmannella vermiformis* amoebas with *Legionella pneumophila* on a potable water biofilm containing *Pseudomonas aeruginosa, Klebsiella pneumoniae,* and *Flavobacterium*

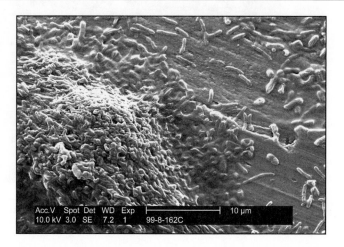

Source: CDC/Janice Carr.

Several genes of *Legionella* encode virulence factors involved in host cell infection. One such gene is *mip*, which codes for a 24 kilodalton homologue of FK506-binding proteins. *Mip* is required for infection of both amoebas and human phagocytic cells. Other such genes belong to the type IV secretion system of the Dot/Icm loci. Their products help in the transfer of plasmid DNA between bacteria by conjugation. Other genes are involved in bacterial survival and growth, such as *pilE*, *pilD*, *mak*, *mil*, and *pmi* that produce proteins found in bacterial flagella, kill macrophages, and allow infection of human and protozoan host cells.

Water systems producing aerosols, sprays, or mists are of health concern because human infection occurs by inhaling the aerosols or aspirating contaminated water, as during choking. Droplets smaller than 5 micrometers are of greatest concern, as they can reach the depths of the lungs. The bacteria are then phagocytized by alveolar macrophages, where they multiply and lyse the host cells. Smokers and individuals with respiratory illness may be defective in mechanisms to prevent aspiration. Nosocomial disease occurs in children and newborns following surgical procedures or using contaminated ventilators. In

RECENT DEVELOPMENTS

Legionella bacteria grow either as intracellular parasites of amoebas or phago-cytic cells of humans or as members of mixed-species colonies in biofilms. Biofilms are assemblages of bacteria encased within extracellular polymeric matrices adhered to surfaces or phase boundaries. Residing in such an adherent, hydrated, structured community confers survival advantages, including anchor-age in favorable locations, protection from biocides and detergents, and avoid-ance of desiccation. One species of *Legionella* was found growing under such extreme conditions as a pH 2.7 geothermal stream in Yellowstone National Park.

A recent study examined how growth conditions affected the composition and growth properties of *Legionella* in biofilms attached to several types of sur-faces. Out of 38 tested species of *Legionella* (including both *L. pneumophila* and *L. longbeachae*), *L. pneumophila* was by far the best able to form biofilms on surfaces such as glass, polystyrene, and polypropylene. This may at least partly explain why this species is the most common cause of human infection. At 37°C or 42°C (human body temperature or higher, which may be encountered in environments such as hot-spring spas or cooling towers during the summer), the bacteria took a form similar to mycelial mats and were composed of mul-tinucleated filamentous cells, whereas at 25°C, the bacteria were rod-shaped. The filamentous forms most likely result from nuclear replication without cell division. Upon being placed in media, these forms rapidly give rise to many rod-shaped bacteria. *Legionella* bacteria also produce filamentous forms in situations of physiological stress, such as exposure to antibiotics or nutrient limitation, where cell division is disrupted. At 37°C or 42°C, bacteria grew best on glass or polystyrene surfaces; growth was best on polypropylene surfaces at 25°C (near room temperature). Mats formed at higher temperatures are also thicker, spread wider, and grow more rapidly.

a 1998 report of 264 hospitals surveyed in the United Kingdom, the United States, and Canada, 12% to 70% contained *L. pneumophila* in their water systems. Person-to-person transmission, however, has yet to be reported.

A greater health hazard is posed by warm-water systems containing areas of water that is stagnant, such as side-arm and dead-leg piping, that resists hyperchlorination, thermal disinfection, or ionization; that has a pH of 5.0 to 8.5; or that contains amoebas, biofilms, scaling, or sediment. Hot-water tanks (particularly those set at lowered temperatures), whirlpools, hot tubs, shower heads, humidifiers, tap water faucets, air-conditioning system cooling towers, ice machines, and grocery store misting machines may all host the bacteria, providing conditions necessary for human infection. The fact that *Legionella* bacteria are associated with building air-conditioners means that disease outbreaks occur most often in the summer and early fall. Of note, these bacteria do not inhabit window or auto air-conditioning systems. Nosocomial transmission shows no seasonal pattern.

In Australia, Japan, and parts of the northwestern coast of the United States, infections have been acquired from open areas of skin coming into contact with contaminated potting soil. In most of those cases, the responsible agent was not *L. pneumophila* but rather **L. longbeachae**, although one case of disease was caused by *L. pneumophila* acquired from nursery soil. Between 1990 and 1999, some 37 incidences of *L. longbeachae* infection in the United States were reported to the CDC. The first such cases arising from potting soil occurred in Oregon, California, and Washington in May and June 2000. In Australia, 73% of tested potting soils contained this species; in Japan in 1998, this figure was 47%. All soils thus far from Europe and the United Kingdom have tested negative for the presence of *L. longbeachae*.

Legionella Life Cycle

Infection of freshwater protozoa (described here for the amoeba *Hartmannella vermiformis*) is initiated by bacterial attachment to filopodia (hairlike projections) on extended amoebic trophozoites. This process involves, in part, tyrosine dephosphorylation of a 170-kilodalton homologue of an *Escherichia coli* lectin that may function as the *Legionella* receptor. Several bacteria enter a single amoebic vesicle via receptor-mediated endocytosis. They subsequently begin to multiply. The infective forms of the bacteria are small, are motile due to the presence of flagella, and have smooth walls and many inclusions of β-hydroxybutyrate; by contrast, multiplicative forms are larger and nonmotile due to the loss of their flagella and have rumpled walls and little β-hydroxybutyrate, if any. After multiplication, bacteria either lyse the host cell, leading to their release, or remain within the now encysted amoeba. It has been proposed that depletion of the host cell's amino acids then occurs, resulting in greater amounts of 3',5'-bispyrophosphate. Levels of the stationary-phase factor σ RpoS increase, initiating expression of stationary-phase genes. The resultant proteins in turn aid in the infection of additional host cells. Flagellin expression appears to be necessary for this process as well.

Human phagocytic white blood cells, monocytes, macrophages, and neutrophils also host *Legionella* species. Entry of the bacterium into host cells occurs via phagocytosis involving a three-component system, including the complement receptors CR1 and CR3. Actin polymerization is required for this process. The bacterium then resides within a unique type of phagosome that does not acidify as normally occurs, protecting the bacterium from death from low pH. A developmentally regulated component of the bacterial membrane temporarily inhibits fusion of the host cell's lysosome with this phagosome. Since lysosomes contain strong digestive enzymes that normally degrade microbes trapped in phagosomes, the internalized bacteria are now able to safely multiply. These early phagosomes do not express alkaline phosphatase, major histocompatibility antigens I or II, the transferrin receptor, Rab 7, LAMP-1, or cathepsin D. After four to six hours, the phagosome associates with the host's rough endoplasmic reticulum.

Host cell death and bacterial release follow. For the amoebic host cell, death occurs by necrosis and involves pore formation. Infected phagocytic cells undergo apoptosis, a form of programmed cell death, before necrosis. In either case, newly produced infective forms of the bacteria are then released to seek out new host cells to continue the cycle.

The Immune Response

The immune response plays an active role in *Legionella* infection. High levels of inflammatory cytokines are produced after infection with virulent but not avirulent bacteria. Other immune cell products, by contrast, are protective. IgG2a antibodies from B lymphocytes protect mice from secondary infection following challenge. The cytokine IFN-γ, derived from the Th1 subset of CD4$^+$ T helper cells and natural killer cells, is also involved in disease resolution by stimulating macrophages to inhibit *L. pneumophila* replication and to kill the bacteria residing within them. The inflammatory cytokine TNF-α acts in concert with IFN-γ. The macrophage-derived cytokine IL-12 is important in this process in that it helps stimulate the production of IFN-γ by Th1 cells. Given the role of IL-12 in IFN-γ production, this cytokine is important for disease resolution. Interestingly, leukocytes from patients with Legionnaires' disease were less able to produce IFN-γ upon stimulation with IL-12 and lipopolysaccharide. The latter is a component of the cell walls of gram-negative bacteria that stimulates the immune response. White blood cells from these persons were able to respond normally to exogenous (added) IFN-γ, however. This suggests that persons with active disease have a reduced ability to produce the protective Th1 cell cytokine IFN-γ but would be able to respond to this cytokine if it were present.

Alveolar macrophages (specialized macrophages that dwell in the air sacs of the lungs) undergo a respiratory burst following phagocytosis of *Legionella* bacteria,

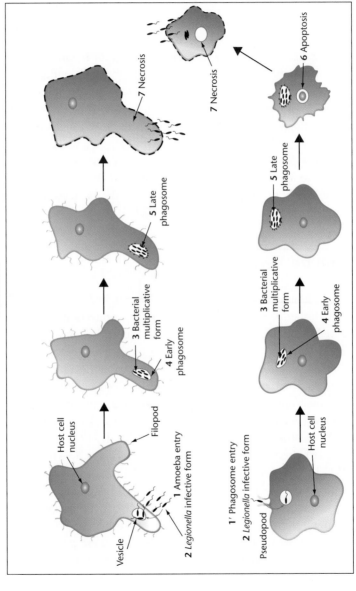

FIGURE 9.4   The life cycle of *Legionella*

Stages of the life cycle:

1. Several bacteria enter the vesicle of a free-living amoeba via receptor-mediated endocytosis involving a 170-kilodalton homologue of an *Escherichia coli* lectin on the amoeba's filopodia. Host protein synthesis is required.

   1'. A bacterium enters a human phagocyte via phagocytosis involving actin polymerization. No synthesis of host proteins is required.

2. The infective form of the bacterium is small, smooth-walled, and motile and contains multiple β-hydroxybutyrate inclusions.

3. The bacterial multiplicative form is larger, has a rumpled wall, is nonmotile, and contains little β-hydroxybutyrate, if any. It resides within the host's cytoplasm.

4. The early phagosome lacks endocytic markers, as well as alkaline phosphatase, major histocompatibility markers I and II, the transferrin receptor, Rab7, LAMP-1, and cathepsin D.

5. After four to six hours, the phagosome associates with the host's rough endoplasmic reticulum but does not acidify or fuse with lysosomes. As the stores of the host cell's amino acids decrease, the levels of 3',5'-bispyrophosphate increase, raising levels of the stationary-phase σ factor RpoS and inducing expression of the stationary-phase genes.

6. The human phagocytes, but not the amoeba, undergo apoptosis.

7. The amoeba and the phagocytes undergo necrosis involving pore formation, releasing more of the newly produced infective forms of the bacterium.

Source: Adapted from B. S. Fields, R. F. Benson, and R. E. Besser, "*Legionella* and Legionnaires' Disease: 25 Years of Investigation," *Clinical Microbiological Reviews*, 2002, 15, 506–526.

inducing the production of toxic reactive oxygen species. Several of these oxidative compounds work together to kill the bacteria; the compounds include superoxide and hydrogen peroxide, as well as the powerful hydroxyl radical generated by the metal-catalyzed interaction of these molecules. IFN-γ stimulates the respiratory burst in macrophages, promoting bacterial killing. Decreased levels of this cytokine may thus allow the bacteria to survive and replicate in these cells.

Several toll-like receptors (TLR) or associated molecules on cells of the innate immune system help to recognize *Legionella bacteria* and to stimulate a protective host response. TLR2 on macrophages and dendritic cells is involved in recognition of *L. pneumophila* and activating the innate immune cells. This receptor recognizes bacterial peptidoglycans, lipoproteins, and lipopeptides. The TLR adapter protein MyD88 works together with TLR9 to stimulate both innate and adaptive immune responses to the bacteria by triggering cells to produce IL-12. TLR9 recognizes bacterial DNA and blocking its activity using chloroquine inhibits production of IL-12 by macrophages and dendritic cells.

Diagnosis

As noted earlier, pneumonia associated with Legionnaires' disease may be detected by chest X-ray, however this technique does not reveal which bacterial species is responsible. Several other techniques may more precisely determine the involvement of *Legionella*. The first of these involves bacterial isolation in culture from respiratory secretions (sputum, bronchial alveolar lavage), serum, and lung biopsy and stool samples. The correct nutrients must be present for growth to occur. *Legionella* bacteria form white colonies on buffered charcoal–yeast extract agar. They use amino acids as a carbon source and require supplemental L-cysteine. Most test positive for catalase and β-lactamase and liquefy gelatin. They do not reduce nitrate and test negative for urease and carbohydrate utilization.

Other diagnostic tests employ detection by antigen-antibody reactions. Some of these tests search for the presence of antibodies in serum. One such commonly used technique is indirect fluorescent-antibody assay (IFA). The U.S. version uses antigens prepared from *L. pneumophila* serogroup 1, Philadelphia 1, while the European version uses *L. pneumophila* serogroup 1, Pontiac 1 instead. A rapid microagglutination test is also used to a great extent in Europe. ELISAs additionally detect the presence of IgG, IgM, and IgA antibodies against *Legionella*. These assays require the testing of paired serum samples collected three to six weeks apart. The urine antigen tests detect bacterial antigen in urine samples and are more commonly used currently. Radioimmunoassay (RIA) was used initially to test urine samples, but this was later replaced by ELISAs.

FIGURE 9.5   Colony isolation on buffered charcoal–yeast
extract (BCYE) agar

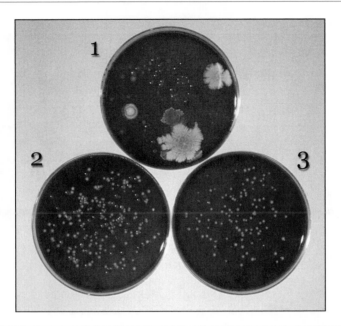

Note: The dish in photo 1 lacks antimicrobial agents—only a few *Legionella* bacteria are present along with many other bacterial colonies. The dish in photo 2 contains the antibiotics polymixin B, anisomycin, and vancomycin—many *Legionella* colonies are present as well as those of several other bacterial species. The dish in photo 3 also contains glycine—the colonies are almost exclusively *Legionella*.

Source: CDC.

The immunochromatographic membrane assay was developed more recently and is similar to home pregnancy tests. Most of these serum and urine tests are both rapid and accurate for *L. pneumophila* serotype group 1 but not sensitive for other *Legionella* species or serotypes, potentially failing to detect as much as 40% of the cases of Legionnaires' disease. The CDC in Atlanta has, however, developed a series of antisera that recognize all known *Legionella* species and subtypes for use in a slide agglutination assay. A broad-spectrum ELISA has also been developed to recognize a larger number of *Legionella* species.

PCR analysis has the potential to spot all infections caused by *Legionella* species. Several of these tests have been developed and recognize random DNA sequences, or the 5S rRNA, 16S rRNA, or the *mip* genes. Samples that have been successfully analyzed by PCR include respiratory secretions, nasopharyngeal swabs, white blood cells, urine, and serum.

FIGURE 9.6 Fluorescent antibody staining to detect the presence of *L. pneumophila*

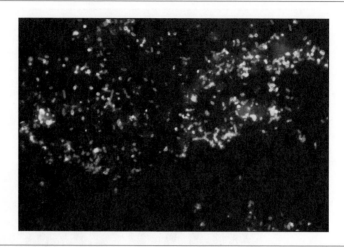

Source: CDC/William Cherry.

Table 9.1 Diagnostic techniques for Legionnaires' disease

Type	Diagnostic Method	Sensitivity[a] (%)	Specificity[b] (%)
Culture	Culture	60	~100
Serology	Slide Agglutination Test	N.D.	N.D.
	Direct Fluorescent Antibody	25–75	>95
	Rapid Microagglutination Test	80	97–99
	IFA—U.S.	78–91	99
	IFA—European	80	N.D.
	ELISA	N.D.	N.D.
Urine Antigen Testing	ELISA	100	100
	Radioimmunoassay	93	100
	Enzyme Immunoassay	90	100
	Immunochromatographic Membrane Test	80	97
Nucleic Acid Testing	Polymerase Chain Reaction—rRNA	31–67	99

Note: N.D. = not determined.
[a]Proportion of positives that are accurately identified (i.e., false negatives avoided).
[b]Proportion of negatives that are accurately identified (i.e., false positives avoided).

Treatment

Due to the generalized antibiotic susceptibility of *Legionella* species , the mortality rate for Legionnaires' disease declined during the 1990s. Drugs commonly used belong to the macrolides or quinolones groups. Of these, erythromycin was the drug of choice. Recently, however, azithromycin drugs have been found to be more active in vitro and have fewer side effects. Azithromycin and fluoroquinolone and levofloxacin are FDA-licensed for use in Legionnaires' disease. Tigecycline is a novel glycylcycline antibiotic that is well tolerated in humans. It is nearly as effective as erythromycin and slightly less effective than azithromycin against intracellular *L. pneumophila* in vitro. Interestingly, unlike erythromycin and azithromycin, this drug is more active against other species of *Legionella* than it is against *L. pneumophila*, suggesting that it may be particularly useful in treating disease caused by infection with these less commonly encountered species. In the guinea pig model of Legionnaires' disease, tigecycline was able to prevent death from pneumonia but was not able to clear the bacteria from the animal's lungs. In vitro data do not support the use of rifampin, doxycycline, or tetracycline, and they are not recommended for the treatment of Legionnaires' disease.

If treatment is begun promptly, the outcome is usually favorable, especially in the absence of underlying illnesses. In individuals with compromised immune responses, delayed treatment may result in prolonged illness or death. Even after discharge from the hospital, many patients continue to experience fatigue and difficulty in concentrating for months, but recovery is usually complete within a year.

Prevention

Legionellosis is often a preventable disease. Three requirements are necessary for human infection to occur: the presence of *Legionella* bacteria in an aqueous environment, bacterial numbers reaching a critical infectious number, and transmission to a susceptible human via aerosol. First, one of the most effective means of preventing the serious consequences of *Legionella* infection is to stop smoking cigarettes. (Pipe and cigar smoking, with their lower levels of inhalation, do not appear to be risk factors.) Cigarette smoking is the primary risk factor in healthy people, increasing their risk of disease to 3.4 times that of nonsmokers. Second, in order to reduce the chance of acquiring infection with *Legionella* bacteria from cooling towers, it is prudent to wear a HEPA-filtered mask when cleaning or collecting water samples from these structures. Third, several means exist for reducing infection by nosocomial routes. For persons using respiratory equipment, rinses should be performed with sterile, not distilled, water. Hospitals may need to raise water temperatures at the fixtures to 48.9°C (120°F) in spite of the increased risk of scalding.

Several methods of water treatment are available that may temporarily eliminate free-living bacteria. Heat-and-flush disinfection involves raising water temperatures in hot water tanks beyond 60°C (140°), followed by flushing through all outlets for up to 30 minutes. This may prove effective for weeks to months. In one medical center in Taiwan, however, 66% of the intensive care units were contaminated ten days after two rounds of heat-and-flush treatment. High levels of chlorine (20–50 mg/L) may be added and flushed through water systems for temporary disinfection; however, this is corrosive to copper and steel pipes. Lower levels (1–2 mg/L) may be used continuously in drinking water, but *Legionella* bacteria are known to survive 10 minutes in the presence of 2.5 milligrams per liter of free chlorine. These lower levels are also of limited effectiveness against bacteria in biofilms. In a recent study of 96 buildings in Florida, chlorine treatment was not as effective as monochloramine (20% of sites colonized with *Legionella* versus 6%). Highly reactive chlorine dioxide gas may also be dissolved in water and is active over a wide pH range. It functions as an oxidizer but is not as harmful to piping as chlorine. It is active on biofilms at concentrations as low as 0.2 milligrams per liter. The major obstacles to its use are cost and the requirement for on-site generation.

Ultraviolet (UV) irradiation (250–280 nm) is used to damage bacterial DNA. UV lamps act as point sources to rapidly kill bacteria in water flowing through the unit. Suspended solids, biofilms, and scaling of the UV lens reduce the effectiveness of this method. Ozone (1–2 ppm) is a strong oxidizer and may be dissolved in water by a generator. It has a very short half-life, however, and may damage piping. Ozone does not work well against bacteria in biofilms or living in protozoa. Another option is to install copper-silver electrode ionization chambers on hot-water lines. When current is applied, these positively charged ions are released to bind to and disrupt negative sites on the bacterial membrane. Scaling and pH levels greater than 8 reduce effectiveness of these chambers. They also cannot be used on cold-water lines.

The following routine practices help decrease contamination of plumbing systems with *Legionella*. Reduce or eliminate dead legs (dead-end pipes not easily flushed with water). Clean hot-water tanks at least once a year. Store hot water at above 60°C (140°F), and set tap water temperature to 50°C (122°F) or higher. Store and deliver cold water at less than 20°C (68°F). Flush the entire water system regularly. Routine treatment of drinking water with biocides may also be useful.

Table 9.2 Water treatment options to decrease
Legionella contamination

Method	Treatment	Drawbacks
Heat-and-flush decontamination	↑ water temperature in hot-water tanks beyond 140°F; flush 30 minutes	Not always effective
High levels of chloride	Flush pipes with 20–50 mg/L	Corrosive to copper and steel pipes
Low levels of chloride	Add 1–2 mg/L to drinking water	Bacteria may survive in biofilms
Monochloramine gas	Dissolve in water	Cost-prohibitive; must be generated on-site
Ultraviolet irradiation	Pass water through units with UV lamps	Suspended solids, biofilms, and scaling reduce effectiveness
Ozone	Use generator to dissolve gas in water	Short half-life, damaging to pipes, limited activity in biofilms
Copper-silver electrode ionization chamber	Apply current to hot-water pipes	Scaling and high pH reduce effectiveness; not useful on cold-water pipes

Surveillance

The United Kingdom began its national surveillance program for Legionnaires' disease in 1977, after the production of serological tests for the bacteria. By 1985, more than 1,200 cases were reported during investigations of outbreaks in England and Wales. Between 1979 and 1985, some 129 to 209 cases were reported per year, resulting in 11 to 37 deaths with an overall case fatality ratio of 6% to 12%. Men were affected more than twice as often as women. Over 40% of the cases of disease occurred in persons over the age of 60 years, an additional 27% occurred in those between the ages of 50 and 59, and few infections occurred in those under the age of 20. Laboratory reports of infection peaked in September, particularly in the 37% of persons infected outside of the United Kingdom. Many of the outbreaks were associated with hotels or hospitals.

Recent surveillance efforts for Legionnaires' disease have focused on rapidly identifying travel-associated cases using an extensive European surveillance network. This has successfully linked cases to specific high-risk premises, such as hotels. This network quickly communicates intelligence concerning suspected clusters and permits timely alerting of the travel industry and national control and enforcement agencies in order to take prompt remedial actions. In 2005, the U.S. Council of State and Territorial Epidemiologists produced a position statement that recommended enhanced surveillance measures for Legionnaires' disease, emphasizing diagnosis and reporting of confirmed travel-associated cases within a seven-day time frame. They found that 23% to 35% of the cases of Legionnaire's disease in the United States during 2005 and 2006 were related to travel. The CDC is notified of all cases of legionellosis through the National Notifiable Diseases Surveillance System, which collects demographic information such as the patients' age and state of residence but not their travel history. After 1980, states had the option of using a supplementary reporting system, which collects information related to diagnostic testing, location of disease acquisition (such as community or hospital), and travel.

Critical reviews of surveillance data indicate the wet cooling towers used by industries as important sources of community-acquired legionellosis. Placing data acquired from individual organizations in a large multiagency intelligence pool may improve the development of strategic policies for long-term prevention efforts. Such data may include the location, type, and state of maintenance of cooling towers in addition to the occurrence of community-acquired cases of Legionnaires' disease. This information may be combined with molecular bacterial-typing methods in order to pinpoint the source of outbreaks or sporadic cases. This may involve proactively asking local health authorities in areas where wet cooling towers are in use to monitor the date of the last satisfactory maintenance inspection.

Summary

Diseases

- Legionnaires' disease   •   Pontiac fever

Causative Agents

- *Legionella pneumophila*   •   *L. longbeachae*

Agent Type

- Gram-negative motile rod form of the γ-2 subdivision of the family *Proteobacteria*

Genome

- DNA

Vector

• None

Common Reservoir

• Amoebas

Modes of Transmission

• Inhaling aerosols or aspirating contaminated water from systems producing aerosols, sprays, or mists, including hot-water tanks set at too low temperature, whirlpools, hot tubs, showerheads, humidifiers, tap-water faucets, air-conditioning system cooling towers, ice machines, grocery store misting machines, ventilators, and nebulizers   • Contact with contaminated potting soil

Geographical Distribution

• Temperate areas, including North America, Europe, Japan, and Australia

Year of Emergence

• 1976

Key Terms

Biofilms Assemblages of bacteria encased in extracellular polymeric matrices adhered to surfaces or phase boundaries

Legionella longbeachae Bacterium in potting soil that may cause Legionnaires' disease

Legionella pneumophila Most common causative agent of Legionnaires' disease and Pontiac fever

Legionnaires' disease Severe multisystem disorder resulting from infection by *Legionella* species, often characterized by pneumonia

Pontiac fever Mild, self-limiting illness resulting from infection by *Legionella* species

Review Questions

1. What are the symptoms of Legionnaires' disease?
2. What type of microbial agent causes Legionnaires' disease? Briefly describe it.

3. How might nosocomial or waterborne transmission of Legionnaires' disease be prevented?

4. What are the roles of IL-12 and IFN-γ in immunity to *Legionella pneumophila*?

5. What types of cells or organisms are involved in the life cycle of *Legionella*?

Topics for Further Discussion

1. IFN-γ is a key to resolving infections with *Legionella pneumophila*. White blood cells taken from infected persons produce lower levels of this cytokine than cells from normal people upon stimulation with the macrophage cytokine IL-12, however, but respond normally to added IFN-γ. Discuss the potential benefits of administering IFN-γ directly to persons with Legionnaires' disease. Research any known adverse effects of such IFN-γ therapy, and include this information in your discussion.

2. Infection with *Legionella longbeachae* may be acquired by exposure to potting soil. Research the ingredients of potting soil, and discuss which of these may harbor the bacteria. Because the route of transmission of this bacterial species differs greatly from that of *Legionella pneumophila*, different areas of the human body may host these bacteria. Research the location of *L. longbeachae* in the body and any diseases with which it is associated.

3. To save money and fossil fuel resources as well as to prevent scalding, homeowners are sometimes urged to lower the temperature of their water heaters. Discuss the potential consequences of this action on human health, particularly for households containing elderly persons, infants, or persons with respiratory disorders, including asthma, chronic bronchitis, and emphysema.

4. The year 1976 was an exceptional one for the emergence of infectious diseases. In addition, many people died that year in massive flooding in China. Discuss potential underlying climatic or geological causes for the large number of human deaths in that year. Were these conditions linked with the emergence or reemergence of other diseases in other years? Explore whether any of these conditions were present during flu pandemic or plague years.

Resources

Archer, K. A., and Roy, C. R. "MyD88-Dependent Responses Involving Toll-Like Receptor 2 Are Important for Protection and Clearance of *Legionella pneumophila* in a Mouse Model of Legionnaires' Disease." *Infection and Immunity*, 2006, *74*, 3325–3333.

Centers for Disease Control and Prevention. "Legionnaires' Disease Associated with Potting Soil: California, Oregon, and Washington, May-June 2000." *Morbidity and Mortality Weekly Report*, 2000, *49*, 777–778.

Chen, Y. S., and others. "Abbreviated Duration of Superheat-and-Flush and Disinfection of Taps for *Legionella* Disinfection: Lessons Learned from Failure." *American Journal of Infection Control*, 2005, *33*, 606–610.

Fernandez-Morcira, E., Helbig, J. H., and Swanson, M. S. "Membrane Vesicles Shed by *Legionella pneumophila* Inhibit Fusion of Phagosomes with Lysosomes." *Infection and Immunity*, 2006, *74*, 3285–3295.

Fields, B. S., Benson, R.F., and Besser, R. E. "*Legionella* and Legionnaires' Disease: 25 Years of Investigation." *Clinical Microbiological Reviews*, 2002, *15*, 506–526.

Koide, M., and others. "Isolation of *Legionella longbeachae* Serogroup 1 from Potting Soils in Japan." *Clinical and Infectious Diseases*, 1999, *29*, 943–944.

McDade, J. E., Brenner, D. J., and Bozeman, F. M. "Legionnaires' Disease Bacterium Isolated in 1947." *Annals of Internal Medicine*, 1979, *90*, 659–661.

Moore, M. R., and others. "Introduction of Monochloramine into a Municipal Water System: Impact on Colonization of Buildings by *Legionella* spp." *Applied and Environmental Microbiology*, 2006, *72*, 378–383.

Murray, S. "Legionella Infection." *Canadian Medical Association Journal*, 2005, *173*, 1322.

Newton, C. A., and others. "Role of Toll-Like Receptor 9 in *Legionella pneumophila*–Induced Interleukin-12 p40 Production in Bone Marrow–Derived Dendritic Cells and Macrophages from Permissive and Nonpermissive Mice." *Infection and Immunity*, 2007, *75*, 146–151.

Piao, Z., and others. "Temperature-Regulated Formation of Mycelial Matlike Biofilms by *Legionella pneumophila*." *Applied and Environmental Microbiology*, 2006, *72*, 1613–1622.

Sporri, R., and others. "MyD88-Dependent IFN-Gamma Production by NK Cells Is Key for Control of *Legionella pneumophila* Infection." *Journal of Immunology*, 2006, *176*, 162–171.

CHAPTER 10

PULMONARY TUBERCULOSIS AND MULTIDRUG RESISTANCE

LEARNING OBJECTIVES

- Define tuberculosis and describe the emergence of drug-resistant forms of the disease
- Describe the mycobacterium responsible for causing this illness
- Discuss modes of infection
- Discuss the host's response to infection
- Describe symptomatology and diagnosis
- Discuss potential methods of treatment
- Discuss methods of prevention

Major Concepts

Incidence

Tuberculosis (TB) is an ancient enemy, plaguing humans for over 7,000 years and affecting every region of the world. Some populations are afflicted more than others, with socioeconomic factors playing a large role in disease prevalence in that crowded living conditions and poor sanitation contribute to transmission of the causative bacterium. Latin America, Africa, and Asia have high incidence of infection. In the United States, residents of homeless shelters, migrant farmworker camps, prisons, some nursing homes, mental health facilities, and large urban centers have higher risk of infection. Infection is also more common among Hispanics and persons of African descent than among Caucasians. Disease incidence dramatically decreased in the 1940s due to increased sanitation, improved general health, higher socioeconomic status, and the discovery of effective chemotherapeutic drugs. The victory was temporary, however, and infection numbers rose again in the mid-1980s. Weakened immune status due to the AIDS pandemic, combined with inadequate health care in many regions of the world and the spread of drug-resistant strains of bacteria, contributed to TB's reemergence. Currently, 2 to 3 million deaths occur each year, making TB the single leading infectious cause of death in persons older than 5 years. One-third of humanity is latently infected with the TB bacilli—a huge reservoir of potential bacterial transmission.

Symptoms

TB is typically acquired by inhaling bacilli found in small aerosolized respiratory droplets produced when persons with active disease cough, sneeze, talk, laugh, or sing. Oral transmission previously played a large role in the spread of disease, but has greatly decreased due to declining numbers of infected cattle and routine pasteurization of milk. Following airborne infection, bacteria enter the lungs, are ingested by alveolar macrophages, escape destruction in the phagolysosome, and multiply in the cell's cytoplasm or extracellularly. The ensuing inflammatory reaction causes immune cells to wall off the area, forming tubercles. Cells and bacilli then disintegrate, forming a homogeneous, coagulated mass that may persist for prolonged periods of time. The area is often encapsulated by collagenous material, slowing bacterial growth and containing the infection, which then passes into a latent form. In 5% to 15% of infected individuals, active disease develops at some later time due to reactivation of formerly dormant tubercles. The lesion's center liquefies and oxygen-rich air may flow into the cavity, rapidly accelerating bacterial growth. Bacilli disseminate throughout the lungs and may spread to other organs, including the lymph nodes, bones and joints, kidneys, or brain. Symptoms of active TB are chronic cough, dull and aching chest pain, coughing up of blood or sputum, shortness of breath, malaise, weakness and fatigue, weight loss, loss of appetite, chills, fever, and severe night sweats. The mortality rate of untreated active disease is 50%.

Infection

TB is caused by several species of mycobacteria, usually *Mycobacterium tuberculosis*, but *M. bovis*, the *M. avium* complex (MAC), *M. africanum*, or *M. microti* may also cause the disease. All these bacteria are nonmotile, noncapsulated, non-spore-forming, acid-fast bacilli that prefer environments similar to alveolar air. Mycobacteria are slow-growing organisms with a unique colony appearance and unusual growth requirements in vitro.

Treatment and Resistance

Treatment of TB involves long-term administration of combination therapy with drugs such as streptomycin, isoniazid, rifampin, pyrazinamide, para-aminosalicylic acid, ethambutol, viomycin, kanamucin, or capreomucin. Drug resistance rapidly arose, first to streptomycin and then to isoniazid and rifampin. Mycobacterial strains resistant to both rifampin and isoniazid and sometimes other drugs are designated as multidrug-resistant TB (MDR-TB). Rates of MDR-TB increased sharply in the early 1990s due to the dismantling of public health infrastructure, increased numbers of persons in homeless shelters or prisons, the AIDS epidemic, inadequate infection control procedures in hospitals, and poor practices in prescribing and compliance with anti-TB medications. MDR-TB is now a global concern. Extensively drug-resistant TB (XDR-TB) is also increasing in prevalence and is resistant to at least rifampin, isoniazid, one of the second-line injectable drugs, and a fluoroquinolone. XDR-TB has a much higher mortality rate than TB or MDR-TB.

Introduction

Tuberculosis (TB; also formerly known as *consumption*) has plagued humankind since antiquity. Once the leading cause of death in the United States, this dreaded disease was dramatically curbed by the discovery of several new drugs in the 1940s. The respite was short-lived, however, and in 1984, TB incidence began to increase again; greater than 25,000 cases were reported in the United States in 1993. The AIDS pandemic and the consequent weakening of large number of persons' immunity have fueled this reemergence, and many TB cases (57%) are found in California, Florida, Illinois, New York, and Texas, where HIV infection rates are high. Throughout the world, 2 to 3 million TB-related deaths occur annually and 8 to 12 million new cases are identified each year. It is currently the single leading cause of death due to infectious disease in individuals over the age of 5 years. Approximately one-third of the world's population is thought to harbor latent TB infection.

TB strikes certain populations more commonly than others. The infection rate in men is twice that in women. Crowded living conditions and poor sanitation contribute to increased incidence of this disease. It is especially common among persons living in homeless shelters, migrant farmworker camps, prisons, and some nursing homes and mental health facilities. TB is particularly problematic throughout Latin America, Africa, and Asia. In the United States, residents of large urban centers are at high risk. In these areas, the infection rate among Caucasians is lower than that among persons of Hispanic or African descent. Socioeconomic factors play an important role, with the least affluent members of society being the most vulnerable.

History

Throughout recorded history, tuberculosis has left its deadly mark. Human bones dating to 5000 B.C. have shown infection. Egyptian mummies also show disease manifestations. Hippocrates described a disease called *phthisis* ("wasting away"), characterized by lung nodules that resembled the tubercles of TB, in 1000 B.C. The major causative bacterium in humans, ***Mycobacterium tuberculosis***, was discovered by Robert Koch in 1882, and two additional species, *M. bovis* and *M. avium*, were recognized by 1900. These also cause disease in cattle and birds. Several other related atypical types of mycobacteria also causing lung disease were discovered by the 1950s.

TB has left a trail throughout the history of the Western world; it was a common cause of death from the Middle Ages until the early 1800s. During the seventeenth and eighteenth centuries, it is believed to have caused 20% to 30% of the deaths in London. Brought to the Americas by European colonists, TB soon wreaked havoc in the New World. In several large U.S. metropolitan areas, TB infection was responsible for 300 to 400 deaths per 100,000 population between 1812 and 1880; the toll decreased to 245 per 100,000 in 1900, 119 in 1920, 69 in 1932, and just 5 in 1970. Much of the decrease in numbers of infected individuals and deaths, especially in developed areas, resulted from increased sanitation, general health, and socioeconomic status followed by the discovery of effective chemotherapeutic drugs. Incidence increased again in the 1990s due in part to the AIDS pandemic, lack of adequate health care in portions of the world, and increased prevalence of drug-resistant strains.

At various times in the nineteenth and twentieth centuries, sanatoriums became popular among people who were able to afford them. Patients in these institutions lived for extended periods of time in isolation, receiving bed rest, sunshine, and nutritious foods. Exposure to fresh, often cool, air was stressed, and sanatoriums were therefore often located in alpine settings, where patients sat outside covered with blankets. Mammoth Cave, with its chill environment, once housed a sanatorium. In 1892, Hermann Briggs, the New York City health commissioner, implemented a program to decrease TB in that city by reporting cases, stressing proper disposable of lung discharges, and education.

TB influenced and affected many aspects of human history. In the arts, the heroines of *La Bohème* and *Moulin Rouge* suffered from this disease. Dostoevski's *Crime and Punishment* and Upton Sinclair's *Jungle* both featured TB. A number of prominent people succumbed to this infection, including Frédéric Chopin, Henry Thoreau, John Keats, Emily Brontë, Elizabeth Barrett Browning, Robert Burns, Alexander Pope, Cardinal Richelieu, John Calvin, Andrew Jackson, Eleanor Roosevelt, Alexander Graham Bell, and Louis Braille.

The Disease

Although TB is usually associated with infection of the lungs, it may attack any part of the body. Because this disease generally relies on airborne transmission, bacteria settle initially in the lungs and may later spread via the circulatory system to other organs, such as the kidneys, lymph nodes, joints, spine, or brain. Transmission usually occurs by inhalation of aerosolized droplets containing the causative species of mycobacteria. Such droplets are produced by individuals with active lesions when they cough, sneeze, talk, laugh, or sing. Those droplets containing viable bacilli, which are only a few micrometers in diameter, may remain suspended in the air for up to 30 minutes. Only a few bacteria are needed to initiate infection via this route. Larger particles tend to deposit in the upper respiratory tract and are often expelled. Other means of transmission are currently much less common, and the bacteria are readily killed by drying or exposure to sunlight. These characteristics inhibit the usefulness of mycobacteria as bioterrorist agents. Crowded living conditions and poor hygienic practices, including failure to cover one's mouth when coughing or sneezing, facilitate transmission. Transmission via the oral route through the ingestion of cow's milk was far more common in the past until tuberculosis in cattle was brought under control and milk was routinely pasteurized. Infection via this route requires ingestion of a large number of bacteria.

Once in the body, bacilli travel to the alveoli of the lungs, where some are phagocytized by alveolar macrophages and multiply in their cytoplasm. Other bacteria multiply outside the cells. Infection induces an inflammatory reaction, and the alveoli fill up with fibrin, additional macrophages, and neutrophils (other phagocytic immune system cells). Bacteria may escape from the local focus and travel via the pulmonary lymph nodes to other areas of the lungs. The neutrophils are later replaced by more macrophages, and lymphocytes are recruited into the area. Small inflammatory lesions then evolve into productive walled-off areas named **tubercles** with a peripheral region of lymphocytes and a central area of Langerhans cells, epithelioid cells, and multinucleated giant cells. The latter two cell types are derived from activated macrophages that have altered their shape to become epithelioid cells, some of which then fuse to form giant cells. The few bacilli present dwell in the epithelioid cells. Formation of multinucleated giant cells also occurs during HIV infection. Later, as a delayed-type hypersensitivity reaction develops, **caseation** may occur, characterized by the disintegration of cells and bacilli and the formation of a homogeneous, coagulated mass with a cheeselike appearance that may persist for years. Often the area undergoes **inspissation**, becoming encapsulated by collagenous material, and bacterial growth rate slows as the infection is contained by the host's immune response. During subsequent years, calcium salts may deposit in these lesions, forming Ghon complexes that may be detected by chest X-rays.

In some individuals, infection may later reactivate in formerly dormant caseous lesions and progress to the liquefaction stage of chronic cavitary pulmonary TB, in which the centers of the tubercles becomes liquid, providing a rich growth medium for the bacteria and accelerating their growth. Often the bronchus erodes as the surrounding lung tissue becomes involved. The liquid contents of the tubercle then drain out of the lesions, and the tubercle may subsequently undergo **cavitation**, in which the center is transformed into an air-filled abscess, the tuberculous cavity, and exposure to oxygen-rich air leads to rapid bacterial growth.

Under normal conditions, primary lesions and noncaseous tubercles heal spontaneously. After caseation, however, lesions seldom resorb. If the primary lesions are not localized, the disease may disseminate, spreading through the lungs. A heavy load of bacilli in the lungs may enter the lymphatic and circulatory systems, spreading throughout the body and leading to the development of **miliary TB lesions** in other organs, including lymph nodes, bones and joints, and the kidneys. When such lesions occur in the brain or meninges, the extremely serious tubercular meningitis may develop.

Most infections with TB assume a latent form, and only 5% to 15% progress to active infection. In its latent form, TB causes no symptoms and the individual does not feel ill. Although these latently infected people do react positively for TB by the commonly used skin test, they are not able to spread the infection. Such individuals may later develop active TB without proper treatment and serve as potential disease reservoirs.

Some individuals rapidly develop an active form of the disease after their initial infection. Such **progressive primary tuberculosis** occurs most commonly in children under the age of 5 years and in persons with weakened resistance to mycobacterial infection. Other individuals progress to an active form of the disease when their immune response is unable to control the bacterial infection adequately. Those at high risk include people who are infected with HIV or have received immunosuppressive therapy and those with diabetes, cancer of the head and neck, leukemia, kidney disease, or low body weight. Active disease has a 50% mortality rate when untreated.

Active TB often causes a number of respiratory symptoms, including a chronic cough (usually productive) lasting more than two weeks, dull and aching chest pain, coughing up of blood or sputum, and shortness of breath. Other symptoms include malaise, weakness and fatigue, weight loss, loss of appetite, chills, fever, and severe night sweats.

FIGURE 10.1   Advanced bilateral tuberculosis

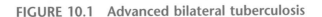

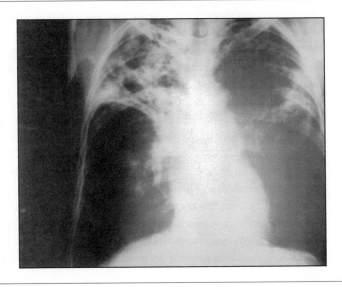

Source: CDC.

The Causative Agents

TB results from mycobacterial infection, most commonly *Mycobacterium tuberculosis;* however, other bacilli, such as *M. bovis,* the *M. avium* complex (MAC), *M. africanum,* and *M. microti,* may also cause this disease. MAC is particularly problematic in HIV-positive individuals. **Mycobacteria** have several unusual properties. *M. tuberculosis* bacteria are nonmotile, noncapsulated, non-spore-forming bacilli, 1 to 4 micrometers long by 0.3 to 0.5 micrometer in diameter. They are **acid-fast bacteria**, requiring the application of heat or surface-acting agents to absorb the dye fuchsin and resisting decoloration by alcohol solutions of mineral acids. Other mycobacteria also cause disease in humans, including leprosy and Buruli ulcer, both of which may disfigure infected persons and, in the case of leprosy, lead to their physical and social isolation and death.

These bacteria are **obligate aerobes** (requiring oxygen for growth) and grow best in environments similar to alveolar air. For growth in the laboratory, the addition of 5% to 10% CO_2 to the air is preferred. *M. tuberculosis* grows very slowly, requiring 18 to 24 hours to divide. (By comparison, *E. coli* divide every 30 minutes.) Rather than becoming grossly visible after one to two days, as is the case for many bacteria, *M. tuberculosis* colonies require three to four weeks. The colonies are cream-colored, dry, and wrinkled. They also undergo cord formation as growth occurs in a serpentine manner and is indicative of virulence.

FIGURE 10.2 *Mycobacterium tuberculosis*

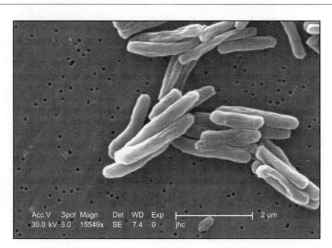

Source: CDC/Ray Butler.

FIGURE 10.3   *M. tuberculosis* with acid-fast stain

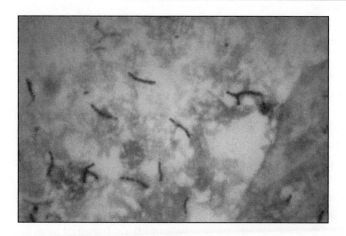

Source: CDC.

Culturing *M. tuberculosis* in the laboratory requires special care. Colonies are cultured in either complex medium containing eggs and potato extract or in Middlebrook 7H-11 agar with oleic acid and albumin.

The Immune Response

During the course of infection, B lymphocytes produce TB-specific antibodies. These appear to have little to no protective activity, arguing for a minimal role of humoral immunity in host defense. Several days after inoculation of an infected individual with extracts of the TB bacteria, however, a vigorous delayed-type (Type IV)hypersensitivity reaction develops, which is the basis of the Mantoux test (described later in this chapter). This response is a double-edged sword, being responsible for both protective immunity and for most of the pathogenic tissue damage. Two cell types that are keys to this reaction are Th1 $CD4^+$ T lymphocytes and macrophages. The Th1 cells encounter TB antigens, proliferate, and produce chemokines and other cytokines, including migration inhibitory factor, which allows macrophages to accumulate in large numbers at the infection site.

Macrophages typically ingest bacteria into phagocytic vacuoles that fuse with acidic lysosomes. The resultant phagolysosomes contain hydrolytic enzymes and reactive oxygen and nitrogen species that normally kill the bacteria within them. In the case of TB, however, macrophages successfully ingest the bacilli but are usually unable to kill them due to their ability to escape destruction in the phagolysosome. Rather than eliminating the mycobacteria, macrophages instead serve as hosts for subsequent intracellular bacterial growth and, upon their lysis, release large numbers of bacteria. Another cytokine produced by T lymphocytes is IFN-γ, which increases phagocytosis and production of hydrolytic enzymes by macrophages, thus aiding in bacterial killing. IL-12 is also present in high levels in the lungs of TB patients and is important in the activation of the Th1 T lymphocytes.

In addition to their role in phagocytosis, macrophages are key players in tubercle formation, which serves to contain the bacteria and prevent their spread to other areas of the lungs. Within these tubercles, macrophages release concentrated amounts of lytic enzymes outside of the cells in order to kill extracellular bacteria. During this process, the surrounding healthy tissue within the tubercle is damaged, resulting in caseation. In individuals with continued, chronic bacterial growth, Th1 cell and macrophage activation persists long-term, and the caseous lesions liquefy, amplifying bacterial growth and spread. One of the major causes for the necrotic inflammatory reaction is the cytokine TNF-α.

Detection and Diagnosis

Because TB is such a prevalent infection throughout the world, rapid, simple means of detection are required to screen large numbers of people in order to clear infection while in the latent form before progression occurs to active disease, which is both pathogenic and contagious. Rapid detection of drug-resistant strains is also important in order to devise correct drug regimens that will inhibit the emergence of MDR-TB and XDR-TB strains. Two large-scale screening procedures are commonly used. The first of these uses chest X-rays to detect lung lesions, which in adults are typically located in the apical or posterior portions of the upper lobes.

The second screening method is the **Mantoux tuberculin skin test**. This immunological reaction uses purified protein derivative (PPD) of bacterial origin. PPD is injected beneath the skin of the lower arm. Individuals exposed to *M. tuberculosis* develop a Type IV hypersensitivity reaction to the bacterial protein which is measured two to three days later. A positive test consists of an area of raised, reddened skin more than 10 millimeters from the injection site. Individuals must have been infected for several weeks to give a positive reaction using this test. Health care workers, especially those in contact with individuals with compromised immune systems, are screened prior to beginning a job and at intervals thereafter. This protects patients from infection and allows detection of infections that the workers may have acquired on the job.

FIGURE 10.4   Mobile tuberculosis testing clinic, 1963

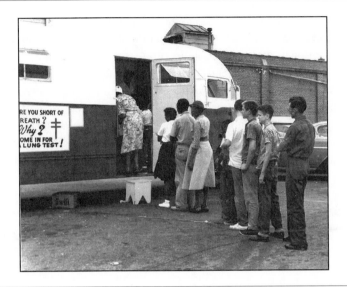

Source: CDC.

FIGURE 10.5   Measuring the extent of the hypersensitivity
reaction during a Mantoux tuberculin skin test

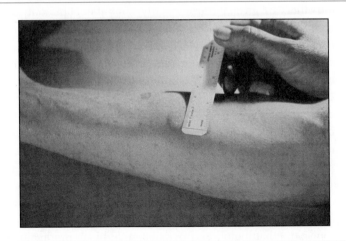

Source: CDC/Gabrielle Benenson.

Bacterial isolation and identification from sputum, body fluids, or tissue are important diagnostic tools based on the culture of correct species of acid-fast bacilli. Infection with *M. tuberculosis* may be differentiated from that of other *Mycobacterium* species based on several criteria. *M. tuberculosis* colonies are rough, grow slowly, and are unable to produce yellow or orange pigment in the dark or after light exposure. *M. tuberculosis* additionally produces niacin and reduces nitrate. They are highly pathogenic for guinea pigs but not rabbits. In strains that are highly resistant to isoniazid, catalase activity and virulence to guinea pigs is reduced or absent, and they exhibit poor cord formation. Mycobacterial species also differ in tests measuring catalase activity and hydrolysis of Tween 80. Serological tests and typing with bacteriophage may also be used in order to differentiate *Mycobacterium* species.

Inexpensive tests are needed to determine drug resistance of a given patient's isolate. One such newly described test is the malachite green microtubule assay (MGMT). This test is based on a change in color as a result of bacterial metabolism. While retaining the sensitivity of other assays, the MGMT assay requires 15 days to complete, compared to 70 days for the standard culture assays, and is less expensive.

Treatment and Drug Resistance

Several drugs have been successfully used to treat TB infection or disease. Treatment regimens are lengthy because the bacilli's intracellular location decreases access to the drugs. Some anti-TB compounds are administered orally and others are given intramuscularly; a number commonly cause nervous system or renal complications. Streptomycin, which inhibits bacterial protein synthesis in the ribosome, was the first practical antibiotic active against *M. tuberculosis* infection. Isoniazid or rifampin is used to prevent latent infections from evolving into active disease. Rifampin blocks bacterial RNA synthesis by inhibiting RNA polymerase. Drug resistance occurs readily as a result of mutations in this enzyme that prevent drug binding. The introduction of this drug allowed treatment regimens to be shortened to nine and then six months, especially for children or adults coinfected with HIV. Consuming alcohol during treatment with isoniazid is dangerous and may be problematic because TB is more prevalent among alcoholics than the general population.

Some other drugs that have been developed to treat TB include pyrazinamide, para-aminosalicylic acid, ethambutol, viomycin, kanamucin, and capreomucin. Isoniazid, ethambutol, and pyrazinamide block production of components of mycobacterial cell walls such as mycolic acid (a lipid) and lipoarabunomannon (a lipopolysaccharide). Mycolic acid is restricted to *M. tuberculosis* and is responsible for much of the disease pathology due to its role in tubercle formation. Isoniazid must be activated by bacteria, and this process involves catalase, which is not present in most other mycobacterial species. Drug-resistant strains have arisen with inactive catalase or with alterations in enzymes involved in mycolic acid synthesis. Pyrazinamide requires bacterial activation by the enzyme PZase. In resistant bacteria, this enzyme has lowered activity levels. In susceptible bacteria, pyrazinamide's activity is increased by the acidic environment of the phagolysosome.

Usually, several drugs must be taken concurrently in order to eliminate all of the bacteria and to decrease the emergence of drug-resistant strains. Acquired drug resistance arises from the enhanced drug-induced selection of resistant bacteria already present at low levels in mycobacterial populations as a result of random mutations. Approximately 1 in 100 million bacilli is naturally resistant to rifampin and 1 in 1 million organisms for isoniazid. Improper drug use or single-agent therapy allows resistant bacteria to proliferate after the more prevalent susceptible organisms have been eliminated, thus allowing the resistant organisms to predominate.

Originally used as a single agent, streptomycin gave rise to resistant strains soon after it became available in 1944. Streptomycin was then paired with isoniazid, whereupon strains resistant to the latter also rapidly appeared in the early 1950s. In the 1970s, rifampin was introduced in the United States, and by the mid-1980s, resistance to that drug was reported in several locations around the world. Strains resistant to both rifampin and isoniazid and sometimes other drugs are designated multidrug-resistant tuberculosis (MDR-TB). A sharp rise in the incidence of MDR-TB and nonresistant TB occurred in the early 1990s in New York City and Florida as the public health infrastructure was dismantled, the numbers of persons occupying homeless shelters and in prison rose, and AIDS became more widespread. Other factors influencing the increased prevalence of MDR-TB include inadequate infection control procedures in hospitals and the faulty prescribing of anti-TB medications.

MDR-TB has become a global concern. A study of the prevalence of this form of the disease in 35 countries conducted by the World Health Organization (WHO) in 1994 found that 7% to 22% of TB cases were MDR-TB. Parts of eastern Europe, China, southern Africa, and the former Soviet Union have a high proportion of such cases. MDR-TB generally has a worse outcome and is more difficult to manage than the ordinary disease. Owing to the fact that the infection rate with TB is quite high in some regions (450 per 100,000 in Delhi, India), the absolute numbers of MDR-TB cases is also high. Prisons in portions of the Soviet Union in 1994 had infection rates of 4,000 per 100,000, and

20% of those were MDR-TB. The frequency of MDR-TB rose in the following decade and continues to rise in many parts of the world. In a 2006 report from South Africa, 41% of the TB cases were classified as MDR-TB and 24% as extensively drug resistant (XDR-TB). The latter form is resistant to at least rifampin, isoniazid, one of the second-line injectable drugs, and a fluoroquinolone. Among individuals in South Africa infected with XDR-TB, 98% rapidly progressed to death. Between 2000 and 2004, the WHO and the CDC found that 2% of the MDR-TB isolates tested throughout the world were XDR-TB, most frequently in eastern Europe, western Asia, and South Korea but also throughout the Americas, including the United States. XDR-TB is not a single strain but multiple strains which have arisen in multiple locations at multiple times.

Contributing to the health risks associated with TB is the fact that no new classes of anti-TB drugs have been introduced since the rifamycins in the 1970s, and little new developmental work is being undertaken. Because the majority of TB cases occur in economically underdeveloped areas of the world, pharmaceutical companies have little incentive to invest the vast sums of money required to develop and test new types of drugs. Vaccines protect persons in affluent areas as well as developing regions, and their development is proceeding.

To decrease the chance of MDR-TB and XDR-TB strains becoming increasingly predominant, it is vital for patients to strictly follow their drug regimen over its entire course. Patients do not always comply due to the length of treatment, complications such as nausea, and the improvement in their general sense of well-being within several weeks of drug initiation. Drug resistance due to noncompliance has become common in Southeast Asia, Latin America, Haiti, and the Philippines and is more likely to occur in HIV-positive persons, who require a much longer treatment regimen, and alcoholics, as isoniazid should not be taken with alcohol. In an effort to prevent noncompliance, directly observed therapy, short-course (DOTS), in which health care providers supervised individuals while taking their medications, was implemented. This led to a cure rate of up to 85% in some settings. MDR-TB strains, however, have reduced responsiveness to standard short-course chemotherapy, resulting in increased periods of transmission as well as increased mortality rates. The WHO has therefore adopted the DOTS-Plus strategy to study feasibility and cost-effectiveness of regimens containing second-line drugs for the treatment of MDR-TB. Factors other than noncompliance that have led to the emergence of MDR-TB and XDR-TB strains include poor prescribing practices and low drug quality or irregular availability. Furthermore, some second-line anti-TB drugs are widely used to treat other infections. Since many individuals have latent infection with *M. tuberculosis*, this practice selects for TB bacteria that are resistant to those drugs and may have serious consequences if the infection subsequently progresses to active disease.

Prevention

Most susceptible to infection are people who live in close quarters with poor sanitary practices, such as those in large, poverty-stricken urban centers; homeless shelters; prisons; nursing homes; mental health care facilities; and refugee camps. Measures that decrease overcrowding, improve housing, and increase general hygiene and health status have been shown to reduce TB transmission.

No truly effective vaccine is currently available to prevent infection with *M. tuberculosis.* One vaccine widely used since 1921 in many areas of the world with high rates of infection is BCG (bacillus Calmette-Guérin), an attenuated strain of *M. bovis.* This vaccine is fairly protective against the development of extrapulmonary TB, but it varies widely in its usefulness in preventing the pulmonary form of the disease, with reported rates of 15% to 80% efficacy. It is not safe for immunosuppressed people, limiting its utility in areas of the world with high numbers of HIV-positive individuals, such as Africa and Southeast Asia. Also, after vaccination with BCG, individuals temporarily score as infected using the Mantoux skin test. This vaccine effectively removes one of the most important means of detecting TB infection from the public health arsenal. For these reasons, BCG is not commonly used in the United States.

RECENT DEVELOPMENTS

A regulatory subset of lymphocytes, Treg, negatively regulates the immune response to various infectious diseases while decreasing inflammation through the production of IL-10 and TGF-β. A recent report found that removal of these cells from *M. tuberculosis*–infected BALB/c mice raised IFN-γ levels. BCG immunization efficacy was increased in mice lacking Tregs. Removal or inactivation of these cells or their cytokines may also increase the usefulness of this vaccine for humans.

Several new vaccines are currently under development. One of these, a genetically altered live BCG vaccine, rBCG30, that overexpresses an immunodominant antigen, is in phase I clinical trials. This is more protective than the parental BCG. Another new vaccine, BCG::RD1, is based on the premise that BCG is "too attenuated." BCG::RD1 has the RD1 region-of-difference gene reinserted. This vaccine induces a stronger immune response but is also more virulent than BCG, which is especially problematic for HIV-positive persons. A third vaccine being tested is rBCG::_ureC-llo_ vaccine, a urease-deficient BCG that is unable to suppress phagosome maturation and is hoped to be less virulent and perhaps safer for use in immunosuppressed individuals. Booster vaccines and postexposure vaccines for those harboring latent infection are also under consideration.

Surveillance

In 1994, the Global Project on Anti-Tuberculosis Drug Resistance Surveillance was established by the World Health Organization and the International Union Against Tuberculosis and Lung Disease. Its mission was to monitor the extent of drug resistance and to chart its trends over time in 58 different geopolitical settings representing 33% of the world's population. Resistance was differentiated as occurring in new cases or previously treated individuals. Work was performed using the Global Network of Supranational Reference Laboratories as well as some national reference laboratories. Estonia had the highest proportion (37%) of MDR-TB among new cases, and Iran had the highest (48%) among previously treated individuals. Drug resistance in a given area was associated with HIV-positive status and inversely correlated with gross domestic product per capita and the proportion of TB cases under DOTS chemotherapy. Several countries, including Iran and the United States, showed significantly higher proportions of MDR-TB in immigrant populations than among indigenous residents.

In a 2007 study, rates of *M. tuberculosis* and HIV infection were determined among residents living in shacks in an overpopulated area of sub-Saharan Africa with an unemployment rate in excess of 50%. Individuals with TB were diagnosed by microscopy of sputum samples and by culture for *M. tuberculosis*. This study identified a number of undiagnosed individuals with TB, the majority of whom were also HIV-positive. Screening for TB based on symptoms was found to be inadequate.

Other epidemiological studies have included examination of TB incidence in immigrant populations, diabetics, residents of former Communist countries, smokers, and heath care workers. These studies used clinical databases, laboratory or molecular diagnosis, questionnaires, and global informational surveys.

Summary

Diseases

- Pulmonary tuberculosis • Multidrug-resistant tuberculosis • Extensively drug-resistant tuberculosis

Causative Agents

- Mycobacterium tuberculosis (most common cause) • *M. bovis*
- Members of the *M. avium* complex • *M. africanum* • *M. microti*

Agent Type

- Nonmotile, noncapsulated, non-spore-forming acid-fast bacillus

Genome

- DNA

Vector

- None

Common Reservoir

- Humans

Modes of Transmission

- Inhalation of aerosolized particles
- Orally via ingestion of contaminated milk (rare)

Geographical Distribution

- Worldwide

Year of Emergence

- Ancient
- Mid-1980s
- Circa 2000

Key Terms

Acid-fast bacteria Bacteria that require the application of heat or surface-acting agents in order to absorb fuchsin and resisting decoloration by alcohol solutions of mineral acids

Caseation Formation of a homogeneous, coagulated mass with a cheeselike appearance during TB

Cavitation Transformation of a TB tubercle into an air-filled abscess in which exposure to oxygen-rich air leads to rapid bacterial growth

Inspissation Encapsulation of a TB tubercle by collagenous material, slowing the bacterial growth rate as the infection is contained by the host's immune response

Mantoux tuberculin skin test Immunologic assay to detect infection with *M. tuberculosis*

Miliary TB lesions Lesions occurring in organs outside the respiratory tract, including lymph nodes, bones and joints, kidneys, and the brain and meninges

Mycobacteria Nonmotile, noncapsulated, non-spore-forming acid-fast bacilli

Mycobacterium tuberculosis Most common causative agent of human tuberculosis

Obligate aerobes Organisms that require oxygen for growth

Progressive primary tuberculosis Active form of disease developing rapidly after the initial infection; occurs most often in children under the age of 5 years and in individuals with weakened resistance to mycobacterial infection

Tubercle Walled-off region of the lungs produced by the immune system to contain growth of *M. tuberculosis*

Tuberculosis Severe, chronic disease that typically affects the respiratory system; characterized by the formation of tubercles containing inactive or active bacilli of *Mycobacterium Tuberculosis* or other similar pathogenic mycobacteria

Review Questions

1. Which populations have the highest incidence of TB infection? What risk factors are involved in these groups?
2. What is the course of progressive tubercular disease?
3. In what ways may the immune response to TB be both protective and pathogenic?
4. What drugs and combinations of drugs are currently used in the treatment of TB?
5. What are MDR-TB and XDR-TB?

Topics for Further Discussion

1. Considering that a very large percentage of the world's population is infected by *Mycobacterium tuberculosis*, what measures might the world health community and national and local health care agencies take to decrease the number of infected individuals and prevent the progression of disease to an active form in individuals already infected?
2. Given the harmful interactions between HIV and *M. tuberculosis* in disease progression and transmission, discuss means of increasing life span and quality of life for persons who are coinfected, especially in regions of the world where infection with both organisms is at epidemic levels, such as sub-Saharan Africa.
3. Numbers of MDR-TB and XDR-TB cases are increasing worldwide. What steps might be taken to halt this ominous development?

4. *Mycobacterium* species have been responsible for much human suffering and many deaths throughout history by causing TB, AIDS-related pathology, and leprosy. These bacteria have several unusual characteristics. How might these be used to develop drugs that specifically target organisms such as *M. tuberculosis*, the *M. avium intracellular* complex, and *M. leprae*?

Resources

Doherty, T. M., and Andersen, P. "Vaccines for Tuberculosis: Novel Concepts and Recent Progress." *Clinical Microbiology Reviews*, 2005, *18*, 687–702.

Farnia, P., and others. "Colorimetric Detection of Multidrug-Resistant or Extensively Drug-Resistant Tuberculosis by Use of Malachite Green Indicator Dye." *Journal of Clinical Microbiology*, 2008, *46*, 796–799.

Harris, H. W., and McClement, J. H. "Pulmonary Tuberculosis." In P. D. Hoeprich (ed.), *Infectious Diseases: A Modern Treatise of Infectious Processes* (2nd ed.). New York: Harper & Row, 1977.

Jaron, B., Maranghi, E., Leclerc, C., and Majlessi, L. "Effect of Attenuation of Treg During BCG Immunization on Anti-Mycobacterial Th1 Responses and Protection Against *Mycobacterium tuberculosis*." *PLoS ONE*, 2008, *3*, e2833.

Kindt, T. J., Goldsby, R. A., and Osbourne, B. A. *Kuby Immunology* (6th ed.). New York: Freeman, 2007.

Lawn, S. D., and Wilkinson, R. "Extensively Drug Resistant Tuberculosis." *British Medical Journal*, 2006, *333*, 559–560.

Salyers, A. A., and Whitt, D. D. *Revenge of the Microbes. How Bacterial Resistance Is Undermining the Antibiotic Miracle*. Washington, D.C.: ASM Press, 2005.

Wood, R., and others. "Undiagnosed Tuberculosis in a Community with High HIV Prevalence: Implications for Tuberculosis Control." *American Journal of Respiratory Critical Care Medicine*, 2007, *75*, 87–93.

World Health Organization. *Anti-Tuberculosis Drug Resistance in the World, Report No.2: Prevalence and Trends*. Geneva, Switzerland: World Health Organization, 2002.

Zager, E. M., and McNerney, R. "Multidrug-Resistant Tuberculosis." *BMC Infectious Diseases*, 2008, *8*, 10.

CHAPTER 11

EMERGING BACTERIAL DRUG RESISTANCE

LEARNING OBJECTIVES

- Define several prominent drug-resistant bacteria and the diseases associated with them

- Describe the processes responsible for drug resistance

- Discuss modes of action of various classes of antibiotics

- Discuss potential methods of treating infection with drug-resistant bacteria

- Discuss methods of preventing the emergence of drug resistance

Major Concepts

Drug Resistance

Drug resistance is becoming a major problem in the treatment of infectious diseases. Several of the important types of resistant bacteria are discussed in this chapter. The first of these are drug-resistant strains of *Staphylococcus aureus*. Some of these bacteria (MRSA) have become resistant to penicillin, methicillin, and cephalosporins, and perhaps to aminoglycosides and fluoroquinones as well. These bacteria may be either hospital-associated or community-associated. The former often affect individuals in a weakened state or the immunosuppressed (persons who are hospitalized; persons undergoing long-term health care, dialysis, or surgery; cancer patients; and the elderly). The latter affect children in day care facilities; athletes, especially those participating in high-contact sports; prisoners; members of the military; and men who have sex with men. Vancomycin-resistant enterococci, especially *Enterococcus faecium*, are responsible for nosocomial infections. Drug resistance is due to factors found on a plasmid. This plasmid has been also acquired by some strains of *S. aureus*. *Escherichia coli* have developed resistance to a number of drugs, including aminopenicillins, narrow-spectrum cepalosporins, and third-generation cephalosporins and monobactams due to their acquisition of β-lactamase and extended-spectrum β-lactamase enzymes. Increasing numbers of *Pseudomonas aeruginosa* isolates are resistant to extended-spectrum cephalosporins, carbapenems, aminoglycosides, and fluoroquinolones. Penicillin resistance is also becoming more common among *Streptococcus pneumoniae* strains.

Modes of Antibiotic Action

Antibiotics use several mechanisms of action to kill bacteria or inhibit their growth. Some of these drugs interfere with synthesis of bacterial cell walls, such as the β-lactams and the glycopeptide agents. Other drugs, such as the macrolides, chloramphenicol, clindamycin, quinupristin-dalfopristin, linezolid, tetracyclines, and aminoglycosides, inhibit protein synthesis by binding to bacterial 30S or 50S ribosomal subunits. Some antibiotics block DNA or RNA synthesis. Such drugs include fluoroquinolones, sulfamethoxalone, the folic acid analogue trimethoprim, and rifampin. Another category of drugs, including polymyxins and daptomycin, acts by disrupting the bacterial plasma membrane.

Processes Leading to Drug Resistance

Drug resistance may arise by several mechanisms. These include the production of enzymes that degrade the drugs, efflux pumps that extrude drugs from the bacteria, changes in the drug's target site, alterations in metabolic pathways, or down-regulation of the expression of the porin gene. Some of the more common resistance elements include β-lactamases, which cleave β-lactam antibiotics; the *mecA* gene, which induces resistance to β-lactam drugs by not binding to them; the *VanX*, *VanH*, and *VanA* or *VanB*, which alter the bacterial cell wall so that it no longer binds vancomycin; *P. aeruginosa* multidrug efflux pumps; and erythromycin ribosomal methylase, which inactivates erythromycin.

Prevention

Overuse or incorrect use of antibiotics is partly responsible for the rapid rise of antibiotic resistance. To avoid giving a survival advantage to resistant bacterial strains, programs need to stress compliance with prescribed drug dosage, frequency, and duration. Decreasing prophylactic use in agriculture and in personal care products may decrease the ability of resistant clones to dominate the bacterial population. The proper use of gloves and gowns, particularly by individuals in acute care settings or in contact with draining wounds, blocks transmission of hospital-associated MRSA. Hand-washing should be stressed following visits to hospitals or long-term care facilities. Covering wounds with dry bandages prevents transmission of community-associated MRSA. Personal care items should not be shared. Athletic equipment shared by multiple individuals should be cleaned with antiseptics before use. New drugs are continuing to be tested for activity against drug-resistant bacteria.

Introduction

The introduction of antibiotics and other antimicrobial compounds revolutionized medical treatment of infectious diseases, leading some observers to declare victory in the lengthy war against these illnesses. The proclamation proved to be premature, for microbes demonstrated impressive abilities to escape killing or inactivation by these drugs. In populations of bacteria and other microbes, various clones exist that are resistant to the actions of different drugs. After exposure or improper exposure to these drugs, the more susceptible organisms are killed and the more resistant organisms tend to survive and may come to dominate the population under certain circumstances due to their increased fitness (greater ability to survive and reproduce). Many bacterial resistance elements are contained either singly or in groups within mobile genetic elements (discussed later in this chapter) that may enable rapid transmission of multiple drug resistance genes. As microbial populations develop resistance to existing drugs, humans have responded by producing new drugs. The microbes subsequently find means of evading these drugs, forcing humans to search for more novel agents in the continuing evolutionary waltz of life.

Increased incidence of drug resistance is currently a rapidly growing phenomenon in many types of organisms, including viruses, bacteria, protozoa, and insects. Separate chapters deal with this phenomenon in several organisms, including HIV, tuberculosis, and malaria. In bacteria, genes encoding products that allow bacteria to escape drug actions (**resistance genes**) often exist on plasmids, circular pieces of extrachromosomal DNA. These genes may also be found in transposons and integrons. These three genetic elements are readily passed between bacteria of the same as well as different species, allowing intra- and interspecies spread of resistance elements.

Bacteria may pass resistance genes to other organisms during the processes of conjugation, transformation, or transduction. During **conjugation** in gram-positive bacteria, DNA is exchanged between a mating pair of microbes. In gram-negative bacteria, plasmids are transferred to nearby bacteria in an act that often involves elongated pili that join the microbes together. **Transformation** involves the acquisition of DNA from other bacteria that have previously lysed and released their DNA into the external environment. During **transduction**, **bacteriophages** (viruses that infect bacteria) transfer genetic material between bacteria. These mechanisms may lead to **multidrug resistance**, the acquisition of resistance to three or more drugs, an increasing cause for concern, especially in health care settings.

Human actions may aid in the development of drug resistance. Such actions include noncompliance with instructions regarding the completion of a course of medication and the overuse of antimicrobial drugs in both humans and agriculture.

History

Antibiotics revolutionized the treatment of infectious diseases of bacterial origin. Older antimicrobial compounds included toxic compounds, such as mercury and arsenic derivatives; gramicidin, discovered by the work of René Dubos and Rollin Hotchkiss; and sulfanilamide. The first antibiotic was penicillin, produced by the fungus *Penicillium notatum* and discovered almost accidentally by Sir Alexander Fleming in 1928. Two Australian scientists, Howard Florey and Ernst Chain, found means of producing penicillin in the large quantities necessary for general use. Widespread use of penicillin began in the 1940s, whereupon morbidity and mortality rates from bacterial diseases fell drastically. Military forces during World War II benefited greatly as the number of deaths due to wounds infected with organisms such as *Staphylococcus aureus* and *Streptococcus pyogenes* diminished. Penicillin is itself attacked (hydrolyzed) by the enzyme **β-lactamase**. This enzyme is carried on a plasmid that resided within most strains of *S. aureus* by the end of that war. Currently, 95% of the clinical isolates of these bacteria are penicillin-resistant.

Bacteria soon began to develop resistance to other antibiotics—in 1961, methicillin-resistant strains of *S. aureus* were reported; during the mid-1970s, strains of *P. aeruginosa* developed resistance to extended-spectrum cephalosporins, carbapenems, aminoglycosides, and fluoroquinolones; in 1983, strains of *E. coli* became resistant to penicillin; and the 1990s saw the advent of vancomycin-resistant enterococci. Resistance genes are often contained within mobile genetic elements, allowing rapid transmission between bacteria of the same or different species. Some of these genetic elements have accumulated resistance genes to several drugs, resulting in multidrug resistance. The increased use of antibiotics in human health and in agriculture combined with noncompliance in completion of the course of medication has fueled and accelerated this natural trend in bacterial evolution.

The Diseases, Causative Agents, and Treatment Options

Methicillin- and Vancomycin-Resistant *Staphylococcus aureus*

Staphylococcus species are common bacteria occurring naturally in the environment and in hospital settings. These gram-positive spherical bacteria reside on the skin or in the nasal or pharyngeal passages of 25% to 40% of the general population. They may enter the body's interior through cuts, sores, catheters, and breathing tubes. *S. aureus* is pathogenic, resulting in a wide spectrum of diseases ranging from minor infections of skin or soft tissues to severe sepsis with a high rate of mortality.

Penicillin was the first antibiotic to be highly effective against *S. aureus* infection. As noted earlier, however, penicillin resistance emerged soon after it became widely used. Other antibiotics effective against the β-lactamase-containing bacteria were introduced in the early 1960s and included methicillin and oxacillin. Within a year of their introduction, however, resistant strains of bacteria were reported in the United Kingdom and later in Europe and Australia, occurring in hospitals throughout the world by the 1980s. These strains came to be known as **methicillin-resistant *Staphylococcus aureus* (MRSA)** and were soon found to be resistant not just to methicillin but to all β-lactams, including many penicillins and cephalosporins. Many strains are also resistant to aminoglycosides and fluoroquinones.

MRSA was first reported in the United Kingdom in 1961. Between the 1970s and late 1990s, MRSA slowly began to spread and cause infections, mostly in medical centers or in patients using these facilities. By 2004, some 69% of the staphylococcal isolates in U.S. intensive care units were of the resistant phenotype. Five MRSA clones are responsible for approximately 70% of the current infections.

Infection with MRSA is especially problematic for individuals in a weakened state or immunosuppressed, such as those who are hospitalized; patients undergoing long-term health care, dialysis, or surgery; cancer patients; and the elderly. This type of MRSA is referred to as hospital-associated (HA-MRSA). Risk factors for developing HA-MRSA include exposure to a hospital or long-term health care facility, use of antibiotics within the past year, chronic disease, IV drug use, or close contact with a person having one of these risk factors. HA-MRSA infections usually involve ventilator-associated pneumonia or

FIGURE 11.1   MRSA

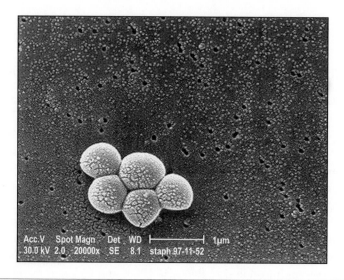

Source: CDC.

bacterial invasion of indwelling venous devices or wounds. Such infections are related to increased length of hospital stay and cost and higher mortality.

Recently, a growing number of MRSA infections have been found in normal, healthy people and are designated community-associated MRSA (CA-MRSA). They are particularly prevalent in Denmark and Switzerland. In one Chicago hospital, the incidence of CA-MRSA rose from 10 cases per 100,000 admissions (1988–1990) to 259 cases per 100,000 (1993–1995). CA-MRSA may be acquired by children in day care facilities and by athletes sharing equipment, including towels and razors. Athletes in high-contact sports, such as wrestling and football, are at particularly great risk. Prisoners, members of the military, and men who have sex with men are also affected. Prison outbreaks may be due to decreased hygiene, limited access to health care, infrequent clothes laundering, and limited access to soap. CA-MRSA predominantly causes infections of pulmonary tissue, bone, and skin and soft tissues and is associated with **Panton-Valentine leukocidin**, encoded by the *pvl* genes and transmitted by bacteriophages. This toxin destroys host neutrophils and causes tissue necrosis. Asymptomatic isolates have a far lower chance of carrying *pvl*.

HA-MRSA and CA-MRSA strains appear to differ. The two have different types of the mobile genetic island, staphylococcal cassette chromosome SCC*mec*, which contains the *mecA* gene conferring methicillin resistance. Due to the frequency of multidrug resistance, HA-MRSA is often treated with vancomycin as a drug of "last resort" despite potential adverse effects, such as nephrotoxicity and "red-man syndrome," a histamine-like reaction. CA-MRSA isolates are often susceptible to non-β-lactam drugs, such as clindamycin, doxycycline, and trimethoprim-sulfamethoxazole. Pathology associated with CA-MRSA infections appears to be somewhat similar to those of community-associated methicillin-susceptible *S. aureus* (CA-MSSA). The *pvl* gene is found in almost all CA-MRSA isolates and 93% of CA-MSSA strains from patients with boils and in 85% of CA-MSSA strains from *S. aureus* pneumonia. These facts have led to the suggestion that CA-MRSA and CA-MSSA share a genetic background, as further evidenced by molecular typing studies.

The range of symptoms of *S. aureus* infection vary widely and include normal infections of the skin, such as red, swollen, or painful areas; abscesses; pus formation; boils; furuncles; and warmth in the affected area. Symptoms of more serious infections include rash, shortness of breath, fever, chills, chest pain, fatigue, myalgia, malaise, and headache. Invasive MRSA infections may result in bacteremia, necrotizing pneumonia, necrotizing fasciitis, cellulitis, endocarditis, **septic shock syndrome** (hypotension, respiratory distress syndrome or failure, and abnormal functioning of the central nervous system, liver, kidneys, or muscles), osteomyelitis, septic thrombophlebitis with pulmonary embolisms,

FIGURE 11.2 Cutaneous lesion due to MRSA infection

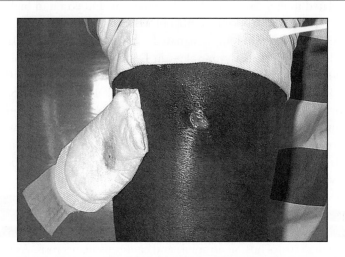

Source: CDC.

septic arthritis, and death. Both HA-MRSA and CA-MRSA infections may be invasive, although the rate is higher with HA-MRSA. Very serious infections may result in MRSA pneumonia or blood poisoning, with high death rates. Influenza virus infection may predispose to lung colonization by CA-MRSA.

MRSA skin infection may be diagnosed by biopsy or by culture of fluid draining from the affected area or the blood. For individuals with pneumonia, cultures of the sputum or urine may be performed. If MRSA is determined to be the cause of a localized skin infection, treatment may involve drainage of the abscess. More serious infections may require intravenous administration of medication, ventilation, or dialysis. Only a few antibiotics effectively treat MRSA infection. Prognosis is dependent on disease severity and the condition of the person's general health. MRSA pneumonia and blood poisoning lead to the highest mortality rates. A number of newer drugs are effective against MRSA infections. These include linezolid, quinupristin-dalfopristin, tigecycline, daptomycin, and cefrobiprole. Dalbavancin and telavancin are two promising new lipogycopeptides.

A troublesome problem has been the development of *S. aureus* strains with an intermediate resistance to vancomycin (VISA). Such isolates contain a thickened cell wall that traps the vancomycin and prevents the drug from reaching its target in the outer plasma membrane. More recently, strains with high-level vancomycin resistance, known as **vancomycin-resistant *Staphylococcus*** *aureus* (**VRSA**), are being reported. Five isolates have been found in the U.S. since 2002. VRSA arises from a determinant carried by a plasmid originating from *Enterococcus faecium*. Several newer drugs that are active against MRSA remain effective against VRSA.

Vancomycin-Resistant Enterococcus

A large increase in the occurrence of infections with **vancomycin-resistant enterococcus** (**VRE**) species occurred in intensive care units in the United States during the 1990s, and VRE species now account for 30% to 70% of enterococcal infections. The bacterial species most often involved is *E. faecium*. VRE species have been fairly uncommon in Europe until recently; however, the incidence of infection with these bacteria is increasing, as evidenced by an outbreak of VanA-type[+] *E. faecium* in a Paris hospital in 2003. These isolates result from nosocomial infection and are not expected to become community-acquired in the future.

As noted earlier, vancomycin resistance is transmitted on a plasmid by genes such as the *vanA* gene and is transferable to other bacterial species, including MRSA strains of *S. aureus*. *VanA* allows alterations to occur in the vancomycin-binding site of the cell wall. Such plasmids have been found in other bacterial species with resistance to many types of antibiotics, leading to multidrug resistance. Usage of extended-spectrum cephalosporins and glycosporins in hospitals may help spread these isolates. VRE infections have a 30% mortality rate.

Several drugs used to treat MRSA retain some usefulness against infection with VRE species. These drugs include linezolid, quinipristin-dalfopristin, tigecycline, and daptomycin, which still have some activity against VRE strains. Lower urinary tract infections are responsive to fosfomycin and nitrofuantoin but are already encountering resistance. Platensimycin, derived from *Streptomyces plantensis*, is active against VRE and MRSA.

Extended-Spectrum β-Lactamase-Producing *Escherichia coli*

E. coli is an intestinal bacterium that is commonly involved in urinary tract infections and bacteremia. Members of this species are frequently resistant to aminopenicillins, such as amoxicillin and ampicillin, and narrow-spectrum cepalosporins as a result of β-lactamases, such as TEM-1, TEM-2, and SHV-1, carried on plasmids. An even more serious development is the bacterial acquisition of **extended-spectum β-lactamase** (**ESBL**), an enzyme that allows resistance to third-generation cephalosporins and monobactams. The **extended-spectrum β-lactamase-producing *Escherichia coli*** may thus survive treatment with a wide range of antibiotics, increasing the difficulty of eliminating some serious urinary tract infections. Resistance to monobactams may have resulted from mutations of a previously acquired β-lactamase; a single amino acid change from aspartate to asparagine in the β-lactamase SHV-1 may have triggered the change in the drug resistance pattern.

Multidrug-Resistant *Pseudomonas aeruginosa*

P. aeruginosa is a gram-negative bacterium of soil and water. These bacteria infect animals and plants and are a major cause of opportunistic infections in immunosuppressed individuals. *P. aeruginosa* infections are normally treated by pseudomonad β-lactams, aminoglycosides, and fluoroquinolones. Recently, however, **multidrug-resistant *Pseudomonas aeruginosa*** (MDR *P. aeruginosa*) have emerged and are becoming increasingly common worldwide. MDR strains are often resistant to expanded-spectrum cephalosporins, carbapenems, aminoglycosides, and fluoroquinolones. These strains are particularly prevalent in Asia, South America, southern Europe, and parts of the Mediterranean. In the United States, 9.9% of *P. aeruginosa* isolates were multidrug-resistant in 2003, compared to 7.1% just two years earlier.

Resistance is partly due to the spread of several types of ESBL from other bacteria, including PER-1 in Turkey, Korea, and China; VEB in South Asia

FIGURE 11.3   Electron micrograph of *Pseudomonas aeruginosa*

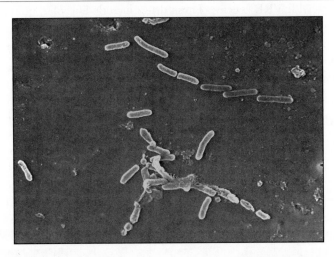

Source: CDC.

and Kuwait; GES in France, Greece, South Africa, and Brazil; and BEL-1 in Belgium. Some of these ESBL are associated with new gene plasticity elements (Re). New strains in South America have the very broad-spectrum carbapenemase enzyme, KPC, from *Enterobacteriaceae*. Another category of carbapenemases that is increasing in frequency consists of members of the metallo-β-lactamase group, present in all inhabited continents. Many of the latter carbapenemases are carried on transmissible elements, such as transposons, integrons, or plasmids. Some isolates have been found to contain both ESBL and metallo-β-lactamase. The β-lactam elements are also found in association with most aminoglycosides. The ARN methylase enzymes are new aminoglycoside resistance genes found in Japan.

Several drugs or drug combinations are being examined for use against MDR *P. aeruginosa*. Colistin is one such drug being tested for use in combination with rifampin. Some derivatives of existing drugs have been considered but have only slightly increased activity against *P. aeruginosa*. These include doripenem and sitafloxacin. Drugs that inhibit efflux pumps are being tested but may prove to be toxic to eukaryotes.

Drug-Resistant *Streptococcus pneumoniae*

S. pneumoniae is a diplococcus that commonly colonizes the pharynx but may invade the lungs, leading to earache in children, infant meningitis, and bacterial pneumonia, the most common cause of death from infectious disease in the United States. Penicillin has been successfully used to treat these diseases, but in 1977 **drug-resistant *Streptococcus pneumoniae*** began to appear that did not respond well to penicillin and other drugs. Drug resistance is increasing, partly in response to their use to treat upper respiratory tract infections. Among adults in the United States, 40% bear penicillin-resistant pneumonococci. Other drugs to which *S. pneumoniae* is developing resistance include erythromycin, trimethoprim-sulfamethoxazole, vancomycin, tetracycline, chloramphenicol, and ofloxacin.

Mechanisms of Resistance

Modes of Drug Action

The mechanisms of action of antibacterial agents fall into five major categories. The first category contains drugs that interfere with synthesis of the bacterial cell walls, such as the β-lactams and the glycopeptide agents. The β-lactams include the penicillins, cephalosporins, carbapenems, and the monobactams.

These drugs interfere with enzymatic activity that synthesizes the bacterial wall's peptidoglycan layer. Glycopeptides include vancomycin and teicoplanin; these inhibit cell wall synthesis by binding to D-alanine-D-alanine residues on the ends of the young peptidoglycan chain, preventing it from cross-linking to form a stable wall structure. The *vanA* resistance determinant changes this terminal structure to D-alanine-D-lactate, lowering vancomycin affinity 1,000-fold.

The second category of drugs function by inhibiting protein synthesis on the basis of differences in structure between bacterial and eukaryotic ribosomes. Eukaryotic ribosomes contain 40S and 60S ribosomal subunits, while bacterial ribosomes bear 30S and 50S subunits. Some drugs, such as the macrolides (erythromycin and azithromycin), chloramphenicol, clindamycin, quinupristin-dalfopristin, and linezolid, bind to the 50S ribosomal subunit, while others, like the tetracyclines and aminoglycosides (streptomycin, amikacin, and neomycin), bind to the 30S ribosomal subunit. Another drug, mupirocin, binds instead to the bacterial isoleucyl-tRNA synthestase.

The third and fourth drug categories interfere either directly or indirectly with nucleic acid synthesis. The fluoroquinolones act by binding to bacterial DNA gyrase, an enzyme that supercoils DNA during its replication. They also target bacterial topoisomerase IV. Sulfamethoxalone and the folic acid analogue trimethoprim inhibit the metabolic pathway for tetrahydrofolic acid synthesis,

Table 11.1   Mechanisms of antibiotic drug action

Major Mechanism of Action	Specific Action	Example of Drug
Interferes with cell wall synthesis	Interferes with cell wall peptidoglycan synthesis	β-lactams
	Prevents cross-linking of peptidoglycans	Glycopeptides
Binds to or interferes with 30S or 50S ribosomal subunits	Binds to 30S subunit	Tetracyclines
	Binds to 50S subunit	Macrolides
Blocks nucleic acid synthesis	Inhibits DNA gyrase and topisomerase	Fluoroquinolones
	Inhibits tetrahydrofolic acid synthesis	Sulfamethoxalone
	Inhibits RNA synthesis	Rifampin
Disrupts bacterial membrane	Increases membrane permeability	Polymyxins
	Depolarizes membrane	Daptomycin

required for DNA production; these two drugs are often used together. Rifampin, by contrast, inhibits synthesis of RNA and may be used in conjunction with trimethoprim and sulfamethoxalone.

Finally, some drugs act by disrupting the bacterial membrane. Polymyxins are believed to increase permeability of the bacterial membrane, causing it to leak the bacteria's contents. Daptomycin is a cyclic lipopeptide that appears to function by causing the membrane to depolarize by inserting its lipid tail into the cell membrane.

Bacterial Resistance Genes

Resistance genes protect bacteria by interfering with drugs' abilities to function. Some encode enzymes that degrade the drugs; others encode efflux pumps that extrude drugs before reaching their targets; still others change the drug's target site or alter a metabolic pathway, enabling the construction of cell walls that lack the drug's binding site. Some mutations also down-regulate the porin gene expression and thus decrease drug access to the intracellular targets.

Several genes and gene products are linked to resistant phenotypes. The β-lactamases cleave and inactivate β-lactam antibiotics, such as penicillin. After developing newer β-lactam drugs with reduced ability to bind β-lactamases, β-lactamases mutated in such a manner as to gain the capacity to degrade the newer drugs. These modified bacterial enzymes are the aforementioned ESBLs. The β-lactamases are inhibited by clavulanic acid. Augmentin is a combination of the β-lactam amoxicillin and clavonic acid.

MRSA strains contain the *mecA* gene on the *SCCmec* genetic island, encoding a modified penicillin-binding protein, PBP2a, allowing resistance to β-lactam drugs by not binding to them. *MecA* is regulated by the MecR1 and MecI proteins. The former binds to the β-lactam antibiotics followed by the proteolytic cleavage of the latter, resulting in derepression and transcription of the *mecA* gene. SCC*mec* type II in HA-MRSA strains contains genes inducing resistance to non-β-lactam antibiotics, such as the *ermA* gene, conferring resistance to erythromycin and either inducible or constitutive resistance to clindamycin. CA-MRSA strains often bear SCC*mec* type IV that contains *mecA*, but not other resistance genes. They may also produce ESBLs and metallo-carbapenemases.

Vancomycin resistance involves the action of three enzymes. VanX removes one D-alanine from the D-alanine-D-alanine that binds vancomycin. VanH converts pyruvate to lactate. VanA or VanB forms D-alanine-D-lactate, which is not bound by vancomycin.

P. aeruginosa bacteria often contain multidrug efflux pumps that work in concert with the limited permeability of this species's outer membrane. The *P. aeruginosa* membrane contains both an outer membrane and a cytoplasmic membrane. Its efflux pump contains three proteins, a pump in the cytoplasmic membrane (such as MexB), a porin in the outer membrane (such as OprM) and a joining protein (such as MexA). Four major efflux systems are found in *P. aeruginosa*: MexAB-OprM, MexXY-OprM, MexCD-OprJ, and MexEF-OprN. The first two of these are associated with intrinsic multidrug resistance, whereas overexpression of MexXY-OprM or MexCD-OprJ is involved in acquired resistance.

Other bacteria have evolved other means of resistance. One example is the erythromycin ribosomal methylase of *Staphylococcus* species, an enzyme that inactivates erythromycin. Another means of drug resistance is the loss of OmpF by *E. coli*, which removes the outer membrane protein porin channel that allows entry of cephalomycins into the microbe.

RECENT DEVELOPMENTS

Under development are new analogues of existing drugs that have lower potential for bacterial resistance. One of these is telavancin, derived from vancomycin. This drug is active against MRSA strains, and its efficacy in the treatment of skin infections is equal or superior to standard drugs.

Another newer drug is daptomycin, derived from fermentation of *Streptomyces roseosporus*. This compound is active against most gram-positive bacteria, including *Listeria,* resistant bacteria like MRSA and VRE, and rarer gram-positive organisms, such as corynebacterium and some bacillus species. It acts in a novel manner by destroying bacterial membrane potential without lysing the cell wall. In the proposed mechanism, calcium binds to daptomycin in the cytoplasmic membrane, leading to conformational changes with insertion into the plasma membrane and oligomerization. This builds channels, inducing membrane leakage and loss of intracellular potassium. Daptomycin appears to be less susceptible to the development of resistance; however, some resistant strains have been seen in vitro by over 20 passages in the presence of the drug. Clinical resistant isolates have been reported with mutations in the *mprF* or the *yycF* genes. Some strains of *Staphylococcus aureus* are also cross-resistant to vancomycin and daptomycin, even though they have not been exposed to the latter drug. Daptomycin has been FDA-approved for infections of skin and soft tissues, bacteremia, and right-side endocarditis and is clinically effective in the treatment of MRSA, VRE, and drug-resistant pneumonococci.

Diagnosis

Antibiotic resistance may be determined by assessing susceptibility of bacteria to a panel of antimicrobial agents. One assay is the disk-diffusion test, in which bacterial growth is recorded on agar plates in the vicinity of disks impregnated with different dosages and types of antibiotics. The D-zone form of this test uses erythromycin and clindamycin disks to detect the presence of an inducible *erm* gene by the appearance of a D-shaped bacterial clearance zone around the latter disk. In the microbroth dilution minimal inhibitory concentration test, a constant number of bacteria are inoculated into wells of a plate containing different dilutions of the antibiotic. Killing is indicated by a decrease in turbidity in the wells. This allows the determination of bacterial susceptibility in a quantitative manner.

Molecular typing techniques are also useful. Pulsed-field gel electrophoresis patterns allow grouping of organisms into types, assessments of relatedness of strains during outbreaks, and examination of rapidly occurring evolutionary events in *S. aureus*. Slower evolution may be assessed by multilocus sequence typing. Polymerase chain reaction may be used to determine the presence of toxicity genes, such as staphylococcal enterotoxins, toxic shock syndrome toxin 1, and Panton-Valentine leukocidin, and resistance genes, such as *mec*.

FIGURE 11.4   Measuring antibiotic resistance: A clearance zone appears around bacteria susceptible to antibiotics on the disks

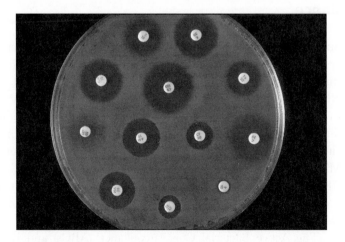

Source: CDC/J. J. Farmer.

Prevention

Prevention of MRSA requires good personal hygiene practices, as close contact with an infected person is a risk factor for infection with microbes such as MRSA. Gloves and gowns should be used by health care workers, especially in acute care setting or when draining wounds. Hands should be washed frequently following visits to hospitals or long-term care facilities. Wounds should be covered with dry bandages, for the presence of skin abscesses or spider bite sites are risk factors for MRSA. Personal care items should not be shared. Athletic equipment shared by multiple individuals should be cleaned with antiseptics before use. In several countries, including France and Belgium, HA-MRSA rates have either stabilized or decreased as a result of implementation of these practices combined with patient isolation and careful decontamination procedures. Use of intranasal mupirocin ointment decreases *S. aureus* colonization of the nose; however, recolonization is fairly rapid, and widespread prophylactic use may induce the development of resistance.

A recent history of antibiotic use is a risk factor for MRSA. Compliance with prescribed drug dosage, frequency, and duration decreases the development of drug resistance. Recent trends of indiscriminate antibiotic use, including prophylactic applications in agriculture and in personal care products such as soaps, may contribute to the selection and outgrowth of resistant bacterial clones.

Surveillance

Surveillance is needed to determine the magnitude of infections with resistant organisms to establish priorities for prevention and control strategies. Such studies of resistance patterns have been conducted by the EMERGEncy ID NET Study Group, among others. In that report, the prevalence of different strains of CA-MRSA were determined in over 400 patients with purulent soft tissue or skin infections from 11 university-affiliated emergency departments in cities from diverse areas in the United States (Oregon, California, New Mexico, Missouri, Pennsylvania, and New York). The majority of the *S. aureus* isolates (78%) were MRSA, and of those, 99% were the CA form. Despite the wide geographical area, 97% of the isolates were represented by one specific type of CA-MRSA, USA300.

The Active Bacterial Core surveillance (ABCs) and Emerging Infections Program Network of the CDC conducted a population-based active-case-finding investigation of the incidence of invasive MRSA in nine sites in California,

Tennessee, Georgia, Maryland, New York, and Connecticut over an 18-month period in 2004 and 2005. Incidence was determined from computerized microbiology databanks and regular telephone calls to microbiology laboratory contacts, census data, and demographic and outcome data. MRSA was considered to be invasive if isolated from a normally sterile body site (blood; cerebrospinal fluid; pleural, pericardial, peritoneal, or synovial fluid; bone; or internal body sites). The CDC identified and stored isolates. From a population of 16.5 million, almost 9,000 cases of invasive MRSA were detected, the majority (85%) of them HA-MRSA and the remainder CA-MRSA. The overall incidence rate was 32 per 100,000. Rates were highest among individuals over the age of 65 years (128 per 100,000) and those of African origin (67 per 100,000). Persons aged 5 to 17 years had the lowest rates of infection (1.4 per 100,000). Another study reported a high risk for children under the age of 2 years, as well as Pacific Islanders and Native Americans. The overall standardized mortality rate was 6 per 100,000, and the populations with the highest incidence rates had the highest mortality rates. Low socioeconomic status and urban residence are associated with higher infection rates. Molecular tests revealed the presence of strains previously associated with CA-MRSA in HA-MRSA cultures in all nine surveillance areas. HA-MRSA strains were most commonly USA100 and USA200, while the CA-MRSA strains were predominantly USA300. Interestingly, 23% of CA-MRSA isolates were USA100 and 16% to 22% of HA-MRSA isolates were USA300.

Summary

Diseases and Causative Agents

- Methicillin- and vancomycin-resistant *Staphylococcus aureus* • Vancomycin-resistant enterococcus • Extended-spectrum β-lactamase-producing *Escherichia coli* • Multidrug-resistant *Pseudomonas aeruginosa* • Drug-resistant *Streptococcus pneumoniae*

Agent Type

- Gram-positive coccus • Gram-negative coccus • Gram-negative rod
- Gram-positive diplococcus

Genome

- DNA

Vector

- None

Common Reservoirs

• None

Modes of Transmission

• Inhalation • Cuts, sores, and catheters

Geographical Distribution

• Worldwide

Years of Emergence

• 1961 • 1990s • 1983 • 1970s • 1977

Key Terms

β-lactamase Enzyme that destroys penicillin and related β-lactam antibiotics

Bacteriophage Virus that infects bacteria

Conjugation Exchange of DNA between bacteria during mating

Drug-resistant *Streptococcus pneumoniae* Any *S. pneumoniae* strain that is resistant to penicillin

Extended-spectum β-lactamase (ESBL) A bacterial enzyme that allows resistance to third-generation cephalosporins and monobactams

Extended-spectrum β-lactamase-producing *Escherichia coli* Any strain of *E. coli* that is resistant to aminopenicillins, narrow-spectrum and third generation cephalosporins, and monobactams

Methicillin-resistant *Staphylococcus aureus* (MRSA) Any strain of *S. aureus* that is resistant to the β-lactam antibiotics

Multidrug resistance Microbes acquire resistance to three or more drugs

Multidrug-resistant *Pseudomonas aeruginosa* Any *P. aeruginosa* strain that is resistant to expanded-spectrum cephalosporins, carbapenems, aminoglycosides, and fluoroquinolones

Panton-Valentine leukocidin Bacterial toxin transmitted by bacteriophages; destroys neutrophils and causes tissue necrosis

Resistance genes Genes encoding products that allow microbes to escape drug actions

Septic shock syndrome Hypotension, respiratory distress syndrome or failure, and abnormal functioning of the central nervous system, liver, kidneys, or muscles

Transduction Bacteriophage transfer of genetic material between bacteria

Transformation Bacteria acquire DNA from other bacteria that have previously released their DNA into the external environment

Vancomycin-resistant enterococcus (VRE) Any strain of *Enterococcus faecium* that is resistant to the antibiotic vancomycin

Vancomycin-resistant *Staphylococcus aureus* (VRSA) Any strain of *S. aureus* that is resistant to the antibiotic vancomycin

Review Questions

1. For *Enterococcus faecium*, (a) name the antibiotics for which resistance has developed, (b) identify the bacterial gene or enzyme responsible for resistance, and (c) discuss the mechanism of resistance for each gene or enzyme.
2. What groups of persons are affected by HA-MRSA and CA-MRSA? How do these strains differ?
3. What are the major methods that bacteria use to escape killing by drugs?
4. What tests are used to detect and quantify bacterial drug resistance?
5. How might the risk of MRSA infection be decreased?

Topics for Further Discussion

1. Seeing that some drug-resistant bacteria use common genetic elements, such as *mecA* and *ermA,* suggest methods that might be used to target the products of those genes and thus defend simultaneously against several resistant isolates.
2. As drug resistance becomes more prevalent, should other means of bacterial control be considered to supplement the drug arsenal? Discuss means of augmenting the immune system, including vaccination, the use of bacteriophages to kill pathogenic bacteria, and disinfectants to eliminate environmental microbial exposure.
3. Poor hygienic practices and low socioeconomic status contribute to the spread of drug-resistant bacteria. What strategies might public health care agencies and workers devise to lower infection rates?
4. The addition of antibiotics to domestic animal feed reduces infection, increases animal health and weight, and boosts food production. It is also believed to contribute to the development of drug resistance. In light of the need to maximize agricultural output to more effectively feed the world's population, is this use of antibiotics wise? What other methods could be practically and affordably used to achieve the desired results without the risks?

Resources

Cottagnoud, P. "Daptomycin: A New Treatment for Insidious Infections Due to Gram-Positive Pathogens." *Swiss Medicine Weekly,* 2008, *138,* 93–99.

Crawford, S. E., Boyle-Vavra, S., and Daum, R. S. "Community-Associated Methicillin-Resistant *Staphylococcus aureus.*" In W. M. Scheld, D. C. Hooper, and J. N. Hughes (eds.), *Emerging Infections* (Vol. 7). Washington, D.C.: ASM Press, 2007.

Klevens, R. M., and others. "Invasive Methicillin-Resistant *Staphylococcus aureus* Infections in the United States." *Journal of the American Medical Association,* 2007, *298,* 1763–1771.

Moran, G. J., and others. "Methicillin-Resistant *S. aureus* Infections Among Patients in the Emergency Department." *New England Journal of Medicine,* 2006, *355,* 666–674.

Nordmann, P., Naas, T., Fortineay, N., and Poirel, L. "Superbugs in the Coming New Decade: Multidrug Resistance and Prospects for Treatment of *Staphylococcus aureus, Enterococcus* spp., and *Pseudomonas aeruginosa* in 2010." *Current Opinions in Microbiology,* 2007, *10,* 436–440.

Salyers, A. A., and Whitt, D. D. *Revenge of the Microbes: How Bacterial Resistance Is Undermining the Antibiotic Miracle.* Washington, D.C.: ASM Press, 2005.

Tenover, F. C. "Mechanisms of Antimicrobial Resistance in Bacteria." *American Journal of Infection Control,* 2006, *34,* S3–S10.

Zhanel, G. G., and others. "Dalbavancin and Telavancin: Novel Lipoglycopeptides for the Treatment of Gram-Positive Infections." *Expert Reviews of Anti-Infectious Therapies,* 2008, *6,* 67–81.

PART
III

VIRAL INFECTIONS

CHAPTER 12

MARBURG AND EBOLA HEMORRHAGIC FEVERS

LEARNING OBJECTIVES

- Define and compare Marburg and Ebola hemorrhagic fevers
- Describe the filoviruses responsible for causing these illnesses
- Discuss modes of infection
- Discuss the host's response to infection
- Describe symptomatology and diagnosis
- Discuss methods of treatment
- Discuss methods of prevention

Major Concepts

Outbreaks

Marburg and Ebola hemorrhagic fevers are diseases of unusual severity and high mortality rates that emerged in the late 1960s and 1970s, respectively. While natural infection of humans and nonhuman primates occurs primarily in Africa, monkeys infected with *Reston ebolavirus* have originated in the Philippines, and their importation led to severe disease in animal colonies in the United States and Italy. Humans contracted fatal cases of Marburg hemorrhagic fever from monkeys brought into Germany and Yugoslavia, and a nonfatal case of infection was reported in the United States in a traveler returning from Africa. Large-scale outbreaks of both Marburg and Ebola hemorrhagic fevers occurred in Africa over the following decades, characterized by fatality rates that at times exceeded 80%, resulting in hundreds of human deaths. Epidemics of Ebola hemorrhagic fever also had a serious impact on populations of some nonhuman primates, such as gorillas, in parts of Africa.

Symptoms

Marburg and Ebola hemorrhagic fevers are similar in clinical presentation and are characterized by chills and high fever; apathy; nausea, vomiting, and diarrhea; disseminated intravascular coagulation leading to depletion of clotting factors; severe hemorrhaging into multiple organs; anemia; multiple organ failure due to loss of tissue oxygenation; shock due to decreased blood pressure; and death. Endothelial cells and monocytes, macrophages, and dendritic cells of the innate immune system are infected by the viruses and produce massive amounts of proinflammatory cytokines that greatly contribute to the pathology. Lymphocyte functions are suppressed by several viral proteins, allowing the viruses to evade the host's defenses. The filoviruses are resistant to killing by IFN-α and IFN-β, two of the key antiviral cytokines, and also inhibit interferon production.

Infection

Marburg and Ebola hemorrhagic fevers are caused by filoviruses. The *Lake Victoria marburgvirus* causes Marburg hemorrhagic fever and the *Zaire, Sudan, Ivory Coast*, and *Reston ebolavirus* species cause Ebola hemorrhagic fever. Infection with *Zaire* and *Sudan ebolavirus* leads to severe disease in humans, whereas *Ivory Coast ebolavirus* has caused only one nonfatal case in humans, and fatal infection with

Reston ebolavirus appears to be restricted to monkeys and apparently does not result in human disease. Filoviruses are enveloped viruses with regularly spaced protruding spikes. Their genome consists of one strand of linear negative-sense single-stranded RNA that contains a unique sequence (UAAUU) at the beginning of start sites and the end of stop sites.

Transmission

Filoviruses are present in high levels in body secretions and may be deposited on the skin by sweating. Marburg and Ebola viruses are transmitted between individuals via droplets of body fluids or through direct contact with infected individuals or objects contaminated with blood or tissue. After recovery, infectious virus may be transmitted sexually for up to seven weeks. Fruit bats are believed be a reservoir host, as infected bats have been captured in western Africa. The indicated species of fruit bats roosts in caves, and many of the outbreaks of Marburg or Ebola hemorrhagic fever have been associated with visits to bat-infested caves or mines.

Protection

Care for persons infected by filoviruses is generally supportive, as proven treatment options are limited. Antiviral compounds have not thus far been effective against these viruses. Administration of heparin, interferon, or human immune serum to patients may or may not increase survival. More recent work has focused on the use of antisense oligonucleotides and short interfering RNA (siRNA) molecules to decrease production of key viral proteins. Other treatment options seek to decrease symptoms such as disseminated intravascular coagulation. Research is progressing in the development of effective antifilovirus vaccines. Other preventive measures involve general improvements in the availability of regional health care and medical supplies and rapid communication to detect and halt outbreaks in their initial stages.

Introduction

Fueled by movies and books such as *Outbreak*, *The Hot Zone*, and *The Coming Plague* and spurred by sporadic media attention, reports of Ebola and Marburg hemorrhagic fevers have generated fear and curiosity among the American public. While such accounts are often presented in a highly dramatic, graphic, and sensational manner, they have succeeded in periodically bringing public attention to the threat of emerging viral infections. Coverage of emerging infections, however, waxes and wanes in accordance with the general populace's attention span, while the threat of emerging diseases continues unabated. The Ebola outbreak of 1995 received a great deal of media coverage, but subsequent large outbreaks in Gabon and Uganda went largely unnoticed by most of the world's press, as were the preliminary stages of the AIDS pandemic in Africa. In addition to the threat of future outbreaks, which may continue to kill hundreds of humans in sub-Saharan Africa, thousands of members of endangered nonhuman primate species, including gorillas, have already died in their sanctuaries in West Africa, further challenging the survival of these animal populations.

History

The first known instance of Marburg hemorrhagic fever (MHF) occurred in 1967 in vaccine production facilities in Marburg and Frankfurt, Germany, and Belgrade, Serbia (at the time, part of Yugoslavia). The outbreak began among 25 persons working with African green (vervet) monkeys from Uganda (primary cases) and later spread to six of their family members or health care workers (secondary cases). Seven of the primary cases died (mortality rate of 28% among primary cases).

Another small outbreak occurred in 1975, originating with a tourist who had a history of recent travel in Zimbabwe and South Africa. Two cases of secondary infection resulted: a traveling companion and a nurse, both of whom survived. In 1980, two persons were infected in western Kenya. These people had visited the Kitum cave, which was believed to be the source of the infection. Later, researchers placed sentinel animals in the cave, but none of them became infected. A large number of different animal species were trapped in the vicinity of the cave (including rodents, bats, insects, grazing animals, and large African cats). These also had no sign of the causative virus. Laboratory tests did find, however, that the virus is able to replicate in experimentally infected bats. *Lake Victoria marburgvirus* (Marburg virus), the causative agent, has subsequently led to disease in several areas of Africa, including Uganda, western Kenya, South Africa, and Zimbabwe. Far more deadly epidemics of MHF occurred among gold miners near Durba in the Democratic Republic of Congo (DRC; formerly Zaire) in 1998–2000, with 154 cases and 128 deaths (mortality rate of 83%) and in the Uige province of Angola in 2004–2005 (374 cases, 88% mortality). An outbreak of MHF also occurred in 2008 in a bat-infested mine in Uganda. Disease spread in many of these outbreaks was amplified by unsanitary injections given in health care centers or private clinics or by self-administration in homes.

RECENT DEVELOPMENTS

Marburg viral RNA and antiviral IgG antibody were detected in a common species of fruit bat, *Rousettus aegyptiacus,* trapped in caves in Gabon in 2005 and 2006. Many of the human cases of MHF have been associated with caves. Unlike most fruit bats, this species is known to roost in caves, and its geographical range includes the locales in which outbreaks of MHF have occurred. This is the first naturally infected nonprimate species thus far identified with this virus and the first detection of the virus in that part of western Africa. This discovery follows the identification of asymptomatic infection of three species of fruit bats with the Ebola virus in Gabon and the Congo Republic in 2004.

The first case of MHF in the United States was detected in a traveler returning to Colorado from a trip to Uganda in January 2008. He had visited the bat-infested "python cave" in Maramagambo Forest, Queen Elizabeth Park, in the western part of that nation. The U.S. tourist recovered; however, another cave visitor from the Netherlands acquired a fatal case of MHF in July of that year. This cave is about 60 kilometers from the Kitaka gold mine, the source of a large disease outbreak in Uganda in 2008. The mine contains large numbers of fruit bats. A band was found in the python cave that had been used to tag a bat from the Kitaka mine, indicating that bats did indeed travel between the two sites.

A similar disease, Ebola hemorrhagic fever (EHF), emerged in 1976 in two simultaneous outbreaks involving over 550 persons in the DRC and Sudan. The mortality rate was very high—88% in Zaire and 53% in Sudan. The outbreak in the DRC began in a missionary hospital in Yambuku, in the vicinity of the Ebola River, and spread rapidly among patients, health care providers, and patients' relatives. The patients were taken to a regional center in Kinshasa. Most of the primary cases (72 of 103, or 70%) were spread by the local hospital via improperly sterilized needles used for multiple patients. Of the persons infected by secondary contact with an infected person, 43% survived, compared to only 7.5% of those infected by a contaminated needle. In that outbreak, the Ebola strain was passed for four generations in humans and then disappeared for no apparent reason.

At approximately the same time, a separate epidemic of this hemorrhagic fever began in Maridi and N'zara in Sudan and rapidly spread to members of the medical staff. This outbreak had a lower mortality rate than that occurring concurrently in the DRC. An investigator in Porton Down, England, was subsequently infected with virus from this outbreak following an accidental injection

FIGURE 12.1   Surveying for infection during the 1976
Ebola outbreak in Zaire

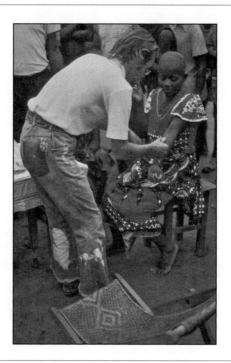

Source: CDC/J. Lyle Conrad.

into his thumb. He was given antifungal medication, interferon, and immune serum and survived the infection. The major risk factors in this outbreak were determined to be the performance of local rituals of preparing relatives' bodies for funerals and association with the regional hospitals (nosocomial spread). Up to 30% of the health care workers became infected in this outbreak. N'zara had a population of approximately 20,000 and was the economic center of the area due to its cotton factory. This factory was infested with bats, rats, boll weevils, and spiders, and all of the early cases were among factory workers. This outbreak passed through at least eight generations in humans. Over 400 miles separated these epidemics in the DRC and Sudan. Due to the extremely poor road conditions at the time, the differences in mortality rates, and differential ability to survive multiple passages in humans, it is unlikely that the disease was spread to Sudan by a person traveling between the two areas; it is more likely that these were separate outbreaks involving different strains of the causative

FIGURE 12.2   Graveyard containing some of the first victims of the Ebola outbreak in Sudan in 1976

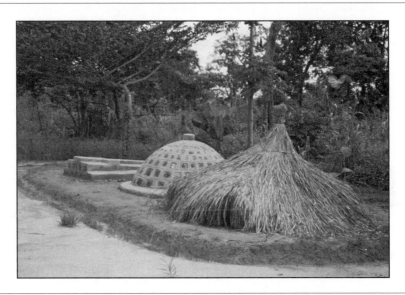

Source: CDC/J. Lyle Conrad.

agent, which were later designated as *Zaire ebolavirus* (Ebola Zaire) and *Sudan ebolavirus* (Ebola Sudan).

A second major epidemic of Ebola Zaire occurred in 1995 in Kikwit, Zaire, about 1,000 kilometers from the site of the previous outbreak. The index case was a surgical patient, and disease spread by nosocomial transmission to health care providers, others in the hospital, and family members, resulting in 245 deaths. In 1996–1997 (Gabon) and 2000–2001 (Gulu, Uganda), large outbreaks involved 98 persons with 66 deaths (67% mortality rate) and 425 people (83% mortality), respectively. EHF has occurred in other parts of Africa, such as the Central African Republic, Nigeria, the Ivory Coast, Liberia, Kenya, Congo Republic, and Cameroon, where antibodies to the virus were found in 15% of the local pygmies. Wild chimpanzees and gorilla populations (including mountain gorillas) have also suffered large losses.

A different subtype of Ebola is named after an outbreak among primates in Reston, Virginia, in 1989. It caused lethal infection of cynomolgus monkeys held in quarantine facilities in Virginia, Texas, and Pennsylvania. Many of the animals became severely ill and died, and the rest were euthanized. Several of the human caretakers were also infected, as evidenced by the production of antibodies, but no humans demonstrated disease symptoms. The monkeys in these outbreaks originated in the Philippines. This strain is known as *Reston ebolavirus* (Ebola Reston), and it is not virulent in humans, although it does share antigenic cross-reactivity with the other Ebola strains. Due to the spread of infection to animals in all parts of the quarantine facility, it is likely that Ebola Reston may have been spread by airborne transmission. On several subsequent occasions during 1989, 1990, and 1996, Ebola Reston killed monkeys in colonies in the United States. These animals had been purchased from the Ferlite Scientific Research monkey farm in the Philippines. Some of the people at the colony in Texas and several of the workers at the facility in the Philippines also produced antibodies to the virus but did not become ill. Ebola Reston was also found in cynomolgus monkeys imported from the Philippines in Italy in 1992.

The fourth subtype of Ebola virus, *Ivory Coast ebolavirus* (Ebola Ivory Coast, formerly Ebola Tai), was found in 1994 in a scientist performing an autopsy on a wild chimpanzee that had died of a hemorrhagic disease in the Tai Forest of the Ivory Coast. She developed a serious acute illness characterized by fever and rash, but no hemorrhage, and survived the infection. No subsequent cases of infection with Ebola Ivory Coast are known to have occurred.

The Diseases

Both the Marburg and Ebola viruses cause serious and often fatal hemorrhagic fever in humans and some nonhuman primates. Pathological responses entail an intense, systemic inflammatory response similar to septic shock, resulting from an overwhelming activation of infected monocytes, macrophages, and dendritic cells, which produce large amounts of proinflammatory cytokines. This hyperactivation of the innate immune system is responsible for much of the subsequent pathology induced by filoviruses. The severity of the symptoms and the high mortality rates associated with these diseases have made them popular topics for the media and for several best-selling movies and books.

Marburg Hemorrhagic Fever (MHF)

Marburg hemorrhagic fever (MHF) has an abrupt onset with severe headache, high fever, chills, and back pain. This is followed by severe watery or bloody diarrhea, abdominal cramping, vomiting, and a rash on the trunk. Severe bleeding (hemorrhaging) occurs from multiple sites, particularly the gastrointestinal tract, gums, eyes, and lungs, within five to seven days of onset. Disease manifestations include jaundice, inflammation of the pancreas, severe weight loss, delirium, central nervous system involvement, terminal shock, liver failure, pulmonary edema, and multiorgan dysfunction. Major lesions may be present in the liver (focal hepatic necrosis), spleen, lymph nodes (follicular necrosis), and kidneys and are accompanied by hemorrhaging in the gastrointestinal tract; the pleural, pericardial, and peritoneal spaces; and the renal (kidney) tubules. Laboratory findings include severe thrombocytopenia, leading to the hemorrhagic manifestations; hemoconcentration; and amylase, blood urea nitrogen, creatinine, and transaminase elevation, with aspartate aminotransferase (AST) greater than alanine aminotransferase (ALT). A profound leucopenia may result from apoptosis of lymphocytes; the resultant drop in immunity may lead to secondary bacteremia. Death may occur after 7 to 16 days due to shock resulting from severe decreases in blood pressure following hemorrhaging. The mortality rate ranges from 23% to 88%. MHF occurs in humans, Old World primates, and guinea pigs but not in mice or New World primates.

Ebola Hemorrhagic Fever (EHF)

Infection with the Ebola Zaire or Ebola Sudan virus results in a disease similar to MHF. Following an incubation period of 2 to 21 days (most commonly, 7 to 14

FIGURE 12.3 Lung pathology due to Marburg virus infection, showing breakdown of alveolar walls, leading to pulmonary edema

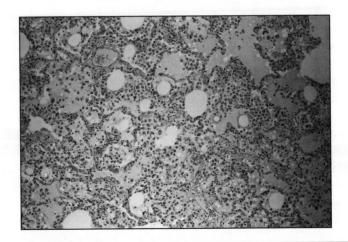

Source: CDC/J. Lyle Conrad.

FIGURE 12.4   Acute tubular necrosis and glomerular fibrin thrombosis in the kidney of a patient with Marburg hemorrhagic fever

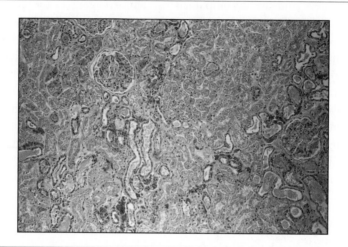

Source: CDC/J. Lyle Conrad.

days), **Ebola hemorrhagic fever (EHF)** begins abruptly and is characterized by fever, chills, anorexia, and muscle aches, followed by nausea, vomiting, sore throat, abdominal pain, nosebleeds, and diarrhea. Affected persons are overtly ill and dehydrated, apathetic, and disoriented. Some patients lose hair, fingernails, and skin. Severe hemorrhaging begins between days 5 and 7, with bleeding from multiple sites, similar to that seen in MHF. Large lesions may be found in the liver, lymph nodes, spleen, and kidneys. Death as a result of shock may occur within one to two weeks in 50% to 90% of infected individuals.

The Ebola viruses interact with liver cells, endothelial cells lining the capillaries, and monocytes, macrophages, and dendritic cells of the innate immune system. Endothelial cells are damaged either directly or via toxic cytokines, such as TNF-α, released from infected macrophages. This causes the capillaries to leak fluids and plasma into the surrounding tissues. **Disseminated intravascular coagulation** may also be present, depleting the blood of platelets and interfering with clotting at other sites. The infected persons then bleed from any orifice, including sites of injection. The loss of fluid from the circulatory system as a result of capillary leakage and hemorrhaging leads to low fluid volume in the blood vessels, decreasing blood pressure and potentially causing the individual to enter into shock. The blood loss also decreases tissue oxygenation and may induce multiorgan failure. In addition to the severe thrombocytopenia resulting

FIGURE 12.5   Histology of liver tissue infected
with Ebola virus

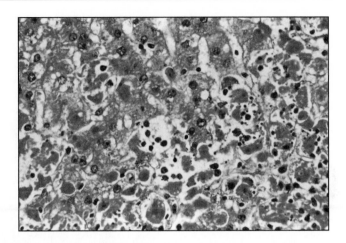

Source: CDC/J. Lyle Conrad.

from disseminated intravascular coagulation, the initial state of lymphopenia may be followed by a dramatic neutrophilia (increased numbers of neutrophils, primarily immature cells).

The Causative Agents

Both Marburg and Ebola viruses belong to the **Filoviridae** family of the order Mononegavirales and are most closely related to paramyxoviruses and rhabdoviruses. Filoviruses are enclosed within a lipoprotein envelope and have pleomorphic shapes ranging from filamentous and branched to simple and, less commonly, spherical. The molecular weight of these viruses is 3 to 6×10^8 kilodaltons. Virion size is 790 to 1400 nanometers in length and 80 nanometers in diameter. Longer virion-related structures approach 10 micrometers. Nucleocapsids contain a dark central space 20 nanometers in diameter surrounded by a helical capsid 50 nanometers in diameter with cross-striations. Knoblike surface projections (7 nanometers) containing the glycoprotein protrude with an even distribution at 10 nanometer intervals over the entire envelope surface. The viral envelope also contains lipids derived from the host cell plasma membrane.

FIGURE 12.6   Electron micrographs of Ebola (left) and Marburg (right) viruses

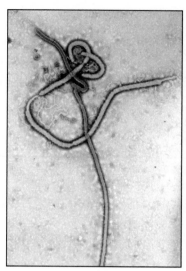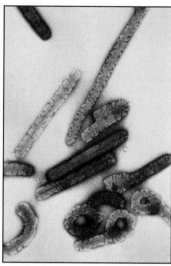

Sources: CDC/F. A. Murphy for Ebola virus image and CDC/Erskine Palmer and Russell Regnery for Marburg virus image.

The viral genome composes 1.1% of the virion and consists of one strand of linear negative-sense single-stranded RNA that is not infectious. The length of the RNA is approximately 19 kilobases, with complementary 5' and 3' sequences. Filoviruses contain the sequence UAAUU at the 5' end of start sites and the 3' end of stop sites; the sequence is unique to this group

Filoviruses contain seven proteins. Four of these are associated with the nucleoprotein complex (the phosphorylated nucleoprotein, L protein, VP35, and VP30). The nucleoprotein is involved in nucleocapsid assembly and budding. The L protein is the filovirus polymerase. It is an RNA-dependent RNA polymerase. VP35 is a component of the transcriptase complex and has a role in evading the immune response. Hexamers of VP30 aid in viral RNA transcription by activating and modulating RNA synthesis and stabilizing the newly formed RNA chain.

The envelope glycoprotein forms the surface projections and mediates viral attachment and entry into host cells. It is also involved in cytotoxicity, down-regulation of host surface proteins, and virus assembly and budding. The glycoprotein is produced in three forms, differing in length, by three different mRNAs. It is a protein that inserts into the plasma membrane of the host cells as a trimer (three protein chains). The carbohydrate portion of this glycoprotein composes over 50% of its molecular weight and consists of N- and O-linked sugars. This glycoprotein does not contain terminal sialic acid residues in the Marburg virus but does in the Ebola virus. The mature form of the surface glycoprotein contains two disulfide-linked subunits, a large extracellular GP1 and a membrane-anchored GP2. A shorter form of the envelope glycoprotein is also produced and is secreted as a homodimer that may have anti-inflammatory properties, while the longer forms of the glycoprotein may instead induce an inflammatory response, similar to the lipopolysaccharide of gram-negative bacteria.

Viruses bind to C-type lectins on host cells; these lectins contain carbohydrate recognition domains. Viral binding to this receptor binding is specific and requires the presence of the calcium ion. When the Ebola virus is grown in some cell types, it lacks the terminal sialic acid but instead ends in galactose. These viruses are able to bind to the asialoglycoprotein receptor on HepG2 liver cells but cannot bind to Vero African green monkey kidney cells, which lack this receptor. The human liver has the asialoglycoprotein receptor; this may explain in part why the Ebola virus is hepatotropic. Marburg and Ebola viruses also use dendritic cell-specific ICAM-3-grabbing nonintegrin (DC-SIGN) and its homologue, L-SIGN, as cellular receptors. The former is expressed on immature dendritic cells and macrophages, and the latter is located on endothelial cells in the liver. These molecules bind high-mannose carbohydrates on a number of viruses, including HIV, and may mediate viral attachment to the cell surface rather than viral entry into the cell. Other C-type lectins believed to bind filoviruses include the human macrophage galactose- and acetylgalactosamine-specific C-type lectin on immature dendritic cell and macrophages and the lymph node sinusoidal endothelial cell C-type lectin on endothelial cells in the lymph nodes and liver.

Filoviruses bind to other receptors on the surface of target cells as well. These include members of the β1 integrin family of adhesion receptors, which mediate attachment of cells to the extracellular matrix as well as to other cells. The viruses also bind to the folic acid receptor α, responsible for transport of folic acid into cells' cytosol. This receptor appears to act as a cofactor for viral entry and is found on many types of cells in a wide variety of species. Other receptors that help mediate cellular infection include the Tyro3 receptor tyrosine kinases Axl, Dtk, and Mer.

Filoviruses apparently use a number of host molecules to attach to and enter target cells, and combinations of these molecules may be required for successful infection of cells. Filoviruses are taken into cells by macropinocytosis or endocytosis, which may or may not involve clathrin- or caveolin-1-coated pits.

Lipid rafts containing cholesterol and glycosphingolipids appear to be involved in the endocytic process. Viruses may also enter macrophages by phagocytosis.

The remaining proteins, VP40 and VP24, compose the matrix. Dimers, hexamers, or octamers of VP40, the major matrix protein, aid in viral assembly and budding by linking the surrounding membrane with viral RNA in the nucleocapsid. They help sequester host RNA as well. VP24 is the minor matrix component but appears to also function in virus assembly and budding.

The amino acid identity between the Ebola viruses and Marburg viruses ranges from 24% to 46%, with the least degree of similarity occurring in the VP40, glycoprotein, and VP30 proteins. Within the Ebola virus subtypes, amino acid identity is higher, ranging from 55% to 81%, with the least amount of similarity found in the glycoprotein.

Filoviruses are present in a number of tissues in the human host, particularly those involved in the immune response. These include the spleen, lymph nodes, liver, and kidney; virus is rarely present in the brain. Replication occurs primarily in monocytes and dendritic cells, key components of the innate immune response. These cells respond by producing large amounts of proinflammatory cytokines. Virus is present in high levels in most body secretions (blood, urine, feces, semen, and vomit) and is deposited on the skin by sweating. It may be isolated from whole blood, sera, throat washes, urine, soft tissues, eye fluid, and serum. Marburg and Ebola viruses are transmitted from person to person via droplets of body fluids or through direct contact with infected individuals or with objects contaminated with blood or tissue. Individuals are most likely to transmit virus late in infection, through vomiting, diarrhea, or hemorrhaging. After recovery from disease, viruses may be transmitted sexually by males in semen for up to seven weeks.

During replication, a full-length positive strand that serves as a template for the production of genomic RNA is synthesized. Budding of the genome occurs at the cell's membrane, which contains inserted viral glycoprotein, by the addition of membrane-associated proteins and the nucleocapsid. Replication requires eight hours.

The five currently recognized filoviruses are **_Lake Victoria marburgvirus_** (strains Musoke, Popp, Ravn, Ozolin, Ratayczak, Voege), **_Zaire ebolavirus_** (strains Eckron, Gabon, Kikwit, Mayinga, Tandala, Zaire), **_Sudan ebolavirus_** (strains Boniface and Maleo), **_Ivory Coast ebolavirus_**, and **_Reston ebolavirus_** (strains Reston, Philippine, Siena, and Texas). These are more commonly known, respectively, as Marburg virus, Ebola Zaire, Ebola Sudan, Ebola Ivory Coast, and Ebola Reston. The six strains of the Marburg virus are serologically distinct and do not demonstrate immunological cross-reactivity. The filovirus groups have distinctive geographical distribution, with Ebola viruses primarily confined to humid rain forests in central and western

FIGURE 12.7 Budding of Ebola virus from the plasma membrane of an infected cell

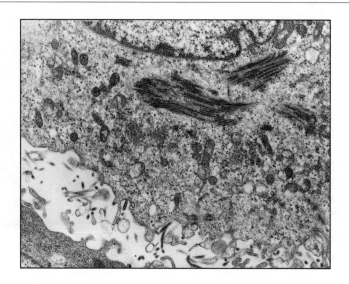

Source: CDC/Fred Murphy.

Africa, while Marburg virus is typically concentrated in drier areas found in central and eastern Africa, although infected bats have also been identified in Gabon and Congo Republic on Africa's west coast. Among the Ebola viruses, Ebola Zaire and Ebola Ivory Coast also appear to be clustered in a different geographical region than Ebola Sudan. Infections with the Zaire and Ivory Coast viruses also rise during periods of low or declining rainfall, whereas infections with the Sudan virus are associated with wet months.

The reservoir hosts for both Marburg and Ebola viruses are unknown, although fruit bats have been suggested to play this role because these animals may be infected experimentally and have been shown to have antiviral antibodies and viral RNA in the wild, indicating that natural infection has occurred. Infection among humans is highest among persons who venture into caves, mines, and forests, where they may encounter these bats. It is not known whether the differences in distribution of different species of filoviruses are related to differences in the reservoir host or hosts. The seasonality patterns for outbreaks may be due to factors that influence either infection of the reservoir host (the rate of seropositivity is higher in pregnant than nonpregnant bats, and higher viral titers may reflect decreased immune system activity during times of food scarcity) or may be due to increased interactions between the reservoir host and

FIGURE 12.8   Sampling animal tissues to determine the reservoir species for Ebola virus, Kikwit, Zaire, 1995

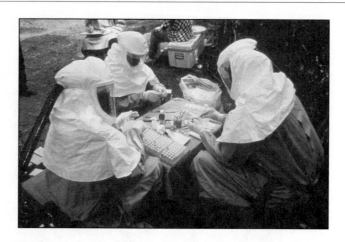

Source: CDC/Robert McLean.

nonhuman primates or humans occurring when competing for food during times of limited availability.

Both viruses are of potential concern for use as bioweapons. In experimentally infected mice, the **lethal dose$_{50}$ (LD$_{50}$)** (number of organisms required to kill 50% of a host) for Ebola Zaire is 1, indicating that an extremely low number of viruses are needed to kill mammalian hosts. Fortunately, Ebola Zaire is not known to be transmitted by any airborne mechanisms.

The Immune Response

The ability of filoviruses to infect monocytes, macrophages, and dendritic cells is the key to many of the pathological effects of infection as well as an aid to the evasion of the host's immune response. As previously mentioned, infected monocytes release large levels of destructive proinflammatory cytokines, such as TNF-α. Monocytes and dendritic cells normally play vital roles in stimulating the adaptive immune responses by lymphocytes, which themselves are not infected. Monocytes and dendritic cells express the MCH II molecules that are required to activate CD4$^+$ T helper cells. Dendritic cells are especially important in initiating a T and B lymphocyte responses to a novel antigen. Infection of dendritic cells leads to decreased maturation and necrotic death, thus decreasing their activation of T helper cells and B lymphocytes. Apoptosis of both CD4$^+$ T helper cells and CD8$^+$ T killer cells is also common during filovirus infections.

While human neutrophils are not themselves infected by filoviruses, they contribute to septic shock–like symptoms by their secretion of proinflammatory cytokines. Viral glycoprotein binds to the neutrophil surface immunorecognition receptor, known as the triggering receptor expressed on myeloid cells (TREM-1), thereby activating neutrophils to produce and release pathogenic cytokines. Cytokine release may be blocked by interfering with this binding.

During MHF, small amounts of antibodies are typically produced by B lymphocytes, primarily against the surface glycoproteins. Host survival following infection with filoviruses is associated with production of antiviral neutralizing IgM. The envelope glycoprotein plays an important role in evasion of the host immune response by down-regulating the expression of MHC I, which is required for recognition of viral antigens by CD8$^+$ T killer cells, and by thus decreasing the activation of these cells, which are the chief effectors of the adaptive immune system against viral infection. The glycoprotein also decreases expression of adhesion molecules on the surface of immune cells, interfering with their ability to home in on the site of infection. Increased levels of IFN-γ and IL-10 often accompany fatal cases of MHF.

Ebola viruses are not affected by host IFN-α and IFN-β (type I IFN). Type I IFN are normally important components of the innate immune response to viral infection and also regulate development of adaptive immunity. Viral VP35, in addition to serving a vital role in RNA synthesis, is also an antagonist of type I IFN. It blocks activation of IFN regulatory factor-3-responsive promoters, thus inhibiting IFN production, and suppresses this pathway, which inhibits viral synthesis, by blocking activity of the host antiviral enzyme double-strand RNA-dependent protein kinase. VP24 also appears to inhibit expression of IFN-induced genes, blocking IFN from effectively inducing an antiviral state. Natural killer (NK) cells are important mediators of the antiviral activity of the innate immune system that are activated to high levels of killing activity by IFN. VP35-induced reduction of IFN activity therefore also diminishes NK cell effectiveness.

Diagnosis

The initial stages of infection with filoviruses share symptoms with other tropical diseases common in the same regions of Africa, such as malaria and typhoid fever. Some diagnostic tests currently in use include antigen-capture ELISA, IgM-ELISA, indirect immunofluorescence, polymerase chain reaction, and viral isolation. For Ebola, virus may be isolated from blood, serum, or homogenates of internal organs and subsequently grown in tissue culture. MA-104 cells are used for Ebola Sudan, Vero cells (African green monkey kidney cells) for Reston. Virus may also be grown in guinea pigs. Diagnosis may also be performed on skin samples using immunohistochemisty.

Treatment

No specific treatment is currently effective against filovirus infection. None of the current antiviral drugs, including ribavirin, has been found to combat filoviruses, even in vitro. Hospital care is generally supportive and involves regulation of the balance of fluids and electrolytes, replacement of plasma albumin, maintenance of O2 status and blood pressure, and the replacement of blood and clotting factors. Administration of heparin has been attempted to block the consumption of clotting factors in order to prevent hemorrhaging; this is controversial, however, because heparin may actually accentuate blood loss.

Human immune serum and IFN have been used, with some degree of success. During the 1976 outbreak of Ebola Sudan, a researcher in England was accidently infected, but his levels of viremia dropped after receiving immune serum, and he recovered. It is not known, however, whether the serum contributed to his recovery because the overall mortality rate in that outbreak was 53%. Other research using a monkey model system suggests that if antiserum is beneficial, it functions in a strain-restricted manner.

More recent research has used several approaches to decrease viral replication. Two of these approaches are the use of antisense oligonucleotides and short interfering RNA (siRNA) molecules to decrease production of key viral proteins. Another approach employs *S*-adenosylhomocysteine hydrolase inhibitors and has been beneficial in infected mice. Other recent work has focused on preventing pathological host responses. Administration of recombinant nematode anticoagulant protein C2, which decreases disseminated intravascular coagulation, reduces mortality in macaques. However, these interventions are beneficial only when given before or soon after viral challenge.

Prevention

The Marburg virus and the four Ebola viruses are considered to be BioSafety Level 4 (BSL4) organisms and may only be grown in BSL4 laboratories. Few such laboratories exist—in the United States, one such lab is housed in the CDC and another in a U.S. Army facility. Care for people infected with BSL4 organisms requires special protective measures, including barrier nursing. Personnel must wear protective gloves, gowns, and masks; patients should be placed in isolation wards, and all material coming into contact with patients or their secretions (such as needles, medical equipment, clothing, and bedding) must be properly sterilized. These viruses may be inactivated by ultraviolet or γ-irradiation, 10% bleach, a 1% solution of formalin, phenolic disinfectants (such as Lysol), or lipid solvents (ether).

Research is being conducted on the development of an effective vaccine to protect against MHF and EHF. One such Marburg virus vaccine uses a slightly truncated glycoprotein whose gene is expressed in a baculovirus vector. This system provides proper N- and O-linked glycosylation. The vaccine construct was partially protective, blocking infection in 80% of animals challenged with same isolate (Musoke) as the vaccine, but was not active against the Ravn strain. An inactivated whole-virus vaccine protected animals against challenge by either strain and did so without inducing plaque-inhibiting antibodies. Cell-free serum from the vaccinated animals was able to transfer protection to previously

FIGURE 12.9   Isolation unit harboring persons with suspected cases of Ebola hemorrhagic fever in 1976

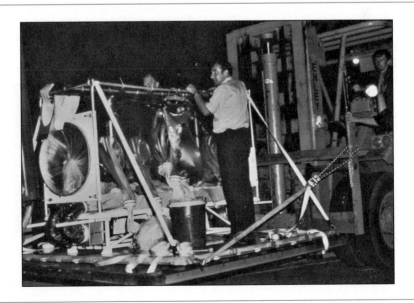

Source: CDC/J. Lyle Conrad.

FIGURE 12.10   Technician in protective field gear, Zaire, 1976

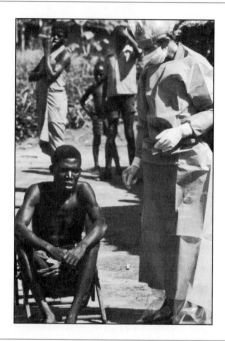

Source: CDC/J. Lyle Conrad.

FIGURE 12.11   Barrier clothing donned prior to entering
an Ebola isolation ward, Kikwit, Zaire, 1995

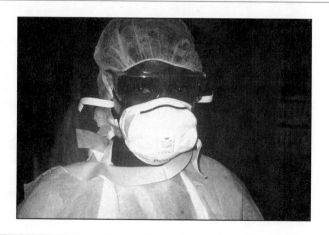

Source: CDC/Ethleen Lloyd.

unexposed guinea pigs. A vaccine composed of Ebola virus DNA followed by boosting with an adenovirus vector containing Ebola genes was found to protect monkeys from subsequent challenge with Ebola Zaire. Virus-specific $CD8^+$ T killer cells and antibodies were produced in the immunized animals. Ebola Zaire VP30 and VP40 proteins can also stimulate protective immune responses, indicating their possible utility in vaccines. Vesicular stomatitis virus and parainfluenza type 3 viruses are being used to produce live, recombinant vaccines that contain various filovirus genes. Another approach employs noninfectious ebolavirus-like particles.

Control of MHF and EHF outbreaks and prevention of disease epidemics may involve improving sanitation conditions in the regions at risk; increasing the availability and quality of health care, supplies, and training required for implementation of barrier nursing procedures; quarantining patients to prevent nosocomial transmission; and decreased travel of potentially infected persons from the area. Some of the major obstacles to these goals are limited local financial resources and civil unrest and violence in the affected areas. Because the international community would be threatened should a large-scale epidemic occur, preventive measures designed to improve public health in sub-Saharan Africa may be a matter for international consideration. Improved communications with health care agencies and experts from around the world and access to online medical journals may be achievable first steps toward modernizing medical care in some of the affected regions.

Surveillance

Epidemiological studies have found that several conditions contribute to the development and spread of MHF and EHF epidemics. These include travel of infected persons; decreased immune responses of the populace due to poor nutritional status, HIV/AIDS, and presence of other debilitating diseases; social customs (funeral rites, multiple sex partners); poor communication between areas of initial outbreak with regional, national, and international health care agencies; difficulty in reaching regions experiencing outbreaks and in transporting required protective equipment and medical supplies; lack of trained medical personnel; similarity of symptoms to those of other endemic diseases; and a lack of public health infrastructure and a reliable electrical supply needed for refrigeration or freezing in remote areas. Nosocomial transmission is one of the most important factors underlying the rapid spread of filovirus infections. Many areas suffer from an inadequate number of hospital beds and health care personnel; due to extremely limited financial resources in some areas, sanitary conditions in local hospitals may be poor, and if syringes and needles are scarce, they may be reused multiple times, often before they have been properly sterilized; personal protective supplies, such as sterile gloves, lab coats, and masks, are in short supply; availability of medications is limited due to expense and difficulties in transportation (poor or muddy roads, swollen rivers, and shortage of vehicles or gasoline); and the populace may be unable to afford medical care. The development of surveillance systems and infrastructure to rapidly report any suspected cases of MHF or EHF to public health authorities is critical to avoiding large-scale outbreaks. Surveillance studies need also to include animals, such as chimpanzees and gorillas, which are highly susceptible to serious infection. The death of these animals signals the potential for an outbreak in human populations in the area. Several outbreaks have already been traced to people eating nonhuman primates found dead in the wild.

Surveillance studies are needed to definitively determine all animal species that serve as viral reservoirs between epidemics and the level of infection of each species in the affected regions. The route by which infection passes periodically to susceptible human and nonhuman primate populations and factors affecting this transmission need to be determined as well, either to prevent epidemics or to prepare for potential outbreaks.

FIGURE 12.12 Vehicles used to cross the rugged roads of Zaire during the 1976 Ebola outbreak

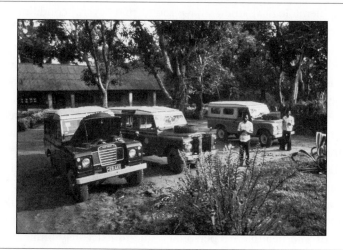

Source: CDC/J. Lyle Conrad.

Summary

Diseases

- Marburg hemorrhagic fever • Ebola hemorrhagic fever

Causative Agents

- Marburg virus • Ebola virus

Agent Type

- Filovirus

Genome

- Single-stranded RNA

Vector

- Unknown

Common Reservoir

- Fruit bats

Modes of Transmission

- Among humans, direct contact with blood, secretions, organs, or semen

Geographical Distribution

- Germany, Yugoslavia, Africa • Africa • United States, Italy, Philippines

Year of Emergence

- 1967 • 1976 • 1989 • 1995

Key Terms

Disseminated intravascular coagulation Widespread clotting of blood in small vessels with subsequent depletion of platelets and interference with clotting at other sites

Ebola hemorrhagic fever (EHF) Disease induced by the *Zaire* or *Sudan ebolavirus*, characterized by high fever, hemorrhagic symptoms, shock, and multiorgan failure

Filoviridae Family of enveloped viruses of the order Mononegavirales consisting of the Marburg and Ebola viruses

Ivory Coast ebolavirus Very rare causative agent of Ebola hemorrhagic fever in humans; found primarily among nonhuman primates in West Africa

Lake Victoria marburgvirus Causative agent of Marburg hemorrhagic fever; found naturally primarily in dry areas of Central and East Africa and occasionally in West Africa

Lethal dose$_{50}$ (LD$_{50}$) Number of organisms required to kill 50% of a host

Marburg hemorrhagic fever (MHF) Disease induced by *Lake Victoria marburgvirus,* characterized by high fever, hemorrhagic symptoms, shock, and multi-organ failure

Reston ebolavirus Ebola virus that induces a hemorrhagic fever with a high fatality rate among nonhuman primates but has not been reported to induce disease in humans; several outbreaks have been reported in primate facilities in the United States and Italy from animals imported from the Philippines

Sudan ebolavirus One of the causative agents of Ebola hemorrhagic fever; found primarily in humid rain forests of Central Africa

Zaire ebolavirus One of the causative agents of Ebola hemorrhagic fever; found primarily in humid rain forests of West Africa

Review Questions

1. What are the symptoms of infection with Marburg or Ebola hemorrhagic fever? What is the mechanism of pathology?
2. What organisms cause Marburg and Ebola hemorrhagic fevers? To what group of microbes do they belong, and what are some of their close relatives?
3. In what countries has infection with Marburg and the various Ebola viruses been reported?
4. What is the natural reservoir for filoviruses? How does human-to-human infection occur?
5. How does the host's immune response contribute to pathology? How do the viruses evade the host's defenses?

Topics for Further Discussion

1. Marburg and Ebola viruses are members of the Filoviridae family of the order Mononegavirales. Their closest relatives are the paramyxoviruses and rhabdoviruses. Identify pathogenic viruses that belong to these latter viral groups and the symptoms of the diseases that they produce in humans and domestic animals.

2. Filoviruses actively suppress protective antiviral activities of B, CD4$^+$ T helper, and CD8$^+$ T killer lymphocytes as well as NK cells. These viruses also induce production of a pathogenic proinflammatory innate immune response. Discuss ways in which the pathogenic immune responses might be minimized and protective immunity maximized.

3. Fruit bats appear to be at least one of the reservoir hosts for filoviruses. Discuss affordable protective measures that might be implemented to decrease transmission of the viruses from bats to mine workers and tourists. Your answer may involve ways of decreasing human contact with infectious bat materials, decreasing the infection rate in bats, or decreasing infectivity of bat-derived material.

4. Limited ability to rapidly transport regional, national, and international health care teams and proper protective equipment and supplies into remote regions during filovirus outbreaks hampers efforts to control epidemics. Limited access to communication with the global medical and health care agencies inhibits rapid identification and response to initial stages of a hemorrhagic fever epidemic and decreases the ability of local clinicians and public health personnel to easily learn of the most recent advances in prevention and treatment of serious microbial infections, including filovirus infections. Suggest ways in which transportation and communications might be improved, keeping in mind relevant local economic circumstances, civil unrest and refugee migrations, and environmental and climatic conditions.

Resources

Ascenzi, P., and others. "Ebolavirus and Marburgvirus: Insight the Filoviridae family." *Molecular Aspects of Medicine*, 2008, *29*, 151–185.

Bausch, D. G., Sprecher, A. G., Jeffs, B., and Boumandouki, P. "Treatment of Marburg and Ebola Hemorrhagic Fevers: A Strategy for Testing New Drugs and Vaccines Under Outbreak Conditions." *Antiviral Research*, 2008, *78*, 150–161.

Chin, J. *Control of Communicable Diseases Manual* (17th ed.). Washington, D.C.: American Public Health Association. 2000.

Dolnik, O., Kolesnikova, L., and Becker, S. "Filoviruses: Interactions with the Host Cell." *Cellular and Molecular Life Science*, 2008, *65*, 756–776.

Groseth, A., Feldmann, H., and Strong, J. E. "The Ecology of Ebola Virus." *Trends in Microbiology*, 2007, *15*, 408–416.

Leroy, E. M., and others. "Fruit Bats as Reservoirs of Ebola Virus." *Nature*, 2005, *438*, 575–576.

Mohamadzadeh, M., and others. "Filoviruses and the Balance of Innate, Adaptive, and Inflammatory Responses." *Viral Immunology*, 2006, *19*, 602–612.

Towner, J. S., and others. "Marburg Virus Infection Detected in a Common African Bat." *PLoS ONE*, 2007, *8*, e762–e765.

CHAPTER 13

AMERICAN HEMORRHAGIC FEVERS

LEARNING OBJECTIVES

- Define and contrast the American hemorrhagic fevers and other hemorrhagic fevers

- Describe the New World arenaviruses responsible for causing these illnesses

- Discuss modes of infection

- Discuss the host's response to infection

- Describe symptomatology and diagnosis

- Discuss methods of treatment

- Discuss methods of prevention

Major Concepts

Diseases

Several types of clinically similar hemorrhagic fevers (HFs) due to New World arenaviruses are found in the Western Hemisphere. These are the Argentine, Bolivian, Venezuelan, Brazilian, Whitewater Arroyo virus, and Chapare virus hemorrhagic fevers, caused by the Junin, Machupo, Guanarito, Sabia, Whitewater Arroyo, and Chapare viruses, respectively. All of these diseases occur in South America, with the exception of Whitewater Arroyo virus HF.

Symptoms

All of the American HFs have a relatively high mortality rate and a low infectious dose and may be acquired by inhalation of infectious rodent excreta or person-to-person contact. Early symptoms include headache, weakness, fever, petechial and erythematous rashes, anorexia, nausea and vomiting, and lymphadenopathy. Later symptoms include bloody diarrhea, enlargement of the spleen, low blood pressure, and shock. Thrombocytopenia may cause small focal hemorrhages, and increased vascular permeability may result in hemoconcentration. Hemorrhagic manifestations are present and may be accompanied by pneumonia, neurological sequelae, deafness, dehydration, and renal, myocardial, and liver involvement. Some of the American HFs are quite rare, with only three to five reported cases, while others, such as the Argentine, Bolivian, and Venezuelan HFs, have infected hundreds to tens of thousands of individuals.

Infection

The American HF viruses belong to the Tacaribe serogroup of the Arenaviridae family and are small, enveloped, single-stranded positive-sense RNA viruses. These organisms are also called "sandy viruses" because they contain multiple particles that are similar in appearance to ribosomes, giving the viruses a sandy appearance. Almost all of the pathogenic New World arenaviruses are found in South America and belong to clade B. The Whitewater Arroyo virus and several nonpathogenic viruses are located in North America and belong to clade A. On the average, a new member of the Tacaribe serogroup is identified every three years. Several Old World arenaviruses also infect humans. These are the lymphocytic choriomeningitis virus, Lassa virus, and a currently unnamed virus found in southern Africa.

Immune Response

Levels of several cytokines increase during American HF, including IFN-α, IL-6, IL-8, IL-10, and TNF-α. IFN-α levels are particularly high in fatal cases, and this cytokine may contribute to pathology. Amounts of the hematopoietic growth factor G-CSF also rise during New World arenavirus infection, and its levels correlate with disease severity. Levels of an erythrocyte growth factor decrease, perhaps contributing to the decrease in red blood cell production. Levels of CD4$^+$ T helper cells are reduced as well.

Treatment

Ribavirin used in combination with convalescent plasma containing virus-specific antibodies has proved effective in the treatment of Argentine, Bolivian, and Brazilian HFs. Ribavirin may also be protective in treating infection with Lassa virus and a novel Old World arenavirus found in South Africa and Zambia. Several newer drugs have been developed as well.

Prevention

Barrier precautions (gloves and masks) protect health care personnel from infection. Rodent control, such as trapping and poisoning of rodents, may reduce disease incidence in the general population. A highly effective live attenuated-virus vaccine is available to protect against infection with Junin virus. It is cross-protective against challenge with Machupo virus in animal model systems.

Introduction

Six naturally occurring types of HFs in humans are currently recognized in the Americas: Argentine, Bolivian, Venezuelan, Brazilian, Whitewater Arroyo virus, and Chapare virus HFs. These are caused by the Junin, Machupo, Guanarito, Sabia, Whitewater Arroyo, and Chapare viruses, respectively, and belong to the **Tacaribe (New World) serocomplex** of the Arenaviridae family. This complex is composed of three clades: clade A consists of the pathogenic Whitewater Arroyo and the nonpathogenic Tamiami and Bear Canyon viruses, all from North America, and Pichinde, Parana, Pirital, Flexal, and Allapahuayo South American viruses; clade B contains the pathogenic Junin, Machupo, Guanarito, Sabia, and Chapare viruses and the nonpathogenic Tacaribe, Amapari, and Cupixi viruses; and clade C contains the nonpathogenic Oliveros, Latino, and Pampa viruses.

However, a recent report places the three North American viruses in a distinct group. On the average, a new member of the serocomplex is found every three years. They are transmitted by sigmodontine rodents, and with the exception of the Whitewater Arroyo virus, pathogenic members are restricted to South America. The Old World arenavirus found in North America is the lymphocytic choriomeningitis virus.

RECENT DEVELOPMENTS

The cellular receptor for the Old World arenaviruses, lymphocytic choriomeningitis virus and the Lassa fever virus, and clade C but not clade A or B New World viruses is α-dytroglycan. The latter two types of New World viruses interact with human target cells by binding to the transferrin receptor, involved in iron transport into the cell. The pathogenic clade B viruses Junin, Machupo, and Guanarito all infected human and nonhuman primate cells to a high level, with lesser infection of rodent cell lines. The opposite is true of the nonpathogenic Amapari clade B member. Using a multiplicity of infection of 10, the pathogenic viruses have been found to be highly effective in establishing infection of HeLa cervical epithelial cells, A549 lung epithelial cells, Huh7 hepatoma cells, HUVEC human umbilical vein endothelial cells, and Thp-1 monocytes and less effective in infection of WIL-2 B and Jurkat T lymphocyte cell lines. Preincubation of cells with inactivated Junin or Guanarito viruses blocks infection by the other pathogenic South American arenaviruses. This is not true of the tested nonpathogenic viruses of any clade. The receptor for these viruses is sensitive to treatments that remove proteins but not phospholipids, N-linked glycosylation, α-N-galactosamine, fucose, galactose, O-linked glycosylation, or sialic acid alone. Removal of both O-glycans and sialic acid leads to a slight enhancement of infection. Neither heparin sulfate nor heparin appears to affect infection. Identification of the chemical composition of the receptors for arenaviruses may allow development of drugs that specifically block these viruses from entering cells, thus preventing infection of humans.

The American HF viruses pose unique challenges: infection with these viruses leads to a high mortality rate, vaccines against the majority of these agents are lacking, and infection may occur via inhalation. These factors, together with the low numbers of organisms required to infect a human, make these viruses good candidates for weaponization and therefore agents of special concern to the world community. Fortunately, several effective treatment options are available for use for individuals afflicted by American hemorrhagic fevers, which is not the case for some of the other hemorrhagic fevers, including one caused by infection by the Old World arenavirus Lassa fever (discussed in Chapter Fourteen).

History

Argentine hemorrhagic fever was first described as a clinical disease in 1955 in an epidemic in Bragado, Argentina, in Buenos Aires Province. The endemic area for this disease is continuing to spread over this province and parts of Sante Fé and Cérdoba provinces. The Junin virus, the causative agent, was subsequently isolated in 1958 in the city of Junín. Between 1958 and 1987, about 21,000 cases of Argentine HF were reported.

Scattered cases of "black typhus" began in the Bolivian Amazon River basin in 1959. The outbreak of this disease, now known as Bolivian hemorrhagic fever, resulted in 470 cases and 142 deaths (30% fatality rate) between 1959 and 1962. In the 1960s, there were large epidemics with many deaths. In one town with 3,000 residents, 600 cases occurred, with 113 deaths recorded in two years (20% incidence, 19% fatality rate). These epidemics were finally stopped by the use of mousetraps and oil-grain baits containing zinc phosphide to eliminate the rodent vector. The causative arenavirus, the Machupo virus, was first isolated in 1963. There were no cases between 1973 and 1992. A familial cluster of patients was reported in 1994.

In September 1989, an outbreak of severe febrile disease was noted in Portuguesa, Venezuela. This outbreak was confined mainly to rural inhabitants in the southern portions of the state. A total of 105 confirmed or probable cases of Venezuelan hemorrhagic fever occurred from September 1989 to May 1995. Many of the cases originated near Guanarito, in the Portuguesa state.

The first reported case of Brazilian hemorrhagic fever occurred in a 25-year-old female agricultural engineer in Sã Paulo state in 1990 and was fatal even after treatment with defoxitin and amikacin. She had worked mainly in an office. A lab worker later became infected, probably via an aerosol, was treated with intravenous fluids, and recovered. A second infected lab worker was put on intravenous ribavirin, an antiviral agent, and the fever disappeared within two days.

Flexal virus has not been reported to cause natural infection in humans yet but has resulted in moderately severe infections in two laboratory workers. It must therefore be regarded as a potential danger.

In 1999 and 2000, three cases of hemorrhagic fever caused by Whitewater Arroyo virus occurred in California. All three were fatal. The virus itself was first isolated from whitethroat woodrats in New Mexico in 1996.

The most recently discovered pathogenic member of the Tacaribe group is the **Chapare virus**. This clade B virus caused a cluster of infections, including one fatal case of hemorrhagic fever in a remote region of the Andes mountains of rural Bolivia in 2008. Little information about this virus is currently available.

The Diseases

The American hemorrhagic fevers closely resemble dengue, yellow fever, idiopathic thrombocytopenic purpura, and other illness whose symptoms include prolonged fever with leukopenia and hemorrhagic signs. The prodrome (early warning signs) includes fever, sore throat, and muscle and retro-ocular pain. The infectious dose for these viruses is one to ten organisms, followed by an incubation period of 7 to 14 days. Symptoms occurring during the early stages of infection include headache, weakness, flushing of the face and thorax, petechial and erythematous rashes, anorexia, nausea and vomiting, and lymphadenopathy.

Later during the course of disease, various vascular abnormalities occur, and many patients are hospitalized. Thrombocytopenia leads to the development of small focal hemorrhages in many organs, particularly the liver (hepatocellular necrosis). The diarrhea is bloody. The number of eosinophils increases, but the total number of white blood cells decreases with both neutropenia and lymphoid depletion and necrosis in the spleen and lymph nodes. Increased vascular permeability may result in hemoconcentration. Hemorrhagic manifestations include

FIGURE 13.1   Petechial lesions

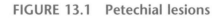

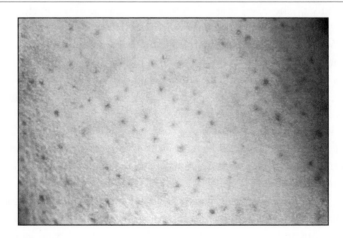

Source: CDC.

nosebleed, bleeding gums, bloody vomit, and massive gastrointestinal hemorrhages. The spleen may enlarge and become congested. Low blood pressure may lead to shock. There is extensive infection of macrophages and, in Argentine HF, dendritic cells as well, but not lymphocytes. Lymphocyte loss in Argentine HF may be due at least in part to apoptosis. There is minimal involvement of the endothelium, with no specific vascular lesions found in infected monkeys. Substantial changes in coagulation and fibrinolysis markers may be found, including complexes of thrombin and antithrombin, prothrombin fragments, protein C, D-dimers, tissue plasminogen activator, and plasminogen activator inhibitor-1. Levels of the acute-phase proteins fibrinogen and von Willebrand factor are also increased. These changes may be caused by the presence of proinflammatory cytokines.

The nitrogen free radical nitric oxide is found in elevated amounts in the serum. This macrophage-produced mediator has both protective and deleterious properties. The latter include lymphocyte apoptosis, tissue damage, hypotension, and loss of vascular integrity, which might lead to the induction of shock. Unlike Ebola and Marburg hemorrhagic fevers, there is no disseminated intravascular coagulation.

In addition to the circulatory system, several other organ systems are affected by the American hemorrhagic fever viruses. Pneumonia may occur, with pulmonary edema and hemorrhaging. In half of a dozen fatal cases studied, secondary bacterial infections were found in the lungs. Neurological findings may include sleepiness, tremors, difficulty walking, tonic-clonic convulsions, and coma. In the case of Venezuelan HF, deafness may occur during convalescence. Other clinical findings are dehydration and renal, myocardial, and liver involvement. The renal manifestations include the presence of albumin, hyaline and granular casts, and Milani cells in the urine. Most patients recover without long-lasting sequelae after an acute illness of 10 days and a two- to three-week period of convalescence.

For patients who recover, the illness persists 10 to 14 days. Fatality rates are rather high, however. In Argentine HF, 25% to 35% of untreated cases result in death; in Bolivian HF, the figure is 30%; in Venezuelan HF, 34%; in Brazilian HF, 33%; and in hemorrhagic fever induced by the Whitewater Arroyo virus, 100%.

Argentine Hemorrhagic Fever

Argentine hemorrhagic fever preferentially strikes young male agricultural workers between the ages of 20 and 50 from the rural areas of the central-east part of Argentina, the Humid Pampa. Disease incidence is greatest in late autumn, during the corn harvest season. It is transmitted by the drylands vesper mouse (*Calomys musculinus*), *Calomys laucha*, *Akodon azarae*, and *Mus musculus* via the airborne route whereby people are infected by inhaling aerosols of mouse urine, feces, or saliva in the dust raised by manual or mechanical harvesting or plowing or by the cutaneous route through abrasions in the skin. The former species of mouse is an opportunistic species whose populations may reach high levels in crop fields, with cornfields having a higher density of rodents than soybean fields. Agriculture (introduced into the Pampa in the late 1800s) may have favored recent range expansion and subsequent introduction of this rodent species into the area. This hypothesis is supported by studies of genetic diversity using mitochondrial DNA. Almost 8% of the principal vectors in this region of Argentina were found to be infected by screening for antibodies using an indirect fluorescence assay. Other species were also infected at a lower level; these were *C. laucha, Bolomys obscurus,* and a predatory carnivore, *Galictis cuja.* Most of the animals are associated with a relatively rare roadside and fence-line habitat, and the infected animals were most likely to be aggressive, older males. Between 100 and 4,000 human cases are reported per year; however, some years have higher infection rates (24,000 cases in 1993).

Rhesus macaques are able to be experimentally infected with this virus via aerosols. They become ill within the third week of infection; half die by day 21, and the remainder within the first month. Virus may be recovered from the visceral organs and the central nervous system. Like infected humans, these animals had high levels of interferon-α in their blood. Person-to-person transmission between couples has also been reported.

Bolivian Hemorrhagic Fever

Bolivian hemorrhagic fever is transmitted by the large vesper mouse (*Calomys callosus*). When suckling mice are infected or if adult mice are inoculated with low amounts of virus, most animals become chronically infected, with growth retardation, splenomegaly, shortened life span, and reduced fertility. The animals are viremic and shed virus in the urine and saliva. The virus may then be contracted by humans via the airborne route, through inhalation of rodent excreta, or by eating contaminated food. In addition to being a zoonotic infection, person-to-person transmission is also found both in health care settings and among family members. In one instance, a person infected two relatives and two health care workers, and three of these died (75% fatality rate). Bolivian HF may be transmitted via inhalation of infected droplets or aerosols.

Venezuelan Hemorrhagic Fever

The natural reservoirs for **Venezuelan hemorrhagic fever** are the cane mouse (*Zygodontomys brevicauda*) and the cotton rat (*Sigmodon alstoni*), which develop chronic infections with the Guanarito virus. Infected rodents have been found in multiple sites in five states of the central plain region: Portuguesa, Barinas,

FIGURE 13.2   Cotton rat

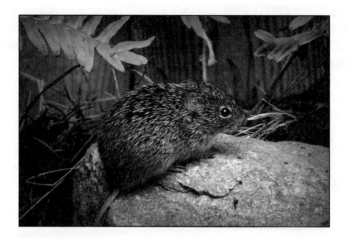

Source: CDC.

Apure, Guarico, and Cojedes. The rate of infection of the cotton rats in these sites ranged from 10% to 55%; fewer than 2% of the humans living in Portuguesa state, however, had developed antibodies to the virus. Transmission is presumed to be via aerosolized mouse urine and saliva, which contain virus for up to five months. No cases have been reported among secondary contacts, such as medical personnel or family members.

Both sexes and all age groups are affected, but the highest rates are seen in individuals between the ages of 14 and 44. Venezuelan HF is found in areas where the forest has been cleared for agriculture plots and cattle ranching. In such areas, forest rodents have been replaced by grassland rodents who have an increase in food supply and human contact. Cases appear sporadically during the entire year, however, more than half occur in the dry season, which lasts from December to March. During these months, agricultural activities, such as land clearing, occur.

Guanarito virus kills suckling mice and adult guinea pigs but not adult mice. Infected rhesus macaques become ill but recover and produce antibody.

Brazilian Hemorrhagic Fever

The route of natural transmission of **Brazilian hemorrhagic fever** is currently unknown but is believed to be contracted from a rodent. There have only been three reported cases, one of them fatal (33% fatality rate).

Hemorrhagic Fever Caused by the Whitewater Arroyo Virus

Hemorrhagic fever caused by the Whitewater Arroyo virus is a related illness that occurs in North America. The vectors for this virus are wood rats (*Neotoma* species) and several types of mice, including *Peromyscus maniculatus*, the deer mouse. Transmission is presumed to be via aerosolized excreta. A 3278 nucleotide fragment of the smaller of the RNA strands that encodes the glycoprotein precursor gene, the nucleoprotein gene, and the 5' and 3' ends was sequenced. When compared to other Tacaribe arenaviruses, the nucleoprotein gene was found to be more similar to A-lineage viruses, while the glycoprotein precursor was more like the B-lineage viruses, suggesting that the Whitewater Arroyo virus may have arisen as a result of recombination between an A- and a B-lineage virus.

The Causative Agents

The American HFs are caused by pathogenic American arenaviruses, which are called "sandy viruses" due to the fact that the virions contain multiple particles resembling host ribosomes, giving them a sandy appearance. **Junin virus** is the causative agent of Argentine HF, **Guanarito virus** causes Venezuelan HF, **Machupo virus** causes Bolivian HF, **Sabia virus** causes Brazilian HF. A relatively rare hemorrhagic fever has also been caused by the **Whitewater Arroyo virus**. This virus has been isolated from New Mexico, Utah, Oklahoma, and Texas, and antibody-positive rodents were found in southern California and southeastern Colorado as well. In Colorado, 26.8% of male and 42.9% of female white-throated wood rats had this antibody.

These are single-stranded RNA viruses, containing almost 11 kilobases of RNA in two segments, and are antigenically related to the Lassa fever virus. The Guanarito virus has diverged about 30% from the other arenaviruses. Nucleotide and amino acid sequence homology of the Whitewater Arroyo and Tamiami viruses are 73.1% and 80.0%, while that among the South American arenaviruses are 54.9% to 76.5% and 47.3% to 86.2%, respectively. They are ambisense, meaning that the RNA segments read in opposite directions. Virions are spherical or pleomorphic in shape, with a diameter of 110 to 130 nanometers. Club-shaped or spiked glycoproteins (GP1 and GP2) are encoded by the smaller of the two RNAs and appear on the virus's lipid envelope, GP1 interacting with the host cell's receptor.

FIGURE 13.3 "Sandy" appearance of New World arenaviruses

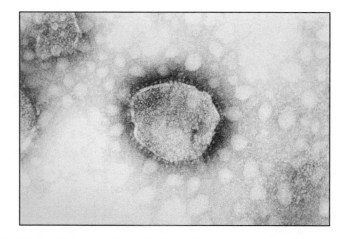

Source: CDC/E. L. Palmer.

FIGURE 13.4 Machupo virus

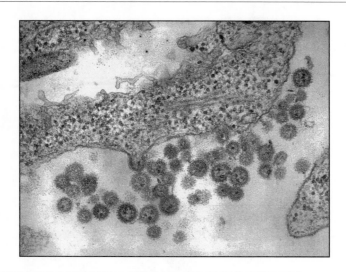

Source: CDC/Fred Murphy and Sylvia Whitfield.

Viremia is acute and long-lasting, with high viral titers. In fatal cases, Junin viral antigens have been found in reticular cells of the hematological system, renal tubular cells, and hepatocytes. Viruslike particles and cytopathic effect have been seen in these cells.

Because infection with the American HF viruses may occur in primates via aerosols, work on these agents must be conducted in a BSL-4 laboratory. These viruses have been considered potential candidates for biological weapons. They are particularly attractive for this use due to the facts that they have a very low infectious dose, they have a high mortality rate, vaccines either aren't available or availability is limited, and the viruses can be readily be grown in large quantities. The former Soviet Union and United States both conducted biological weapon research on these viruses, as well as the Lassa fever and yellow fever viruses and a number of other viruses or bacteria (further discussed in Chapter Thirty).

FIGURE 13.5   Working in a Biosafety Level 4 laboratory

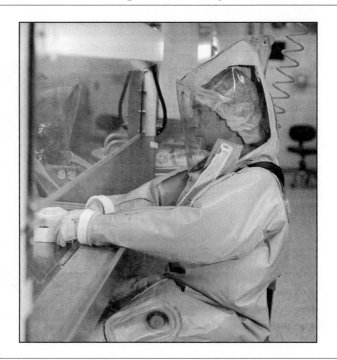

Source: CDC.

The Immune Response

Cytokine activation may occur during American HF, as is seen during infection with Ebola, Marburg, hantavirus, Lassa, and yellow fever viruses. For Argentine HF, these cytokines include IFN-α, IL-6, IL-8, IL-10, and TNF-α. Levels of IFN-α are unusually high, more so in the cases of fatal infections than in those of survivors, and this cytokine may play an important role in viral pathogenesis, perhaps leading to inhibition of megakaryocyte maturation and the resulting thrombocytopenia. IL-6 and TNF-α are active in blood coagulation, and IL-6 also induces liver acute-phase proteins and is involved in hematopoiesis. Furthermore, 10% to 25% of patients have elevated levels of soluble IL-6 receptor. IL-8 is a chemotactic and activating factor for neutrophils and plays a causal role in acute respiratory distress syndrome. Neutrophil lysosomal degranulation with the release of toxic compounds may be confirmed by detection of elastase complexed with its inhibitor, α1-antitypsin, levels of which are also increased, particularly during severe disease. IL-10 is an anti-inflammatory cytokine that reduces production of IL-1, IL-6, IL-8, and TNF-α in a regulatory fashion, perhaps reducing damage.

A recent study examined bone marrow functions in 48 patients with Argentine hemorrhagic fever. Erythroblastopenia (low numbers of erythrocyte precursors) was observed, together with low levels of granulocytic precursors with abnormal maturation. Nevertheless, normal red blood cell count, hematocrit, and hemoglobin levels are seen during the acute phase of the disease, suggesting a transient, early maturational arrest in the erythrocyte precursors that is not reflected in the periphery due to the length of red blood cell survival. Decreased levels of erythropoietin (Epo) were found in 62% of the patients, but it increased upon recovery. High levels of granulocyte colony-stimulating factor (G-CSF) was found in 63% of the patients, and 91% had increased amounts of thrombopoietin (Tpo), but most patients had normal levels of IL-3, granulocyte-macrophage colony-stimulating factor (GM-CSF), and TGF-β. Epo is an erythroid growth factor; TGF-β has the opposite effect. G-CSF, GM-CSF, and IL-3 function as growth factors for granulocytes, and Tpo, GM-CSF, and IL-3 serve a similar function for megakaryocytes, the precursors of platelets. Seeing that Junin virus was not detected in the bone marrow, it is likely that the decreased amounts of Epo contributed to the noted erythroblastopenia. The amount of G-CSF showed a positive correlation with disease severity. High levels of G-CSF have been noted in other viral and bacterial infections as well. This increase in the levels of G-CSF and Tpo might be a countermeasure by the body to restore homeostasis in the face of ongoing acute neutropenia and thrombocytopenia, respectively.

Immunosuppression is commonly associated with American HF, including decreased numbers of CD4$^+$ T helper cells but not CD8$^+$ T killer cells.

Table 13.1 Cytokines active during New World hemorrhagic fevers

Cytokine or Growth Factor	Type of Factor	Action
IL-1	Proinflammatory cytokine	Induces fever
IL-3	Hematopoietic growth factor	Increases numbers of stem and progenitor cells
IL-6	Proinflammatory cytokine	Stimulates production of acute-phase proteins; helps coagulate blood; increases hematopoiesis
IL-8	Chemokine	Induces neutrophil chemotactic activity
IL-10	Anti-inflammatory cytokine	Negatively regulates the immune response
IFN-α	Antiviral agent	Interferes with viral replication; reduces platelet production
TNF-α	Proinflammatory cytokine	Induces fever; wasting and shock
TGF-α	Anti-inflammatory cytokine	Negatively regulates the immune response
Epo	Hematopoietic growth factor	Increases erythrocyte production
Tpo	Hematopoietic growth factor	Increases platelet production
G-CSF	Hematopoietic growth factor	Increases production of granulocytes (neutrophils, eosinophils, basophils)
GM-CSF	Hematopoietic growth factor	Increases production of granulocytes and of monocytes

Hematopoiesis is transiently inhibited. Antibodies are detected late during the convalescence period, four to six weeks after symptoms occur. No antibodies are found in fatal cases, suggesting that these immune mediators may have a protective function.

Diagnosis

Diagnostic procedures include several antibody-dependent techniques, including antigen-capture ELISA or IgM-specific ELISA, indirect immunofluorescence, and plaque reduction neutralizing antibody tests, but not complement fixation. RT-PCR and virus isolation from blood or organs may also be performed; the latter must be carried out in BSL-4 labs with complete protective gear. Viruses may be grown in Vero cells, blood mononuclear cells, or suckling mice or hamsters.

Treatment

Ribavirin, a nonimmunosuppressive nucleoside analogue, is effective in the treatment of Argentine and Brazilian HF and is used together with immune plasma. However, it does not cross the blood-brain barrier and thus will probably not be efficacious in treating neurological manifestations of the diseases. IFN-α and IFN-β are antiviral agents produced by the host that have not proved useful in treating these diseases. Administration of convalescent plasma containing neutralizing antibodies, whole blood, or immune globulin has been beneficial in the treatment of both Argentine and Bolivian HF, provided that treatment is begun within eight days after disease onset, reducing the mortality rate 20-fold in the former case. Coadministration of ribavirin and immune plasma proved effective in the recovery of two of three individuals infected with the Machupo virus and in the case of marmosets infected experimentally with Junin virus. Use of immune plasma is associated with a late but rarely severe neurological syndrome in 8% to 10% of patients treated.

Several agents are active against the Junin virus in cell culture. These include the antiemetic chloroprornazine and the antipsychotic trifluorperazine and disulfide-based compounds, such as intermolecular aromatic disulfides and sulfur-containing dithianes, which inactivate Junin viruses in culture rapidly and in a concentration- and time-dependent manner. Two inosine monophosphate dehydrogenase inhibitors, ribamidine and 5-ethynyl-1-β-D-reibofuranosylimidazole-carboxamine, are effective in killing viruses in cell culture and in animal models.

Prevention

Rodent control was the primary method used to halt the outbreaks of Bolivian HF in the 1960s. This includes trapping and poisoning rodents, particularly by immune individuals. Barrier precautions, such as gloves and masks, should be used by health care personnel.

A live, weakened (attenuated) virus vaccine (Candid #1) was developed for use against Argentine HF in 1989. It was derived from the XJ strain after 44 passages through mouse brains and 19 times through the FRhL-2 cell line. In a prospective, placebo-controlled efficacy trial, this vaccine was found to have a protective rate of 95% and to confer resistance for about nine years after a single inoculum. Between 1991 and 1999, more than 200,000 people were vaccinated with Candid #1, and only 0.1% reported an adverse reaction, none of which

FIGURE 13.6   Baiting a rodent trap with peanut butter

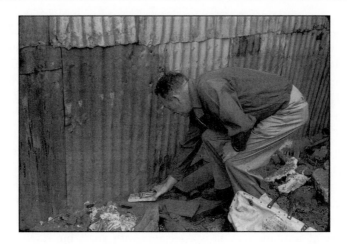

Source: CDC.

was severe. Vaccine efficacy was 98%, and all cases of Argentine HF in vaccines were mild. This vaccine is also effective in prophylaxis against Bolivian, but not Venezuelan, HF in primates.

Surveillance

A control program to monitor and eliminate the rodent vector of Bolivian HF (large vesper mouse) operates in a portion of the Department of Beni covering approximately 28,000 square kilometers. This area is home to 50,000 residents whose primary occupations are cattle raising and subsistence agriculture. The surveillance consists of regular visits to many less inhabited localities once each year. Over the course of two nights, 50 to 150 Sherman traps are operated. If some of the rodent vectors are found but none are infected with Machupo virus (evidenced by enlarged spleens), supplies of warfarin are left as mouse poison. Observations are then repeated at three months, six months, and annually after elimination of all of these mice. When a case of human Bolivian HF is found, all neighboring farms and ranches are surveyed until a perimeter area that is not infested by the vesper mice is determined. The area within this parameter is systematically poisoned and surveyed by trapping until no more infected mice are detected. The program costs about $30,000 per year and has reduced the numbers of infected humans to fewer than 50 per year.

Arenaviruses and human hemorrhagic fever are found only in parts of the geographical range of the vector species. Ongoing surveillance programs are needed to monitor the changing areas in which the viruses are located within the vector populations. For example, in 1955, the Argentine HF-endemic area was about 10,000 square kilometers in the Buenos Aires province. By 1985, the endemic area had expanded to more than 150,000 square kilometers in four provinces. The virus may periodically become extinct in local mouse populations and be reintroduced later from neighboring locales. Thus while a single cross-sectional survey may delineate the range of infection, repeated or longitudinal studies are required to determine temporal and spatial patterns.

Surveillance of infection in mouse populations may additionally provide a clearer view of potential disease-endemic areas than human disease surveillance, particularly in diseases such as Argentine HF, where vaccine administration may mask true human exposure. Vector surveys may also pinpoint habitat preferences. Such studies found that the drylands vesper mouse vector of Argentine HF is rarely located in the cornfields but instead is found in the more stable, weedy fence lines and roadsides bordering the fields. Such studies suggest that removing vegetation in these locations may decrease the incidence of this disease.

Other studies have clearly linked climatic activity to vector abundance and incidence of human disease. Mark-and-recapture studies found that unusually mild weather leads to mouse reproduction throughout the winter, high overwinter survival, and high vector numbers at the beginning of the spring reproductive season. Abundant rainfall during summer months allows vegetation to remain green, stopping the typical midsummer decline in mouse populations. These factors permit increased mouse populations and numbers of infected mice, followed by unusually severe epidemics of hemorrhagic fever. Careful monitoring of rodent populations may allow for the development of predictive models for human infection or programs to prevent rodent infection or interaction with humans.

Summary

Diseases

- Argentine hemorrhagic fever • Bolivian hemorrhagic fever
- Venezuelan hemorrhagic fever • Brazilian hemorrhagic fever
- Hemorrhagic fever caused by the Whitewater Arroyo virus or Chapare virus

Causative Agents

- Junin virus • Machupo virus • Guanarito virus • Sabia virus
- Whitewater Arroyo virus • Chapare virus

Agent Type

- Arenaviridae virus of the Tacaribe (New World) serocomplex

Genome

- Single-stranded RNA virus

Vector

- Woodrats and mice

Common Reservoirs

- *Calomys musculinus, Calomys laucha, Akodon azarae,* and *Mus musculus* • *Calomys callosus* • *Zygodontomys brevicauda* and *Sigmodon alstoni* • Unknown • *Neotoma* spp. and *Peromyscus maniculatus* • Unknown

Modes of Transmission

- Airborne route by inhaling aerosols of rodent urine, feces, or saliva • Ingestion of food contaminated by rodent excreta • Cutaneous route through abrasions in the skin • Person-to-person contact

Geographical Distribution

- South America and parts of southern North America

Year of Emergence

- 1955 • 1959 • 1989 • 1990 • 1999 • 2008

Key Terms

Argentine hemorrhagic fever Hemorrhagic fever with a high fatality rate caused by an arenavirus in Argentina

Bolivian hemorrhagic fever Hemorrhagic fever with a high fatality rate caused by an arenavirus in Bolivia

Brazilian hemorrhagic fever Hemorrhagic fever with a high fatality rate caused by an arenavirus in Brazil

Chapare virus Causative agent of hemorrhagic fever in the Andes region of Bolivia

Guanarito virus Causative agent of Venezuelan hemorrhagic fever

Hemorrhagic fever caused by the Whitewater Arroyo virus Hemorrhagic fever with a high fatality rate caused by an arenavirus in California

Junin virus Causative agent of Argentine hemorrhagic fever

Machupo virus Causative agent of Bolivian hemorrhagic fever

Sabia virus Causative agent of Brazilian hemorrhagic fever

Tacaribe (New World) serocomplex Complex of the Arenaviridae family that contains viruses causing hemorrhagic fevers in the Americas

Venezuelan hemorrhagic fever Hemorrhagic fever with a high fatality rate caused by an arenavirus in Venezuela

Whitewater Arroyo virus Causative agent of hemorrhagic fever in parts of the southwestern United States

Review Questions

1. What are the six pathogenic arenaviruses found in the Americas? What disease does each cause?
2. What are the vectors for these viruses?
3. What are the symptoms of American hemorrhagic fever?
4. What are the functions of erythropoietin, thrombopoietin, G-CSF, GM-CSF, and IL-3? How are the levels of these cytokines affected by infection with New World arenaviruses?
5. What agents effectively kill the Junin virus in cell culture?

Topics for Further Discussion

1. Pathogenic arenaviruses are found in mainly in Africa and South America, with one member of this group occurring in the southwestern United States. Speculate on the ecological, geographical, and historical reasons for this distribution. Given the rate of discovery of arenaviruses, do you believe that other members of this group will be found in other areas of the world?
2. What characteristics make New World arenaviruses attractive targets for bioweapons research? What other microbes have been studied for such use? What are several ways in which the world community may protect itself against such weapons?
3. Discuss factors that may be driving the emergence of hemorrhagic fever in the Americas. In which other areas of the world are these factors currently occurring?

4. In addition to diseases caused by the New World arenaviruses, what other type of hemorrhagic fever is present to a great extent in South America? What other viral HFs are found throughout the world?

Resources

Bronze, M. S., and Greenfield, R. A. "Preventive and Therapeutic Approaches to Viral Agents of Bioterrorism." *DDT*, 2003, *8*, 740–745.

Carballal, G., Cidela, C. M., and Merani, M. S. "Epidemiology of Argentine Hemorrhagic Fever." *European Journal of Epidemiology*, 1988, *4*, 259–274.

Coimbra, T. L., and Nassar, E. S. "New Arenavirus Isolated in Brazil." *Lancet*, 1994, *343*, 391–392.

Enria, D. A., and Oro, J.G.B. "Junin Virus Vaccines." *Current Topics in Microbiology and Immunology*, 2002, *263*, 239–261.

Fulhorst, C. F., and others. "Isolation and Characterization of Whitewater Arroyo Virus, a Novel North American Arenavirus." *Virology*, 1996, *224*, 114–120.

Fulhorst, C. F., and others. "Bear Canyon Virus: An Arenavirus Naturally Associated with the California Mouse (*Peromyscus californicus*)." *Emerging Infectious Diseases*, 2002, *8*, 717–721.

Geisbert, T. W., and Jahrling, P. B. "Exotic Emerging Viral Diseases: Progress and Challenges." *Nature Medicine*, 2004, *10*, S110–S121.

Kilgore, P. E., and others. "Prospects for the Control of Bolivian Hemorrhagic Fever." *Emerging Infectious Diseases*, 1995, *1*, 97–100.

Marta, R. F., and Molinas, F. C. "Relationship Between Hematopoietic Growth Factor Levels and Hematological Parameters in Argentine Hemorrhagic Fever." *American Journal of Hematology*, 2000, *64*, 1–6.

Marta, R. F., and others. "Proinflammatory Cytokines and Elastase-α-1-antitrypsin in Argentine Hemorrhagic Fever." *American Journal of Tropical Medicine and Hygiene*, 1999, *60*, 85–89.

Peters, C. J. "Human Infection with Arenaviruses in the Americas." *Current Topics in Microbiology and Immunology*, 2002, *262*, 65–72.

Rojek, J. M., Spiropoulou, C. F., and Kunz, S. "Characterization of the Cellular Receptors for the South American Hemorrhagic Fever Viruses Junin, Guanarito, and Machupo." *Virology*, 2006, *349*, 476–491.

Salas, R., and others. "Venezuelan Hemorrhagic Fever (VHF)." *Epidemiology Bulletin*, 1995, *16*, 1–2.

Tesh, R. B., Jahrling, P. B., Salas, R., and Shope, R. E. "Description of Guanarito Virus (Arenaviridae: Arenavirus), the Etiologic Agent of Venezuelan Hemorrhagic Fever." *American Journal of Tropical Medicine and Hygiene*, 1994, *50*, 452–459.

CHAPTER 14

LASSA HEMORRHAGIC FEVER

LEARNING OBJECTIVES

- Define Lassa hemorrhagic fever and compare and contrast it to similar hemorrhagic fevers in the New World

- Describe the arenavirus responsible for causing this illness

- Discuss modes of infection

- Discuss the host's response to infection

- Describe symptomatology and diagnosis

- Discuss methods of treatment

- Discuss methods of prevention

Major Concepts

Symptoms

Lassa virus causes Lassa hemorrhagic fever (LHF) in approximately 20% of infected persons. Although the mortality rate is only 1% overall, it climbs to 15% to 20% in hospitalized patients and 60% in persons who are untreated. Symptoms include joint and lower back pain, severe muscle pain, headache, a nonproductive cough, epigastric pain, vomiting and diarrhea, abdominal discomfort, myocarditis, and hemorrhagic manifestations. Severe cases of disease may report edema of the face and neck, conjunctival hemorrhaging, mucosal bleeding, central cyanosis, bradycardia, pleural effusions, hepatitis, and encephalopathy with neurological manifestations. Large amounts of blood loss result from hemorrhaging and movement of fluid into the tissues, potentially leading to shock or death. Unlike most other hemorrhagic fevers, pathology during LHF is not associated with the production of large necrotic lesions or inflammation but rather results from loss of function of platelets, endothelial cells, monocytes and macrophages, and lymphocytes. Approximately 25% of individuals with LHF develop some degree of hearing loss, which is often permanent. Infection during pregnancy usually results in death of the fetus or the mother (or both).

Infection

Lassa virus is an Old World arenavirus. It is considered a BioSafety Level 4 organism and is closely related to the New World arenaviruses responsible for the American hemorrhagic fevers as well as several nonpathogenic Old World viruses that infect humans. Lassa virus is endemic to several West African countries, where the annual incidence of infection is 100,000 to 500,000, resulting in approximately 5,000 deaths per year. A rodent, the multimammate rat, serves as the reservoir host for Lassa virus, as is the case for other pathogenic arenaviruses. Humans may be infected by internalization of rat excreta via inhalation or ingestion, by being bitten by an infected rat, or during the preparation or eating of rats. Human-to-human transmission also occurs via exposure to body fluids or clinical samples or by sexual contact with an infected male. Nosocomial infection is also common.

Immune Response

Lassa virus inhibits production of proinflammatory cytokines and chemokines such as IL-6, TNF-α, and IL-8. This state of immunosuppression appears to aid in viral evasion of the immune response. Lassa virus infection of monocytes and macrophages is responsible, in part, for decreased immunity because infected cells are less able to produce proinflammatory cytokines or to express major histocompatibility complex type I molecules. These latter aid in activation of $CD8^+$ killer T lymphocytes, which are among the most important forces behind host antiviral activity. Other arenaviruses that do not alter cytokine production are not pathogenic to humans.

Protection

Ribavirin is the drug of choice in the treatment of LHF and is fairly efficacious when administered early after the beginning of symptomatic disease. A newer drug, T-705, appears to be less toxic and is effective when given to patients with advanced disease. Several candidate vaccines have been developed. Some of these use live, avirulent viruses, while other vaccines incorporate Lassa virus glycoprotein or nucleoprotein genes (or both) into a vaccinia virus vector. This latter approach may be problematic in that inoculation with vaccinia-based vaccines may prove fatal to immunosuppressed individuals, and HIV infection is common in regions endemic for the Lassa virus.

Introduction

Lassa virus, the causative agent of **Lassa hemorrhagic fever** (LHF), is a member of a family of viruses, the arenaviruses, which cause severe hemorrhagic fevers with high fatality rates in people from Africa and the Americas. Lassa virus is the most prevalent member of the family that infects humans: it is estimated to infect 100,000 to 500,000 people in West Africa annually. Most infections are asymptomatic, but LHF causes a severe and potentially fatal disease in individuals who do report symptoms. Many residents in some regions have developed antibodies to the virus, suggesting past undetected infection. The reservoir for Lassa virus is a rodent that is common in large areas of Africa, including many areas in which LHF has not yet been reported. Because the rodent frequently enters human habitations and is considered a delicacy among inhabitants of the region, contacts between humans and this rodent are very common. The large geological range of the viral reservoir, the frequency of interactions with humans, the low rate of overt disease, and the presence of other causes of hemorrhagic fever in Africa suggest the possibility that asymptomatic or otherwise undetected infections may be occurring in other areas of Africa. Furthermore, a new arenavirus that causes hemorrhagic fever in humans has recently been identified in South Africa and Zambia. Arenaviruses and arenavirus-associated hemorrhagic fevers

FIGURE 14.1 Lassa witch doctors

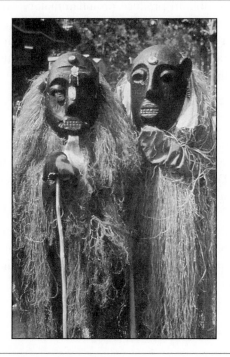

Note: The causes of infectious diseases are often not understood by residents of developing areas of the world who may turn to traditional healers for treatment. *Source:* CDC.

may thus pose a more serious threat to the health of residents of Africa than previously suspected.

A small number of cases have been found in people from Europe and North America after they have visited West Africa. LHF has been tested by some groups for use as a bioweapon, as has been the case for other related viral hemorrhagic fevers. Nonendemic regions of the world thus need to be prepared to deal with potential outbreaks of this disease in the future.

History

The first reported cases of LHF occurred during 1969 in a missionary hospital in Nigeria in western Africa. A nurse became infected while manually clearing secretions from the mouth of the first known Lassa fever patient. Infectious

FIGURE 14.2   Serum from a nurse who contracted
Lassa fever in Nigeria, 1969

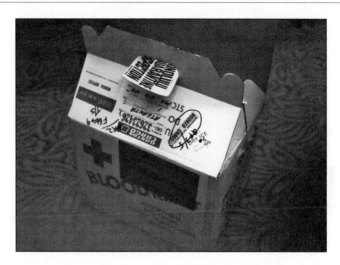

Source: CDC/Lyle Conrad.

material entered her body through a cut on her finger. Within a week, she was acutely ill and died three days later. Sixteen secondary infections were reported at that time.

A larger outbreak occurred in 1996 in which 470 persons became ill in Sierra Leone and the fatality rate among the hospitalized was 23%. In the first four months of 1997, a total of 328 persons were hospitalized, with a 14.6% fatality rate. The 1997 epidemic originated by human consumption of food that had been contaminated by rodent urine and later cases resulted from human-to-human transmission. In that year, the blood of health care workers from six centers in Nigeria was screened for the presence of antibodies to Lassa virus: 12.3% of those tested showed signs of past infection, the highest rate being among ward aides. Cases of Lassa fever have also been seen in the United States, Canada, the United Kingdom, Germany, the Netherlands, Japan, and Israel. Some infected individuals were residents of Africa who were transported to Europe or North America for medical care. Other infected persons had traveled to western Africa as students, soldiers, or members of a peacekeeping force in Sierra Leone.

In September and October 2008, an outbreak of a new type of viral hemorrhagic fever occurred in Zambia and South Africa caused by the **Lojo virus**. This is the only Arenavirus reported to cause disease in southern Africa. The first known cases involved a paramedic (the index case), the person cleaning his room, and the nurse caring for the index case. These reports were followed by the infection of a safari agent and her nurse. Four of the five infected individuals died. The nurse caring for the paramedic received ribavirin and recovered. None of the other patients received this antiviral drug.

The Disease

Infection with the Lassa virus is usually asymptomatic or mild, and the proportion of infected individuals who become ill ranges from 9% to 26%. Among those who become symptomatic, many will develop a severe, multisystem disease that may result in death or permanent disability. Hundreds of thousands of infections occur annually in western Africa, resulting in approximately 5,000 deaths. In some areas of Sierra Leone, LHF is responsible for 10% to 16% of hospital admissions, and as much as 40% of the general population has antibody to the virus, indicating previous exposure or infection.

FIGURE 14.3   Treating a child with Lassa fever in Sierra Leone

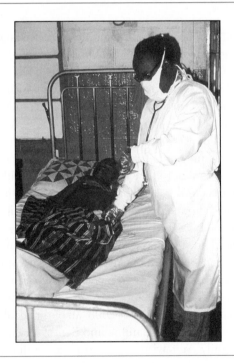

Source: CDC.

Disease severity is related to viral load. Pathogenic manifestations differ from those of filovirus-induced hemorrhagic fevers (Marburg and Ebola hemorrhagic fevers) and appear to result from alteration of cellular functions rather than an inflammatory response or the presence of lesions. Endothelial cell, platelet, and lymphocyte functions are suppressed, resulting in loss of fluid from blood vessels, decreased blood coagulation, hemorrhaging, and reduced antiviral immunity, including suppressed production of proinflammatory cytokines.

The virus initially replicates at the site of infection, generally the lungs or the bloodstream, if acquired through a break in the skin. During later stages of the disease, high levels of virus are found in the lymphatic system, including the spleen, liver, lymph nodes, and bone marrow. Very high viral titers have been reported in the mammary glands and placenta, and the ovaries, lungs, kidneys, adrenal glands, and myocardium of the heart are also infected. Unlike the case of Marburg and Ebola hemorrhagic fevers, infection of these organs does not result in significant production of lesions. After an incubation period of one to three weeks, infected individuals present with chills and high fever, exudative pharyngitis, weakness, and generalized malaise. This is followed by the gradual onset of joint and lower back pain, severe muscle pain, headache, a nonproductive cough, epigastric pain, vomiting and diarrhea with abdominal discomfort, myocarditis, and hemorrhagic manifestations, such as bleeding from the gums, nose, and lungs. Petechiae, pinpoint skin lesions, may be found on the upper chest, shoulders, and neck. Laboratory findings often include early lymphopenia, late neutrophilia, abnormal platelet functions, hemoconcentration as fluid leaves the circulatory system, and proteinuria (the presence of protein in the urine) due to kidney dysfunction. Jaundice and skin rash are rare.

After one week, individuals with mild infections begin to recover and the more severe cases begin to deteriorate. The most severe cases may be accompanied by edema of the face and neck, conjunctival hemorrhaging, mucosal bleeding, central cyanosis (bluish color), bradycardia (slowed heart rate), pleural effusions, hepatitis, and encephalopathy. Neurological manifestations may include intention tremors of the tongue, pharynx, larynx, and later, the extremities, followed by generalized convulsions. Loss of blood volume due to hemorrhaging and fluid entering the tissues may result in shock or death. In some of the early cases of LHF, death occurred about a week after the development of symptoms. Findings during the autopsy of those individuals included fluid in the lungs; enlarged pale livers; congestion of the heart, spleen, and kidneys; and a low number of lymphocytes. Although the overall mortality among infected persons is 1%, the mortality rate among hospitalized patients is much higher (15% to 20%) and approaches 60% among those who are not treated. Transient hair loss and ataxia (unsteady movement) may occur during recovery. Unlike the

FIGURE 14.4   Hepatitis caused by Lassa virus

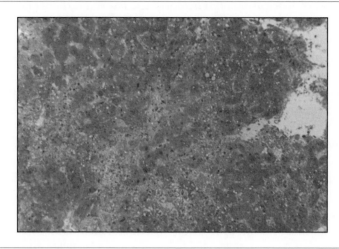

Source: CDC / W. Winn.

case with other hemorrhagic fevers, 25% of persons developing LHF experience some degree of unilateral or bilateral eighth cranial nerve deafness. Only half of these recover some degree of function after one to three months.

LHF is particularly severe for pregnant women and their fetuses. If infection occurs during the first trimester of pregnancy, a spontaneous abortion will usually result. If infection takes place during the third trimester, however, both mother and fetus typically will die. This unusual severity may result from the extremely high viral titer found in the placenta. The precise cause of death in these cases remains unknown as pathological lesions are not found in infected fetuses.

The Causative Agent

Lassa virus is a member of the Old World group of **Arenaviridae**. It is named after the town, about 100 miles south of the Sahara, in which the first case of LHF was detected. Other pathogenic members of this group include the cosmopolitan lymphocytic choriomeningitis virus and the Lojo virus from Zambia and South Africa. Other pathogenic members of the Arenaviridae are the New World Junin, Machupo, Guanarito, Sabia, and Chapare viruses (from South America) and the Whitewater Arroyo virus (from North America) in humans. These viruses cause hemorrhagic fevers in the Americas with high fatality rates (described in Chapter Thirteen). Other Old World viruses in this family include Ippy and Mobala viruses from the Central African Republic and **Mopeia virus** from Mozambique and Zimbabwe, all of which lead to non-pathogenic infections of humans. Interestingly, 75% of the amino acids from the nonpathogenic Mopeia virus and the pathogenic Lassa virus are the same. It may be useful to determine if Lassa virus isolates from patients with severe disease differ from those from persons with asymptomatic infection. In 2008, a novel Old World virus, the Lojo virus, caused an outbreak of hemorrhagic fever in South Africa and Zambia in which of the five persons infected, four died. The surviving individual had been treated with the antiviral compound ribavirin. **Pichinde virus** infection of hamsters or guinea pigs is frequently used as an animal model system for LHF due to the safety issues associated with working with Lassa virus.

Lassa virus and the American hemorrhagic fever viruses are all classified as BSL-4 microorganisms because they induce illnesses with a high mortality rate, are highly transmissible, and lack either an effective treatment or a useful vaccine. Work on these organisms, as well as other BSL-4 microbes, such as the Marburg and Ebola hemorrhagic fever viruses and variola (the smallpox agent), must be conducted under the tightly controlled conditions of a BSL-4 labora-tory, of which few exist throughout the world. Some groups have attempted to use the Lassa virus as a bioweapon.

Lassa virus is generally spheroidal but may be pleomorphic (assume many shapes). As is the case with the American hemorrhagic fever viruses, Lassa virus incorporates host ribosomes into the viral particle, giving it a "sandy" appear-ance. The viral envelope contains essential lipids, and its surface is studded with 10-nanometer projection spikes. Due to the presence of lipids in their envelopes, Lassa viruses are inactivated by either ether or chloroform. The genome of Lassa virus is single-stranded, negative-sense, bisegemented RNA consisting of a large and a small segment. The 3' and 5' portions of the RNA are transcribed to pro-duce proteins in opposite orientations. Replication of the genome occurs in the cytoplasm, followed by budding of infectious virions from the plasma membrane.

The large RNA segment encodes an RNA-dependent RNA polymerase and a small RING finger protein Z, which is a viral matrix protein. The small RNA segment encodes viral glycoprotein precursor and nucleoprotein. The former is processed to produce two mature glycoproteins, GP1 and GP2. GP1 is found on the top of the glycoprotein spike and allows viral interaction with the host cell's surface receptors. It is the target of host antibodies. GP2 is located next to the viral membrane and is similar to other viral membrane proteins involved in fusion with the host cell. GP1 of the Old World arenaviruses uses host **α-dystroglycan** (a cellular receptor for extracellular matrix proteins) as their receptor, whereas New World arenaviruses use the transferrin receptor 1 for this purpose. Following

FIGURE 14.5 Budding of Lassa viruses from an infected host cell

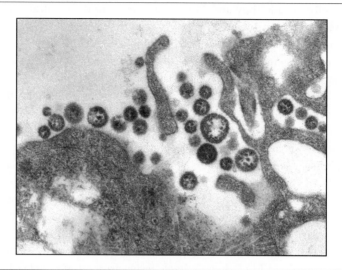

Source: CDC/C. S. Goldsmith, P. Rollin, and M. Bowen.

receptor binding, all known arenaviruses are taken into the cell by endocytosis into acidified endosomes, where GP2 mediates a pH-dependent fusion between the viral and host cell membranes. Lassa and the closely related lymphocytic choriomeningitis virus, however, enter target cells in a manner distinct from that of the New World viruses. The latter enter cells by clathrin-dependent endocytosis, whereas the former gain entry by a process that is independent of the human cell surface proteins clathrin, dynamin, and caveolin, which are typically involved in endocytosis. The pathway used by Old World arenaviruses requires cellular microtubules but not actin. This apparently rules out viral entry via macropinocytosis or the other clathrin- and caveolin-independent pathway used for trafficking of glycosylphosphatidylinositol-anchored proteins, as both rely on actin. Old World arenaviruses also undergo membrane fusion at an unusually low pH of less than 4.5. Viral delivery to late endosomes with this low pH does not require the Rab5 and Rab7 proteins, which transport some other viruses (New World arenaviruses and the influenza virus) to endosomes. Understanding the unusual entry and fusion mechanisms of these viruses may provide a key to blocking the early stages of infection. Target cells for Lassa virus infection and replication are the monocytes and macrophages of the innate immune system and endothelial cells lining blood vessels. Monocytes must mature into macrophages before viral replication may occur. Macrophages and endothelial cells are not damaged by Lassa virus infection.

The natural reservoir host of Lassa virus is *Mastomys natalensis* (the **multi-mammate rat**). The range of this rat covers the majority of Africa, but LHF is found only in West Africa (Nigeria, Sierra Leone, Liberia, and Guinea, and perhaps Senegal, Mali, the Central African Republic, and the Congo Republic). It should be noted that the American hemorrhagic fever viruses also have rodent reservoir hosts. Rat urine and droppings contain shed viruses, which may be transmitted to humans via direct contact with excretions on floors or in beds or by ingestion of contaminated food and water, breathing dried and aerosolized urine, being bitten by a rat, or during preparation or consumption of infected rats. Rats of this species are plentiful in many poorer regions of Africa and are commonly used as a food source. The virus does not cause disease in the rodent host. Transmission from rats to humans is highest during the dry season. Human-to-human transmission occurs via contact with secretions such as blood, saliva, pharyngeal secretions, urine, and semen or by contaminated medical equipment.

The Immune Response

The host immune response is responsible for both host protection and much of the pathology. Individuals who survive acute infection develop antibodies that persist for years after recovery. Immunity is protective against reinfection by the virus. CD8$^+$ T killer cells appear to be the most important component of a protective immune response against many viruses, including Lassa virus. To recognize the virus, they require that viral proteins be "presented" to them by other cells. Lassa virus has evolved mechanisms of avoiding such host immune responses.

Monocytes and macrophages are part of the innate immune system, producing inflammatory cytokines and, via expression of major histocompatibility class I molecules (MHC I), aid in presenting antigen to and activating CD8$^+$ T killer cells. Infection of monocytes and macrophages occurs early in infection. Macrophages are among the major host cells infected by Lassa virus. Infection of these cells by either virulent or avirulent Pichinde virus in the animal model of LHF leads to production of inflammatory cytokines, such as IL-6 and TNF-α; however, the avirulent form produces higher levels of these cytokines, indicating a potential role for these cytokines in host defense. Synthesis of both cytokines and MHC I is induced by some forms of the transcription factor nuclear factor kappa of B lymphocytes (NF-κB) and is influenced by different forms of another transcription factor, RBP-Jκ. Infection with avirulent, but not virulent, arenaviruses leads to production of stimulatory forms of both transcription factors and a higher degree of macrophage activation, stressing the beneficial role of macrophage activity in preventing arenavirus disease. Lassa virus decreases production of the proinflammatory **chemokine** IL-8 by macrophages and endothelial cells by inhibiting transcription of its mRNA. IL-8 increases adherence of immune cells to endothelial cells, extravasation of cells from blood vessels, and migration of these cells into the areas of active Lassa virus replication. Interestingly, Mopeia virus, a closely related but nonpathogenic Old World arenavirus, does not suppress IL-8 production.

In later stages of the infection, CD8$^+$ T killer cells may initiate harmful allergic responses. These cells, however, are also beneficial to the host in that they are responsible for the majority of viral clearance. Decreased MCH I expression by macrophages infected with virulent viruses may result in reduced CD8$^+$ T killer cell activity and viral evasion of the immune response. Furthermore, Lassa viruses are fairly resistant to host IFN-α and IFN-β; in fact, IFN levels are generally higher in patients with fatal versus nonfatal infections.

Diagnosis

Diagnosis may involve direct detection of the virus. Lassa virus may be isolated from blood or urine samples or from throat washings. It may be detected by polymerase chain reaction analysis of whole blood or serum. Alternatively, more indirect means of diagnosis may be employed, such as detecting the presence of antibodies to the virus. ELISA may be used to detect the presence of anti-Lassa virus IgM antibody. Infection is also indicated by a fourfold rise in the titer of antiviral IgG antibody between samples of acute and convalescent-phase serum as detected by ELISA or indirect fluorescent-antibody assay.

Laboratory abnormalities associated with LHF include proteinuria and elevated liver enzymes in which aspartate aminotransferase (AST) levels exceed those of alanine aminotransferase (ALT). Adverse prognostic factors are an AST exceeding 150 units per liter and a high level of viremia. Lassa virus–contaminated patient samples are a biohazard and should be handled under BSL-4 conditions; this is frequently not possible since no BSL-4 laboratories are present in the endemic regions. Heating serum for one hour at 60°C (140°F) inactivates the majority of the viruses and allows determination of heat-stable material.

Treatment

Treatment for LHF is generally supportive and may include renal dialysis and mechanical ventilation. Fluid and electrolyte balance and blood pressure must be carefully monitored and regulated to prevent shock, particularly if proteinuria

FIGURE 14.6 Receiving plasma to maintain blood volume during Lassa fever

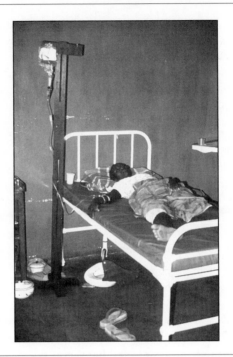

Source: CDC.

or rising hematocrit is detected. Seizures must be controlled. Intervention may be needed to treat secondary bacterial infections.

Administration of convalescent plasma has been attempted in the treatment of individuals with LHF but was not found to be beneficial; on the contrary, its use may lead to the transmission of bloodborne pathogens, such as HIV or the hepatitis B or hepatitis C viruses, which are common in the affected area. This is in contrast to American HF, which often responds favorably to convalescent plasma. Ribavirin has been the antiviral drug of choice but appears to be effective only when administered during the first six days of illness. It also has significant toxicity to humans, with hemolytic anemia being the major side effect. This destruction of red blood cells may be particularly problematic for persons with hemorrhagic diseases in which large amounts of blood are lost through excessive bleeding. A newer drug being tested for use during arenavirus infections is T-705 (6-fluoro-3-hydroxy-2-pyrazinecarboxamid), which is less toxic than ribavirin. This compound appears to be effective in killing several

RECENT DEVELOPMENTS

Stampidine (stavudine-5'-[p-bromophenyl methoxyalaninyl phosphate]) is a pyrimidine nucleoside analogue derived from the reverse transcriptase inhibitor d4T. It appears to have a greater degree of antiviral activity against immunodeficiency-causing retroviruses than AZT. It is effective against organisms such as the feline immunodeficiency virus, HIV-1 and HIV-2, including drug-resistant strains of HIV-1 and a variety of clinical isolates from various regions of the world. It also has a good safety profile with little to no detectable toxicity in mice and dogs and rapidly reaches therapeutic levels in the plasma that are maintained for hours. This drug was recently reported to decrease seizures and mortality in Lassa virus–infected mice. Stampidine is able to cross the blood-brain barrier to kill viruses that have been able to enter the central nervous system. Given the interest among some parties for developing hemorrhagic fever viruses, including Lassa virus and the American hemorrhagic fever arenaviruses, as agents of biowarfare, the development of new treatment strategies for these viruses that have little toxicity to mammals is encouraging.

types of RNA viruses and is under clinical development for influenza. T-705 proved more effective than ribavirin at decreasing mortality in the animal model of LHF (Pichinde virus–infected hamsters), even when administered during the advanced stage of infection.

Prevention

Patients diagnosed with LHF should be confined to strict barrier isolation in a private room separated from traffic patterns. Room entry should be restricted to essential personnel. Care must be used in handling patient samples and material contaminated with excretions or coming into contact with the patient. Solutions such as sodium hypochlorite (bleach) or phenol plus detergent or formaldehyde fumigation may be used on material unable to withstand boiling, incineration, or autoclaving. Male patients should abstain from unprotected sexual activity for three months or until their semen is shown to be virus-free. Bodies of the deceased should not be embalmed but should instead be sealed in leakproof material prior to cremation or buried promptly in a sealed casket.

Several lines of research are being pursued in the hope of developing a protective, affordable vaccine for LHF. One avenue of attack employs a similar

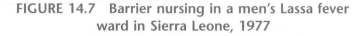

FIGURE 14.7   Barrier nursing in a men's Lassa fever
ward in Sierra Leone, 1977

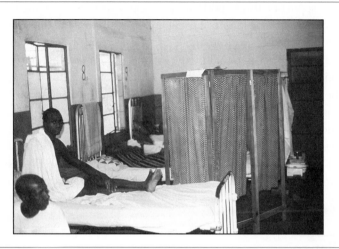

Source: CDC.

virus, the Mozambique virus, which is nonpathogenic. This approach is similar
to that of Edward Jenner, who used the nonpathogenic cowpox virus to immunize people against infection with the highly pathogenic variola (smallpox) virus.
Another vaccine candidate is the ML29 live, attenuated, reassortment virus
containing the nucleoprotein and glycoproteins of Lassa virus and the Z and
L proteins of the nonpathogenic Mopeia virus. Live vaccines are better able to
induce a CD8$^+$ T killer cell response than are vaccines that use dead material
or viral proteins alone, and this type of immunity appears to be most important
in stopping Lassa virus infections. The ML29 vaccine was safe for use in common marmosets, a nonhuman T primate species, and completely protected them
against challenge with virulent Lassa virus. The vaccine elicited production of
the cytokines TNF-α and IFN-γ. Considering that TNF-α production is inhibited by virulent arenaviruses but not by avirulent strains, this cytokine may be
important for host protection.

A number of researchers have developed viral vectors containing Lassa virus
genes incorporated into nonpathogenic viruses. One group used vaccinia as a
viral vector for the Lassa virus nucleoprotein and glycoprotein. This vaccinia
construct induced antibody production in mice and was protective to monkeys
after challenge with intact Lassa virus. Other researchers administered a whole,
killed Lassa virus vaccine to rhesus macaques following inactivation by gamma
radiation. The vaccine successfully induced antibody production in the monkeys;

however, the animals died after challenge with active virus. This may indicate that antibodies may not be the most useful component of the host immune response. In support of this hypothesis, a vaccinia vector expressing both Lassa virus glycoproteins induced only a small antibody response in animals; nevertheless, 88% of the animals survived challenge. Conversely, if the vaccinia vector contained Lassa nucleoprotein, all of the animals developed high levels of antibodies, but only 20% survived challenge. It is thus believed that $CD8^+$ T killer cells may be a more important part of the host immune response to Lassa virus infection than antibodies produced by B lymphocytes. One major problem with most of these lines of research is that administration of vaccines based on the vaccinia virus has the potential to kill HIV-infected persons. In light of the fact that much of the population of the area threatened by LHF is HIV-positive, this approach would produce vaccines that could not be safely administered to the majority of the people.

Surveillance

Surveillance of the incidence of LHF revealed that civil disruption, such as that occurring around the turn of the century in Sierra Leone, may alter patterns of disease transmission. Although incidence had been highest during the dry season, infection rate rose during the change from the dry to wet season. Unrest among civilians may lead to disruption of food production, destruction of crops and loss of livestock, and population displacement and relocation to refugee centers, resulting in overcrowding. These conditions may lead to increased dependence on rats as a food source, facilitate the spread of infectious diseases, and place increased stress on an already overburdened health care system, with consequent amplification of nosocomial spread.

Given the recent (2008) discovery of the Lojo virus, an arenavirus that causes hemorrhagic fever with a very high fatality rate in southern Africa, as well as discoveries of new members of the New World group of the family, some of which cause hemorrhagic fever in the Americas, efforts need to be made to identify other arenaviruses that may produce severe or fatal disease in humans. Lassa virus is confined to West Africa, but the detection of a new hemorrhagic fever virus in southern Africa calls into question whether other pathogenic arenaviruses may exist undetected in the African continent. Infections with such viruses may be currently attributed to other, more common organisms, such as *Plasmodium* species (agents of malaria) or dengue virus, which cause serious febrile illness in the region. Considering that ribavirin may be effective in the treatment of infections caused by both the Lassa and Lojo viruses but not other microbes causing

FIGURE 14.8   Viewing tissue samples during a Lassa fever investigation

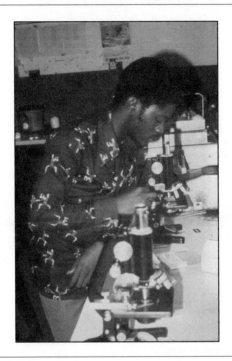

Source: CDC/P. A. Webb.

similar symptoms, it is crucial to determine the causative agent correctly in order to administer potentially lifesaving therapy. Surveillance efforts may include determination of the causative agent for all outbreaks of potential hemorrhagic fever in Africa and studies of the incidence of infection and transmission patterns for the rodent reservoir hosts.

Summary

Disease

- Lassa hemorrhagic fever

Causative Agent

- Lassa virus

Agent Type

- Virus of the Old World Arenaviridae family

Genome

- Single-stranded RNA

Vector

- None

Common Reservoir

- Multimammate rat

Modes of Transmission

- Direct contact with contaminated rat urine or droppings, ingestion of contaminated food, inhalation of aerosolized urine, rat bite, or during preparation or consumption of rats as food   • Human-to-human transmission via contact with contaminated blood, saliva, and semen or from medical equipment

Geographical Distribution

- West Africa

Year of Emergence

- 1969

Key Terms

α-dystroglycan Cell surface receptor for extracellular matrix proteins that binds to Lassa virus glycoprotein during infection of its target cells

Arenaviridae Family of enveloped RNA viruses that contain the causative agents for Lassa hemorrhagic fever and the American hemorrhagic fevers

Chemokine Immune messenger molecule that attracts specific white blood cells to areas of infection

Lassa hemorrhagic fever Potentially fatal illness characterized by high fever, hemorrhagic manifestations, severe muscle and bone pain, deafness, and shock

Lassa virus Causative agent for Lassa hemorrhagic fever in West Africa

Lojo virus Causative agent for hemorrhagic fever in southern Africa

Mopeia virus Old World arenavirus that causes a nonpathogenic infection in humans

Multimammate rat *Mastomys natalensis*, the reservoir host for Lassa fever virus

Pichinde virus Old World arenavirus used to model Lassa hemorrhagic fever in guinea pigs and hamsters

Review Questions

1. To what family does the causative agent of Lassa hemorrhagic fever belong? What other members of this family cause disease in humans, where are they found, and with which diseases are they associated?
2. What symptoms occur during severe cases of Lassa hemorrhagic fever?
3. What are several ways in which infection with Lassa hemorrhagic fever differs from that caused by closely related New World viruses?
4. What components of the host immune response are inhibited during Lassa virus infection? What are the underlying causes of this loss of immunity?
5. What are the methods of treatment for Lassa hemorrhagic fever? What are the possible deleterious effects of these methods?

Topics for Further Discussion

1. Explore the potential significance of the important differences between the pathogenic mechanisms and cellular receptors used by hemorrhagic fevers induced by Lassa virus and other arenaviruses and filoviruses. Postulate how these differences might affect the development of drugs to combat these diseases.
2. Lassa virus enters its target cells using an unusual type of endocytosis that differs from the mechanism human cells typically employ in the internalization of nutrients and other macromolecules. Learn more about the normal endocytic process, and discuss how it differs from that used by Lassa virus. How do you think these differences might possibly be exploited to block Lassa virus infection of human cells?
3. Knowing that a number of serious infectious diseases in sub-Saharan Africa result in fever, blood loss, and death and that the number of emerging infectious diseases is continuing to increase, discuss the possibility that other as yet unknown arenaviruses causing human illnesses may be discovered and then, based on your findings, describe the geographical areas and populations most likely to be at risk.

4. The animal reservoir for Lassa virus is the multimammate rat. This animal is very common in Africa and has a large range. It also interacts frequently with humans. Find out more about this rodent's habits and habitat and the ways in which it interacts with humans throughout its range. Use this information to suggest practical and affordable means of preventing viral transmission to humans. Discuss reasons why Lassa hemorrhagic fever is found in only a small portion of the range of this rat.

Resources

Briese, T., and others. "Genetic Detection and Characterization of Lojo Virus, a New Hemorrhagic Fever–Associated Arenavirus from Southern Africa." *PLoS Pathogens*, 2009, *4*, 1–8.

Chin, J. *Control of Communicable Diseases Manual* (17th ed.). Washington, D.C.: American Public Health Association, 2000.

Fennewald, S. M., Aronson, J. F., Zhang, L., and Herzog, N. K. "Alterations in NF-κB and RBP-Jκ by arenavirus infection of macrophages in vitro and in vivo." *Journal of Virology*, 2002, *76*, 1154–1162.

Gowen, B. B., and others. "Treatment of Late Stage Disease in a Model of Arenaviral Hemorrhagic Fever: T-705 Efficacy and Reduced Toxicity Suggests an Alternative to Ribavirin." *PLos ONE*, 2008, *3*, 1–11.

Johnson, K. M. "Epidemic Hemorrhagic Fevers." In P. D. Hoeprich (ed.), *Infectious Diseases*. Hagerstown, Md.: Harper & Row, 1977.

Keeton, C. "South African Doctors Move Quickly to Contain New Virus." *Bulletin of the World Health Organization*, 2008, *86*, 912–913.

Lukashevich, I. S., and others. "Lassa and Mopeia Virus Replication in Human Monocytes/Macrophages and in Endothelial Cells: Different Effects on IL-8 and TNF-α Gene Expression." *Journal of Medical Virology*, 1999, *59*, 552–560.

Lukashevich, I. S., and others. "Safety, Immunogenicity, and Efficacy of the ML29 Reassortant Vaccine for Lassa Fever in Small Non-Human Primates." *Vaccine*, 2008, *26*, 5246–5254.

Rojek, J. M., and others. "Different Mechanisms of Cell Entry by Human-Pathogenic Old World and New World Arenaviruses." *Journal of Virology*, 2008, *82*, 7677–7687.

Uckun, F. M., and others. "Stampidine Prevents Mortality in an Experimental Mouse Model of Viral Hemorrhagic Fever Caused by Lassa Virus." *BMC Infectious Diseases*, 2004, *4*, 1–7.

Walker, D. H., and others. "Pathologic and Virologic Study of Fatal Lassa Fever in Man." *American Journal of Pathology*, 1982, *107*, 349–356.

CHAPTER 15

DENGUE FEVER AND DENGUE HEMORRHAGIC FEVER

LEARNING OBJECTIVES

- Define and contrast dengue fever, dengue hemorrhagic fever, and dengue shock syndrome

- Describe the flavivirus responsible for causing these illnesses

- Discuss modes of infection

- Discuss the host's response to infection

- Describe symptomatology and diagnosis

- Discuss potential methods of treatment

- Discuss methods of prevention

Major Concepts

Symptoms

Infection with dengue virus leads to either dengue fever (DF), dengue hemorrhagic fever (DHF), or dengue shock syndrome (DSS). DF is an extremely painful febrile illness likened to the pain of having many broken bones. It is self-limiting and typically resolves within ten days except for transient fatigue and depression. DHF is a severe, life-threatening form of the disease that primarily affects children under the age of 15 years. Its symptoms include fever, profound abdominal pain, liver damage, petechial rash, hemorrhaging, increased vascular permeability, and capillary leak syndrome. DSS is characterized by the DHF symptoms as well as dangerously low blood pressure and shock, which may result in death if fluid volume is not promptly restored. DHF and DSS have mortality rates of up to 30%.

Emergence of DHF and DSS

Dengue fever has been known in tropical areas of the world since 1770, with increasing numbers of epidemics occurring over time as the disease spread throughout Asia, Africa, and the Americas. The incidence of DHF and DSS are rapidly increasing as well. Dengue is now pandemic, due in part to events beginning during World War II when large-scale movement of vehicles and infected personnel, trapping of water in tires, and increased numbers of water storage areas brought the virus into areas with many new, susceptible human hosts and provided breeding habitat for the principal vector, *Aedes aegypti*, a day-biting mosquito whose preferential hosts are humans. Although *A. aegypti* numbers were once greatly reduced in much of the Americas due to large-scale mosquito elimination programs, vector numbers rebounded when the programs were halted during the 1970s. An additional mosquito vector, *A. albopictus*, is able to survive colder temperatures, including those found in many U.S. states.

Infection

Dengue virus is a single-stranded RNA member of the flavivirus group and is closely related to the causative agents of yellow fever and Japanese encephalitis. Four viral serotypes exist that are currently expanding their ranges. Several serotypes coexist in many parts of the world, triggering increasing numbers of DHF and DSS, as these disease manifestations usually occur following an individual's secondary infection with a serotype differing from that first encountered. Host factors that affect disease severity include age, sex, and racial background: DHF and DSS are more common in female children and less common in those of African origin or persons suffering from malnutrition. Secondary infection with viruses of the DEN-2 serotype or strains originating in Asia is more likely to cause severe disease.

Immune Response

The immune response to dengue virus either may be protective or may increase pathology. DHF and DSS often result from antibody-dependent enhancement, a process in which nonneutralizing antibodies to one viral serotype decrease to low levels at the time of infection with dengue viruses of a different serotype. Low levels of these cross-reacting IgG antibodies lead to the formation of large immune complexes that are ingested by macrophages; these cells then act as hosts for replicating viruses. Inflammatory cytokines released by immune cells cause much of the pathology associated with infection, including increased vascular permeability, loss of fluid from capillaries, and destruction of platelets. Other cytokines, such as IFN-γ, may have dual roles during the illness, blocking viral replication but also increasing infection of macrophages. One viral protein blocks cellular responses to interferons in an attempt to evade the immune response.

Introduction

Dengue fever (DF) and its more serious correlates, **dengue hemorrhagic fever (DHF)** and **dengue shock syndrome (DSS),** are currently found throughout the world, causing great pain and many deaths. It is the most common vectorborne infection of humanity, with 50 to 100 million cases of DF reported per year, mostly in tropical regions. Several hundred thousand cases of DHF occur as well, with a fatality rate of 5% in treated individuals. This severe condition is most common in children and young adults. Over time, the epidemics have become larger and more frequent due to population increases in urban centers and to rapid dissemination via air travel. The largest single epidemic involved 370,000 cases in Vietnam in 1987. In addition to the toll in human suffering and lives, dengue heavily taxes economic systems, often in regions that can ill afford this burden. The costs of medical intervention, mosquito eradication programs, and lost tourist revenues place a great strain on developing regions and health care systems already struggling under a host of other infectious diseases.

We are currently in the midst of a dengue pandemic as DHF spreads to countries in which it was previously unknown. In 1980, DHF was not endemic in any country in the Americas. By 1995, some 250,000 confirmed cases of DF and 7,000 cases of DHF were reported spread among 18 countries in the Americas. Dengue remains relatively rare are in United States, although over 400 confirmed cases have been brought into the country by travelers. This situation is likely to change, however, as the correct mosquito vectors are present in the United States. At least three cases are known to have been transmitted endogenously in Texas since 1980.

Four serotypes of the dengue virus have been reported from various locales around the globe. Each of these serotypes contains multiple viral strains that differ in virulence and in antigenicity. Areas of hyperendemicity (where more than one strain of dengue is endemic) are increasing, complicating epidemiological studies.

History

The first epidemics of dengue fever were reported in 1770 in Asia, Africa, and North America. Infections thereafter were periodic and infrequent, and intervals of 10 to 40 years often separated epidemics due to their slow spread by sailing vessels. Since the early 1980s, however, dengue has been at pandemic levels, its rapid spread fueled by an expansion of the geographical range of both the mosquito vector and all of the virus serotypes. Hyperendemicity is growing as multiple serotypes occupy the same region, resulting in the emergence of the more deadly manifestations of infection, dengue hemorrhagic fever and dengue shock syndrome.

The modern DF pandemic began in Southeast Asia during the Second World War as a result of the movement of military equipment that trapped rainwater and led to the spread of the mosquito vector to previously uninfected regions. During the war, many water systems were destroyed and the number of water storage facilities increased, providing new niches for mosquito larvae to exploit. The outbreak was further spurred by the transit of hundreds of thousands of uninfected Japanese and Allied soldiers into infected areas. Mosquito hosts moved into most of the central and southern islands of the Pacific, although their isolation and small human populations kept dengue epidemics brief. Larger Pacific islands were also affected, and in 1953 and 1954, an epidemic of DHF occurred in Manila in the Philippines, having previously appeared in Bangkok, Thailand, in 1950. Earlier clinical reports of illnesses similar to DHF and DSS appear in medical records from northeastern Australia in 1897 and Greece in 1928.

Several decades after World War II, DHF again struck Asia in Sri Lanka, India, Pakistan, Taiwan, China, and Singapore as the range of the virus and its mosquito vector spread. Multiple serotypes were present during this epidemic, with the DEN-3 serotype predominating. The responsible viral strain was distinct from previous isolates. By 1975, DHF was the leading cause of hospitalization and death in children. About 900,000 cases of DHF and DSS occurred in Thailand between the years of 1958 and 1990. Since then, the incidence of dengue diseases in Southeast Asia has continued to increase in intensity as the presence of multiple viral serotypes in a given area became more frequent. Four times as many cases of DHF were reported in the past 15 years than were reported during the previous 30 years.

In Africa, dengue-related disease is also increasing. The surveillance system in the area is imperfect, but the number of DF epidemics has been rising since 1980, most notably in East Africa (Kenya, Mozambique, Sudan, Djibouti, and Somalia) and in Saudi Arabia. All four serotypes are active in these regions. Although sporadic cases of DHF have been reported in several of these countries, no epidemic of severe disease has occurred. In western Africa and parts of Southeast Asia, dengue virus also circulates in monkey populations.

Dengue was unknown in the Western Hemisphere until the advent of European colonization and the African slave trade. In the Americas, programs directed by the Pan-American Health Organization wiped out the mosquito vector, virtually eliminating yellow fever and decreasing the incidence of dengue until only sporadic cases of DF occurred in island areas that failed to eradicate the vector entirely. During the 1970s, these mosquito control programs were abandoned; as a result, the incidence of DF is now greater than before the vector control program began. In 1970, the DEN-2 and DEN-3 serotypes were found in the Americas, and the latter caused several epidemics in Puerto Rico and Colombia in the mid-1970s. DEN-1 was introduced into the area in 1977, resulting in epidemics of DF in Jamaica, Cuba, Puerto Rico, and Venezuela in 1977 and 1978 before spreading throughout the Caribbean, north into Mexico and Texas, and south into Central America and northern South America. DEN-4 was imported into the eastern Caribbean in 1981 and caused major epidemics throughout the surrounding areas. The same year, a new strain of DEN-2 originating in Southeast Asia (most likely in Vietnam) was imported into Cuba, leading to the first major epidemic of DHF in the Americas. Over 10,000 cases of DHF occurred during this outbreak; however, large-scale hospitalization and effective fluid replacement therapy limited the number of deaths to 158 people. The next major epidemic of DHF began in Venezuela in 1989 and 1990, resulting in more than 6,000 cases of disease and 73 deaths. Between 1990 and 1995, DEN-2 led to a series of smaller epidemics in Colombia, Brazil, Puerto Rico, and Mexico. By 1997, 18 countries in the region had reported DHF cases. A novel strain of DEN-3 from Sri Lanka appeared in 1994 and led to an outbreak of DF in Costa Rica and Panama and DHF in Nicaragua. Yellow fever incidence has increased in the tropical areas of the Americas as well.

FIGURE 15.1 Female *Aedes aegypti* taking a blood meal

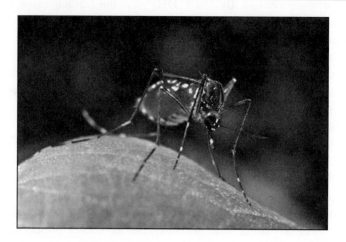

Source: CDC/Frank Hadley Collins.

The United States has seen a small number of imported cases of dengue in Texas in 1980, 1986, 1995, and 1997. Although the virus has not yet established a foothold in the country, the United States is home to two species of suitable mosquito vectors, most notably ***Aedes aegypti***, which abides in the Gulf Coast states from Texas to Florida. The other potential vector species, ***Aedes albopictus***, entered the United States in the early 1980s and has spread to 25 states.

Several factors account for the spread of dengue. Numbers of mosquito vectors rise as the extent of urbanization in a region increases and adequate access to sewage treatment facilities decreases. The presence of pools of standing water also fuels the growth of mosquito populations. Aggressive vector control programs eliminated many of the dengue vectors from most of Latin America during the 1940s and 1950s, but subsequent increases in urbanization led to reinfestation of many areas during the 1970s. Air travel has also rapidly spread the virus to new locales with susceptible hosts. Between 1983 and 1995, the number of international travelers leaving the United States increased from 20 million to 40 million. Half of these people were bound for tropical regions.

The Diseases

The name *dengue* is derived from the Swahili *ki denga pepo*, which means "seizure caused by an evil spirit."

The illness may manifest itself in three different forms: dengue fever, dengue hemorrhagic fever, or dengue shock syndrome. All forms may present with generalized vascular damage. Diffuse hemorrhage, edema, and congestion of organs also occur in DHF and DSS. In these two serious disease manifestations, antibodies produced in response to a prior infection may lead to the formation of large immune complexes containing antibody bound to microbial components, leading to the production of disseminated intravascular coagulation or hemorrhagic lesions with potentially lethal results.

Dengue Fever (DF)

Dengue fever, also known as **breakbone fever**, generally occurs in older children and adults. Infection may be asymptomatic or result in painful but short-term illness. After an incubation period of 3 to 14 days (usually 4 to 7 days), an infected person may present with fever of sudden onset, severe frontal headache, myalgia, and loss of appetite. This is followed by decreased numbers of neutrophils and platelets; severe eye, bone, and muscle pain; change in taste perception; nausea and vomiting; rapid heartbeat; and anxiety and depression. The extreme pain has been equated to that resulting from a multitude of broken bones. Later during the course of the infection, petechial rashes may be found on the extremities, underarms, and mucous membranes as a result of hemorrhaging of small blood vessels in the skin. This might be due to a host antibody response to the virus. Acute illness persists for eight to ten days. The infection is self-limiting and, though very painful, is seldom fatal in this form and is mild in comparison to DHF or DSS. Following treatment for DF, persons generally recover completely with the exception of some postinfection fatigue and depression. In rare cases, DF progresses to the more serious DHF or DSS.

Dengue Hemorrhagic Fever (DHF) and Dengue Shock Syndrome (DSS)

DHF and DSS constitute the severe dengue virus–associated diseases. More than 500,000 cases of DHF and DSS occur each year, with fatality rates ranging from 1% to 10%. If untreated, these rates may approach 30%. DHF and DSS are generally confined to children under the age of 15 years, with a fatality rate of up to 8%. Early disease manifestations include upper respiratory symptoms, anorexia, vomiting, and facial flush. Worsening of disease is accompanied by the onset of weakness, severe restlessness, facial pallor, profound abdominal pain, cyanosis (bluish hue to the skin), liver enlargement and damage, petechial rash, and bleeding gums. Serious pathology is linked to hemorrhaging two to six days after the onset of fever. Increased vascular permeability with capillary leak syndrome and fluid loss from the circulatory system, low white blood cell and platelet numbers, elevations in hematocrit of over 20%, and hemoconcentration accompany DHF. Decreased platelet levels may interfere with blood clotting, contributing to hemorrhaging. Large decreases in blood pressure, shock, and death may rapidly occur if the loss of plasma is not corrected and quickly countered by fluid replacement. Spontaneous hemorrhaging may be fatal if occurring in the gastrointestinal tract or the inner cerebral region of the brain.

DSS may occur as a result of a decrease in blood pressure and hemoconcentration as plasma leaks from the circulatory system into the tissues. It may present as a weak, rapid pulse; narrow pulse pressure (difference in systolic and diastolic pressures); hypotension; cold, clammy skin; and restlessness. DSS occurs in one-third of severe dengue cases and is most commonly seen in children. Platelet numbers are low, and bleeding times are prolonged. Major bleeding may occur from several sites on the body with or without the presence of shock. Treatment may include administration of intravenous fluids to increase blood volume and raise blood pressure to more optimal levels.

Factors Influencing the Development of DF Versus DHF or DSS

Several factors combine to determine whether a given individual infected with the dengue virus develops the relatively mild DF or the more severe DHF or DSS. Several of these factors relate to the immune system: antibody-dependent enhancement and the types of MHC molecules expressed on surface of the person's cells (discussed later in this chapter). These factors increase the likelihood of developing severe disease in people who have a history of prior dengue infection after secondary infection with viruses of a different serotype than the original virus.

Table 15.1 Factors influencing the development of DHF and DSS

Immune factors	Antibody-dependent enhancement (↑ risk)
	Major histocompatibility complex types
Viral characteristics	DEN-2 (↑ risk)
	Strains of Asian origin (↑ risk)
Population characteristics	Female (↑ risk)
	Child (↑ risk)
	Caucasian or Asian (↑ risk)
Presence of other disease conditions	Peptic ulcer (↑ risk)
	Moderate to severe malnutrition (↓ risk)

Severe disease is partly dependent on the virulence of the infecting strain. Strains of the virus in the DEN-2 serotype are often more virulent than those of other serotypes. Differing degrees of virulence also exist within a serotype: the DEN-2 strain present in Puerto Rico in 1969 was mild, whereas the strain introduced into Cuba during the early 1980s was associated with a higher incidence of DHF and /DSS. The latter strain was more closely related to virulent strains found in SE Asia than to the Puerto Rico strain. Secondary infection with viruses of Southeast Asian origin is typically associated with DHF or DSS.

Gender and racial origin also affect disease severity. Girls are more susceptible than boys to developing lethal DSS. Caucasians and Asians are more likely to have severe infection than individuals of African descent. These differences may be related to major histocompatibility complex (MHC) molecule expression, as these immune system identifiers are genetically determined and the prevalence of each varies among racial groups. The decreased virulence in people of African origin as well as the relative rarity of DHF and DSS in Africa has led to the suggestion that a "dengue resistance gene" may be present in some populations. Whether such a resistance gene is linked the MHC complex has yet to be determined.

Other host factors may also affect disease severity. Children with moderate to severe protein malnutrition are less likely to develop DHF or DSS. Persons with peptic ulcers (usually caused by infection with *Helicobacter pylori*, often in the impoverished) and menstruating females are also more susceptible to dangerous, severe bleeding during dengue infection.

The Causative Agent

Dengue virus is responsible for all three diseases: dengue fever, dengue hemorrhagic fever, and dengue shock syndrome. This member of the ***Flavivirus*** genus is closely related to two other agents of serious disease, the yellow fever virus and the Japanese encephalitis virus, both of which cause substantial morbidity and mortality in the world. The genome of the dengue virus is single-stranded, positive-sense RNA that encodes ten genes. The viral outer membrane contains lipoprotein.

Several types of cells are infected by dengue viruses, including dendritic cells such as Langerhans cells, monocytes and macrophages, lymphocytes, endothelial cells, and hepatocytes. Interestingly, many of these target cells are part of the immune system. Langerhans cells are dendritic cells in the skin that protect the host against invasion via that route. In the case of dengue virus, Langerhans cells are hijacked to serve as hosts for viral replication and to allow travel to distant sites. Langerhans cells are approximately ten times more permeable to infection as are monocytes and macrophages in blood and tissue. DC-SIGN is a molecule on the surface of several types of immune cells, including Langerhans cells and monocytes and macrophages. Dengue virus binds to this molecule either alone or in the presence of a coreceptor prior to infecting host cells. Other viruses also use this immune molecule to begin the cellular infection process, most notably Marburg, Ebola, and hepatitis C viruses. Marburg and Ebola viruses also cause life-threatening hemorrhagic fever, as described in Chapter Twelve. After infection, Langerhans cells travel to regional lymph nodes, where they may interact with and infect T lymphocytes. Dendritic cells also produce matrix metalloproteinases, enzymes that degrade extracellular matrix, enhancing vascular permeability and plasma leakage.

Dengue virus exists in four serotypes (DEN-1, DEN-2, DEN-3, and DEN-4), which emerged approximately 2,000 years ago. The nucleoside sequences of the different serotypes' genomes vary by as much as 40% in the envelope genes, the major targets for antibody-mediated and T cell–mediated immune responses. DEN-1 and DEN-3 are most closely related of the group; DEN-4 has the greatest genetic diversity. No immunological cross-reactivity exists between the various dengue serotypes, thus allowing hyperendemicity to arise. The four serotypes have undergone an explosion in genetic diversity over the past 200 years, in some ways similar to the more recent explosion of HIV strains (another RNA virus). This is likely due to the increased availability of new groups of susceptible hosts that had not previously been exposed to the virus, perhaps reflecting increases in and interactions between human populations. The ability of persons to rapidly travel and relocate, including movement by air and ship, and intermingling of these groups of vulnerable hosts, may have facilitated this process.

Dengue virus is transmitted to humans primarily by the bite of female *Aedes aegypti* or *A. albopictus* mosquitoes. Outbreaks of dengue correlate to the size of the vectors' population and usually occur during the wet season and following a heavy rain, as these events increase the number of potential mosquito breeding sites. *A. aegypti* is a black-and-white mosquito, generally domestic and day-biting, that prefers humans for its blood meals. Biting activity increases in the two hours after sunrise and before sunset. These insects adapt well to urban settings and lay their eggs in small stagnant pools of water or in water that has collected in vessels used to trap and store rainwater, flower vases, pet water bowls, and urban cast-offs, such as nonbiodegradable plastic containers, cellophane, and discarded tires. *A. aegypti* are found south of 35° north latitude.

Aedes albopictus is a rural mosquito originating in Asia that has been adapting itself to urban settings. It was introduced to the United States in the 1980s through Asian truck tires brought into the country to be retreaded. These mosquitoes

FIGURE 15.2 Cemetery in New Orleans serving as an urban breeding site for *A. aegypti*

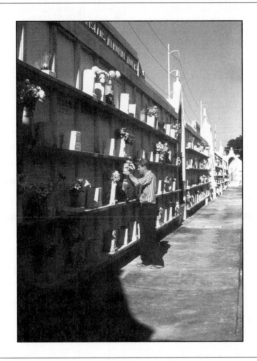

Source: CDC.

are more cold-tolerant than *A. aegypti*, allowing them to extend their range by 7° of north latitude. The increased tolerance to cold results from **diapause**, a suspension of egg hatching during winter months that is similar to hibernation. *A. albopictus* infestations are currently found in many eastern U.S. states. Humans are less of a target for these mosquitoes than for *A. aegypti*. Among other *Aedes* species, *A. scutellaris* serves as the viral vector in Polynesia, and *A. niveus* in Malaysia and *A. furcifer-taylori* in West Africa maintain the mosquito-monkey cycle.

Once a mosquito has ingested the virus from an infected person, it remains infective to humans for the remainder of its life without suffering any ill effects due to its viral passenger. In addition to acquiring the virus during blood meals on human hosts, female mosquitoes may pass dengue virus to their offspring through eggs or to their mates through sexual transmission.

Other than mosquito-to-human transmission, relatively rare instances of human-to-human transmission have been reported. Several cases of vertical transmission from infected mother to newborn have occurred. Nosocomial transmission is also possible from needlesticks of material from infected patients. Rare instances of infection have been reported following renal or bone marrow transplantation, and two instances of transmission via blood transfusion have occurred. Many countries require a deferral period from blood donation following dengue infection.

The Immune Response

The disease manifestation resulting from infection by dengue virus is affected by both the individual's immune response and the serotype of the virus involved. Antibodies to the initial serotype prevent reinfection with that serotype, and this protection may be lifelong. These antibodies also protect briefly (for less than three months) against infection with other serotypes. As antibody concentrations decrease over time, they begin to increase the replication of viruses of other serotypes in the process of **antibody-dependent enhancement (ADE)**. This enhancement is eventually lost as antibody levels fall even further. ADE increases the likelihood of developing the serious forms of infection (DHF and DSS). Interestingly, children are also at higher risk of DHF or DSS during the first year of life due to the lingering presence of maternal antibody acquired transplacentally.

Low levels of nonneutralizing antidengue IgG antibodies produce large immune complexes in combination with viral components. These complexes then bind to antibody receptors present on monocytes, leading to increased infection of these immune system cells and augmentation of viral replication. $CD4^+$ T helper cells may contribute to this process by secreting IFN-γ, a cytokine that increases the number of antibody receptors, but these cells may also protect against dengue virus–related illness. T helper cells are stimulated by viral antigens in the presence of MHC molecules. As mentioned earlier, the type of MHC produced by an individual is genetically determined, varies by racial group, and is related to the severity of infection.

The chances of ADE occurring are greater when viruses of the DEN-2 serotype initiate the second infection. During the 1977 epidemic of DEN-1 in Cuba, 4.5 million cases of DF were reported without any cases of DHF or DSS. After an epidemic of DEN-2 in 1981, however, more than 10,000 people developed severe disease: 95% of these were infected for their second time. Disease in 1981 was minimal in young children who had not been previously infected in 1977.

As noted, females are more prone than males to develop severe disease manifestations. This tendency may also be linked to the immune response, as T and B lymphocyte activities are influenced by estrogens (female sex hormones) and the difference in immune responses between the sexes has been shown to heavily influence the increased prevalence of several autoimmune conditions in women (most notably, systemic lupus erythematosus).

The immune system during dengue infection contributes to both host protection and disease development. Many of the cells infected by dengue virus are part of the immune system: dendritic cells, monocytes and macrophages, and lymphocytes, particularly B cells. Infection of these leukocytes often results in increased production of several interleukins and other cytokines such as TNF-α. IL-8, IL-10, IL-13, and IL-18 may be involved in the development of DHF and increase its severity. IL-6 and perhaps IL-10 may increase vascular permeability and possibly capillary leakage. IL-10 levels are higher in persons with DHF than in those with DF. IL-12, a potent inducer of Th1 immunity, by contrast, appears to moderate DHF severity. IL-12 levels decrease during infection and the T helper cell-mediated immunity shifts from a Th1 to a Th2 response. TNF-α may contribute to disease by stimulating IL-6 production and by inducing thrombocytopenia. This cytokine also induces fever. Persons inheriting a gene that permits production of higher levels of TNF-α are at greater risk of developing DHF. Treating mice with serum containing antibodies to this cytokine reduces mortality by 60%, further underscoring the role of TNF-α in the pathological process.

IFN-γ is a Th1 cytokine that functions both in protection and disease induction. Its levels are increased during infection: this cytokine has antiviral

Table 15.2   Roles of immune mediators in dengue infection

Immune Mediator	Protective or Pathogenic?	Role
IL-12	Protective	↑ production of Th1 cytokines (IFN-γ)
IFN-γ	Protective	Decreases viral replication
	Pathogenic	↑ production of IL-6, IL-8; ↑ infection of macrophages
IL-6, IL-10	Pathogenic	↑ vascular permeability
IL-8	Pathogenic	Recruits target cells into area
TNF-α	Pathogenic	↑ production of IL-6; induces fever
Neutralizing antibody	Protective	↓ reinfection by viruses of same serotype
Low levels of nonneutralizing IgG	Pathogenic	↑ infection of macrophages
Complement components	Pathogenic	Destroy platelets; produce shock via anaphylatoxins

activity but boosts IL-6 and IL-8 production as well. IFN-γ also increases expression of the antibody receptor of macrophages, allowing them to be more easily infected by the virus. One of the dengue viral proteins decreases cells' responses to IFN-γ and IFN-β. Interestingly, when T helper cells are exposed to the viruses of the same serotype as the original infecting strain, they produce much IFN-γ, whereas exposing these cells to a differing serotype leads to greater production of TNF-α instead. IFN-γ may thus be linked to long-lasting immunity against reinfection by viruses of the same serotype, while TNF-α may lead to the pathogenic response induced by secondary infection by viruses of a different serotype.

The type of lymphocyte response to infection may help determine the severity of disease. High-affinity CD8$^+$ T killer cells may aid in controlling viral expansion. Numbers of these cells as well as B lymphocytes and natural killer cells are lower in individuals who develop DHF than in those who do not develop severe disease. Furthermore, T cells in persons with serious disease manifestations are less able to divide when stimulated. Natural killer cells and T killer cells normally provide the best host defense against viral infections. B lymphocytes produce the neutralizing antibodies that provide lifelong protection against a second infection with the same viral serotype. Rather than protect the host, low-affinity T cells against dengue virus may instead contribute to immune-mediated pathology by secreting inflammatory cytokines, whereas B lymphocytes producing nonneutralizing antibody may contribute to disease causation via ADE. Other antibodies against viral antigens appear to cross-react with human platelets, leading to their aggregation and destruction by the complement cascade and to their ingestion and killing by macrophages in a manner similar to that occurring in the autoimmune disease thrombocytopenic purpura. By-products of complement activation, the anaphylatoxins, may lead to shock and death during DSS.

Table 15.3   Roles of leukocytes in dengue infection

Cell Type	Protective or Pathogenic?	Role
NK cells, high-affinity T killer cells	Protective	Kill virally infected cells
Low-affinity T helper cells	Pathogenic	Produce inflammatory cytokines
B cells	Protective	Produce neutralizing antibodies
	Pathogenic	Produce low-affinity nonneutralizing antibodies
Macrophages	Pathogenic	Serve as target cells; kill platelets

Diagnosis

Diagnostic tests may determine the presence of antibodies reactive to the dengue virus if the person has no history of a prior infection with a similar virus. Such tests include the IgG and IgM ELISAs, hemagglutination, and complement fixation assays. The presence of IgM antibody indicates recent or current infection and may be detectable within six to seven days of infection.

Other diagnostic techniques include polymerase chain reaction and viral isolation. Virus may be isolated from blood samples after inoculating mosquitoes or by cell culture. Isolation of viruses from organs is more difficult.

Treatment

Prompt oral or intravenous isotonic fluid replacement therapy is recommended by the World Health Organization to counter the results of plasma leakage from capillaries and the resultant hemoconcentration and dangerous drop in blood pressure during DHF and DSS. Fatality rates of 40% to 50% may occur if shock is untreated; adequate fluid replacement lowers this to 1% to 2%. Platelet transfusions are used in individuals with severe bleeding. Blood transfusions should be administered with extreme caution due to the risk of fluid overload.

New treatment modalities are being developed to strike the virus at several key points:

1. Blockage of viral binding to and entry of their target cells—polyanions like heparin derivatives and hyaluronic acid, seed extracts, and agents that block cellular adhesion of bacteria, algae, and fungal spores

2. Inhibition of RNA polymerase by nucleoside analogues—barbituric and thiobarbituric acid analogues; some of these agents are effective against RNA polymerase of other flaviviruses, such as hepatitis C virus

3. Blockage of production of nucleotides or nucleotide depletion—mycophenolic acid, 6-azauridine, and urea VX-497

4. Inhibition of viral helicase or nucleotide triphosphatase enzyme

5. Inhibition of viral serine protease, which produces active viral proteins from a long precursor polyprotein, using compounds derived from various plants, including members of the ginger family

6. Inhibition of α-glucosidase I enzyme that is vital to correct glycoprotein folding, using alkaloids derived from black bean or the Moreton Bay chestnut tree

7. Inhibition of viral kinases involved in cellular signaling events such as evasion of the host immune response

RECENT DEVELOPMENTS

The antiviral compound ribavirin works well in vitro but has not been effective in animal models of disease. Moreover, ribavirin can be toxic in vivo, causing hemolytic anemia. A new agent, 1-β-d-ribofuranosyl-3-ethynyl-[1,2,4]triazole (ETAR), is structurally related to ribavirin. It has shown promising results in blocking infection of cultured cells and is effective at much lower concentrations than ribavirin (EC50 of 9.5 micromolar for ETAR versus 73.2 micromolar for ribavirin). Both of these agents function by depleting levels of guanosine triphosphate (GTP), an important agent of signaling within organisms. ETAR is active against all four dengue serotypes as well as several other flaviviruses. It has comparable toxicity for cultured cells as ribavirin. In vivo studies are needed to determine whether ETAR is more effective in blocking flavivirus infection of cells than ribavirin *in vivo*.

Another compound that appears to be promising for the treatment of dengue virus diseases is the nucleoside analogue beta-D-2'-ethynyl-7-deaza-adenosine triphosphate. This compound inhibits the viral polymerase that enables replication of the RNA genome. It is also active against all four dengue serotypes and is effective at even lower concentrations than ETAR (EC_{50} = 1 micromolar).

Prevention

Vector control programs have been very effective in the control of dengue and other insectborne diseases. Such programs, however, are currently almost non-existent in countries with endemic dengue. Even more unfortunate, some of the species of mosquito vectors have developed resistance to commonly used insecticides. Development and implementation of vector control programs are vital to control not only diseases spread by insects such as mosquitoes, ticks, and fleas but also rodents that serve as both vectors and disease reservoirs. In the absence of effective vector control, individuals may attempt to avoid being bitten by the use of screening, protective clothing, and insect repellents.

One of the ways employed to decrease the number of infected *A. aegypti* mosquitoes is peridomestic spraying in which droplets of insecticide are sprayed in and around houses of dengue-positive cases. Either thermal fogs or cold fogs are used and may be dispensed from vehicle-mounted or handheld equipment. This method is an emergency procedure used to attempt to eliminate adult mosquitoes. It is politically attractive due to the high visibility of the process but may lull area residents into a false sense of security due to several shortcomings such as the need for people to open doors and windows of their homes to permit the droplets to enter the dwelling and the need for periodic reapplication. Another preventive method that may be more effective at reducing *A. aegypti* numbers in homes is the treatment of materials such as window curtains, water container covers, and bed nets with insecticides. This may prove more useful than the indoor residual spraying that has been effective in the campaign against malaria because *A. aegypti* often rest on nonsprayable materials such as hanging clothes. By modifying insect control measures that have proved successful against other arboviruses, methods may be developed to reduce vector numbers and decrease the extent of the current dengue pandemic.

Vaccination is another powerful means of preventing infection by many pathogenic microbes. In the case of dengue virus, vaccine development is more complicated than for other diseases. Due to the risk of ADE, whereby antibodies to one serotype of dengue virus often enhance the pathogenicity of other serotypes, the research community may need to design a vaccine that provides immunity to all four dengue serotypes simultaneously. Phase 1 clinical trials of a yellow fever–dengue 2 combination vaccine (ChimeriVax-DEN2) have shown it to be safe, unaffected by preexisting immunity to the yellow fever virus, and able to induce a long-lasting, cross-neutralizing antibody response to all dengue serotypes.

Surveillance

Groups at high risk for infection with dengue virus include people residing in large tropical urban centers. Such centers in Southeast Asia have undergone rapid, unplanned growth since World War II, resulting in insufficient housing, water, sewage, and waste management systems as well as the crowding of large numbers of potential viral hosts into a small area. Multiple dengue serotypes are present in these sprawling megacities. Mass population movement brought serotypes into new regions with large numbers of previously unexposed hosts. Children in these environments are more likely than adults to develop severe or fatal disease manifestations. Surveillance of the dengue pandemic is critical in the tropical regions of the world, where 2.5 billion persons live in at-risk areas.

Brazil has been home to 70% of the 3 million cases of dengue fever recorded in the Americas between 2000 and 2005. It had no reported cases of dengue before 1976, due to the successful eradication of its *A. aegypti* vector. The mosquito later returned and entered urban areas. The dengue virus subsequently followed in 1981.

Between 1994 and 2002, more than 2.8 million cases were noted in Brazil, with an incidence rate of 454 cases per 100,000 population. The largest outbreaks occurred during the rainy season; however, almost half a million cases were reported during the dry season. The majority of the disease cases were in the large metropolitan areas of the country. DHF first appeared in Brazil in 1990, after the introduction of DEN-2 serotype into the region. Over the course of the next ten years, 893 cases occurred, resulting in 44 deaths. In 2001, DHF incidence was 2.9 cases per 100,000 population, and this grew to 12.9 cases per 100,000 the following year. DEN-3 entered the country in 2002, further increasing the incidence of DF and DHF. Until 2006, disease was primarily in adults in the Rio de Janeiro state, while children were targeted in the Amazonas state. Interestingly, persons of mixed African ancestry appeared to be protected

FIGURE 15.3   Testing water from a tree hole for the presence of mosquito larvae

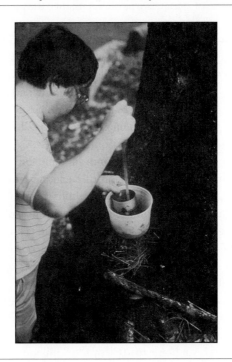

Source: CDC.

against the development of DHF. By 2002, the number of deaths from DHF exceeded those due to malaria for the first time. This rapid explosion of severe disease in the Americas demands close surveillance and effective regional and international epidemiological communication systems in the coming years in order to stem the tide and expansion of this deadly infection.

Summary

Diseases
- Dengue fever • Dengue hemorrhagic fever • Dengue shock syndrome

Causative Agent
- Dengue virus

Agent Type
- Member of the *Flavivirus* genus

Genome
- Single-stranded positive-sense RNA

Vectors
- *Aedes aegypti* and *Aedes albopictus* mosquitoes

Common Reservoirs
- Humans and monkeys

Mode of Transmission
- Mosquito bite

Geographical Distribution
- Worldwide, especially tropical regions

Year of Emergence
- 1770 (dengue fever) • 1953 (dengue hemorrhagic fever)

Key Terms

Aedes aegypti Day-biting, urban mosquito that serves as the primary vector for dengue and yellow fever viruses in humans

Aedes albopictus Rural mosquito that may serve as a vector for dengue virus in humans

Antibody-dependent enhancement (ADE) Worsening of disease manifestations that occurs due to the presence of preexisting low levels of antiviral antibodies that aid in the infection of host macrophages

Breakbone fever Descriptive name for dengue fever, with reference to the severe bone pain associated with this condition

Dengue fever (DF) Self-limiting viral infection characterized by fever and severe headache and eye, bone, and muscle pain

Dengue hemorrhagic fever (DHF) Serious, life-threatening viral infection characterized by fever, increased vascular permeability and capillary leak syndrome, elevated hematocrit, and hemoconcentration

Dengue shock syndrome (DSS) Serious, life-threatening viral infection characterized, in addition to the symptoms of dengue hemorrhagic fever, by a profound drop in blood pressure and shock

Diapause Suspension of insect egg hatching during winter months; similar to hibernation

Flavivirus Viral genus whose members include the causative agents of dengue, yellow fever, Japanese encephalitis, hepatitis C, and West Nile encephalitis

Review Questions

1. What is antibody-dependent enhancement (ADE) during dengue virus infection? What causes ADE?
2. What are the symptoms of dengue fever and dengue hemorrhagic fever?
3. What are the roles of IL-6 and TNF-α during dengue virus infection?
4. What methods can be used to decrease numbers of the dengue vectors?
5. What are some of the processes targeted by drugs used to treat dengue?

Topics for Further Discussion

1. The *Flavivirus* genome contains the causative agents of several serious human diseases. Several of these viruses are closely related to dengue virus (yellow fever virus, Japanese encephalitis virus), and several others are more distantly related (West Nile virus, Saint Louis encephalitis virus, hepatitis C virus). Discuss how the similarities between these viruses might be exploited to develop treatment options effective against multiple flavivirus species.

2. Examine the ways in which various species of mosquitoes have been eliminated from an area or have been prevented from infecting human targets. Discuss which of these methods might be most useful in developing tropical nations and in wealthier, temperate countries.

3. Discuss an "ideal vaccine" to prevent dengue infection in developing countries.

4. Discuss reasons why DF, DHF, and DSS may or may not spread to the United States and cause high mortality.

Resources

Chin, J. *Control of Communicable Diseases Manual* (17th ed.). Washington, D.C.: American Public Health Association, 2000.

Esu, E., Lenhart, A., Smith, L., and Horstick. O. "Effectiveness of Peridomestic Space Spraying with Insecticide on Dengue Transmission: Systematic Review." *Tropical Medicine and International Health*, 2010, *15*, 619–631.

Fink J., Gu, F. and Vasudevan, S. J. "Role of T Cells, Cytokines and Antibody in Dengue Fever and Dengue Haemorrhagic Fever." *Reviews of Medical Virology*, 2006, *16*, 263–275.

Gubler, D. J. "Epidemic Dengue and Dengue Hemorrhagic Fever: A Global Public Health Problem in the 21st Century." In W. M. Scheld, D. Armstrong, and J. M. Hughes (eds.), *Emerging Infections* (Vol. 1). Washington, D.C.: ASM Press, 1998.

Halstead, S. B. "Emergence Mechanisms in Yellow Fever and Dengue." In W. M. Scheld, W. A. Craig, and J. M. Hughes (eds.), *Emerging Infections* (Vol. 2). Washington, D.C.: ASM Press, 1998.

Holmes. E. C., Bartley, L. M., and Garnett, G. P. "The Emergence of Dengue: Past, Present, and Future." In R. M. Krause (ed.), *Emerging Infections*. San Diego, Calif.: Academic Press, 1998.

Latour, D. R., and others. "Biochemical Characterization of the Inhibition of the Dengue Virus RNA Polymerase by Beta-D-2'-ethynyl-7-deaza-adenosine Triphosphate." *Antiviral Research*, 2010, doi:10.1016/j.antiviral.2010.05.003.

Mathew, A., and Rothman, A. L. "Understanding the Contribution of Cellular Immunity to Dengue Disease Pathogenesis." *Immunological Reviews*, 2008, *225*, 300–313.

McDowell, M., and others. "A Novel Nucleoside Analog, 1-β-d-ribofuranosyl-3-ethynyl-[1,2,4]triazole (ETAR), Exhibits Efficacy Against a Broad Range of Flaviviruses In Vitro." *Antiviral Research*, 2010, doi:10.1016/j.antiviral.2010.04.007.

Nielsen, D. G. "The Relationship of Interacting Immunological Components in Dengue Pathogensis." *Virology Journal*, 2009, *6*, 211.

Smart, K., and Safitri, I. "Evidence Behind the WHO Guidelines: Hospital Care for Children: What Treatments Are Effective for the Management of Shock in Severe Dengue?" *Journal of Tropical Pediatrics*, 2009, *55*, 145–147.

Stevens, A. J., Gahan, M. E., Mahalingam, S., and Keller, P. A. "The Medicinal Chemistry of Dengue Fever." *Journal of Medicinal Chemistry*, 2009, *52*, 7911–7926.

Teixeira, M. G., Costa, M. da C. N., Barreto, F., and Barreto, M. L. "Dengue: Twenty-Five Years Since Reemergence in Brazil." *Cadernos de Sáde Pblica*, 2009, *25* (Suppl. 1), S7–S18.

Teo, D., Ng, L. C., and Lam, S. "Is Dengue a Threat to the Blood Supply?" *Transfusion Medicine*, 2009, *19*, 66–77.

CHAPTER 16

THE HUMAN IMMUNODEFICIENCY VIRUS AND ACQUIRED IMMUNE DEFICIENCY SYNDROME

LEARNING OBJECTIVES

- Define the various disease categories associated with HIV infection
- Describe the retrovirus responsible for causing these illnesses
- Discuss modes of infection
- Discuss the host's response to infection
- Describe symptomatology and diagnosis
- Discuss potential methods of treatment
- Discuss methods of prevention

Major Concepts

Outbreaks

Awareness of the acquired immune deficiency syndrome (AIDS) began in 1981 among young gay men in the United States with unexpectedly high numbers of cases of unusual diseases, such as Kaposi's sarcoma and *Pneumocystis carinii* pneumonia. These and other serious diseases were linked to faulty immune responses and later grouped together as AIDS. AIDS was subsequently found to occur in other populations in the United States and throughout the world, especially sub-Saharan Africa, Southeast Asia, and Latin America.

Symptoms

HIV-associated disease is divided into three categories of illness. Initially, individuals infected with the causative virus are asymptomatic or present with swollen lymph nodes. Later, thrush, night sweats, and persistent fever and diarrhea occur, and women may develop pelvic inflammatory syndrome, cervical cancer, or vaginal candidiasis. The disease then progresses to the final stage, full-blown AIDS. This stage is characterized by wasting syndrome, several cancers, opportunistic infections (including blindness induced by cytomegalovirus, atypical pneumonia, disseminated *Mycobacterium avium* complex, diarrhea due to *Cryptosporidium*, and *Toxoplasma* infection of the brain), AIDS dementia, and low numbers of CD4$^+$ T helper cells.

Infection

AIDS is caused by the human immunodeficiency virus (HIV), a retrovirus of which two species are known. HIV-1 is widespread and causes rapid, severe illness. HIV-2 is slower-acting and found predominantly in West Africa. Two other retroviruses infect humans, human T lymphotropic virus I and II, and simian immunodeficiency viruses (SIVs) infect several species of nonhuman primates. Most species of SIV cause nonprogressive disease in their natural hosts; however, rhesus macaques develop a fatal illness similar to AIDS in humans. Retroviruses use the reverse transcriptase enzyme to form viral double-stranded DNA from their genomic single-stranded RNA as an essential step in their life cycle. This enzyme is highly error-prone, leading to an extremely high mutation rate. HIV infects CD4$^+$ T helper cells and macrophages by binding viral gp120 to CD4 plus a coreceptor on host target cells. After entering the cell, HIV uncoats and produces viral DNA. Viral integrase enzyme integrates the DNA into the host chromosome, forming a latent provirus. Events that stimulate the infected cell reactivate the virus, which forms viral RNA and long viral polyproteins. The polyproteins are cleaved by the protease enzyme into their constituent, functional proteins. Viral genomic RNA and several proteins are packaged together as numerous new viruses bud from the surface of the T helper cell, killing the host cell in the process. Viruses are transmitted between people sexually, via blood, or from mother to child.

Immune Response

Most of the pathology resulting from HIV infection is due to the effects of the virus on the immune system. Death or loss of function of $CD4^+$ T helper cells weakens the entire immune response, allowing for the outgrowth of opportunistic pathogens. Excessive production of TNF-α may lead to wasting syndrome. B lymphocyte function is compromised as useful antibody production decreases during the course of infection and B cells become infected with other viruses, leading to malignancies. HIV evades killing by $CD8^+$ T killer cells by mutating the viral surface proteins.

Treatment

Several antiretroviral compounds have been developed. These include drugs that inhibit the activity of reverse transcriptase, protease, or integrase, as well as agents that block viral fusion to target cells or binding of gp120 to its coreceptor. HIV's extremely rapid mutation rate allows it to avoid killing by these drugs, so they are used in various combinations. Combination therapy is not curative but extends life span and quality of life. It is very expensive, but the effects of many groups and individuals have increased its availability in developing nations.

Prevention

No effective vaccine has been developed yet, so other measures must be used to prevent infection with HIV. These include reducing exposure to infected secretions by encouraging safer sexual practices, caution when coming into contact with human blood, and administration of antiviral agents to HIV-positive pregnant women to reduce the risk of transmission to their unborn children.

Introduction

Since awareness of illnesses and deaths due to **acquired immune defi-ciency syndrome (AIDS)** began in 1981, millions of persons throughout the world have died and tens of millions more have become infected. The causative agent was found to be the **human immunodeficiency virus (HIV)**, later differentiated into two species, HIV-1 and HIV-2. A number of drugs have been developed to combat this virus, but its extensive ability to mutate allowed it to avoid killing by both drugs and the immune system. Combination therapy has greatly extended the life span of many infected individuals who are able to afford it, and the world community has pulled together to increase access in developing nations, the hardest-hit regions. Nevertheless, these drugs are not available to all in need, and a preventive vaccine is not yet is sight. Educational programs may have slowed the progress of the pandemic, but large numbers of new infections are still occurring, as well as many deaths. The economic fabric of some regions of the world has been severely stressed due to extensive morbidity and mortality among young adults and the burden of caring for "AIDS orphans," many of whom were born of infected mothers and are HIV-positive themselves.

A total of 33 million persons were reported to be HIV-positive in 2007; in that year, there were 2.5 million new infections and 2.1 million AIDS-related deaths. Nations in southern Africa are particularly affected by HIV/AIDS, reporting 22.5 million infected persons in 2007 and 1.6 million deaths; the

Table 16.1   HIV transmission

Transmission Category	Estimated Number of Aids Cases, 2007		
	Adult and Adolescent Males	Adult and Adolescent Females	Total
Male-to-male sexual contact	16,749	0	16,749
Use of injected drugs	3,750	2,260	6,010
Male-to-male sexual contact and use of injected drugs	1,664	0	1,664
High-risk heterosexual contact	4,011	7,100	11,111
Hemophilia, blood transfusion, perinatal exposure, or unknown risk	181	220	401

Source: CDC.

Table 16.2   Total number of AIDS cases in nine U.S. states
and Puerto Rico through 2007

Area	Cumulative Number of Aids Cases		
	Adults and Adolescents	Children Under the Age of 13	Total
New York	179,116	2,345	181,461
California	148,274	675	148,949
Florida	107,980	1,544	109,524
Texas	72,434	394	72,828
New Jersey	49,907	787	50,694
Pennsylvania	35,120	369	35,489
Illinois	34,783	283	35,066
Georgia	33,607	240	33,847
Maryland	31,611	320	31,931
Puerto Rico	30,333	403	30,736

Source: CDC.

highest numbers are found in Botswana, Lesotho, and Swaziland. Southeast Asia reported 4.0 million infected persons and 270,000 deaths in 2007, and Latin America, 1.6 million HIV-positive persons and 58,000 deaths. Other countries reporting very high numbers of HIV-positive adults were Thailand, Estonia, the Russian Federation, Ukraine, Sudan, six Caribbean nations, Belize, Guyana, Panama, and Suriname.

The greatest number of AIDS cases in the United States occurs in individuals aged 25 to 50 years, and a large proportion are African American or Latino. In 2007, the majority of cases in the United States resulted from either male-to-male sexual contact or high-risk heterosexual contact, although transmission via IV drug use was formerly more common than heterosexual contact. California, New York, Florida, and Texas reported the highest number of AIDS cases in the United States. More than half a million Americans had died of AIDS by the end of 2007.

History

The first reports of severe, unusual diseases later associated with HIV-1 infection surfaced in the United States in New York and California in the spring of 1981 among young and otherwise healthy homosexual men. At least eight cases of an unusually aggressive form of Kaposi's sarcoma were seen in this population in New York in March. Kaposi's sarcoma in the United States had until then been a mild malignancy restricted primarily to the skin that occurred in older men of Jewish or Mediterranean origin. Soon afterward, a number of cases of *Pneumocystis carinii* (now *P. jiroveci*) pneumonia were reported in young homosexual men from Los Angeles. These diseases resulted from opportunistic infections by microorganisms that had previously acted in a commensal fashion and were linked to defective immunity. By December of that year, this immune deficiency disease (later designated AIDS) was recognized in intravenous drug users. The following year, AIDS was also seen in large numbers in Haitians and in hemophiliacs and was found to be transmitted sexually and via contaminated blood or blood products. Cases of AIDS were turning up in Europe, and "slim disease," a fatal wasting syndrome, was reported in Uganda. Slim disease was later found to have been present in parts of Africa, including the Democratic Republic of Congo (Zaire), since the late 1970s.

In 1983, the lymphadenopathy-associated virus (LAV) was isolated by Luc Montagnier of the Pasteur Institute in France while American researcher Robert Gallo isolated a similar virus at nearly the same time that was designated human T lymphotropic virus III (HTLV-III). After determining that the viral isolates were of the same species, the causative agent was renamed the human immunodeficiency virus (HIV, later HIV-1). Amid reports of rapidly increasing numbers of AIDS cases in the United States, Europe, and Africa, the widespread outbreak was declared a pandemic. An antibody-based test was developed to screen blood from potential donors in 1985, an important step in the protection of the blood supply.

FIGURE 16.1   Chemical structure of AZT (zidovudine)

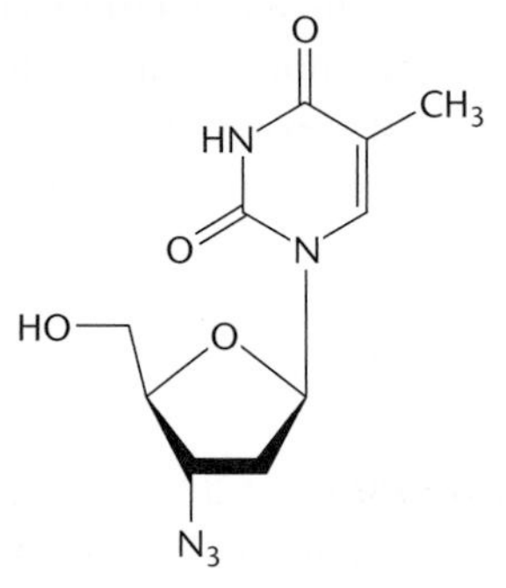

By 1986, the first beneficial antiretroviral drug, zidovudine (AZT), was used to treat AIDS. HIV quickly developed resistance to this drug and other, newer antiviral agents. As the pandemic grew, tens of millions of people became infected with HIV, and millions died of AIDS. Extensive educational programs, distribution of free condoms, and the advent of highly active antiretroviral therapy (HAART), using combinations of three or more drugs, extended the life span of individuals who were able to afford it and slowed the progress of the pandemic. Later, governments, aid organizations, corporations, and individuals contributed to programs to reduce the spread of HIV and to make the expensive antiviral agents more readily available in developing nations.

The Diseases

The diseases associated with HIV infection have been divided into three broad categories.

Category A HIV Infection

During the early stage of infection, HIV-positive persons are placed in category A. During this stage, individuals are either asymptomatic or have lymphade-nopathy (swollen lymph nodes). **Category A HIV infection** may be as short as several weeks or months but typically persists for years, even more than a decade in some cases.

Category B HIV Infection

Category B HIV infection was formerly known as AIDS-related complex (ARC). This phase of infection includes conditions such as thrush (infection of the oral cavity with the yeast *Candida*), fever or diarrhea persisting for more than a month, night sweats, and shingles (*Herpes zoster*, due to reactivation of the varicella virus, the causative agent of chickenpox). Women have additional manifestations, including persistent vaginal candidiasis, cervical cancer, and pelvic inflammatory disease.

Category C HIV Infection

The final stage is **category C HIV infection**, the acquired immune deficiency syndrome (AIDS), and may be subdivided into several categories. During this stage, immune system functions are severely compromised.

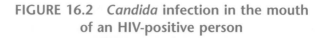

FIGURE 16.2 *Candida* infection in the mouth
of an HIV-positive person

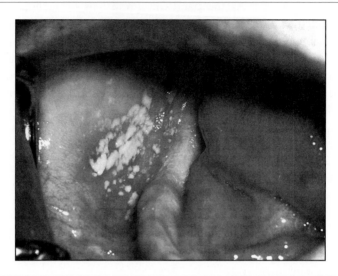

Source: CDC.

Wasting syndrome causes profound weight loss and severe emaciation. This disease manifestation appears to be related to excessive production of the cytokine TNF-α, previously known as cachetin because it may cause cachexia (wasting).

Opportunistic Infections The lack of a properly functional immune response allows a number of **opportunistic infections**, infections with microorganisms that typically have a commensal relationship with humans, to become pathogenic. *Candida albicans* yeast may invade the interior of the body, resulting in respiratory or esophageal candidiasis. Cytomegalovirus may infect the eye, resulting in retinitis and blindness. Individuals may develop chronic infections with herpes simplex virus. Life-threatening pneumonia may result from infections with *Pneumocystis jiroveci* (formerly *P. carinii*). Members of the *Mycobacterium avium* complex may become disseminated in the blood. The protozoan parasite *Toxoplasma gondii* may also cause severe infection of the brain or heart. This parasite also threatens fetuses, and expectant mothers are advised to avoid changing cat litter boxes because this protozoan is transmitted to humans via cat feces.

FIGURE 16.3   *Toxoplasma* infection of the heart

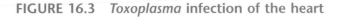

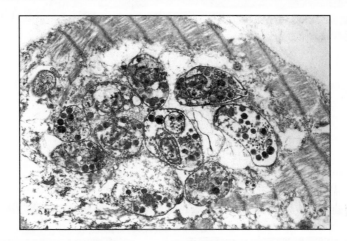

Source: CDC/Edwin P. Ewing Jr.

A number of other infectious diseases are very serious or life-threatening in HIV-positive persons, including babesiosis, bacillary angiomatosis (caused by *Bartonella* species), Chagas' disease, cryptosporidiosis, ehrlichiosis, hepatitis, malaria, tuberculosis, and infection with *Cyclospora* species. Another AIDS-associated illness is progressive multifocal leukoencephalopathy due to infection of the brain by the JC virus. This condition results in severe decline of mental and physical functions. Infections of immunocompromised individuals, including those with AIDS, are discussed in Chapter 30.

AIDS-Associated Malignancies Several malignancies occur with higher frequency in HIV-positive persons. One very dangerous cancer specific for AIDS patients is HIV-related Kaposi's sarcoma (see Chapter Seventeen). Kaposi's sarcoma results from infection with human herpesvirus-8. In immunocompetent individuals, the cancer is usually restricted to the skin and may be removed surgically, by radiation, or with chemotherapy. In HIV-positive and other immunosuppressed persons, the malignancy invades internal organs, with poor prognosis and often fatal results. Those with very low $CD4^+$ T helper cell numbers are particularly vulnerable. Burkitt's lymphoma is more common among HIV-positive persons than the general population. This cancer of B lymphocytes results from infection of these cells with Epstein-Barr virus, the causative agent of mononucleosis, another condition associated with high levels of B cell proliferation.

AIDS Dementia HIV infection affects central nervous system activity. This results in what is known as **AIDS dementia**, characterized by impaired short-term memory, concentration, and fine motor skills; tremors; social withdrawal; and irritability.

Low CD4$^+$ T Helper Cell Numbers HIV-positive persons with less than 200 CD4$^+$ T Ly per microliter are also placed into category C.

The Causative Agent

HIV belongs to the **lentivirus** (slow virus) family of **Retroviridae**. The genome of retroviruses consists of two copies of single-stranded RNA. These viruses also contain the enzyme **reverse transcriptase**, which is required for viral replication. Very few exogenous retroviruses infect humans: the other such naturally acquired viruses are human T lymphotropic virus-1 (HTLV-1) and HTLV-2. These pathogens are responsible for the very aggressive adult T cell leukemia and HTLV-1-associated myelopathy and tropical spastic paraparesis. A similar group of retroviruses is the simian immunodeficiency viruses (SIV) of sooty mangabeys, African green monkeys, mandrills, chimpanzees, and macaques. Most types of SIV cause nonprogressive illness in their natural hosts, and the infected primates live a normal life span. SIV infection of the majority of these animals results in a high level of viremia but little drop in CD4$^+$ T helper cell numbers in the peripheral blood. Mucosal T helper cell numbers, in contrast, do decrease severely. SIV does cause progressive, fatal illness in rhesus macaques. In humans and rhesus macaques, a state of chronic immune activation occurs that is not found in the better adapted sooty mangabeys. Several important differences are seen in the immune response of sooty mangabeys to SIV in comparison to the responses of rhesus macaques to SIV and humans to HIV (these will be discussed later in this chapter).

There are two known members of the HIV group, HIV-1 and HIV-2. HIV-1 is more common and widespread than HIV-2. It also causes a much more rapid and aggressive illness. HIV-2 is confined primarily to West Africa and is less virulent than HIV-1. The genome of HIV-2 is very similar to that of SIV from sooty mangabeys. SIV may be transmitted between nonhuman primates through biting, leading to the hypothesis that HIV-2 and the SIV of rhesus macaques may have evolved from SIV of mangabeys acquired following a mangabey bite or through contact with mangabey blood. Nonhuman primates have a large amount of contact

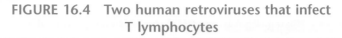

FIGURE 16.4   Two human retroviruses that infect
T lymphocytes

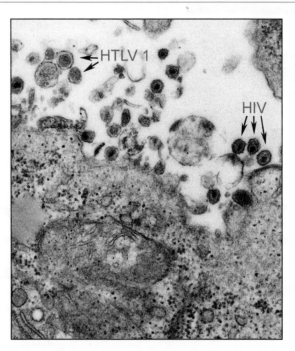

Source: CDC.

with humans in some regions of Africa because they raid farmers' plots and may attack the humans defending their crops. Humans also hunt and eat nonhuman primates (which as food are known as bushmeat). People may come into contact with primate blood during the skinning and preparing of meat for consumption.

HIV does not naturally infect other species of animals, but chimpanzees may be artificially infected. They are not commonly used as an animal model of infection because they are an endangered species and the virus does not appear to often produce disease similar to that seen in humans. Infection of several species of macaques with SIV is the most frequently used model of human HIV infection. These animals are not endangered and develop an immunodeficiency disease within a useful time frame. An alternative animal model of infection is HIV infection of SCID-hu mice. These mice have no functional adaptive immune system and have undergone immune reconstitution with human hematopoietic stem cells. They therefore have human lymphocytes and macrophages that bear human CD4 plus the appropriate HIV coreceptors.

HIV virions exist in two variant forms, the R5 and the X4 forms. **R5 variants** use the chemokine receptor CCR5 as a coreceptor during infection of cells, primarily macrophages. They grow slowly and reach only low titers in culture. They are most common during the initial stages of disease and are believed to be the type of virus that is responsible for the infection of individuals. The **X4 variants**, by contrast, use the chemokine receptor CXCR4 as a coreceptor during infection of cells. They infect CD4$^+$ T helper cells primarily but may also infect macrophages. Viruses of this type grow rapidly and reach high titers in culture. They are found during later stages of infection and are believed to be responsible for disease progression.

HIV Structure, Genome, and Proteins

HIV is surrounded by a lipid bilayer envelope that is primarily derived from the host plasma membrane. It contains host phospholipids, cholesterol, and some host cell surface proteins, including major histocompatibility complex (MHC) molecules used in immune recognition. Some glycoproteins of viral origin are also present as part of gp160. Gp160 is composed of two chains: gp41 spans the envelope and associates with **gp120**. Both are involved in infection of host cells. A protein nucleocapsid surrounds the viral genome.

The HIV genome contains a number of genes; some are structural, some are involved in infection, and several are regulatory genes. Structural genes include *gag* (encoding the nucleocapsid polyprotein) and *env* (encoding the gp160 envelope proteins, gp120 and gp41). The *pol* gene encodes the viral reverse transcriptase, **integrase**, and **protease**, which are produced as a single transcript and a long nonfunctional polyprotein. Regulatory genes include *nef* (enhances virulence) and *tat* (transactivator, which activates viral transcription). The ends of the RNA are flanked by a pair of long-terminal repeats (LTR) that contain a weak promoter. This is converted into a strong promoter by binding to the HIV Tat protein or to host NF-κB. The production of the latter is induced by an immune response to other viruses, such as herpes simplex, cytomegalovirus, or Epstein-Barr virus. These viruses are thus able to stimulate HIV activation.

The HIV Life Cycle

HIV has a complex life cycle that uses several enzymes not present in humans. These present themselves as potential targets for drug intervention. HIV's life cycle begins with infection of a human host. The infecting virus is usually an R5 variant.

Infection of Target Cells The most common cellular targets for HIV infection are cells of the immune system, CD4$^+$ T helper lymphocytes and macrophages, including the microglia of the brain, all of which express CD4$^+$ on their surface. Other cells, such as bowel epithelium, are much less frequently infected.

The first step in cellular infection is the binding of HIV to the target cell, which is accomplished by the gp120 portion of the gp160 viral envelope component attaching to the CD4 molecule located on the surface of T helper cells and macrophages. CD4 is usually used by T helper cells to bind to MHC class II molecules during immune activation. Infection also requires the binding of gp120 to either the CCR5 or CXCR4 chemokine receptor as a coreceptor. Inhibition of viral binding to either CD4 or the correct chemokine receptor blocks the HIV life cycle.

Binding is followed by fusion of the viral envelope with the host cell membrane. This is mediated by the gp41 portion of viral gp160, which protrudes through the viral envelope. The envelope remains on the surface of the cell, and the viral nucleocapsid containing viral RNA is internalized, followed by the uncoating of the RNA.

Replication of the Viral Genome and Integration into Host Chromosomes The initial step in the replication of HIV RNA is reverse transcription, during which reverse transcriptase first copies single-stranded viral RNA into single-stranded DNA. This is then converted into double-stranded viral DNA. This process is very error-prone, and approximately five to ten mistakes occur with each replication. HIV has no mechanism to repair these errors, so the mistakes become permanent, leading to a very high mutation rate for the virus. Due to its accelerated mutation rate, an individual is host to a "swarm" of related HIV viruses soon after the initial infection.

The double-stranded viral DNA is then inserted into a host chromosome by the viral integrase protein. This results in the formation of a latent form of HIV, the **provirus**. Proviruses are inactive and do not produce viral RNA or proteins, thus remaining invisible to surveillance by the immune system and not providing a target for most of the antiviral drugs. HIV proviruses may persist in this safe, hidden state for years until activated.

Activation of the Provirus, Viral Assembly, and Release from Target Cells Proviruses may be activated by signals that stimulate the infected T cells, such as binding to antigen during an immune response. Intracellular signaling molecules, including NF-κB, may convert the weak promoter located in the viral LTR into a strong promoter, thus allowing transcription of viral genes. The viral Tat

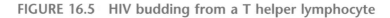

FIGURE 16.5   HIV budding from a T helper lymphocyte

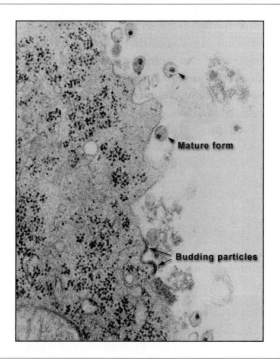

Source: CDC/Edwin P. Ewing Jr.

protein further triggers production of viral RNA. Viral polyproteins are translated from the RNA and cleaved by the viral protease enzyme, producing active structural and regulatory proteins as well as viral genomic RNA.

The viral gp41/120 complex is inserted into the host cell plasma membrane. Genomic RNA and several other proteins are brought into the area, and many new virions are released from the stricken cell during the process of budding. T helper cells bud HIV to the outside of the cell, while macrophages bud HIV internally into vacuoles.

HIV Transmission

Because HIV does not naturally infect animals other than humans, no other reservoir or vector species exists, and the virus must therefore be transmitted by some human-to-human route. HIV infects blood cells and is present in high numbers in whole blood and plasma. During the early stages of the HIV pandemic, high numbers of hemophiliacs became infected via clotting factor, which was prepared using the blood of many donors. Preventive measures have since greatly decreased infection via this route. Viruses are present in secretions such as semen, milk, and vaginal fluid in concentrations that permit transmission. Low levels of HIV are also found in saliva, tears, and spinal fluid.

The most common route of HIV transmission throughout the world is sexual contact. Heterosexual transmission is the primary route of transmission in Africa and Asia, the areas with the highest number of infected persons. Heterosexual transmission often involves the prostitute trade. Some regions of Southeast Asia are hot spots for this activity, and brothels in those regions are often frequented by visiting businessmen. In Africa, recent trends in urbanization have led many men to seek employment in large cities during the week, and many visit prostitutes while there. They subsequently return to their wives and families on the weekends and bring home any sexually transmitted diseases they have contracted. Disease among prostitutes in large urban areas thus spreads in a cross-generational manner from rural husbands to their wives and may also be passed on to some of the children born of infected mothers. The building of a major east-west highway system across Africa also attracted many prostitutes to areas bordering this route, seeking to enlist truckers as clients. Poverty in the developing regions of Africa and Asia is often a key factor that forces women or their female children into the prostitute trade if the alternative is potential starvation for themselves or their family members. In some regions, more than seven in ten prostitutes are HIV-positive.

Homosexual transmission between males remains the major route of infection in the United States, although transmission by the heterosexual route is rapidly increasing. The tissue of the anal region is delicate and may easily be torn or otherwise damaged during anal intercourse. The homosexual population also has a higher number of other sexually transmitted microorganisms that increase the risk of infection and subsequent disease both by damaging the anal tissue to allow viral entry and by stimulating an immune response by infected CD4^{+} T helper cells, thus activating HIV proviruses following infection. Areas with high numbers of sexual contacts, such as bathhouses, increased the spread of disease in the early stages of what became the AIDS pandemic.

One of the other major routes of HIV infection throughout the world is the administration of illegal intravenous (IV) drugs, such as heroin. Given the difficulty of obtaining needles and syringes for such activity, most IV drug users reuse the injection material at least several times, usually without adequate sterilization. Virus present in any blood remaining within this equipment may infect the next user. In an effort to prevent transmission by this route, some countries have provided users of illegal drugs with sterile needles and syringes.

In addition to IV drugs, other drugs such as crack cocaine and alcohol may play a role in HIV infection by decreasing a person's judgment concerning sexual activity. Sexual activity may also be performed in exchange for expensive drugs. Illegally administered material such as steroids may also lead to HIV transmission if the needles or syringes are reused. Other activities that involve the potential sharing of unsterilized needles may transmit HIV as well, including piercing ears, body piercing, and tattooing. Caution should be used in selecting reputable, conscientious sites for such activity.

Because HIV inhabits blood cells, viral transmission may also occur following blood transfusion or organ or bone marrow donation. Administration of questionnaires to potential donors reduces the chance of acquiring blood or organs from persons at high risk of infection. In developed nations, routine screening of blood and clotting factors for antibodies to HIV or for viral components further safeguards the blood supply and has greatly reduced transmission via this route. The entry of contaminated material into the blood supply is now extremely rare (less than 1 in 2 million in the United States). Furthermore, most developed areas of the world, including the United States, use only new needles and tubing during the collection of blood, making blood donation in these areas completely safe for the donor.

HIV may be passed from an infected mother to her child. Such transmission may occur transplacentally or during labor. Treating the mother with antiviral compounds reduces the risk of subsequent transmission to the child. Milk from infected mothers contains virus that may infect children during breast-feeding. This poses a great dilemma for HIV-infected women in some areas of the world where the supply of safe water for preparing a milk substitute or formula is limited or uncertain. Formula may be financially unobtainable, and it lacks the protective IgA antibodies found in mother's milk. The risk of an HIV infection, which is typically lethal in the very young, especially under economic conditions that place medical care or expensive antiviral medications out of reach, must take these additional factors into account.

Despite public fears, HIV is not transmitted through casual contact such as touching doorknobs or phones or shaking hands or hugging. The virus is also not transmitted through food or drink or by mosquitoes or other blood-sucking insects.

The Immune Response

Most of the manifestations of AIDS are due to two interactions of HIV with the immune system: escape from killing by $CD8^+$ T killer cells and viral killing of $CD4^+$ T helper cells, which orchestrate most of immune response actions. The virus also affects other components of the immune response as well.

Escape from Killing by CD8$^+$ T Killer Cells

CD8$^+$ T killer cells play a critical role in controlling a number of viral infections, including HIV and the closely related HTLV-1 viruses. Approximately 0.3% of HIV-positive persons, designated as "elite controllers" or "nonprogressors," maintain a consistently low plasma viral load (fewer than 50 copies per milliliter) for extended periods of time. Elite controllers appear to retain active HIV-specific CD8$^+$ T killer cells for long periods, indicating the vital role of these cells in decreasing HIV viral burden. Interestingly, CD8$^+$ T killer cell activity does not appear to play an important role in controlling the nonprogressive SIV infection seen in sooty mangabeys.

Several factors decrease the ability of CD8$^+$ T cells to kill HIV. The virus itself frequently produces "escape mutants" that alter recognition by T killer cells, allowing the virus to avoid killing and increase its numbers. A loss of HIV-specific T killer cell activity is thus associated with disease progression. T killer cells require help in the form of cytokines produced by CD4$^+$ T helper cells. T helper cell numbers are severely decreased during disease progression, and these cells are unable to adequately aid T killer cell functioning. CD8$^+$ T killer cells themselves may undergo changes during disease progression. These cells increase their expression of the surface receptors Programmed Death-1 (PD-1; CD279) and CTLA-4 (CD152), both of which block T cell proliferation and cytokine production and reduce killing of microbes by these cells. Engagement of PD-1 with its ligand also induces apoptosis of both CD8$^+$ and CD4$^+$ T cells. Expression levels of PD-1 are increased by viral Nef and correlate with HIV viral load and disease progression. HIV infection decreases expression of the IL-7 receptor α, a T cell growth factor receptor. Alteration in regulatory T cell types also occurs as numbers of CD4$^+$CD25$^+$ Treg cells increase in lymphoid tissues during HIV infection. These cells suppress activity of both CD4$^+$ T helper cells and CD8$^+$ T killer cells. Removal of Treg increases HIV-specific immune responses. Treg levels in the nonprogressive SIV infection of sooty mangabeys are increased to a greater extent than that seen in HIV-positive humans and in these animals trigger production of immunosuppressive IL-10, which prevents pathogenic chronic immune activation.

Destruction of CD4$^+$ T Cells

During most of the course of HIV infection (8 to 12 years), numbers of CD4$^+$ T cells decrease while numbers of CD8$^+$ T cells increase, numbers of total T cells remaining constant. This results in inversion of the CD4:CD8 ratio, which is normally 2:1, and decreases to considerably less than 1:2. The decline in numbers of CD4$^+$ cells correlates with a rise in numbers and severity of AIDS-associated diseases. Very late during the course of disease, levels of all T cells decrease as the immune system collapses. Several mechanisms have been proposed to explain the loss of CD4$^+$ T helper cells during HIV infection.

T helper cells may be killed as a result of HIV infection. T helper cells express membrane CD4 and coreceptors for CXCR4 HIV variants, thus allowing their infection. The budding of large numbers of viruses from the cell membrane as HIV leaves the T cells lyses these cells, leading to their death. Expression of viral gp120 glycoprotein on the plasma membrane also makes them targets for killing by anti-HIV CD8$^+$ T killer cells. Macrophages are also infected by HIV but are not killed in this manner, perhaps due to intrinsic differences in the cell types or due to the fact that different viral variants infect these cells. Increased PD-1 expression in CD4$^+$ T helper cells may lead to their apoptotic death as it does in CD8$^+$ T killer cells.

Another means by which HIV leads to T cell death is via formation of syncytia (**cytopathic effect**). Viral gp120 travels to the surface of infected T cells and binds to CD4 found on uninfected T cells, leading to fusion of the cells. This results in the production of giant multinucleated cells with a hollow, balloonlike appearance (syncytia). Syncytia contain as many as 500 cells, which soon die.

FIGURE 16.6   Multinucleated giant cell formed during HIV infection

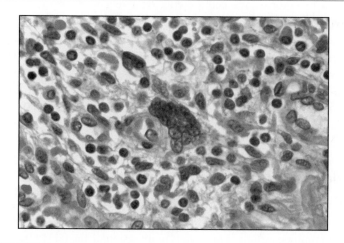

Source: CDC/Edwin P. Ewing Jr.

HIV also induces inappropriate apoptosis of T cells. The rate of apoptosis of both $CD4^+$ and $CD8^+$ T cells is much higher in HIV-positive persons than in uninfected individuals and increases with disease progression toward AIDS.

Other Immunological Abnormalities Occurring During HIV Infection

Lymph Nodes Soon after infection, high numbers of viruses are found in the blood. This number increases during category A, subsequently decreases, and again rises late during infection. Levels of viruses are high in lymph nodes throughout the course of infection due to vigorous replication, resulting in extensive damage to lymph node structure and functional activity.

$CD4^+$ T Helper Lymphocytes In addition to a severe drop in numbers of T helper cells, the remaining cells have decreased responsiveness to antigenic and polyclonal activation. T helper cell numbers decrease soon after infection: the rate of decline slows during category A infection and increases rapidly late in infection, triggering disease progression to AIDS.

B Lymphocytes B cells undergo nonspecific polyclonal activation during HIV infection, decreasing their ability to mount effective specific antibody responses to pathogens. Late in the course of infection, anti-HIV antibodies are lost during the catastrophic collapse of adaptive immunity.

Cytokine Production Some research suggests that the presence of a predominantly Th1 cytokine response is associated with category A infection, while Th2 cytokines are present during the later stages of disease. This situation is similar

Table 16.3 Viral and immunological characteristics during different stages of HIV infection

| | Stage of Infection | | |
Characteristic	Early infection	Asymptomatic Stage	Late Infection
Virus levels	High	Low in blood, high in lymph nodes	High
$CD4^+$ cells	Decrease	Slow decrease	Rapid decrease
Anti-HIV antibodies	Low	High	Low

to that seen in mild cutaneous versus severe visceral leishmaniasis or in tuberculoid (mild) versus lepromatous (severe) leprosy, in which the presence of predominantly Th1 cytokines correlates with protection against infectious disease while the presence of Th2 cytokines correlates with susceptibility to more serious disease manifestations. It is not known whether a cause-and-effect relationship exists between production of Th2 cytokines and disease progression. Viral Nef inhibits transcription of IL-12 by infected monocytes. IL-12 is vital to the development of a functional Th1 cytokine response. HIV Tat protein increases monocyte production of IL-10, a regulatory cytokine that decreases Th1 responses.

Levels of several inflammatory cytokines are increased during HIV infection. These include IL-1 (induces fever), TNF-α (induces fever and wasting), and inflammatory IL-6. Levels of GM-CSF are elevated as well. All of these cytokines increase HIV replication, and most stimulate growth of Kaposi's sarcoma cells.

Monocytes and Dendritic Cells Monocytes host latent viruses, and mature tissue-dwelling macrophages, including microglia of the brain, function as viral reservoirs. Monocyte precursor cells in the bone marrow also serve as HIV reservoirs and may transmit infection to their progeny. Monocyte maturation into macrophages can lead to viral reactivation and production of infectious viruses. Infection alters monocyte functions. Surface expression of PD-1 ligand is increased on monocytes as on the other antigen-presenting cells, dendritic cells (DCs) and B lymphocytes. Interactions between the high levels of PD-1 on T cells and PD-1 ligand on antigen-presenting cells may be responsible for the high levels of apoptosis seen in both CD4$^+$ and CD8$^+$ T cells during HIV progression. HIV Tat protein reduces monocyte death by inducing production of the antiapoptotic molecule Bcl-2 in these cells. The HIV matrix protein p17 stimulates release of the chemokine monocyte chemotactic protein-1 by monocytes, thus recruiting these cells to sites of HIV infection and increasing the available pool of cells for infection.

Dendritic cells also host latent HIV and may aid in the infection of CD4$^+$ T helper cells through the formation of a "virological synapse" that transmits the virus to T helper cells during their stimulation by DCs. Viral Nef stimulates T cell infection via this route. Langerhans cells (DC-like cells in the skin and mucous membranes) are normally fairly resistant to HIV infection. Abrasion occurring during anal sex or coinfection with *Neisseria gonorrhoeae* (causative agent of gonorrhea) or the yeast *Candida* lowers the resistance of Langerhans cells to HIV infection. The use of methamphetamine increases DC susceptibility to infection. The less virulent HIV-2 infects DCs less readily than HIV-1.

Viral infection of dendritic cells induces their production of indoleamine 2,3-deoxygenase. This molecule suppresses functions of CD4$^+$ T helper cells and stimulates differentiation of CD4$^+$ cells into regulatory Treg cells rather than T helper cells. DC production of the antiviral cytokine IFN-α is also reduced during HIV infection. Induction of Treg production and decreased expression of IFN-α by DCs may function as protective mechanisms designed to decrease chronic, pathogenic immune activation. Animals with nonprogressive SIV infection, such as sooty mangabeys, produce very low levels of IFN-α in response to viral infection.

Diagnosis and Detection

Several types of tests have been developed to permit detection of HIV. These tests are used diagnostically and to screen the blood supply in order to remove any contaminated units. Some of these tests rely on immunological detection. ELISA is used to identify either antibodies to HIV gp120 or viral antigens themselves in the blood. Due to the length of time required to mount an adaptive immune response that produces antibodies, such tests may not detect the presence of HIV in blood until six months after infection. Western blot assays test for the presence of viral proteins and may be used in a confirmatory manner. The polymerase chain reaction detects HIV genes. The latter two tests allow detection of the virus much sooner after infection than immunological tests and often scan for the presence of more than one HIV gene product to avoid false-positive results. Thanks to the use of these tests, the number of infections via the blood supply in developed countries is now extremely low.

Molecular detection of HIV load in plasma has been used to predict disease severity. Individuals with a low steady-state number of viral copies in the plasma tend to progress to severe disease more slowly than those with high numbers of plasma viruses. The ratio of CD4:CD8 T lymphocytes in the blood is also used as a marker of disease progression: this ratio drops as disease progresses.

Treatment

Several types of antiretroviral agents, in the form of 26 drugs, are licensed for the treatment of HIV infection. The earliest drugs acted as reverse transcriptase inhibitors and include AZT and stavudine, which are nucleoside analogues. In addition to killing HIV, these drugs are also toxic to the mitochondria in human cells and may cause muscle pain, weakness, fatigue, loss of body fat, and lactic acidosis. Non-nucleoside reverse transcriptase inhibitors, such as etravirine and efavirenz, are also available. These may cause rash and liver toxicity. Replication of human chromosomal DNA does not involve reverse transcription; however, several reverse transcriptase enzymes are present in humans, including the telomerase enzyme that is present in restricted cell types, including stem cells, germinal cells, and lymphocytes: this enzyme allows sustained cell division. Toxic side effects of reverse transcriptase inhibitors may be due to their actions on human reverse transcriptase enzymes.

Protease inhibitors were developed later and include indinivar, squinavir, and ritonavir. These enzymes block the cleavage of viral polyproteins into their active constituent proteins. One such polyprotein contains the proteins reverse transcriptase, protease, and integrase. Protease inhibitors may induce nausea, bloating, and diarrhea. Newer drugs, such as raltegravir, block the ability of viral integrase to insert viral DNA into host chromosomes. Miraviroc and vicriviroc are compounds that block HIV from binding to the CCR5 coreceptor on macrophages. These drugs may lead to upper respiratory tract infections, rash, abdominal pain, and dizziness. Use of intracellular antibodies against CCR5 and RNAi to block CCR5 transcription is also being explored. Enfuvirtide is a member of a new class of drugs that act by blocking viral fusion with the host cell membrane by binding to HIV gp41.

The extremely rapid rate of mutation and replication of HIV allows the virus to produce offspring resistant to antiviral agents soon after their introduction into a population or to an individual's treatment regimen. To forestall drug resistance, a program of combination therapy is often used. **Highly active**

Table 16.4 Categories of anti-HIV agents

Class	Drugs	Adverse Effects
Reverse transcriptase inhibitors: Nucleoside analogues	AZT, stavudine	Muscle pain, weakness, fatigue, loss of body fat, lactic acidosis
Reverse transcriptase inhibitors: Non-nucleosides	Etravirine, efavirenz	Rash, liver toxicity
Protease inhibitors	Indinivir, squinavir, ritonavir	Nausea, bloating, diarrhea
Integrase inhibitors	Raltegravir	None
Inhibitors of coreceptor binding	Miraviroc, vicriviroc	Upper respiratory tract infections, rash, abdominal pain, dizziness
Viral fusion inhibitors	Enfuvirtide	None

antiretroviral therapy (HAART) combines the administration of several reverse transcriptase and protease inhibitors. This extremely effective approach has greatly extended the life span of HIV-positive individuals. The high cost of HAART and the strict time schedule required for proper protection present challenges for its use in areas of the world that have limited economic resources or poor drug delivery infrastructure. HAART costs $10,000 to 15,000 a year in the United States and $350 a year in developing countries. The latter areas are among those with the highest incidence of infection and need. HAART reduces the numbers of opportunistic infections and hospitalizations and permits many persons to return to the workforce, increasing productivity and aiding the economy of these regions. Because widespread use of HAART reduces the overall cost of care while positively affecting employment, it has a positive impact on the economy and may be a cost-effective strategy.

Prevention

Preventive measures center on avoiding contact with the body fluids or organs of infected persons. Safer sexual practices are vital to reducing the risk of AIDS and other sexually transmitted diseases. These practices reduce or eliminate the exchange of body fluids during sexual activity and include the proper use of latex condoms and dental dams. Individuals need to carefully weigh decisions concerning sexual activities in a clear mental state that is not clouded by the use of substances that affect good judgment. Safer sex practices are highly effective in reducing the risk of HIV transmission; however, infection may nevertheless occur. Abstinence is the only sure way to prevent HIV transmission via the sexual route. Moreover, infected persons should tell prospective sexual partners about their HIV-positive status. HIV-positive women should seek counseling concerning the risk to unborn children and to their partners prior to becoming pregnant. If the women do decide to have a child, medications that greatly decrease transmission during pregnancy or delivery are available. HIV-positive mothers should not breast-feed their babies due to the presence of the virus in breast milk. Circumcision reduces the risk of HIV infection of males by 50% and also decreases the risk of acquiring other sexually transmitted diseases.

Because HIV is transmitted via contaminated needles and syringes, the use of illegal injected drugs should be avoided. If IV drugs are used, however, needles and syringes should not be shared. Some communities have free needle exchange programs, which also provide referrals for addiction treatment. Care should be taken to only receive body piercings or tattoos from businesses that use new or properly sterilized needles.

FIGURE 16.7 Proper disposal of a used needle in a "sharps" container

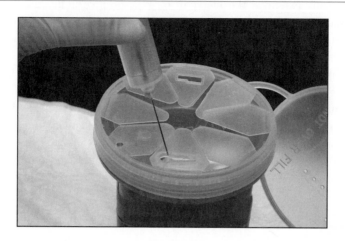

Source: CDC/Jim Gathany.

Contact with blood and other body fluids from all persons, regardless of known HIV status, should be avoided through strict, continuous adherence to universal precautions practices. These include the use of protective clothing and gloves by medical personnel and those caring for injured or ill persons. Masks or goggles may be required in some situations. Materials coming in contact with human body fluids or other human-derived materials need to be properly decontaminated before disposal. Special care must be taken when handling and disposing of "sharps" (objects such as needles, scissors, scalpels, and broken glass). Persons known to be HIV-positive or at high risk of infection should not attempt to donate blood, plasma, body organs, or sperm.

Surveillance

To track the course of the pandemic, discover trends, and monitor the effectiveness of intervention measures, accurate surveillance data were needed. By April 2004, all of the U.S. states had adopted a system for reporting HIV diagnoses to the CDC in Atlanta. Four years later, all U.S. states, the District of Columbia,

RECENT DEVELOPMENTS

A highly effective, inexpensive HIV vaccine could greatly decrease the occurrence of new infections and protect large numbers of people, particularly in areas of high incidence, such as sub-Saharan Africa and Southeast Asia. The extremely high mutation rate of the virus, however, has hampered production of a useful vaccine. Most vaccine development efforts have focused on the surface glyco-protein gp120 or p24. These vaccines have thus far led to incomplete protec-tion, protection effective only against the vaccine strain, or protection against a low-dose challenge. Most of these vaccines induced antibody responses but no activation of CD8$^+$ T killer cells, one of the most important components of antiviral defense.

Some promising results have been obtained using vaccines containing live SIV strains engineered with large deletions in three virulence genes, including *nef*. Monkeys infected with these vaccines were protected against challenge with unrelated virulent SIV strains. These types of live vaccines have not been well received by the biomedical community due to the possibility of back-mutation and fears that insertion of the vaccine strain viruses into host chro-mosomes might induce cancer. Other vaccine studies have triggered CD8$^+$ T killer cell responses in rhesus macaques by injecting naked HIV DNA followed by a booster with a recombinant viral vector containing selected HIV genes. In light of the fact that the majority of infections occur via sexual transmission, care needs to be taken to ensure production of mucosal immunity.

and five U.S. dependencies (American Samoa, Guam, the Northern Marianas, Puerto Rico, and the U.S. Virgin Islands) used a similar confidential name-based reporting system to collect HIV and AIDS data. This system was found to provide reliable and secure information. The CDC subsequently produced the *HIV/AIDS Surveillance Report for 2006* based on data from 33 states and the five dependencies. When compiling this report, it was necessary to discrimi-nate between new HIV infections and older, ongoing infections. The Serologic Testing Algorithm for Recent HIV Seroconversion (STARHS) was developed to analyze HIV-positive blood samples and ascertain whether the HIV infection was recent or ongoing. These surveillance efforts determined that AIDS inci-dence and deaths decreased in the United States during 1996 for the first time since the beginning of the epidemic in 1981. The trend is believed to be due to the early use of combination antiretroviral therapy, which slows progression to AIDS and death for HIV-positive persons. Administration of antiretroviral drugs to pregnant women and their newborns also reduced mother-to-child HIV transmission.

Another source of surveillance information is the HIV/AIDS Surveillance Database, a product of the Center for International Research of the U.S. Bureau of the Census. The data are compiled from information concerning HIV in developing countries as reported in medical and scientific literature, presented at international and regional conferences, or published in the press.

Summary

Disease
- Acquired immune deficiency syndrome (AIDS)

Causative Agents
- Human immunodeficiency virus-1 (HIV-1)   •   HIV-2

Agent Type
- Lentivirus group of Retroviridae

Genome
- Two copies of single-stranded RNA

Vector
- None

Common Reservoir
- Humans

Modes of Transmission
- Sexual contact   •   Blood or blood products   •   Mother-to-child transmission (transplacentally, during childbirth, via mother's milk)

Geographical Distribution
- Worldwide

Year of Emergence
- 1981

Key Terms

Acquired immune deficiency syndrome (AIDS) Usually fatal final stage of infection with the human immunodeficiency virus; characterized by low numbers of CD4$^+$ T helper cells, wasting, opportunistic infections, malignancies, and in some cases dementia

AIDS dementia Decreased central nervous system functions due to HIV infection

Category A HIV infection Asymptomatic infection or swollen lymph nodes

Category B HIV infection Formerly known as AIDS-related complex (ARC); includes conditions such as thrush, fever or diarrhea persisting for greater than a month, and shingles

Category C HIV infection Acquired immune deficiency syndrome (AIDS); includes conditions such as wasting, serious infections with opportunistic pathogens, cancers, dementia, and low CD4$^+$ T helper cell numbers

Cytopathic effect Formation of syncytia, multinucleated giant cells formed by fusion of HIV infected and noninfected cells, followed by cell death

gp120 Envelope glycoprotein that binds to CD4 on human T helper cells prior to cellular infection; primary target of many HIV vaccines

Highly active antiretroviral therapy (HAART) Anti-HIV treatment regimen that combines the administration of several reverse transcriptase and protease inhibitors

Human immunodeficiency virus (HIV) Either of the retroviruses responsible for causing AIDS, known as HIV-1 and HIV-2

Integrase Viral enzyme that catalyzes integration of HIV DNA into host chromosomes

Lentivirus Retrovirus associated with a slowly progressing disease

Opportunistic infection Pathogenic infection by microorganisms that typically have a commensal relationship with their human host

Protease Viral enzyme that cleaves HIV polyproteins into their individual components

Provirus Latent form of HIV that is integrated into the host chromosomes

R5 variants Form of HIV that uses CCR5 as a coreceptor; infects primarily macrophages and may be responsible for the initial infection of new human hosts

Retroviridae Group of viruses that use the enzyme reverse transcriptase during replication of their single-stranded RNA genome; members that infect humans include HIV, human T lymphocytic and leukemia viruses 1 and 2, and simian immunodeficiency virus

Reverse transcriptase Enzyme responsible for production of viral DNA by reverse transcription of RNA in retroviruses, including HIV

Wasting syndrome Physical condition characterized by profound weight loss and severe emaciation

X4 variants Form of HIV that uses CXCR4 as a coreceptor; infects primarily T helper cells and may be responsible for disease progression

Review Questions

1. What are criteria for the three categories of HIV infection? What major types of illnesses characterize those in category C?
2. What geographical regions have the greatest numbers of HIV-positive persons? Which groups are at highest risk for infection?
3. What human and nonhuman primate viruses are most closely related to HIV? What diseases are associated with these?
4. How may HIV kill $CD4^+$ T helper cells?
5. What is HAART, and how does it alter the course of HIV infection?

Topics for Further Discussion

1. Programs have been in place for many years in areas such as the Netherlands and some U.S. cities to distribute clean needles and syringes to intravenous drug users and provide addiction counseling. Explore the effect of these programs on the incidence of infection by HIV and hepatitis C virus and the number of illegal drug users.
2. Educational programs concerning safer sexual practices have targeted the gay community in the United States and some hard-hit regions of Africa. Free condom distribution programs have sometimes accompanied the latter. Explore the immediate effects of these programs on the rate of new infections, and determine whether these results were sustained over a period of years. Discuss which educational strategies have succeeded and which have not. Suggest new means of educating populations at high risk of infection.
3. Sub-Saharan Africa and portions of Southeast Asia have very high rates of HIV infection and deaths. Many inhabitants of these areas live in extreme poverty and cannot afford the expensive but effective antiretroviral medications now available, nor are the affected regions equipped to treat large numbers of persons with life-threatening opportunistic infections. Sickness and death of many young men in these parts of the world have severe economic consequences, as does the death of mothers, which often leaves young

children as orphans in poverty-stricken areas. Many of these children or their siblings are themselves HIV-positive. Corporations including those in the pharmaceutical industry, the governments of developed countries such as the United States, and individuals have facilitated distribution of antiretroviral drugs to developing nations at greatly reduced cost. Explore the effects of these low-cost drug programs on the HIV/AIDS morbidity and mortality rates as well as the economic and social consequences of these programs. Do the drugs reach all populations in need, or do local governments control access? Discuss other practical means of decreasing HIV infection rates or increasing life span or quality of life for infected individuals in developing nations.

4. Examine the literature concerning HIV vaccine development. What setbacks have occurred? What strategies currently seem promising? Suggest some innovative methods of developing an effective vaccine that would provide long-term protection to large numbers of persons with little risk.

Resources

Bangham, C.R.M. "CTL Quality and the Control of Human Retroviral Infections." *European Journal of Immunology,* 2009, *39,* 1700–1712.

Coleman, C. M., and Li, W. "HIV Interactions with Monocytes and Dendritic Cells: Viral Latency and Reservoirs." *Retrovirology,* 2009, *6,* 51–62.

Dhami, H., and others. "The Chemokine System and CCR5 Antagonists: Potential in HIV Treatment and Other Novel Therapies." *Journal of Clinical Pharmacology and Therapeutics,* 2009, *34,* 147–160.

Donnenberg, A. D., and others. "Apoptosis Parallels Lymphopoiesis in Bone Marrow Transplantation and HIV Disease." *Research in Immunology,* 1995, *146,* 11–21.

Emery, S., and Winston, A. "Raltegravir: A New Choice in HIV and New Chances for Research." *Lancet,* 2009, *374,* 764–766.

Gonzalo, T., Goñi, M. G., and Muñoz-Fernández, M. A. "Socioeconomic Impact of Antiretroviral Treatment in HIV Patients: An Economic Review of Cost Savings After Introduction of HAART." *AIDS Reviews,* 2009, *11,* 79–90.

Kaufman, D. R., and Barouch, D. H. "Translational Mini-Review Series on Vaccines for HIV: T Lymphocyte Trafficking and Vaccine-Elicited Mucosal Immunity." *Clinical and Experimental Immunology,* 2009, *157,* 165–173.

Paiardini, M., Pandrea, I., Apetrei, C., and Silvestri, G. "Lessons Learned from the Natural Hosts of HIV-Related Viruses." *Annual Reviews of Medicine,* 2009, *60,* 485–495.

Rinaldo, C., and others. "High Levels of Anti–Human Immunodeficiency Virus Type 1 (HIV-1) Memory Cytotoxic T-Lymphocyte Activity and Low Viral Load Are Associated with Lack of Disease in HIV-1-Infected Long-Term Nonprogressors." *Journal of Virology,* 1995, *69,* 5838–5842.

CHAPTER 17

HUMAN HERPESVIRUS 8 AND KAPOSI'S SARCOMA

LEARNING OBJECTIVES

- Define Kaposi's sarcoma, primary effusion lymphoma, and multi-centric Castleman's disease

- Describe the herpesvirus responsible for causing these illnesses

- Discuss modes of infection

- Discuss the host's response to infection

- Describe symptomatology and diagnosis

- Discuss potential methods of treatment

- Discuss methods of prevention

Major Concepts

Diseases

Human herpesvirus 8 (HHV-8) is a gamma-2 herpesvirus that is present in people presenting with all five forms of Kaposi's sarcoma (KS). These types are *classic KS*, affecting elderly men of Mediterranean or European Jewish ancestry; *endemic KS*, affecting younger men, very young children, and women in East Africa; *iatrogenic KS*, affecting individuals receiving immunosuppressive therapy; *epidemic KS*, affecting HIV-positive persons, especially gay men; and *nonepidemic gay-related KS*, found among HIV-negative gay men. KS is a cancer of endothelial cells lining blood vessels and begins as a skin cancer. It may remain confined to the skin, causing mild disease, or in more aggressive forms, such as epidemic KS, may travel to mucocutaneous areas or internal organs, resulting in life-threatening illness. HHV-8 infection appears to also play an important role in causing primary effusion lymphoma (PEL), a non-Hodgkin's lymphoma with poor prognosis, and multicentric Castleman's disease, a nonmalignant proliferative disorder of B lymphocytes. Individuals with sarcoidosis, multiple myeloma, and pemphigus may also be infected with HHV-8.

Infection

HHV-8 is closely related to the oncogenic *Herpesvirus saimiri* of monkeys and Epstein-Barr virus, which causes mononucleosis and Burkitt's lymphoma in humans. Other herpesviruses cause herpes simplex, chickenpox and shingles, sixth disease (roseola), and a severe infection of the liver and central nervous systems of immunosuppressed persons. HHV-8 is a large, enveloped DNA virus whose genome contains an extensive unique region encompassing approximately 25 genes, many of which appear to have been pirated from human chromosomes. These viral homologues to cellular genes include viral interleukin-6, viral Bcl-2, a receptor for vascular endothelial growth factor, and several viral chemokines. These genes help bring potential viral host cells into the area and trigger their excessive growth and survival. Other HHV-8 genes aid the virus in escaping death by $CD8^+$ T killer cells and inhibit the activity of the antiviral cytokine IFN-γ.

Immune System

HHV-8 has a complex relationship with the host immune response. Virally infected cells are killed by $CD8^+$ T killer cells and natural killer cells, but B lymphocyte–derived antibodies are less protective. HHV-8 infects monocytes and B lymphocytes, leading to the B cell proliferative disorders, PEL, and multi-centric Castleman's disease. Host inflammatory cytokines stimulate the growth of KS and PEL cells.

Protection

Several antiherpes drugs effectively kill lytic viruses but do not kill latent viruses. A number of anticancer medications, particularly those used to treat leukemia and lymphoma, decrease the size of KS lesions and slow disease progression. These medications are not without their drawbacks—relapses often occur, many of the drugs are expensive, and some have potentially dangerous side effects, including damage to the heart and bone marrow, decreased neutrophil numbers, fever, muscle inflammation, anemia, diarrhea, nausea, and depression.

Introduction

Kaposi's sarcoma (KS) is one of several diseases definitively linked to infection by the gamma-2 herpesvirus HHV-8. KS is a cancer of endothelial cells lining the blood vessels and may present as a mild skin cancer or may be aggressive, spreading to internal organs and causing death. Several other cancers or proliferative disorders, including those of B lymphocytes, have been linked to HHV-8 infection. Prior to the early 1980s, the majority of cases of KS were found among discrete populations, including elderly men of Mediterranean or Ashkenazi (eastern European) Jewish ancestry, younger men and very young children in restricted areas of Africa, and immunosuppressed persons. Between 1981 and 1982, an unusual number of cases of life-threatening KS began to turn up among young homosexual men in California. This population with aggressive KS was soon found to be HIV-positive, and the discovery of KS in these men was one of the first indications that a new virus (HIV) was spreading through the United States and later the world. Persons with all forms of KS were subsequently found to be infected with HHV-8, discovered in 1994. HHV-8 appears to play a causal role in primary effusion lymphoma and multicentric Castleman's disease and perhaps several other diseases. KS in HIV-positive persons and primary effusion lymphoma are very dangerous diseases, and the latter usually results in death within 60 days of initial diagnosis. Other gamma herpesviruses, such as Epstein-Barr virus, are linked to cancers in humans and monkeys, and the beta herpesvirus, cytomegalovirus, may cause severe pathology in HIV-positive persons. It is possible that HHV-8 or other presently unknown herpesviruses may contribute to other malignancies. More widespread screening for herpesvirus infection may aid in determining the extent of infection among different populations and may help define cofactors, such as coinfection with HIV-1, that may trigger HHV-8 to cause serious disease.

History

In 1872, a Viennese dermatologist, Moritz Kaposi, recognized an unusual pigmented skin cancer in elderly men of the area. This disease was later named classic Kaposi's sarcoma. Two other forms of KS were subsequently identified: one is endemic in some regions of Africa and affects younger men and children, and the other occurs among persons receiving immunosuppressive therapy, often following organ or bone marrow transplantation. In the early 1980s, an unusually aggressive form of KS was increasingly reported in young, otherwise healthy homosexual men from California. Between June 1982 and April 1983, eight cases of this disease turned up in Los Angeles and Orange Counties. They were linked to infection of at least 11 other men from eight additional cities. This new form of the disease spread beyond the skin, affecting internal organs and often resulting in death. This group of young men was later found to have other unusual conditions, including life-threatening infections with normally harmless commensal microbes. These men were subsequently found to be infected with a new human retrovirus, later named HIV-1. HIV-positive men with this aggressive form of KS were later found to be coinfected with a novel gamma herpesvirus, HHV-8, that is related to the oncogenic Epstein-Barr virus. HHV-8 was first identified in 1994 in KS tissues from an AIDS patient but was later detected in lesions and other tissues from all types of KS, including those occurring in HIV-negative persons. HHV-8 infection is also associated with many of the cases of primary effusion lymphoma and one subtype of multicentric Castleman's disease.

The Diseases

Infection with the human herpesvirus HHV-8 leads to several cancers of cells lining blood vessels or malignancies of B lymphocytes. Some of these diseases are mild, treatable skin malignancies, while others cause progressive illnesses that terminate in death. The most common of these cancers is Kaposi's sarcoma, but several other diseases are also linked to HHV-8 infection. Other members of the herpesvirus group may also cause malignancies, as seen by the link between infection with Epstein-Barr virus (EBV) and B cell lymphomas and nasopharyngeal carcinoma.

Table 17.1   Types of Kaposi's sarcoma

Type	Individuals Affected	Symptoms
Classic	Men over 50 years old of Mediterranean or Ashkenazi Jewish ancestry	Red, purple, or brownish lesions on legs and feet
Endemic	Men and young children in East Africa	Mild to aggressive cancer, with a tendency to metastasize to bone or internal organs
Iatrogenic	Persons receiving medical immunosuppressive treatment	Fever, rash, flulike symptoms, marrow aplasia, diarrhea; graft rejection in transplant recipients
Epidemic	HIV-positive persons, especially gay men	Very aggressive; begins as skin lesions leading to mucocutaneous and visceral lesions of lungs and digestive tract; difficulty in eating and swallowing, restriction of food passage, shortness of breath
Nonepidemic gay-related	HIV-negative gay men	Lesions primarily on arms, legs, and genitals

FIGURE 17.1   Skin lesions of Kaposi's sarcoma

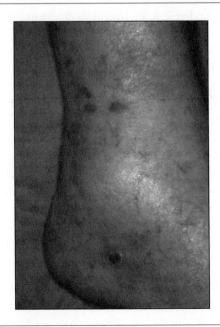

Source: National Institutes of Health.

Kaposi's Sarcoma

Five forms of Kaposi's sarcoma have been described. These are commonly found in the skin, where they appear as flat, painless purple-red spots that do not blanch when pressure is applied to them. They also occur in the lining of the mouth, nose, and eyes. More serious or life-threatening disease results when these cells spread to the lungs, liver, stomach, intestines, or lymph nodes.

Classic KS Classic KS typically occurs primarily in men over the age of 50 years who are either of Mediterranean (particularly Italian) or Ashkenazi Jewish ancestry. Corticosteroid usage and infrequent bathing increase the risk of developing this form of the disease. Classic KS is limited to the skin as one or more red, purple, or brownish lesions usually on the legs and feet, especially the ankles and soles. Lesions grow slowly in both size and number but rarely result in death, although affected persons have an increased risk of developing lymphomas, and lesions may form internally in areas such as the stomach and intestines, leading to gastrointestinal bleeding. Approximately 300 to 400 cases of classic KS are diagnosed each year in the United States. Prior to 1986, this was the predominant form of KS in the United States.

Endemic KS Endemic KS is the prevalent form found in East Africa, particularly in northeastern Democratic Republic of Congo, Tanzania, and western Uganda and was known prior to the advent of HIV infection in the continent. It was responsible for 8% of all cancers in Ugandan men during the mid-1960s. Endemic KS is more common in men and very young children than women; however, it occurs more frequently in women than other forms of KS. The average age of affected men is 35 years.

Endemic KS presents itself in four clinical forms, one of which has a mild course similar to that seen in classic KS but affecting younger adults. The other three forms are more aggressive, particularly in infected Africans as opposed to Americans or Europeans, with an increased tendency to spread to bone or other tissues. A variant found in some young African children spreads via the lymphatic system to internal organs, with rapidly fatal results. In recent years, the incidence of endemic KS has increased among the HIV-negative population in Africa.

Iatrogenic KS Iatrogenic KS is found in persons receiving medically related immunosuppressive regimens, especially organ or bone marrow transplant recipients. Renal transplant patients and those receiving cyclosporine (frequently used following this type of transplantation) are particularly vulnerable. Iatrogenic KS occurs equally in females and males. The immunosuppressive regimens required to prevent rejection may reactivate latent virus, often leading to serious visceral involvement, which may result in graft rejection and the death of the recipient. In patients receiving bone marrow transplants, fever, rash, flulike symptoms, marrow aplasia, diarrhea, and increased viral load have been reported, followed by death.

Epidemic (HIV-Associated) KS This form of KS emerged rapidly in California at the beginning of the AIDS epidemic, and its appearance was one of the first indications of a serious condition sweeping the gay community. It is the most common cancer in HIV-positive men, affecting approximately 20% of HIV-positive people. The decline in $CD4^+$ T helper cell numbers during the progression of HIV infection increases the chances of developing KS, and the Th1 subset of $CD4^+$ lymphocytes appears to protect the host against HHV-8-associated disease (described later in this chapter). Although HHV-8 infection is similar among those coinfected with HIV-1 and HIV-2, epidemic KS is almost exclusively restricted to those who test positive for HIV-1.

Epidemic KS is particularly common in the gay population of HIV-positive men, especially those who have multiple sex partners; it is less common in individuals who acquired HIV via heterosexual contact, IV drug use, or blood transfusion; and it is much less common in HIV-positive women or HIV-positive hemophiliacs. Women who contracted HIV through heterosexual contact with bisexual men are at higher risk for developing KS. In 1990, the incidence of KS in the United States was 300 times more common in AIDS patients than in other immunosuppressed persons and 20,000 times that of the general population. In areas of Africa that are severely affected by the AIDS pandemic, such as Uganda, it is the most common cancer of men and one of the most common in women. The number of KS cases in that region rose tenfold between the 1950s and 1991. HIV-positive children are also afflicted with this cancer.

HIV-associated KS is a very aggressive form of cancer that most commonly begins as small lesions on the face and trunk. The lesions initially appear to be bruises with discolored edges and later become scaly, brown, and elevated. These often then develop into mucocutaneous and visceral lesions involving the lungs and digestive tract. If the disease is restricted to the skin, it is not life-threatening. The prognosis is far worse if the lesions spread to internal organs. These may lead to difficulty in eating or swallowing if lesions are found in the esophagus, restriction of food passage if found in the intestines, shortness of breath if found in the lungs, and lymphadenopathy if found in the lymph nodes. HIV-associated KS appears to consist of a large number of primary lesions rather than metastases from a single initial lesion.

FIGURE 17.2   Kaposi's sarcoma of the hard palate of an HIV-positive person

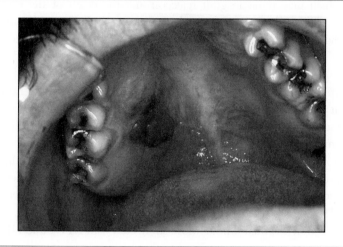

Source: CDC/Sol Silverman Jr.

Nonepidemic Gay-Related KS Nonepidemic KS occurs in homosexual men who are HIV-negative. Its progression is slow, and new lesions appear every few years, most often on the arms, legs, and genitals, but can form anywhere on the skin.

Primary Effusion Lymphoma

Primary effusion lymphoma (PEL), an AIDS-associated non-Hodgkin's lymphoma, contains primary malignant lymphomatous effusions of the pleural, pericardial, or peritoneal cavities with large-cell immunoblasts or anaplastic large cells. The morphology of these cells differs from Burkitt's lymphoma, although they may contain the Epstein-Barr virus. They do not have oncogenic rearrangements in *c-myc*, *bcl-2*, or *p53* oncogenes but do have clonal immuno-globulin rearrangements, similar to B lymphocytes. The cells express the CD45 antigen of dividing B cells. No tumor is present, and the lymphoma cells do not leave the body cavity in which they originated. These cells do not have other B lymphocyte or T lymphocyte antigens, nor do they rearrange DNA encoding the T cell antigen receptor. PEL frequently occurs in men, particularly men who have sex with men (MSM). The prognosis is poor, with a length of survival after diagnosis of approximately 60 days.

Multicentric Castleman's Disease

Multicentric Castleman's disease (MCD) is a rare, polyclonal nonmalignant atypical lymphoproliferative disorder of B lymphocytes in germinal centers. It is more common in men and is often accompanied by malignancies, such as KS or non-Hodgkin's lymphoma. MCD takes two forms, the more common of which presents as a tumor mass in the mediastinum of the thoracic cavity or in the retroperitoneum. It is not associated with HHV-8 infection. The less common form involves infiltrates of plasma cells (B lymphocytes producing antibody) and is associated with HHV-8 infection. This form is characterized by immune system dysfunction, generalized lymphadenopathy, autoimmune disorders, rashes, and generalized symptoms. HHV-8-associated MCD is most common among HIV-positive persons, especially MSM.

Other Diseases Potentially Associated with HHV-8 Infection

Sarcoidosis **Sarcoidosis** is a multisystem disease of unknown origin that may affect a number of organs, including the lungs, lymph nodes, and skin. It is characterized by the presence of noncaseous granulomas in more than one tissue. Conflicting reports have either found an increased association of HHV-8 infection in persons with sarcoidosis or failed to find such an association.

Multiple Myeloma **Multiple myeloma** is the most common lymphoid cancer in persons of African origin and the second most common in persons of European origin. It is a clonal B cell cancer in which plasma cells secrete monoclonal antibody. Growth of these cells involves autocrine and paracrine stimulation by cytokines such as IL-6, TNF-α, and IL-1. As with sarcoidosis, some studies have reported increased incidence of HHV-8 in persons with multiple myeloma, while other studies have not.

Pemphigus **Pemphigus vulgaris and pemphigus foliaceus** are autoimmune skin diseases in which the epidermal and dermal layers separate. KS is the most frequent cancer in individuals with pemphigus, and HHV-8 is often detected in the affected areas.

The Causative Agent

All forms of Kaposi's sarcoma are caused by the sexually transmitted microbe **human herpesvirus 8 (HHV-8)**, also known as **Kaposi's sarcoma–associated herpesvirus**, discovered in 1994. This virus is necessary but not sufficient to cause the disease. It is found in spindle cells in almost all KS skin lesions, in endothelial cells lining the blood vessels, and in B lymphocytes and monocytes of the immune system. Infection of cultured endothelial cells induces a transformation from a cobblestone appearance to a spindle-shaped morphology. The HHV-8 K8.1 envelope glycoprotein binds to heparin sulfate and uses this cell surface molecule as its receptor prior to entering its target cell. The virus is also present in secreted materials, such as saliva, nasal secretions, serum, and semen. Recently, HHV-8 DNA and latent phase proteins have been detected in placental cells from infected women. These cells express heparin sulfate on their surface. Other herpesviruses also infect the placenta, leading to miscarriage, premature delivery, low birth weight, and major congenital abnormalities.

HHV-8 is transmitted sexually, including via oral sexual practices, through contact with infectious secretions; it may also be transmitted transplacentally. Risk factors for infection include having a high number of sexual partners and history of a previous sexually transmitted disease. HHV-8 seropositivity is highest in HIV-positive gay men with documented KS (80%), is only 18% in HIV-positive gay men without KS, and is very low in HIV-positive hemophiliacs and HIV-negative persons in the United States. An unusually high number of cases of KS have also been reported in young otherwise healthy HIV-negative MSM in New York City, suggesting that exposure to fecal material during sexual contact may increase the risk of developing KS. HHV-8 is much more common among the general population in Africa, where 50% of the people have antibodies to HHV-8 (correlating with past or present infection), whether or not they are infected with HIV. Although transmission is primarily via sexual intercourse, infants born to HIV-positive women may develop KS. Transmission also occurs through the use of shared equipment by IV drug users.

HHV-8 is a large, enveloped DNA virus that is a member of the ***Rhadinovirus* (gamma-2) herpesviruses**, as is its close relative, the oncogenic *Herpesvirus saimiri* of squirrel monkeys. Rhadinoviruses also infect spider monkeys, African green monkeys, macaques, chimpanzees, gorillas, drills, and mandrills. These primates include both Old and New World species. Other pathogenic herpesviruses of humans are the alpha human herpesviruses, which include herpes simplex 1 and 2, which cause genital lesions and cold sores, and human herpesvirus 3 (varicella-zoster virus), which causes chickenpox; human (beta) herpesvirus 5 (human cytomegalovirus), which causes severe infection of the liver and central nervous system, particularly among immunosuppressed persons; and human herpesvirus 7, which causes roseola infantum (sixth disease). Human herpesvirus 4 is the Epstein-Barr virus (gamma-1 herpesvirus), which causes mononucleosis and is associated with some cases of Burkitt's lymphoma. HHV-8 DNA is double-stranded and is found within a capsid in a dark central core. While inside the capsid, viral DNA is linear but later becomes circular after being released from the capsid following infection of the cell. The capsid is icosadeltahedral (having 16 surfaces) with a twofold symmetry and a diameter of 100 to 120 nanometers. Outside of the capsid is the tegument, an amorphous proteinaceous material surrounded by the viral envelope, which is studded with short glycoproteins.

HHV-8 has been divided into several major subtypes and at least 13 clades based on differences in the DNA of the K1 gene. Subtype distribution shows geographical preferences. A and C variants dominate samples from persons with epidemic KS in the United States, Europe, Asia, and Saudi Arabia, while the B variant is most common in samples from Africa. The D subtype is uncommon, being restricted to classic KS patients from the Pacific region. An E subtype is found in Amerindians from Brazil and Ecuador, and the Z subtype is unique to Zambia. The presence of several viral groups does not appear to account for differences in disease manifestations in different groups of infected individuals.

Viral infection of cells may be divided into an initial latent and a later lytic stage. A small viral RNA transcript is produced during prolonged **latent viral infection** that is found in most of the cells present in lesions during all stages of KS, while a slightly larger RNA transcript is found during lytic infection and is primarily present in only 10% of the cells in late lesions. During the latent phase, HHV-8 itself does not reproduce but its genes act to increase division of host cells, prevent cell death by apoptosis, and aid in viral evasion of the immune response. All herpesviruses establish latency, although in different types of host cells. Greater than 99% of the cells from KS tissues are latently infected. This stage is followed by **lytic viral infection**, which occurs after reactivation of the virus and results in death of the host cell and release of infectious viral particles. Virus may be artificially induced to the lytic state by the tumor-promoting agent phorbol myristol acetate, which activates the cellular protein kinase C signaling pathway and is involved in normal B lymphocyte functioning.

The genome of HHV-8 contains approximately 95 genes, 25 of which are located within an extensive region (K region). The K region extends over 100 kilobases and is unique to this virus, being absent from the closely related gamma herpesvirus, the Epstein-Barr virus. A number of the gene products are believed to have been originally derived by duplication of parts of host DNA followed by their transfer into the viral genome. Many of these genes aid in growth or survival of HHV-8 in B cells or endothelial cells or contribute to outgrowth of infected cells. Nearby uninfected cells are also stimulated to divide in a paracrine manner in response to the viral proteins, resulting in cancer. HHV-8's K2 gene produces a homologue to the host cytokine IL-6 that is constitutively produced by KS spindle cells and PEL cells and during MCD. Host IL-6 serves as a B cell growth factor,

RECENT DEVELOPMENTS

One of the proteins expressed during the latent stage of cellular infection is the latency-associated nuclear antigen (LANA). LANA prolongs the latent stage by inhibiting production of a protein required for the switch to the lytic phase. It also serves as a viral oncogene by cooperating with the Ras oncogene to transform the cell into a cancerous form while inhibiting the activity of the tumor suppressor genes p53 and Rb, which inhibit cancer development. The immune cell cytokine TGF-β protects the host against tumor growth and survival by binding to its receptor; stimulating pathways that inhibit cancer cell division; and inducing the cell to undergo apoptosis, programmed cell death. Dysregulation of either TGF-β or its receptor enables cancer cells to survive and continue to grow.

Some of the effects of LANA result from its ability to prevent transcription of RNA from the DNA template. The addition of a methyl chemical group to either DNA of a gene or to the surrounding histone proteins around which that section of DNA is wrapped often blocks transcription. LANA has recently been found to stimulate host cell genes that either add methyl groups to DNA or histones or inhibit the cellular genes that remove methyl groups. The TGF-β receptor gene is one of those in which LANA increases methylation, blocking production of the receptor's RNA and protein during PEL, and allowing the malignant B lymphocytes to avoid death by apoptosis and to grow unchecked.

and viral IL-6 acts in a similar manner, stimulating cell division, hematopoiesis, and angiogenesis of IL-6-dependent cell lines, encouraging growth of PEL cells, and inducing production of **vascular endothelial growth factor (VEGF)**, a key host molecule that encourages formation of new blood vessels by stimulating growth of endothelial cells. HHV-8 also encodes a receptor for this growth factor.

Two viral proteins function as chemokines (cytokines that chemically attract immune cells into an area) and have homology to the host chemokine MIP-1α. These viral chemokines have both been found to be angiogenic in vitro (increasing growth of endothelial cells of blood vessels). HHV-8 encodes an interferon regulatory factor homologue via the K9 gene (discussed under "Immune Response"). The virus also contains a B cell leukemia protein-2 (Bcl-2) homologue. **Bcl-2** is a cellular survival factor that inhibits the programmed cell death process of apoptosis, which normally eliminates cells with dysregulated growth, including cancer cells. Unlike its cellular homologue, viral Bcl-2 activity is not down-regulated by proapoptotic proteins. Viral genes also encode a cyclin D homologue similar to cellular Bcl-1. **Cyclins and cyclin-dependent kinases (CDKs)** are proteins that positively regulate passage through the cell cycle, terminating in cell division. The viral cyclin homologue activates CDK6 and blocks functioning of the **retinoblastoma (Rb) protein**, an important tumor suppressor gene that mediates cell cycle arrest in cells with damaged or abnormal DNA. The Rb protein is mutated in several types of human cancers. Viral cyclin D induces degradation of p27^{kip}, an inhibitor of CDK6, thus blocking the normal feedback mechanisms that prevent excessive cell growth. HHV-8 also encodes dihydrofolate reductase, an enzyme that participates in production of folate, which is necessary for nucleic acid production during cell division.

The HHV-8 K12 gene produces **kaposin**, a viral protein found in KS and PEL. This protein induces tumorogenic transformation. This process leads to the expression of telomerase and allows anchorage-independent growth, both common features of malignant cells. **Telomerase** is an enzyme that allows cells to escape the normal capping of cell growth at 40–60 divisions.

The HHV-8 open reading frame 74 gene encodes a **viral G protein-coupled receptor (vGPCR)** that is a homologue of the human IL-8 chemokine receptor. This vGPCR serves as a viral oncogene that transforms endothelial cells and fibroblasts into a cancerous state by stimulating the mitogen-activated protein kinase (MAPK) intracellular signaling pathway that is involved in division of many human cell types. However, vGPCR has also been shown to decrease division of infected B lymphocytes in PEL. It also appears to either increase or decrease production of other proteins involved in virally mediated cell lysis, depending on the stage of viral infection. Thus the functions of vGPCR may vary during the course of infection of a cell.

KS cells secrete angiogenic growth factors such as VEGF, fibroblast growth factor, TNF-α, and oncostatin M. The binding of VEGF to its receptor on an infected endothelial cell triggers cell division and also reproduction of the virus within. Using its various gene products, HHV-8 is thus able to encourage the growth of the B cells and endothelial cells that serve as the virus's cellular homes (IL-6, viral chemokines, VEGF receptor, cyclin D). These factors also encourage their target cells to move to the area of infection (viral chemokines, IL-8 receptor) and enable them to survive once there (Bcl-2 homologue).

The HIV *tat* protein also stimulates KS growth due to its similarity to VEGF. In vitro, normal endothelial cells are stimulated to divide in the presence of *tat* plus the host cellular growth factor, basic fibroblast growth factor; the resulting cells have the appearance of KS cells (spindle cells). This property of *tat* plus the immunosuppression induced by HIV may at least partially explain why the most aggressive form of KS occurs in HIV-positive persons.

Table 17.2   HHV-8 proteins that increase viral growth or survival

Viral Protein	Action
IL-6 homologue	↑ B cell division, hematopoiesis; induction of angiogenesis via production of VEGF
MIP-1α homologue	Induction of angiogenesis; movement of target cells to site
Bcl-2 homologue	↓ apoptosis and ↑ target cell survival
Cyclin D homologue	↑ target cell division, ↓ tumor suppressor gene activity
Dihydrofolate reductase	Production of folate required for nucleic acid synthesis during cell division
Kaposin	Tumorogenic transformation; ↑ expression of telomerase and stimulation of anchorage-independent cell growth
IL-8 receptor homologue	↑ cell division; movement of target cells to site of infection
VEGF, fibroblast growth factor, TNF-α, oncostatin M	Angiogenic growth factors; ↑ growth of B cells and endothelial cells

The Immune Response

HHV-8 infects B lymphocytes, monocytes, and some hematopoietic stem cells but not $CD8^+$ T killer cells. The viral K1 protein activates intracellular tyrosine kinases, mimicking normal B cell activation by the B cell antigen receptor. These infected B cells may then proliferate, leading to a B cell cancer such as PEL or MCD. The growth of KS cells is augmented by the presence of the inflammatory cytokines IL-1, IL-6, and TNF-α, most of which are produced by the infected cells themselves and thus serve as autocrine growth factors.

Protective immunity appears to not be related to the levels of neutralizing antibody but rather to the activity of $CD8^+$ T killer cells and NK cells, which are stimulated in response to several viral proteins. $CD4^+$ T helper cell activity against HHV-8 is lower in infected persons who develop KS than in those who do not; this activity decreases during infection as antibody production increases. Levels of the host inflammatory cytokine IFN-γ, produced by the Th1 subset of $CD4^+$ T helper cells, rise in KS patients. Production of this cytokine is a double-edged sword because it stimulates activation of T killer cells and NK cells but also aids in viral reactivation from the latent to the lytic state in both infected B lymphocytes and monocytes.

HHV-8 employs several K region genes to escape death by $CD8^+$ T killer cell and NK cells. The K3 and K5 genes encode the viral MIR-1 and MIR-2 proteins that aid HHV-8 in escaping from CD8$^+$ T killer cell activity. MIR-1 and MIR-2 enhance the endocytosis of MHC class I molecules and their degradation within lysosomes. MCH I molecules are necessary for the killing of virally infected cells by CD8$^+$ T killer cells. The MIR-2 protein also down-regulates the expression of cellular ICAM-1 and B7.2. The former is a cellular recognition molecule used by immune cells, and the latter is a cell surface receptor of T lymphocytes that is required for their proper stimulation. Viral K13 encodes the **v-FLICE inhibitory protein (vFLIP)**, which allows escape of infected cells from apoptosis induced by host NK cells. vFLIP prevents the formation of caspase-8, a protein involved in the apoptotic cascade.

The K6, K4, and K4.1 genes encode three HHV-8 chemokines, vCCL1, vCCL2, and vCCL3, which help activate Th2-type responses through their respective cellular receptors and are antagonistic to receptors responsible for the chemotaxis of Th1 T helper cells and NK cells. Th2 activity leads to the production of cytokines that polarize the immune response toward a predominantly antibody type of immune reaction as opposed to a CD8$^+$ T killer cell and NK cell response induced by Th1 T helper cells. The K14 gene encodes OX-2, a neural cell adhesion-like protein that stimulates Th2 immune responses and production of IL-6, which acts as a growth factor for KS and PEL cells. The K9 gene product interferes with signaling by the Th1 cytokine, IFN-γ. Together these viral products encourage the production of a Th2 cytokine environment that is favorable to their survival while inhibiting an antiviral Th1 immune response.

Diagnosis

Accurate, practical methods are needed to detect the presence of HHV-8 in blood and tissues prior to their use in transfusions or transplantation as well as to correctly diagnose individuals with KS. HHV-8 may be detected from nodular skin lesions by polymerase chain reaction (PCR) or nested PCR, in which virus is detected in 87% to 91% of the samples tested. The rate of detection is somewhat lower in lesions from the patch and plaque stages and is much lower in lymph node tissue from KS patients. HHV-8 may also be detected in blood lymphocytes from about half of HIV-positive KS patients. Routine use of PCR in screening is hampered by the expense, the time required, and its lack of sensitivity in samples of plasma and peripheral blood cells.

Antibodies to HHV-8 may be detected using IgG or IgM ELISA, indirect fluorescent-antibody assay (IFA), Western blot, or immunohistochemistry. Detection of HHV-8 antigens may also be performed by IFA in which one may

FIGURE 17.3   Polymerase chain reaction (PCR)

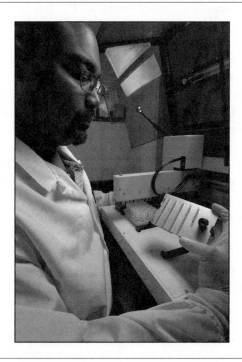

Source: CDC/Hsi Liu and James Gathany.

assess the presence of latent virus antigens (nuclear antigens such as LANA) or lytic virus antigens (cytoplasmic antigens). Detection of the latter may be used to predict the risk of developing KS.

Diagnosis of KS and determination of the extent of the disease includes several nonspecific tests, such as screening the skin and lymph nodes, biopsies of these organs, and chest X-rays, bronchoscopy, and endoscopy to ascertain lung, tracheal, and gastrointestinal involvement.

Treatment

HHV-8 is resistant to killing by acyclovir (a commonly used antiviral agent), but the lytic form is susceptible to several other antiviral compounds, including cidofovir (a nucleoside analogue), ganciclovir, and foscarnet (antiherpesvirus drugs). Because these agents inhibit the viral polymerase used only during viral reproduction, they do not affect latent viruses. Antibiotics are ineffective against HHV-8 because it is a virus.

KS skin lesions may be removed physically using liquid nitrogen, radiation, or surgery. These lesions may be injected with anticancer drugs, such as vincristine or vinblastin, as well. Intralesional use of human chorionic gonadotropin (hCG) was found to be successful in the treatment of KS skin lesions after observing that these lesions disappear during pregnancy due to increased levels of hCG. Subcutaneous administration of hCG in men also leads to stabilization or regression of lesion size. KS often flares up again once treatment is stopped, but in some cases, the remission has persisted for over one year. Therapy with hCG is rather expensive, and its side effects include increases in weight, energy, and appetite. Another newer method used in the treatment of KS skin lesions is topical application of panretin gel (9-cis retionic acid). Up to half of patients treated noted improvement in lesion size. Panretin is a natural hormone that interacts with three receptors that stimulate cell growth and three other receptors that cause apoptosis. Because these treatments do not actually remove HHV-8, relapses often occur.

For persons with HIV-associated KS, lesions in internal organs may be treated by combination chemotherapy with the anticancer drugs adriamycin, bleomycin, and vincristine (ABV). Combination therapy may lead to serious side effects, including damage to the heart or bone marrow, decreased number of neutrophils leading to increased vulnerability to bacterial infections, and nerve damage. Thalidomide, a drug that inhibits the growth of blood vessels, either halts the growth of lesions or leads to their regression. This drug was notorious for causing limb deformities in fetuses when given to pregnant women but is receiving increasing attention for chemotherapy in persons who are not and will not become pregnant. Its side effects include sedation, rash with fever, muscle inflammation, and depression.

A newer approach used to treat advanced KS in patients who do not respond to standard treatments or are unable to tolerate the side effects employs liposomal drugs. Two standard antileukemia medicines, doxorubicin and daunorubicin, are encased within fat droplets (liposomes) to form the liposomal drugs Doxil and DaunoXome. These fat-encapsulated drugs are retained for longer times in the body, pass more readily through the lipid-rich cell membrane, and result in fewer side effects. Many patients receiving Doxil report improvement; however, only 2% to 3% achieve a complete response. The major side effect for these liposomal drugs is neutropenia (decreased neutrophil numbers, which increases the risk of bacterial infection); this condition may be reversed by administration of the hematopoietic growth factor, granulocyte colony stimulating factor. Liposomal drugs do not provide a long-lasting benefit, and the duration of response is approximately four months, after which time KS resumes and retreatment is necessary. These drugs have not been shown to increase survival time in persons with advanced KS.

Two other drugs are being tested for use in patients with HIV-associated KS after progression to AIDS. The first of these is IFN-α, which is used for patients whose CD4$^+$ T helper cell count is less than 200 per cubic centimeter. It is used in combination with nucleoside analogues, such as AZT. Using this combination, KS regression occurs in 30% of treated individuals but may cause chills and headaches. IFN-α makes the KS cells better targets for elimination by T killer cells. The other drug under development is the anticancer drug Taxol. Taxol is being tested for used in persons with very advanced AIDS (CD4$^+$ T helper cell count of around 16) and KS involving internal organs. Taxol is effective but very toxic. Side effects include leukopenia (low white blood cell levels), anemia, hair loss, diarrhea, nausea, muscle pain, and peripheral neuropathy.

For individuals who have the epidemic form of KS, triple drug treatment with HAART is beneficial. HAART has been successfully used to prolong the lives of HIV-positive individuals (discussed in Chapter Sixteen).

A new approach to the treatment of PEL focuses on blocking the action of viral LANA using the drug Nutlin-3a. LANA blocks the activity of the tumor suppressor pathway triggered by p53. p53 is degraded by the host murine double minute 2 (MDM2) protein. LANA binds to and forms a complex with p53 and MDM2, leading to the destruction of the former and permitting PEL cells to avoid the host's antitumor defense system. Nutlin-3a inhibits MDM2, allowing the p53 pathway to remain functional and specifically kill the cancerous PEL cells but not normal B lymphocytes.

FIGURE 17.4   The chemical structure of Taxol

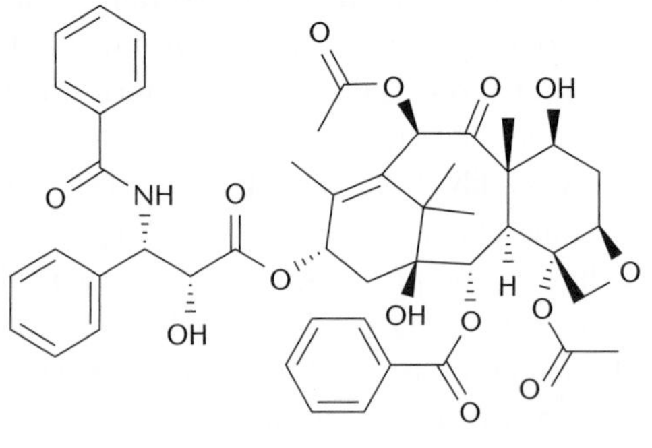

Prevention

The most severe type of KS is the epidemic form found primarily in HIV-positive men, particularly those who acquired the disease via sexual contact with other men. Because transmission of HHV-8 occurs predominantly via homosexual contact between men, avoiding such contact or using safer sex practices lowers the risk of infection. Women who are the sexual partners of bisexual men are also at increased risk for developing epidemic KS and should also practice safer sex. A much lower number of persons acquire infection through illicit IV drug use. The risk of transmission in this population may be decreased by using sterile needles and syringes.

Other forms of HHV-8-associated illnesses appear to be due to nonsexual means in persons living in the Mediterranean region and Africa. Protection against disease for these persons may include testing any unusual skin lesions to allow prompt treatment.

Surveillance

Surveys of the prevalence of HHV-8 antigens reveal differing rates of infection in different areas of the world, with rates higher in areas where KS is more common and among some indigenous populations in various locales throughout the world. When detecting either latent or lytic viral antigens, infection rates were found to be low in U.S. adults (0% to 1.4% and 20%, respectively). In Central Africa, where endemic KS is found, latent antigens were detected in 11% to 53% of the populace and lytic antigens in 32% to 82%. Incidence is also high in all populations in sub-Saharan Africa. The infection rate in southern Italy, where classic KS occurs, is approximately 3.5 times that of northern and central Italy. The rate in Sicily is approximately 10% higher than the rest of southern Italy. HHV-8 appears at a higher rate among indigenous populations of South America, with an incidence rate of 53% in Brazilian Amerindians and 36% in Amerindians from Ecuador, while the rate of HHV-8 among Brazilian blood donors is less than that in the United States. The Uygur people in northwestern China and the indigenous population of New Guinea also have a higher incidence of infection than the general population of Asia and the Pacific Islands.

Age, the presence of coinfections, and other factors contribute to the prevalence of HHV-8 infection. In U.S. children, lytic antibodies were detected in 2% of 3- to 5-year olds, 8% in 6- to 10-year olds, 4% in 11- to 15-year olds, and

18% in persons aged 16 to 20. This trend is also present in Europe, Africa, and Asia. Individuals infected with hepatitis B or syphilis have increased rates of HHV-8 coinfection. Infection occurs primarily among sexually active persons, particularly MSM, whose incidence of infection ranged from 20% to 38%. Among HIV-positive persons or persons with AIDS in North America, the rate of infection with HHV-8 was 30% to 48%. IV drug users had a higher rate of infection than nonusers, which increased with the length of time spent using these drugs.

Summary

Diseases
- Kaposi's sarcoma • Primary effusion lymphoma • Multicentric Castleman's disease • Possibly sarcoidosis and multiple myeloma

Causative Agent
- Human herpesvirus 8

Agent Type
- Gamma herpesvirus of the *Rhadinovirus* genus

Genome
- DNA

Vector
- None

Common Reservoir
- Humans

Modes of Transmission
- Sexually • Through blood and other secretions • From mother to child

Geographical Distribution
- Worldwide

Year of Emergence
- 1872 • 1981

Key Terms

Bcl-2 Cellular survival factor that inhibits programmed cell death, apoptosis, which normally eliminates cells with dysregulated growth, including cancer cells

Cyclins and cyclin-dependent kinases (CDKs) Proteins that positively regulate passage through the cell cycle, resulting in cell division

Human herpesvirus 8 (HHV-8) Gamma herpesvirus infecting humans; the causative agent of Kaposi's sarcoma, primary effusion lymphoma, and multicentric Castleman's disease

Kaposin HHV-8 protein that induces tumorogenic transformation

Kaposi's sarcoma (KS) Cancer associated with infection by human herpesvirus 8; typically involves skin lesions, which may become internalized, leading to fatal disease, particularly in HIV-positive individuals

Kaposi's sarcoma–associated herpesvirus Human herpesvirus 8

Latent viral infection Stage in which a virus coexists with its host cell; may exist for prolonged periods of time

Lytic viral infection Active stage in which a virus lyses its host cell and is released to infect other cells

Multicentric Castleman's disease (MCD) Nonmalignant atypical lymphoproliferative disorder, one form of which is associated with infection by human herpesvirus 8

Multiple myeloma Common cancer of antibody-producing B lymphocytes

Pemphigus vulgaris and pemphigus foliaceus Autoimmune skin diseases in which the epidermal and dermal layers separate

Primary effusion lymphoma (PEL) AIDS-associated non-Hodgkins lymphoma induced by infection of B lymphocytes with human herpesvirus-8

Retinoblastoma (Rb) protein Important tumor suppressor gene that arrests the cell cycle in cells with damaged or abnormal DNA

***Rhadinovirus* (gamma-2) herpesviruses** Genus containing human herpesvirus 8, the causative agent of Kaposi's sarcoma, primary effusion lymphoma, and multicentric Castleman's disease, as well as an oncogenic virus of monkeys

Sarcoidosis Multisystem disease that is characterized by the presence of noncaseous granulomas in a number of organs, including the lungs, lymph nodes, and skin

Telomerase Enzyme that allows cells to escape the normal capping of cell growth

Vascular endothelial growth factor (VEGF) Molecule that encourages formation of new blood vessels by stimulating growth of endothelial cells that line the vessels

v-FLICE inhibitory protein (vFLIP) HHV-8 protein that allows virally-infected cells to escape apoptosis induced by host NK cells by preventing formation of the apoptotic caspase-8 enzyme

Viral G protein-coupled receptor (vGPCR) Homologue of the human IL-8 chemokine receptor that functions as a viral oncogene and transforms endothelial cells and fibroblasts into cancerous cells

Review Questions

1. What are the five types of Kaposi's sarcoma? What groups of people are affected by each?
2. What are the characteristics of primary effusion lymphoma (PEL)? What is the prognosis for this disease?
3. Which cells and body fluids may contain human herpesvirus 8 (HHV-8)?
4. Which herpesviruses of humans and nonhuman primates are similar to HHV-8? With which diseases are they associated?
5. What are some of the anticancer drugs used to treat KS? What are other approaches used to remove skin lesions?

Topics for Further Discussion

1. Some antiviral drugs are able to kill the lytic forms of viruses like HHV-8 but not the latent form because they target the viral polymerase, which is expressed only during lytic infection. Suggest how drugs might be formulated to kill latent viruses and not host cells.
2. HHV-8 infection has been linked to several vascular skin cancers or cancers of B lymphocytes. Could HHV-8 have as yet undetermined links to other cancers? Research other skin malignancies and B cell cancers that occur in humans, especially those populations known to be infected with HHV-8 (elderly men of Mediterranean or southern European ancestry, immunosuppressed persons, persons from East Africa, gay men).
3. Speculate as to why indigenous populations of various, widely separated areas of the world have an unusually high rate of infection with HHV-8. These groups include Amerindians, residents of parts of Africa, the Uygur people in

northwestern China, and the indigenous population of New Guinea. Discuss why KS has not been detected at a high rate in these populations.

4. Some anticancer drugs have been shown to be effective for the treatment of KS and PEL. These cancers often relapse over time, perhaps due to continued activity of HHV-8. Discuss whether combination therapy using antiviral drugs plus anticancer drugs may be beneficial. What is a potential problem with this approach?

Resources

Ablashi, D. V., Chatlynne, L. G., Whitman, J. E., Jr., and Cesarman, E. "Spectrum of Kaposi's Sarcoma–Associated Herpesvirus, or Human Herpesvirus 8, Diseases." *Clinical Microbiology Reviews*, 2002, *15*, 439–464.

Chin, J. *Control of Communicable Diseases Manual* (17th ed.). Washington, D.C.: American Public Health Association, 2000.

"A Cluster of Kaposi's Sarcoma and *Pneumocystis carinii* Pneumonia Among Homosexual Male Residents of Los Angeles and Range Counties, California." *MMWR Weekly*, 1982, *31*, 305–307.

Di Bartolo, D. L., and others. "KSHV LANA Inhibits TGF-β Signaling Through Epigenetic Silencing of the TGF-β Type II Receptor." *Blood*, 2008, *111*, 4731–4740.

Di Stefano, M., and others. "In Vitro and In Vivo Human Herpesvirus 8 Infection of Placenta." *PLoS ONE*, 2008, *3*, e4073.

Edelman, D. C. "Human Herpesvirus 8: A Novel Human Pathogen." *Virology Journal*, 2005, *2*, 78–110.

Sarek, G., and others. "Reactivation of the p53 Pathway as a Treatment Modality for KSHV-Induced Lymphomas." *Journal of Clinical Investigation*, 2007, *117*, 1019–1028.

Spira, T. J., and Jaffe, H. W. "Human Herpesvirus 8 and Kaposi's Sarcoma." In W. M. Scheld, W. A. Craig, and J. M. Hughes (eds.), *Emerging Infections* (Vol. 2). Washington, D.C.: ASM Press, 1998.

CHAPTER 18

HEPATITIS C

LEARNING OBJECTIVES

- Define hepatic and extrahepatic diseases resulting from infection with hepatitis C virus

- Describe the flavivirus responsible for causing these illnesses

- Discuss modes of infection

- Discuss the host's response to infection

- Describe symptomatology and diagnosis

- Discuss potential methods of treatment

- Discuss methods of prevention

Major Concepts

Diseases

Infection with hepatitis C virus (HCV) is very common throughout the world, involving 3% of humans, especially those from the western Pacific, Southeast Asia, and Africa. Chronic infection may result in hepatic or extrahepatic disease manifestations. The hepatic diseases are primarily cirrhosis of the liver and hepatocellular carcinoma. Liver damage may be intensified by alcohol consumption. Extrahepatic diseases include essential mixed cryoglobulinemia (a noncancerous lymphoproliferative disease of B cells), porphyria cutanea tarda (abnormal sensitivity to sun exposure and liver damage due to excessive iron deposition in the liver), Sjögren's syndrome (an autoimmune syndrome in which production of tears and saliva are decreased), lichen planus (an autoimmune disease with chronic dermal or intraorbital keratinization), rheumatoid arthritis (an autoimmune disease in which synovial tissues are damaged), several malignancies, and renal and myocardial impairments. Most persons infected by the virus, however, remain asymptomatic.

Infection

Hepatitis C virus is a flavivirus, a small, enveloped, single-stranded RNA virus that infects primarily liver cells but may also grow in lymphocytes and monocytes. Several genotypes exist that respond differently to treatment. HCV has a very high mutation rate due to the error-prone nature of its RNA polymerase. Rapid mutations allow the virus to escape killing by CD8$^+$ T killer cells.

Transmission and Populations at Risk

HCV infection usually involves intravenous (IV) drug use, blood transfusion, organ donation, or mother-to-child transmission. The virus survives for long periods of time outside of the body, even on surfaces in a dried condition. Some groups of people have higher rates of infection or develop more severe disease manifestations. These groups include persons of African descent, Hispanics, Asians, older persons, the obese, and alcoholics. Coinfection with HIV also increases disease severity. The reasons for these differential effects are complex and involve socioeconomic factors as well as genetic differences in enzymatic activity and susceptibility to other diseases.

Immune Response

CD8$^+$ T killer cells and NK cells are the most important components of the immune response to HCV. The virus's high mutation rate allows it to escape killing by T killer cells, which recognize very specific amino acid sequences on their targets. HCV down-regulates expression of stimulatory receptors on NK cells while increasing expression of inhibitory receptors on both NK cells and T killer cells, thus decreasing the cytotoxic activity of both immune cell types. Treg activity is increased in persons infected with HCV. These cells produce TGF-β that blocks activation of other T lymphocytes and inhibit production of the antiviral agent IFN-γ.

Protection

To prevent infection, IV drug use should be avoided, or the injecting supplies should be decontaminated. Health care workers should carefully follow the universal precautions guidelines and disinfect work surfaces and biohazard spills promptly. If infection were to occur, alcohol consumption should be halted. Patients require plenty of rest and may consider receiving a hepatitis A vaccine to decrease further liver damage. The most commonly used treatment regimen is combination therapy with IFN-α and the antiviral agent ribaviran. This regimen is associated with several side effects, some which are severe.

Introduction

The number of new infections with **hepatitis C virus** (**HCV**) in the United States has been decreasing. In the 1980s, 240,000 new infections occurred per year; by 2004, this number had fallen to 26,000. Most HCV infections result from illegal IV drug use. Of the 4.1 million Americans affected by HCV (1.6% of population), 3.2 million have chronic infection.

HCV is the second most common chronic viral infection in world, affecting approximately 3% of the world's population (180 million people). The areas of the world that are hardest hit are the western Pacific region, Southeast Asia, and Africa. In the United States, infection rates vary from 1% to 2%, while in parts of the developing world, prevalence may reach as high as 7%. This virus contributes to more than 100,000 deaths per year either directly or in connection with alcohol abuse or coinfection with HIV or hepatitis B virus. The number of HCV-related deaths is projected to triple between 2008 and 2020 in the United States. It is estimated that over half of the individuals infected with HCV are not aware of their condition and contribute to the spread of the disease.

In addition to HCV, several other types of hepatitis viruses have been found—A, B, D, and E. Type A is transmitted by being in close contact with infected persons or by contaminated food. This infection is often resolved within six months. Type B is most commonly spread via blood but also via semen or from mother to child. As with HCV, there is an increased risk of liver disease and hepatocellular carcinoma. Effective vaccines have been developed for both type A and type B hepatitis viruses. Hepatitis D virus is able to survive and reproduce only in cells that are coinfected with hepatitis B virus. Approximately 5% of individuals with type B virus also are infected with type D. Hepatitis E virus is most often contracted by consuming contaminated food or water. This virus does not cause chronic infection. Type E infection is rare in the United States and more common in South Asia and North Africa.

History

Initially, HCV was named **"non-A, non-B" hepatitis** and was seen in IV drug users and recipients of blood transfusions in the 1970s. The virus was described by two research groups in the *Lancet* in 1984. Five years later, the Chiron biotech corporation cloned HCV RNA. A test was developed to screen the blood supply in 1990, and an improved test was introduced in 1992, vastly increasing the safety of blood transfusion. The current test detects 95% to 99% of positive blood samples. It is not as widely available in the developing world, where the risk of iatrogenic infection is higher.

Several famous Americans have contracted HCV. This virus curtailed the career of country singer Naomi Judd, who was infected by a needle prick while she was a nurse. Actress Pamela Anderson was infected via a tattoo needle. Motorcycle daredevil Evel Knievel acquired hepatitis C, most likely through a blood transfusion following an accidental spill. He received a liver transplant to replace his damaged organ. Newsman Frank Reynolds and actor-singer Jim Nabors also contracted this disease. Baseball great Mickey Mantle is believed to have been a victim of the unfortunate combination of HCV infection and cirrhosis of the liver induced by excessive alcohol consumption.

The Diseases

For approximately 60% to 85% of persons infected with HCV, infection will become chronic. The long-term nature of this illness is due to the rapid rate at which the virus mutates, allowing continual evasion of antibodies directed against its components. Spontaneous resolution occurs in 0.5% to 0.7% of those with chronic disease; death from hepatic or extrahepatic damage occurs in 1% to 5%.

The majority of individuals infected with HCV (80%) are asymptomatic. For the remaining 20%, symptoms include jaundice, fatigue, dark urine, pain in the right abdominal quadrant, loss of appetite, nausea, vomiting, low-grade fever, pale or clay-colored stools, generalized itching, ascites (fluid in abdominal cavity), and dilated veins in the esophagus. The diseases associated with this viral infection may be broken down into hepatic diseases (involving the liver) and extrahepatic diseases (involving other areas of the body).

Hepatic Diseases

Chronic liver diseases affect 70% to 80% of symptomatic persons. Due to the large number of people affected and the severity of the hepatic damage, HCV infection is the leading cause of liver transplantation in the United States.

FIGURE 18.1   Primary causes of chronic liver disease

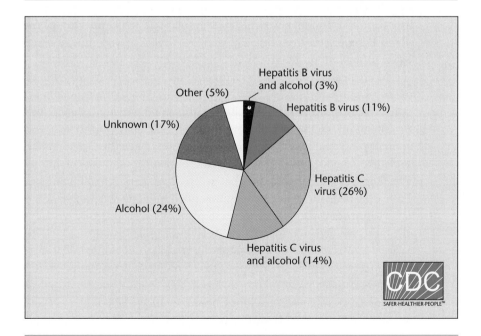

Note: Based on data for Jefferson County, Alabama.
Source: CDC/NCID.

FIGURE 18.2   Cirrhosis of the liver

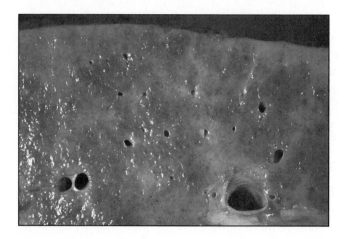

Source: CDC/Edwin P. Ewing Jr.

Following transplantation, however, HCV may infect the new liver and damage it as well. This has led some researchers to examine the possibility of using baboon livers instead of human livers for the transplants. Such **xenotransplants** (transplants using organs from other species) are almost always rapidly rejected, even when strong immunosuppressive drugs are administered.

Many people with hepatic manifestations (20% to 30%) develop **cirrhosis of the liver** (irreversible liver scarring) after 20 to 30 years. Alcohol consumption increases the risk of developing this condition and should be avoided. Symptoms of cirrhosis include jaundice, weakness, weight loss, nausea and vomiting, swelling of the legs, bleeding hemorrhoids, the development of small spiderlike blood vessels in the skin, and impotence and loss of interest in sex. The damage to the liver cannot be repaired, nor can its functioning be restored. Liver transplantation may be recommended in life-threatening cases.

Hepatocellular carcinoma, a form of liver cancer, occurs in 1% to 5% of chronically infected individuals. It is responsible for 80% to 90% of all liver cancers and is seen more commonly in men than in women. The disease typically affects persons in their fifties and is present in Africa and Asia to a greater extent than other areas of the world. If this form of cancer is detected early, small or slow-growing tumors may be successfully treated by aggressive surgery or liver transplantation. Early diagnosis is, however, unusual. Chemotherapy and radiation treatments are not usually curative but may shrink large tumors prior to surgery. Sorafenib toslate may inhibit tumor growth.

Extrahepatic Diseases

Areas other than the liver may also be adversely affected by HCV. Chronic HCV infection has been linked to insulin resistance and can lead to type 2 diabetes. The development of insulin resistance is associated with a rapid progression to fibrosis and cirrhosis, resulting in hepatocellular fibrosis or liver failure. Individuals with insulin resistance often respond poorly to antiviral therapy.

Some of the pathology of the extrahepatic diseases results from inappropriately stimulated immune responses and involves excessive growth of lymphocytes or excessive lymphocyte activation. **Essential mixed cryoglobulinemia (EMC)** is one such extrahepatic disease associated with HCV infection. This condition is a noncancerous lymphoproliferative disease characterized by abnormally high levels of B cell growth that may be associated with decreased apoptosis resulting from a rearrangement of the antiapoptotic protein bcl-2 and Ig JH due to a t(14;18) chromosomal translocation, which leads to the constitutive production of the former. These B cells produce unusual types of antibodies called cryoglobins due to their tendency to precipitate out of solution at temperatures below that of the human body (37°C or 98.6°F). They are of a mixed nature in that both polyclonal IgG, monoclonal IgM, or polyclonal IgM with rheumatoid factor activity antibodies are involved. EMC symptoms include weakness, arthralgia, kidney disease progressing to renal insufficiency, purpura, **Raynaud's phenomenon** (extremities become whitish-blue when exposed to cold), peripheral neuropathy, and lung and liver damage. These symptoms are secondary to systemic vasculitis due to vascular deposition of immune complexes. Cryoglobins may be detected in 70% of individuals with chronic HCV infection.

Another HCV-related condition is **porphyria cutanea tarda**, which results from excessive iron deposits in the liver. Excess iron decreases uroporphyrinogen decarboxylase activity and increases urinary excretion of several porphyrins. Symptoms of this disorder include abnormal sensitivity to sun exposure and liver damage.

Various types of renal impairments are associated with HCV. These include membranoproliferative glomerulonephritis, membranous nephropathy, mesangial proliferative glomerulonephritis, Henoch-Schönlein purpura nephritis, and tubulointerstitial nephritis. The underlying cause of these conditions may be the formation of immune complexes of IgM κ chains with rheumatoid factor activity. These impairments may occur in 2.7% (membranous nephropathy) to 17.6% (mesangial proliferative glomerulonephritis) of persons infected with HCV virus and indicate a poor prognosis.

Several types of cancers are associated with infection with HCV. One of these involves abnormal growth of infected lymphocytes, B cell non-Hodgkin's lymphoma, which may be found in sites such as the salivary glands and the liver. Splenic lymphoma, diffuse large B cell lymphoma, and monoclonal gammopathies of uncertain significance are other associated lymphoproliferative disorders. Other malignancies linked with HCV infection include oral and thyroid cancers and cervical squamous cell carcinoma.

Myocardial impairments may also result from HCV infection. The heart damage may result from an immune response to HCV, whose RNA has been detected in cardiac muscle tissue.

HCV infection has been linked to several autoimmune and inflammatory diseases. In one of these, **Sjögren's syndrome**, production of tears and saliva is decreased due to exocrine lymphocytic infiltration. This leads to dryness of the eyes and mouth and sometimes connective tissue damage. HCV RNA may be found in salivary glands. **Lichen planus**, characterized by chronic dermal or intraorbital keratinization, has been linked to HCV and virus-specific T cell responses. Early treatment is recommended, as lichen planus is a precancerous condition.

Development of type 2 diabetes, with its associated insulin resistance and insulin secretory deficiency, correlates with HCV infection. The cytokine TNF-α, found in conjunction with hepatic inflammation and fibrillation, increases glucose uptake by tissues and may induce insulin resistance by promoting gluconeogenesis. HCV infection is also associated with development of autoimmune

FIGURE 18.3   Lichen planus

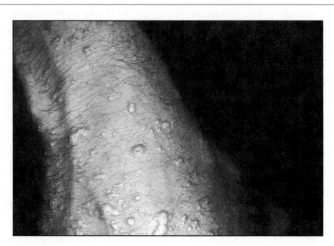

Source: CDC/Richard S. Hibbets.

thyroid disease (hypothyroidism, characterized by lower levels of free thyroxin and triiodothyronine, decreased metabolism, fatigue, and weight gain), idiopathic interstitial pneumonitis, and **rheumatoid arthritis** (autoimmune damage to synovial tissues lubricating the joints).

The Causative Agent

Hepatitis is an infection caused by several distinct groups of viruses. Hepatitis C virus (HCV) is a **flavivirus**. It is a small (50-nanometer), enveloped, single-stranded positive-sense RNA virus. This virus may be divided into six genotypes, more than 50 subtypes, and quasispecies, varying in representation in different areas of the world. Type 1a is most common in North America, type 1b in Europe, and types 4 and 5 are restricted to Africa. Correct typing of the viral population infecting an individual is important for treatment purposes because

FIGURE 18.4   Electron micrograph of hepatitis viruses

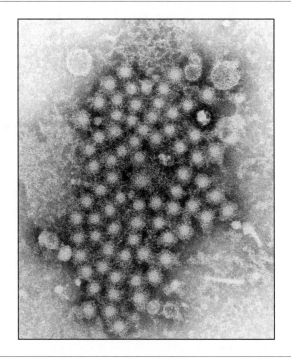

Source: CDC/E. H. Cook Jr.

genotypes 1 and 4 are not as responsive to IFN therapy as the other genotypes. The existence of quasispecies increases the difficulty of isolating a purified viral strain for study and reduces the effectiveness of the immune response. Furthermore, an individual is not protected against reinfection and hence may harbor several genotypes.

HCV replicates quickly; approximately 1 trillion viruses are produced per day. Similar to HIV, this virus has a very high mutation rate. This results in part from both viruses' use of RNA as their genomic material. Viral RNA polymerases do not proofread and correct mistakes produced during reproduction, as occurs in human cells. Thus any errors in the production of the viral genome remain and are passed on to viral progeny. Because the adaptive immune response is extremely specific, the change of a single amino acid may cause antibodies or T cell receptors to lose their ability to recognize and respond to the virus.

In humans, HCV inhabits and replicates primarily in liver cells but may also grow in lymphocytes and monocytes. It binds to CD81, scavenger receptor class B1, low-density lipoprotein receptor, glycosaminoglycans, and claudin-1 on human cell membranes and uses these host proteins to gain access to its target cells. The RNA genome has one open reading frame of 9.6 kilobases flanked by 5' and 3' untranslated regions. Once inside liver cells, a 3011 amino acid polyprotein is translated and cleaved by proteases into ten functional proteins. The structural proteins are C (nucleocapsid) and E1 and E2 (envelope glyco-proteins), and the nonstructural proteins are NS1, NS2 (transmembrane), NS3 (serine protease), NS4A (protease cofactor), NS4B, NS5A (IFN-resisting protein), and NS5B (RNA-dependent RNA polymerase). NS5B synthesizes a negative-strand RNA to act as a template for positive-strand viral genomic RNA. E1 and NS3 proteins down-regulate the immune system by inducing dendritic cells to decrease secretion of the Th1 cell activator IL-12 and increase that of the immunosuppressive IL-10.

HCV has a very narrow host range: the only good animal model is the chim-panzee. This primate is difficult to use in studies of viral pathogenesis because it reproduces slowly and is an endangered species. Among humans, variation in infection rate and disease severity is common; this variation appears to be due to combined biological and socioeconomic differences. Men and obese patients tend not to respond well to IFN therapy. Racial differences also exist. HCV affects older African Americans (over 40 years of age) at twice the level of white Americans, despite a lower lifetime incidence of IV drug use. This could be due to increased likelihood of developing chronic infection (95% versus 33% in whites). This group is less likely to have a sustained virological response follow-ing treatment and is less likely to receive a liver transplant; among individuals who do receive a transplant, graft survival is lower than in whites even after adjustment for socioeconomic status. This may reflect a higher incidence of diabetes mellitus among African Americans and the fact that African American transplant recipients often have more advanced disease. HCV prevalence rate among Hispanics is also high, and disease course more aggressive, with a higher rate of cirrhosis than in any other ethnic group. The variation in severity of liver damage may be partly due to inherent differences in liver enzyme levels, as African Americans and Hispanics normally have higher levels. Alcohol consumption widens the racial gaps in these enzyme levels. Rates of progression to hepatocellular carcinoma are higher in African Africans, Hispanics, and Asians. Societal factors also play a role, for the former two groups are less likely to be referred to specialists for treatment.

HCV may be acquired by humans through transfusion with infected blood or by organ transplantation. The risk of infection via the blood supply in the United States is quite low (less than 1 per 2 million units). Individuals undergoing long-term kidney dialysis are at higher risk, as are health care workers who have contact with blood samples. Approximately 2% of health workers who are stuck with a needle contaminated with HCV become infected. Children born to infected mothers have a 4% rate of infection, which increases to 19% if the mother is coinfected with HIV. Breast-feeding is not believed to be a risk factor unless the nipples are cracked or bleeding. Persons involved in IV drug use are at much greater risk of infection than the general population. HCV may rarely be transmitted sexually or through use of contaminated razors or toothbrushes. It is not transmitted by mosquitoes or other blood-sucking insects. Similarly, HCV is not spread via food or water, sharing drinking glasses or utensils with an infected individual, sneezing, hugging, or casual contact. Accordingly, there is no need to isolate infected persons from others at work, school, or in day care centers.

HCV is able to survive outside the body or cells for at least 16 hours and as long as four days, even in dried blood. This period of infectivity is much longer than that of HIV. People working with human blood must therefore take great care to thoroughly disinfect blood spills or any materials or surfaces that may have becoming contaminated.

The Immune Response

To establish a chronic state of infection, a microbe needs to evade the host's immune response. $CD8^+$ T killer cells play a vital role in containing viral infections, including HCV. These cells recognize and are stimulated by a small specific region of a viral protein. One manner in which viruses escape T killer cell activity is by altering the amino acid sequences of their proteins. HCV has a high mutation rate (1.5–2.0 mutations for each thousand viral replications for each RNA base in the genome per year: HCV RNA contains over 9,000 bases). A recent study demonstrated that mutations associated with escaping T killer cell activity were found at a greater frequency in the early, acute stage of infection and that the mutation rate in nonenvelope proteins decreased during the course of infection. Interestingly, many reversion-type mutations (mutations that restore the RNA to its original form) were also found to occur, perhaps to increase fitness of the viral population in the face of dysfunctional T cells.

RECENT DEVELOPMENTS

Effective vaccines are now widely available for protection against hepatitis A and B but not C. Production of a protective vaccine against HCV has the potential to greatly improve the health of large numbers of people throughout the world. Antibodies do not appear to be the most critical component of protective immunity against HCV; however, an early vaccine approach attempted to induce neutralizing antibodies using recombinant HCV envelope glycoproteins E1 and E2. This approach provided only short-term protection and did not protect against high-dose viral challenge or challenge with other viral genotypes. It did, however, reduce the risk of developing chronic infection. CD8$^+$ T killer cells are an important part of host immunity to viral infections. Vaccine attempts have incorporated HCV genes into plasmids or viral vectors, such as adenovirus or vaccinia virus, in order to stimulate these cells. One such vaccinia virus–based vaccine induced production of IFN-γ in chimpanzees and effectively stimulated resolution of infection following challenge with a combination of viral genotypes. In HCV infection, T killer cells work together with CD4$^+$ T helper cells to prevent the development of chronic disease. The absence of T helper cells tends to promote production of viral escape mutants. Vaccine strategies thus need to stimulate T killer and T helper cells in order to be protective. Strong responses from both of these cell types were induced by a vaccine regimen consisting of priming with nonstructural proteins 3, 4, and 5 given in combination with phospholipid-cholesterol particles containing purified saponins to stimulate Th1-like responses together with CpG oligonucleotides (double-stranded RNA intermediate) to stimulate innate immunity, such as IFN-α production, followed by boosting with chimeric, defective alphaviral particles (Sindbis and Venezuelan equine encephalitis viruses) encoding E1 and E2. This approach also stimulated production of neutralizing antibodies reactive with several genotypes.

NK cell functions are also reduced during HCV infection. Persons with chronic hepatitis C, but not those who had cleared the infection, had a lower percentage of NK cells expressing the stimulatory receptors NKp46 and NKp30. Expression of the natural cytotoxicity receptor (NCR) was reduced as well, paralleled by decreased NCR-mediated target cell killing. The numbers of NK cells and $CD8^+$ T killer cells expressing the inhibitory NKG2A receptor increased. These factors combine to decrease antiviral cytotoxic activity of NK cells and T killer cells.

Treg cells may also protect HCV from the immune response because they function to suppress responses of many immune system cells, including $CD4^+$ T helper cells, $CD8^+$ T killer cells, B cells, NK cells, and dendritic cells. Frequencies of Treg in the circulation are higher in people with chronic HCV infection than in those who resolved infection. Treg suppresses growth and production of the antiviral cytokine IFN-γ by HCV-specific T helper and T killer cells, possibly disabling the functioning of the immune cells best suited to eliminate the virus. The Treg product TGF-β is expressed by hepatocytes of all persons with chronic HCV infection. Removal of this cytokine returns IFN-γ levels to normal. Expression of the COX-2 enzyme, which produces leukotrienes and prostaglandins, is increased in persons with chronic infection and is especially high in those with cirrhosis or hepatocellular carcinoma. Prostaglandins are proinflammatory, and COX-2 plays a role in the early stages of carcinogenesis in the liver.

Diagnosis

There are two general means of diagnosing an infection with HCV. The first of these assays detects the immune response to the virus by testing for the presence of anti-HCV antibodies by EIA or CIA, with confirmation by recombinant immunoblot assay (RIBA). These antibodies are detectable in 70% of infected persons at the time when symptoms appear, but the results do not differentiate between acute, chronic, and past infections. Both false positive and false negative tests may occur. The second type of tests searches for the presence of the virus itself by detecting viral RNA by polymerase chain reaction (PCR). A person is deemed to be infected on the basis of one positive PCR test result. One negative test, however, does not rule out the possibility of infection, and the result needs to be confirmed by repeating the test. Viral RNA is detectable within one to two weeks following infection.

Diagnostic testing is recommended for all people who ever used illegal IV drugs, received clotting factors before 1987, or had a blood transfusion or organ transplant before 1992; long-term dialysis patients; anyone having signs of liver disease; health care workers following a needle stick or splash to the eye by infected blood; and children of HCV-positive women. If a person is found to be infected, often levels of alanine aminotransferase (ALT) liver enzyme are next determined. Elevated levels of this enzyme occur in 30% of the chronically infected and may indicate liver inflammation or even chronic liver disease. It is possible to have chronic disease without elevated ALT levels, so if the levels are normal, they need to be rechecked several times within 6 to 12 months. A positive test result for either hepatitis B or hepatitis C prohibits the individual from ever donating blood again.

Treatment

There is currently no cure for HCV infection; however, two medications are used therapeutically. Pegylated IFN-α-2a, a longer-lasting form of a cytokine produced by the immune system to block viral replication, may be used alone if a person cannot tolerate the other drug, ribavirin. Side effects of this monotherapy include flulike symptoms and tiredness, hair loss, low blood count, difficulty in thinking, and depression. More severe problems occur in fewer than 2% of people, including decreased production of white blood cells and platelets by the bone marrow, thyroid disease, suicidal ideation, seizures, cardiac or renal failure, hearing loss, infection of the blood, and the potential to severely worsen the liver disease. Dosages of this drug eventually need to be reduced in 40% of treated individuals due to these side effects, and 15% of patients must stop taking IFN completely. This treatment is not approved for use in pregnant women.

Combination therapy with IFN and ribavirin may be quite effective. In this regimen, IFN-α is used in conjunction with the antiviral compound ribavirin to

FIGURE 18.5   The chemical structure of ribavirin

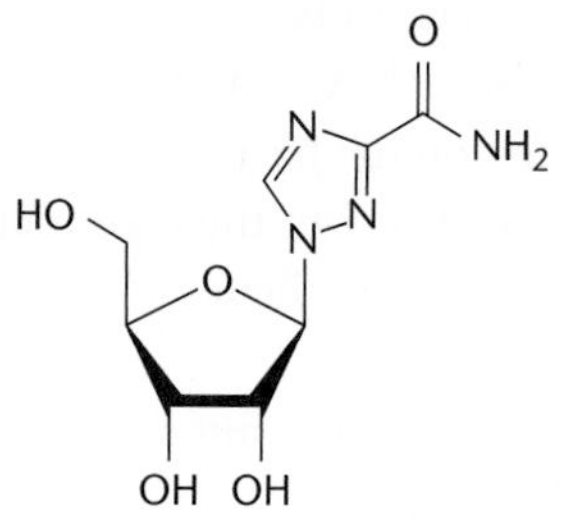

produce a sustained response in 40% to 80% of patients treated. Response rates of up to 50% may be seen in individuals infected with genotype 1, and rates may be as high as 80% in those with genotype 2 or 3. Side effects of combination therapy, in addition to those listed, are severe anemia and possible kidney failure. The side effects are generally more problematic if the person has heart or blood vessel disease. Ribavirin may also cause birth defects.

Some newer anti-HCV drugs inhibit the RNA polymerase, including nucleoside-based and non-nucleoside-based RNA replicase inhibitors (NRRIs and NNRRIs, respectively). The former category includes valopicitabine and 2'-methyl- or 4'-fluoro-substituted nucleosides, which interact with the enzyme's catalytic site. The latter group interacts with a number of sites and includes structurally different compounds, among them indole-*N*-acetamine, phenylanlanine, thiophene, and benzofuran derivatives. Other drugs target the serine protease (NS3/4A). These include ciluprevir, telaprevir, boceprevir, and SCH446211. Telaprevir may reduce viral RNA levels by as much as 10,000-fold in cell cultures, and the addition of IFN inhibited the emergence of resistance mutations. Ciluprevir-resistant mutants remained susceptible to telaprevir as well. Another drug target is cyclophilin B, a stimulatory regulator of the viral RNA polymerase. This stimulation is decreased by cyclosporine A and by its nonimmunosuppressant derivative, Debio-025.

Prevention

The best strategy to prevent or reduce the risk of infection is to avoid high-risk situations. This is particularly true for users of IV drugs. If unable to curtail this activity, care must be taken to use injecting supplies (including water and spoons) that are not contaminated. Health care workers are also at substantial risk and need to carefully follow the universal precaution guidelines when working with blood or patient samples. This includes the wearing of gloves, proper disposal of patient samples and contaminated materials, and proper handling of needles and other sharps, being sure to not recap needles. Surfaces should be cleaned thoroughly after use, and biohazard spills must be disinfected promptly, preferably with a 10% bleach solution. This is vital to the safety of anyone using the work area because HCV remains viable on surfaces for some time, even after the blood or tissue sample has dried.

For people who are infected, in order to prevent liver damage, it is very important to stop drinking alcohol and not to start using any new prescription medicines, herbal treatments, vitamins, or over-the-counter medication without first consulting a physician. Regular doctor appointments are important to

FIGURE 18.6   Disposing of blood-contaminated material

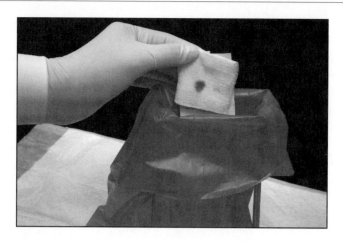

Source: CDC.

monitor disease progression. Patients should get plenty of rest and should consider receiving a hepatitis A vaccine so as to reduce the chances of additional liver damage.

Surveillance

In many parts of the world, the majority of cases of HCV infection are linked to IV drug use. Besides reuse of syringes or needles, other paraphernalia used in drug injection may be contaminated and should be considered during intervention. Surveillance in this demographic group may be challenging but is important in the identification of transmission practices that pose the greatest risk to aid in local and nationwide prevention programs. There now exists a valid testing instrument with standardized content and construct to measure risk practices associated with injection, sexual contact, and skin penetration. The *Blood Borne Virus Transmission Risk Assessment Questionnaire* has been translated into eight languages by the World Health Organization and examines hepatitis B virus, HCV, and HIV risk factors.

HCV infection has been a nationally notifiable disease in the United States since 2003. The Centers for Disease Control and Prevention is sponsoring enhanced surveillance in eight areas, including New York State. This program is particularly concerned with identifying recent infections by prioritizing follow-up studies with infected individuals under the age of 30 years. For example, as part of this program, a group of infected individuals was identified who were IV drug users and attended the same high school. This method may allow agencies to detect outbreaks and clusters, allowing preventive measures to be instituted.

Summary

Diseases
- Cirrhosis of the liver • Hepatocellular carcinoma • Essential mixed cryoglobulinemia • Porphyria cutanea tarda • Renal impairment • Lymphoproliferative disorders • Cardiomyopathy • Autoimmune and inflammatory diseases

Causative Agent
- Hepatitis C virus

Agent Type
- Flavivirus

Genome
- Single-stranded positive-sense RNA virus

Vector
- None

Common Reservoir
- None

Modes of Transmission
- IV drug use, blood transfusion, organ transplantation, mother-to-child
- Rarely, transmitted sexually or via contaminated razors or toothbrushes

Geographical Distribution
- Worldwide

Year of Emergence
- 1970s

Key Terms

Cirrhosis of the liver Scarring of the liver

Essential mixed cryoglobulinemia (EMC) Noncancerous lymphoproliferative disease characterized by abnormally high levels of B cells; associated with infection with hepatitis C virus

Flavivirus Small, enveloped, single-stranded positive-sense RNA virus group to which the hepatitis C virus belongs

Hepatitis C virus (HCV) Flavivirus responsible for hepatitis C disease

Hepatocellular carcinoma Form of liver cancer associated with infection with hepatitis C virus

Lichen planus Autoimmune disease characterized by chronic dermal or intraorbital keratinization

"Non-A, non-B" hepatitis Former name of hepatitis C

Porphyria cutanea tarda Abnormal sensitivity to sun exposure and liver damage due to excessive iron deposition in the liver

Raynaud's phenomenon Extremities become whitish-blue when exposed to cold

Rheumatoid arthritis Autoimmune condition leading to damage to the synovial tissues that lubricate joints

Sjögren's syndrome Autoimmune syndrome characterized by decreased production of tears and saliva

Xenotransplants Transplants using organs from other species

Review Questions

1. What are the names and routes of transmission of the agents responsible for viral hepatitis?
2. What types of liver damage are induced by HCV? Describe several of the extrahepatic conditions associated with chronic HCV infection.
3. What cells are infected by HCV? What receptors does it use to bind to these cells?
4. What preventive measures might be used to reduce the risk of infection by HCV?
5. What are the most common methods being currently used to treat HCV infection, and how does viral genotype affect treatment?

Topics for Further Discussion

1. What are the similarities between the life cycles of HCV and HIV? What impact might these similarities have in the associated diseases and in potential therapeutic agents?
2. HCV is one of a number of diseases found at high frequency in individuals who use IV drugs. How might public health agencies effectively reduce the incidence of these types of infections without encouraging illegal drug use?
3. Severity of HCV-associated illness differs among genders and racial groups. Some of the underlying reasons for these differences are biological, and others are socioeconomic. How might the scientific and medical community and health agencies address these differences?
4. Currently, no vaccine is available to prevent infection by HCV. Explore the effects of HCV on the medical community in terms of numbers of infected health care workers as well as numbers of fatal infections in developed and developing nations. Discuss the potential effects of a protective vaccine.

Resources

Berzofsky, J. A., and others. "Progress on New Vaccine Strategies Against Chronic Viral Infections." *Journal of Clinical Investigation*, 2004, *114*, 450–462.

Centers for Disease Control and Prevention. "Use of Enhanced Surveillance for Hepatitis C Virus Infection to Detect a Cluster Among Young Injection-Drug Users, New York, November 2004–April 2007." *MMWR Morbidity and Mortality Weekly Report*, 2008, *57*, 517–521.

Craxì, A., Laffi. G., and Zignego, A. L. "Hepatitis C Virus (HCV) Infection: A Systemic Disease." *Molecular Aspects of Medicine*, 2008, *29*, 85–95.

De Clercq, E. "The Design of Drugs for HIV and HCV." *Nature Reviews: Drug Discovery*, 2008, *6*, 1001–1018.

Douglas, M. W., and George, J. "Molecular Mechanisms of Insulin Resistance in Chronic Hepatitis C." *World Journal of Gastroenterology*, 2009, *15*, 4356–4364.

El-Bassiouny, A. E. I., and others. "Expression of Cyclooxygenase-2 and Transforming Growth Factor-Beta1 in HCV-Induced Chronic Liver Disease and Hepatocellular Carcinoma." *Medscape General Medicine*, 2007, *9*, 45.

Kuntzen, T., and others. "Viral Sequence Evolution in Acute Hepatitis C Virus Infection." *Journal of Virology*, 2007, *81*, 11658–11668.

Lin, Y., and others. "Induction of Broad CD4$^+$ and CD8$^+$ T-Cell Responses and Cross-Neutralizing Antibodies Against Hepatitis C Virus by Vaccination with Th1-Adjuvanted Polypeptides Followed by Defective Alphaviral Particles Expressing Envelope Glycoproteins gpE1 and gpE2 and Nonstructural Proteins 3, 4, and 5." *Journal of Virology*, 2008, *82*, 7492–7503.

Manigold, T., and Racanelli, V. "T-Cell Regulation by CD4 Regulatory T Cells During Hepatitis B and C Virus Infections: Facts and Controversies." *Lancet Infectious Diseases,* 2007, *7,* 804–813.

Nattermann, J., and others. "Surface Expression and Cytolytic Function of Natural Killer Cell Receptors Is Altered in Chronic Hepatitis C." *Gut,* 2006, *55,* 869–877.

Okuse, C., Yotsuyanagi, H., and Koike, K. "Hepatitis C as a Systemic Disease: Virus and Host Immunologic Responses Underlie Hepatic and Extrahepatic Manifestations." *Journal of Gastroenterology,* 2007, *42,* 857–865.

Rodriguez-Torres, M. "Latinos and Chronic Hepatitis C: A Singular Population." *Clinical Gastroenterology and Hepatology,* 2008, *6,* 484–490.

CHAPTER 19

EPIDEMIC AND PANDEMIC INFLUENZA

LEARNING OBJECTIVES

- Define and contrast the various influenza pandemics that have occurred

- Describe the orthomyxovirus responsible for causing the flu

- Discuss modes of infection

- Discuss the host's response to infection

- Describe symptomatology and diagnosis

- Discuss potential methods of treatment

- Discuss methods of prevention

Major Concepts

Outbreaks

Influenza infections typically occur as sporadic cases, local outbreaks, and seasonal epidemics resulting from antigenic drift. Pandemics arise by antigenic shift and are rare but typically much more pathogenic. Four human influenza pandemics have occurred since 1900. Several regions of the world have recently experienced sporadic outbreaks of H5N1 avian influenza in humans. H5N1 infection is associated with a high mortality rate, especially in Southeast Asia. Almost all of the human infections resulted from contact with ill or dead birds or contaminated material from them. Due to differences between the cellular binding sites of human and avian influenza viruses, avian influenza viruses are very rarely able to be transmitted between humans. Beginning in 2009, a new strain of H1N1 virus spread rapidly throughout the world. This virus contained genetic information from influenza viruses of swine, birds, and humans and generated great concern that it would result in death rates similar to those experienced in the devastating 1918 pandemic. Fortunately, this did not occur, and the 2009–2010 H1N1 pandemic resulted in a fatality rate slightly lower than that of a typical year. The massive mobilization of health care resources and enormous associated expenses may nevertheless serve to alert the medical profession and the public to the necessary actions that must be taken when a true public health emergency does occur.

Symptoms

Influenza is usually self-limiting, with rapid and complete recovery from uncomplicated infections. Serious or fatal complications may occur in some populations, including secondary bacterial pneumonia, Reye syndrome, encephalitis, and myocarditis. Persons at high risk include the elderly, individuals with chronic health problems, and the immunosuppressed.

Prevention

Vaccinations are recommended for at-risk populations as well as young children, health care workers, residents of long-term care facilities, and pregnant women. Rapid mutation by influenza viruses allows them to escape immune responses against strains to which an individual was previously exposed via infection or vaccination. Annual immunization is therefore recommended to defend against newly arising viral variants. Other means of preventing infection include personal hygienic practices.

Infection

Influenza is caused by single-stranded RNA viruses of the *Orthomyxoviridae* family. They are divided into three general types: A, B, and C. A and B types are responsible for human epidemics and cause more severe disease symptoms than type C. Type A viruses also infect animals other than humans, including pigs and birds, and are solely responsible for pandemics. They are divided into subgroups based on differential expression of the hemagglutinin and neuraminidase surface glycoproteins.

Protection

Treatment for influenza often entails bed rest, aspirin, and supportive care. Several types of antiviral compounds may also be used. Adamantanes may have neurological side effects, and the avian H5N1 strains have developed resistance to them. Most H5N1 isolates retain susceptibility to neuraminidase inhibitors, and these drugs are becoming more widely available.

Introduction

Influenza viruses infect the respiratory tract, causing the familiar symptoms of fever, cough, sore throat, muscle aches, and general malaise. While most individuals usually recover in a week or two, some 20,000 to 40,000 deaths occurred in each of 11 recent epidemics in the United States alone, making this illness a very important public health care concern. Infection rates are highest among school-aged children; however, the elderly and individuals with chronic health problems (including cardiac, pulmonary, renal, and metabolic diseases, and anemia) and immunosuppressed individuals are particularly susceptible to severe disease manifestations and death. The most dangerous forms of influenza outbreaks are the periodic **influenza pandemics**. In the not-so-distant past, these have occurred in 1889, 1918, 1957, and 1968. Since then, the H3N2 type (the same general type prevalent in 1968) has killed 400,000 Americans, 80% to 90% of whom were over the age of 65 years. H1N1 type (the general type prevalent in 1918) reappeared in 1976 and again in 2009, both times promoting fears of massive loss of life that, fortunately, did not materialize.

History

Sporadic cases of influenza, localized outbreaks, and epidemics occur frequently, and individuals with chronic illnesses or compromised immune systems are at greatest risk. Epidemics are most frequent in the winter months in temperate climates and in the rainy season in tropical regions. Pandemics recur infrequently, are more pathogenic, and often strike wider segments of the population. These require major antigenic changes in viral surface glycoproteins, the ability to sustain high levels of human-to-human transmission, and pathogenicity in humans. People residing in closed environments, such as nursing homes, mental health facilities, and boarding schools, generally have higher rates of infection. Ten pandemics are believed to have occurred in the past 300 years. Several of the most recent are discussed here.

1918 "Spanish Flu" Pandemic (Type H1N1)

The **"Spanish flu" pandemic of 1918** caused the largest numbers of recorded deaths from an infectious disease in this short of a period of time. It is believed to have begun as a viral infection of pigs in the American Midwest.

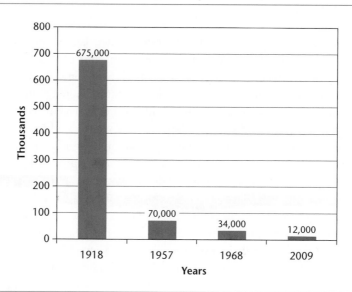

FIGURE 19.1   Annual mortality rate during recent influenza pandemics

A mild form of this disease then occurred in humans in March 1918. The virus responsible is believed to have arisen as a result of a reassortment of genomic RNA from human and pig influenza viruses. This form of influenza struck troops gathered in an American army base in Kansas prior to transport to France for service in World War I. Due to the speed of transportation at the time and to the state of enhanced travel due to the worldwide military conflict, the infection was able to circle the globe within four months. By August of that year, major outbreaks were reported in France, Sierra Leone, and Boston.

The loss of life was massive and was most pronounced among young adults. Half of the soldiers who died during World War I died of influenza. In one Alaskan village, 85% of the population died within one week. Some South Pacific islands suffered mortality rates of 20%. More than 675,000 deaths occurred in the United States and 20 to 50 million more throughout the world.

1957 "Asian Flu" Pandemic (Type H2N2)

This pandemic originated in central China in 1956 or 1957, migrated to Hong Kong, and then spread to other areas of the world. It entered the United States in June 1957 with the arrival of naval personnel at Newport, Rhode Island, or San Diego, California. The first recognized outbreak in the country was during a conference of high school girls in Davis, California. From there, the flu was transported to another large conference of students from 43 states in Grinnell, Iowa. Attendees soon spread the epidemic throughout the country. An estimated 70,000 deaths occurred in the United States.

1968 "Hong Kong Flu" Pandemic (Type H3N2)

This pandemic originated in Hong Kong in early 1968 and reached the United States later that year. It was responsible for 34,000 deaths in the nation. Variants of the H3N2 subtype remain in circulation.

1976 "Swine Flu" (Type H1N1)

In 1974, a swine influenza virus was found in autopsied lung tissue of a young farmer after treatment for Hodgkin's lymphoma. In February 1976, five cases of human infection with a swine influenza virus were found among army recruits at Fort Dix, New Jersey. It was apparently transmitted between humans, for about 500 other people in that part of the state were also infected. This particular influenza strain caused a great deal of concern because of its host species of origin and because it was of the H1N1 type responsible for the massive destruction

FIGURE 19.2   Boxes of "swine flu" vaccine, stored in connection with the National Influenza Immunization Program

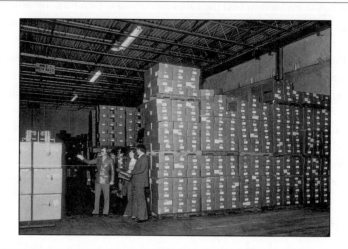

Source: CDC.

in 1918. A national movement was initiated in the United States to immunize all Americans against this variant via the National Influenza Immunization Program. This program began in October 1976, and 40 million people were vaccinated before the program was halted in mid-December. The vaccine had proved to be dangerous, and by January 1977, more than 500 cases of **Guillain-Barré syndrome** had been reported, resulting in 25 vaccine-related deaths. This syndrome is a neurological disorder, potentially resulting from an immunopathological response to the vaccine. Its primary symptom is weakness, with potential for the involvement of respiratory muscles. Most affected individuals recover within three months. Fortunately, the feared pandemic did not occur, confirmed cases during this outbreak being confined to New Jersey.

The Disease

Influenza is typically characterized by fever of 102°F to 104°F and chills, sore throat, dryness of the nasopharyngeal area, cough that aggravates substernal pain, headache, retro-orbital pain, severe myalgia (muscle aches) that may particularly affect the back and limbs, fatigue, prostration, and general malaise. Gastrointestinal involvement, including nausea, vomiting, and diarrhea, is present in up to 25% of infections of schoolchildren. Due to rapid antigenic changes in the virus (to be discussed shortly), individuals may be infected by slightly different influenza variants every year and hence develop disease repeatedly. In uncomplicated cases, infection is usually self-limiting and resolves completely within one week. In susceptible persons, serious complications may occur, including infection with bacteria, especially *Staphylococcus aureus*, *Haemophilus influenzae*, *Streptococcus pneumoniae*, or *Streptococcus pyogenes*, resulting in pneumonia. Encephalitis, with confusion, delirium, and coma, may occur, as well as myocarditis.

Much of the danger arising during influenza epidemics results from their rapidity, the prevalence of morbidity, and the severity of complications. **Reye syndrome**, a serious complication affecting the central nervous system and liver, may occur in children receiving aspirin or other salicylates. It is more common in those infected with type B influenza. During pandemics of type A influenza, the viral strains may be considerably more pathogenic. In 1918, infected persons' lungs filled with blood and body fluids, potentially drowning the person within two to three days. Dark areas frequently occurred on the skin as well.

The Causative Agent

Viral Types

Influenza results from infection with influenza virus of the *Orthomyxoviridae* family, first isolated in 1933. The virus particles are spherical to ovoid, 80 to 120 nanometers in diameter, surrounded by a lipid bilayer outer membrane obtained from the host cell. Inside of the envelope, the inner matrix surrounds the nucleocapsid containing single-stranded, negative-sense genomic RNA and several proteins, including the RNA polymerase needed for replication. The genome consists of eight single-stranded RNAs encoding ten proteins.

Viruses may be divided into three major categories—A, B, and C—based on antigenic differences in viral nucleoproteins and matrix proteins. Types A and B cause winter epidemics; C viruses cause only mild illness. Type A influenza viruses cause disease in humans, pigs, birds, horses, mink, seals, and whales. They have been responsible for all of the recorded pandemics. Bird reservoirs are present for all known A subtypes. Type B viruses affect only humans. They cause some of the regional epidemics but not pandemics.

Type A viral subtypes are differentiated on the basis of two surface molecules, **hemagglutinin** (H) and **neuraminidase** (N). As stated earlier, the Spanish flu, the Swine flu, and the 2009–2010 flu strains were of the H1N1 type. Several types of hemagglutinin have been reported in humans—H0, H1,

FIGURE 19.3   H3N2 "Hong Kong flu" virus showing spikes of hemagglutinin and neuraminidase on the surface

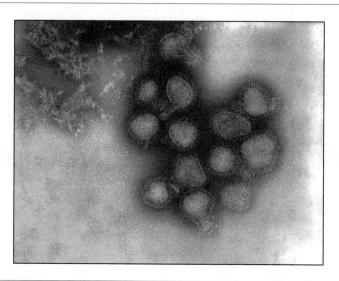

Source: CDC/Fred Murphy.

H2, H3, H5, and H7; H5 and H7 are less common and were derived from avian viruses. Two types of neuraminidase commonly occur in humans—N1 and N2; infection with N7 is rare. Influenza variants are named according to their site of isolation, culture number, year of isolation, and, for A strains, the H and N type. Several such variants include A/Singapore/1/57 (H2N2), A/Hong Kong/1/68 (H3N2), A/New Jersey/8/76 (H1N1), and B/Yamanashi/166/98.

Life Cycle

Influenza viruses typically enter a host by inhalation, but infection may also occur by direct contact with infectious material, which may persist in this state for 48 hours, especially under conditions of low humidity or cold. The viruses primarily infect tracheobronchial epithelial cells of the upper respiratory tract and major airways but may also infect the lower respiratory tract. This process involves several glycoproteins on the viral surface. Trimers of the viral hemagglutinin bind to a sugar, sialic (*N*-acetylneuraminic) acid, found on glycoproteins and glycolipids of the target cell's surface, allowing viral entry into the cell. The virus subsequently travels to the nucleus, where it produces new viral genomic RNA, mRNA, and proteins. The viral progeny then buds outward from the cell membrane, in the process becoming coated with sialic acid, which is cleaved and removed by neuraminidase. The new viral particles bind to and infect new host cells to continue their life cycle.

Antigenic Variation

Influenza viruses mutate rapidly, being second only to HIV in the pace of this activity. This allows them to change frequently the surface antigens that are the targets of the immune system. Due to the alterations of genetic material resulting from this process of **antigenic variation**, a person may be infected annually because the adaptive immune response is extremely specific and is sensitive to very small changes in the antigens expressed by microbes. These rapid genetic changes are accomplished through two mechanisms: antigenic drift and antigenic shift. **Antigenic drift** is a gradual, spontaneous production of point mutations (changes in a single RNA base) over time. It is very common and produces small (less than 1%) changes in amino acid sequence of the resulting proteins. Persons generally retain some diminished level of immunity to the new viral variants.

Antigenic shift is rare and results in large and rapid changes in either hemagglutinin or neuraminidase. Shift may result from interspecies transmission and **genetic reassortment** of the eight RNA strands of influenza viruses of different species, frequently viruses originating from birds, pigs, and humans. If a pig is infected with an influenza virus of pig and bird origin, both species of virus may infect a single cell and exchange parts of their RNA. This occurs only for type A influenza viruses since type B viruses do not infect animals other than humans. Subsequent human infection with the hybrid virus may lead to a pandemic.

Because the virus resulting from genetic reassortment is composed of proteins from viruses of several species, it is very different from previously encountered influenza strains, and most people have no immunity to it. Due to the lack of immunity, the infections may be unusually severe, resulting in a higher than normal mortality rate. These shifts often occur rapidly and originate most often in regions in which fowl (domestic chickens and geese) are in close contact with pigs and humans. In some parts of Asia and Africa, all three species may be housed in a single building. For this reason, pandemic strains often originate in the Far East. The 1957 and 1968 pandemics resulted from genetic reassortment between low-pathogenicity avian and human influenza viruses.

Another means of producing antigenic shift is the entry of an influenza virus from another animal species directly infecting humans. This occurred in 1918 and again in 1997 and 2003–2006, leading to the human cases of avian influenza ("bird flu").

Avian Influenza and Human Disease

The H5N1 **avian influenza** was first detected in terns in South Africa in 1961 and later became widespread in other species of domestic or wild birds, such as ducks and other waterfowl, which served only as carriers, and chickens and pigeons in which it caused a fatal illness. In May 1997, H5N1 influenza A was reported in a small number of humans. No cases were detected from May to November, when 18 cases occurred in Hong Kong. The patients ranged in age from 1 to 60 years, with half of the individuals under the age of 12. The mortality rate was unusually high—6 of the 18 died, and mortality was higher in adults (57%) than in children (18%). The age spread of the persons with fatal disease was also unusual—3, 13, 25, 34, 54, and 60 years old, rather than the elderly, who are generally most susceptible to severe influenza. The symptoms included persistent fever above 39°C (102.2°F), malaise, myalgia, sore throat, and cough, sometimes evolving into viral pneumonia, respiratory distress syndrome, and multiorgan failure. This strain was sensitive to the antiviral compounds amantadine and rimantadine, but such treatment was often associated with serious neurological side effects.

Humans were primarily infected by contact with contaminated chickens or their feces, and human-to-human transmission was very inefficient. People did not become infected by contact with raw or frozen meat. Due to the strong association of human disease with infected birds, a massive program to eliminate infected or potentially infected birds was undertaken in Hong Kong. On three days in December 1997, a total of 1.6 million chickens, ducks, and geese were killed in that territory; 19% of the chickens had influenza prior to the slaughter. This effort halted the epidemic.

Another wave of avian influenza struck humans beginning in 2003. The influenza-related deaths of domestic poultry throughout the East Asia spread to the human communities in Cambodia, China, Hong Kong, Japan, Laos, South Korea, Thailand, and Vietnam. A total of 143 cases of human H5N1 influenza occurred during the next three years, with 76 deaths (53% fatality rate). As in the previous outbreak, the disease initially presented as typical influenza, and patients often later developed pneumonia or respiratory failure requiring intubation. Some infections resulted in cardiac or renal impairment. This epidemic was not associated with secondary bacterial infections or gastrointestinal involvement.

The 2003 strain differed genetically and antigenically from that found in 1997. The viral species responsible for the human infections appeared to be solely of avian origin, since all of the genes were from influenza viruses of birds and not a result of genetic reassortment associated with pandemics. Few, if any, human cases appear to have resulted from human-to-human contact. Avian H5N1 viruses preferentially attach to type II pneumocytes, alveolar macrophages, and ciliated cuboidal epithelial cells with -2,6-linked sialic acids found in the terminal bronchioles of the human lower respiratory tract. Human H3N2 viruses, in contrast, prefer nonciliated cells whose sialic acid residues use -2,3 linkages. The highly pathogenic H5N1 viruses do not attach to cells of the human upper respiratory tract, which may limit their direct spread between humans. The poor transmissibility among humans has been a critical factor in preventing the development of an H5N1pandemic in humans. Should this viral strain acquire that ability, widespread human infection and death could occur. The virus has shown no tendency to gain such a characteristic during the years since its first infection of humans.

During the 2003 influenza outbreak, many of the cases of influenza in birds resulted from infections of migratory birds spreading to domestic species, such as chickens, ducks, and geese. These animals play vital roles in the lives of many families living in developing countries, both economically and as a much needed source of protein in the form of meat and eggs. One of the preferred means of preventing human disease is to kill domestic fowl en masse. This is very effective at halting epidemic disease spread, but it is a great hardship in terms of the loss of so many animals. The new avian influenza strain is susceptible to killing by oseltamir but resistant to amantadine and rimantadine.

In 2006, human infections with H5N1 influenza were first detected outside of Southeast Asia. In Turkey, four deaths were reported in children, several of whom had used the head of a deceased ill chicken as a soccer ball. A total of 12 cases were eventually found in that country. Outside of Southeast Asia, 32 other cases and 17 deaths (53% mortality rate) occurred in 2006 in Azerbaijan, Djibouti, Egypt, and Iraq. Within Southeast Asia in 2006, 73 cases and 58 deaths (79%) occurred. From 2007 until January 24, 2008, 27 cases and 11 deaths (41%) were found in Egypt, Nigeria, and Pakistan and 63 cases and 53 deaths (84%) in Southeast Asia. From 2003 to 2008, the majority of infections and deaths have occurred in Southeast Asia, in the countries of Cambodia, China, Indonesia, Laos, Myanmar, Thailand, and Vietnam. Overall mortality rates are highest in this region as well. In the avian influenza epidemic, a total of 387 confirmed human cases and 245 deaths (63%) occurred throughout the world, restricted to portions of Eurasia, the Middle East, and Africa, as of September 2008. The two countries most affected were Indonesia (137 cases, 112 deaths) and Vietnam (106 cases, 53 deaths). Members of the feline family, including zoo animals and domestic cats, have also died of avian influenza. Some of these animals were infected by consuming infected poultry, but intraspecies transmission has occurred among tigers. Infections in pigs are asymptomatic.

Table 19.1 Incidence and mortality: Human cases of avian influenza, 2003–January 2008

Country	Number of Deaths/Number of Cases (%)						
	2003	2004	2005	2006	2007	September 2008	TOTAL
Southeast Asia							
Cambodia	—	—	4/4 (100)	2/2 (100)	1/1 (100)	—	7/7 (100)
China	1/1 (100)	—	5/8 (63)	8/13 (62)	3/5 (60)	3/3 (100)	20/30 (67)
Indonesia	—	—	13/20 (65)	45/55 (82)	37/42 (88)	17/20 (70)	112/137 (82)
Laos	—	—	—	—	2/2 (100)	—	2/2 (100)
Myanmar	—	—	—	—	0/1 (0)	—	0/1 (0)
Thailand	—	12/17 (71)	2/5 (40)	3/3 (100)	—	—	17/25 (68)
Vietnam	3/3 (100)	20/29 (69)	19/61 (31)	—	5/8 (63)	5/5 (100)	52/106 (50)
Subtotal	4/4 (100)	32/46 (70)	43/98 (44)	58/73 (79)	48/59 (81)	25/28 (89)	210/308 (68)
Other Countries							
Azerbaijan	—	—	—	5/8 (63)	—	—	5/8 (63)
Bangladesh	—	—	—	—	—	0/1 (0)	0/1 (0)
Djibouti	—	—	—	0/1 (0)	—	—	0/1 (0)
Egypt	—	—	—	10/18 (56)	9/25 (36)	3/7 (43)	22/50 (44)
Iraq	—	—	—	2/3 (67)	—	—	2/3 (67)
Nigeria	—	—	—	—	1/1 (100)	—	1/1 (100)
Pakistan	—	—	—	—	1/3 (100)	—	1/3 (33)
Turkey	—	—	—	4/12 (33)	—	—	4/12 (33)
Subtotal	—	—	—	21/42 (50)	11/29 (38)	3/8 (38)	35/79 (44)
Total	4/4 (100)	32/46 (70)	43/98 (44)	79/115 (69)	59/86 (69)	28/36 (78)	245/387 (63)

Source: Data from the CDC.

Other highly pathogenic strains of avian influenza have infected humans and some have resulted in illness. In the Netherlands in 2003, H7N7 viruses infected poultry, which shed viruses in their saliva, nasal secretions, and feces. Pigs and later humans became infected. Eighty-nine people became ill, 79 with conjunctivitis and 6 with flulike illnesses; a veterinarian died. Three of the cases of human infections may have resulted from poultry workers transmitting disease to family members. In 2004, two individuals in Canada developed a mild illness associated with infection by an avian H7N3 variant after having close contact with infected birds. In January 2008, 77 human infections with H5N2 avian influenza occurred among poultry workers in Japan. None of those infected developed any symptoms of disease.

The Immune Response

Following infection with influenza viruses, the host rapidly mounts a humoral immune response, producing antibodies recognizing viral hemagglutinin, particularly the areas surrounding the sialic acid–binding cleft. These antibodies provide protection by blocking viral binding to its target cells and subsequent cell entry. Antibody titers peak within several days of infection and decline over the following six months. Antibodies are not essential for protection, because individuals lacking them still recover from infection. Their major role may be in preventing reinfection with the same viral strain. Cell-mediated immunity may also be protective due to the action of $CD8^+$ cytotoxic T cells.

The adoptive immune response is highly specific, meaning that the emergence of new viral variants by antigenic drift may greatly reduce immune recognition, depending on the extent of change involved. Both children and individuals previously infected with other viral subtypes are affected to a differing degree. Antigenic shift occurring during pandemics produces novel viral antigens that are not responsive to people's preexisting immunity. These strains are accordingly highly pathogenic and strike wide segments of the population. The immune system may contribute to pathology during human infection with the avian H5N1 influenza virus by inducing higher levels of proinflammatory cytokines and chemokines than are normally produced in response to human H1N1 viruses.

Diagnosis

Confirmation of influenza infection may entail isolation of the virus from nasal or pharyngeal secretions or washings by intra-amniotic inoculation of chick embryos or in primary cultures of mammalian cells, including those from monkey kidneys. Immunological assays, such as immunofluorescent analysis (IFA) or ELISA, may identify viral antigens in exfoliated nasopharyngeal epithelial cells or fluids or detect at least a fourfold increase in titer of specific antibodies in paired or convalescent serum samples. Polymerase chain reaction (PCR) may be used to amplify viral RNA. The microneutralization assay uses live viruses and should be confirmed by Western blotting. All tests that involve live H5N1 virus need to be performed in enhanced BioSafety Level 3 conditions.

Treatment

In uncomplicated cases of influenza, treatment is often restricted to supportive care and alleviation of symptoms. Bed rest is important and usually desired by the affected individual. Pain relievers, such as aspirin, are useful in fever reduction and to decrease the discomfort caused by headache and muscle aches. Codeine may be used to combat dry cough and substernal pain. For those with severe respiratory complications, oxygen therapy and artificial ventilation may be used.

Because influenza is a viral disease, it is not directly treatable by antibiotics, although these may be prescribed to prevent complications from secondary bacterial infections. Recently, a number of effective antiviral compounds have been developed. Several of these that are used in the treatment of type A influenza include adamantanes (amantadine and rimantadine) and neuraminidase inhibitors (oseltamir and zanamivir). Amantadine use may lead to side effects of central nervous system in 5% to 10% of recipients that can be particularly severe for the elderly and individuals with kidney disorders. Rimantadine poses less risk to the nervous system. Neuraminidase inhibitors are safe and partially effective for influenza prevention and treatment. These are becoming more widely available and are commended for treatment of H5N1 infections.

Prevention

Vaccines are available to either prevent infection or reduce disease severity to defined strains of influenza by inducing strain-specific antibody production. These are typically grown in eggs or bird cell cultures.

The typical vaccine contains two or three killed viral strains predicted to be most problematic in the coming flu season. These vaccines are administered by subcutaneous or intramuscular injection. Protective immunity is achieved in 65% to 70% of vaccinated individuals and persists for three to six months. Due

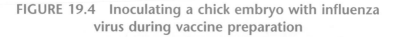

FIGURE 19.4   Inoculating a chick embryo with influenza
virus during vaccine preparation

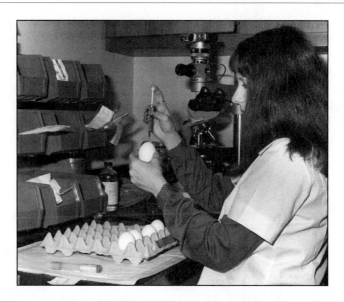

Source: CDC.

to the ability of influenza strains to rapidly vary their antigens and to the highly specific mechanisms used by the immune system to recognize pathogens, vaccines are altered yearly and persons need to be immunized annually. Successful vaccines are produced against defined viral strains; unknown viral variants are not good vaccine candidates, as researchers would not be able to predict the structure of unknown antigens for inclusion in a vaccine. For this reason, it would be extremely difficult to produce a useful vaccine against a future pandemic influenza strain or against mutants of existing strains before their emergence. This includes potential future strains of avian or pandemic influenza viruses, which may at some point mutate to become readily transmissible among humans or cause significant morbidity or mortality. While vast amounts of money have been poured into vaccine development, efforts to produce antiviral agents that are effective against most, if not all, viral subtypes and do not lead to serious side effects may prove to be more profitable.

Several groups of people are urged to be vaccinated. These are children aged 6 to 24 months, adults over the age of 65 years, and persons residing in nursing homes or who have chronic disorders of pulmonary or cardiovascular systems or other chronic conditions, the immunosuppressed, health care workers,

RECENT DEVELOPMENTS

A recent live attenuated influenza vaccine has been licensed as FluMist. The vaccine strain is adapted to the cold, living at lower than human body temperatures. It is administered intranasally and transiently infects cells of the upper respiratory tract, eliciting a vigorous nasal mucosal IgA immune response. This is desirable because the typical injected vaccines often do not induce large amounts of this type of immunity that specifically targets microbes infecting mucosal tissues. This vaccine-strain virus cannot colonize the lower respiratory tract due to the higher temperature in this locale, greatly reducing the potential for pathogenicity.

FIGURE 19.5   Administration of a live attenuated intranasal H1N1 vaccine

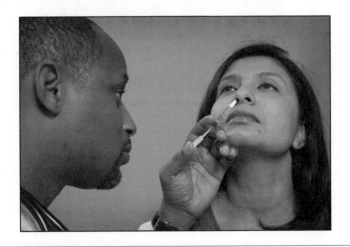

Source: CDC/Bill Atkinson.

and women who are more than three months pregnant. This vaccine may be combined with that against pneumococcal pneumonia although multiple vaccinations with the latter are not recommended. Decreases in hospitalization rates of 30% to 50% have been seen among immunized adults over age 65. Vaccination may also be recommended for children taking long-term aspirin therapy to decrease the risk of developing Reye syndrome. Individuals with hypersensitivity (allergic) reactions to egg proteins or other vaccine components should not receive this vaccine.

More general means of preventing infection involve public education concerning personal hygiene. Infected individuals should be urged to avoid unprotected coughs and sneezes. Following hand contact with mucous secretions, one should wash one's hands to avoid infecting others by shaking hands or touching surfaces such as doorknobs, radios, or phones. Uninfected persons should practice frequent hand-washing, particularly before eating food or touching their faces and especially after potential contact with infected individuals or their nasopharyngeal secretions.

To decrease the risk of human acquisition of avian influenza, people are instructed to avoid contact with ill or dead birds in areas in which H5N1 is infecting wild or domestic species of birds. Farmers should report any suspected cases of avian influenza among their flocks and should not butcher the animals or take them to market. Many governments have chosen to slaughter and incinerate massive numbers of both ill and healthy fowl in affected areas by personnel wearing protective clothing in an attempt to eliminate disease reservoirs and potential hosts, halting the spread of infection. This may be followed by disinfection of the environment. Other efforts include vaccinating domestic birds with H5N1 vaccines and improving sanitary conditions in the live-poultry markets and prohibiting the mixing of different bird species there. These measures have stretched the resources of governments of the affected countries, especially if the poultry owners are partially compensated for their losses. Extensive surveillance programs are also required for this effort.

Surveillance

Following the outbreak of avian influenza among humans in Hong Kong in 1997, surveillance programs were instituted to detect similar infections in birds and humans to allow rapid institution of protective measures and to track shifts in viral constitution and behavior. To be considered a confirmed case of avian influenza in Vietnam in 2004, laboratory testing by the World Health Organization was required to demonstrate at least one of the following conditions: a positive culture for H5N1, positive PCR findings, a positive IFA test, or a fourfold rise in H5N1-specific antibody titer using paired serum samples. The WHO discovered that human infection with avian H9N2 viruses had occurred in 1999 and 2003. Additional outbreaks of H5N1 among poultry were found sporadically that enabled prompt action by authorities to prevent its spread to humans by culling poultry and closing markets. H5N1 was found to have emerged in China in 1996 and led to outbreaks among domestic birds in other countries, including Indonesia, Vietnam, and Thailand, which were unreported until December 2003, when South Korea notified the WHO of the presence of H5N1 in poultry farms. In 2004, other Asian countries reported similar infections among farm birds. In 2005, Asian migratory birds were also discovered to be infected, and by 2006, avian infections had been noted in Africa, the Middle East, and Europe. The spread of avian influenza among birds is believed to have involved migratory waterfowl and movement of poultry. Hong Kong, South Korea, and Japan have subsequently controlled poultry outbreaks of highly pathogenic avian influenza. Continuing surveillance has revealed that H5N1 infection of birds increases during cooler months with low humidity.

H5N1 viruses have evolved since emerging in humans in 1997 and differ in their antigenic profile. Genetic analysis of avian influenza isolates has further revealed that human infections from 1997 to 2005 were from clades 1, 1', and 3 of the Z genotype. In 2005, humans cases caused by clade 2 viruses were detected in Indonesia and China. Similar careful viral typing of persons infected with pandemic or suspected pandemic influenza viruses would be useful in identifying which strains are the most pathogenic, tracking their prevalence and spread, and detecting the emergence of more pathogenic viral mutants. Such typing may allow an accurate assessment of the true risk of the potential advent of a large-scale infection with a highly pathogenic influenza strain. A case-control study of the 1997 outbreak indicated that the major risk factor for human acquisition of avian influenza was visiting a live-poultry market and found no association with eating poultry or preparing it at home, exposure to other bird species, contacting individuals with respiratory illness, or traveling. A 10% seroprevalance rate was found among workers in Hong Kong poultry markets. Very limited human-to-human transmission has been confirmed.

Summary

Disease

- Influenza

Causative Agent

- Influenza virus

Agent Type

- Virus in the *Orthomyxoviridae* family

Genome

- Single-stranded RNA

Vector

- None

Common Reservoirs

- Wild aquatic waterfowl and humans (normal outbreaks and epidemics)
- Birds and swine (pandemics)

Modes of Transmission

- Primarily airborne • Direct contact with infectious secretions
- Contact with sick or dead birds

Geographical Distribution

- Worldwide (normal outbreaks and epidemics) • Asia and Africa (human cases of avian influenza)

Year of Emergence

- Present throughout history • Pandemics emerge periodically

Key Terms

Antigenic drift Minor, frequent changes in the amino acid sequence of proteins recognized by the immune system as a result of point mutations

Antigenic shift Large, rare changes in the amino acid sequence of proteins recognized by the immune system as a result of genetic reassortment; major factor in influenza pandemics

Antigenic variation Changes in the amino acid sequence of proteins recognized by the immune system

Avian influenza Influenza of birds that rarely infects humans; high fatality rate in both species

Genetic reassortment Exchange of portions of genomic RNA between influenza viruses, including viruses originating in different host species

Guillain-Barré syndrome Serious neurological complications associated with the 1976 swine flu vaccination program

Hemagglutinin Viral surface glycoprotein that binds to sialic acid; one of the major viral antigens recognized by the immune system

Influenza pandemics Worldwide outbreaks of type A influenza

Neuraminidase Viral surface glycoprotein that cleaves sialic acid; one of the major viral antigens recognized by the immune system

Reye syndrome Disease of the central nervous system and liver that occasionally affects children infected with type B influenza when using aspirin

"Spanish flu" pandemic of 1918 Pandemic resulting in the largest loss of human lives (20 to 50 million deaths) from an infectious disease in a very short period of time

Review Questions

1. What were the three major pandemics of the twentieth century? What are four differences between influenza pandemics and seasonal epidemics? What populations are typically at highest risk for developing severe disease manifestations in each?

2. What are the symptoms of uncomplicated influenza? What are Reye syndrome and Guillain-Barré syndrome, and what causes each?

3. What are the three major types of influenza virus? What are the disease severity, susceptible animal species, and relationship to epidemics and pandemics for each? How are isolates of type A virus classified?

4. What viral surface molecules are the principal targets of the immune response? What is the role of each in the viral life cycle? What makes up the viral genetic material?

5. What are antigenic drift and antigenic shift? How does each arise? What are their contributions to the emergence of influenza pandemics?

Topics for Further Discussion

1. Compare current and potential future health impacts of human seasonal influenza epidemics and a possible human avian influenza pandemic, taking into account current numbers of human and bird infections and deaths and the mortality rates of each. How might this affect the level of government funding for research and public education for each?

2. Discuss why H5N1 viruses have not currently been able to cause a human pandemic or sustained epidemic. What are several methods by which a highly pathogenic human pandemic of H5N1 avian or H1N1 type of influenza might be averted?

3. Discuss past and current methods to decrease the spread of highly pathogenic strains of avian influenza to domestic birds in affected regions and prevent its

emergence in other areas. How might these affect local and national economies and the livelihoods of residents? Discuss other methods that might be developed which have less impact on people's lives.

4. Discuss the role of World War I in the 1918 Spanish flu pandemic. How did the pandemic affect the course of the war and human history?

Resources

Belshe, R. B., and others. "Comparative Immunogenicity of Trivalent Influenza Vaccine Administered by Intradermal or Intramuscular Route in Healthy Adults." *Vaccine,* 2007, *25,* 6755–6763.

Chin, J. *Control of Communicable Diseases Manual* (17th ed.). Washington, D.C.: American Public Health Association, 2000.

Kindt, T. J., Goldsby, R. A., and Osborne, B. A. *Kuby Immunology* (6th ed.). New York: Freeman, 2007.

Liu, C. "Influenza." In *Infectious Diseases* (2nd ed.), ed. P. D. Hoeprich. New York: HarperCollins, 2007.

Ortiz, J. R., and Uyeki, T. M. "Avian Influenza A (H5N1) Virus." In *Emerging Infections* (Vol. 7). W. M. Scheld, D. C. Hooper, and J. M. Hughes (eds.). Washington, D.C.: AMS Press, 2007.

Taubenberger, J. K., and Morens, D. M. "The Pathology of Influenza Virus Infections." *Annual Reviews of Pathology,* 2008, *3,* 499–522.

Thompson, C. I., Barclay, W. S., Zambon, M. C., and Pickles, R. J. "Infection of Human Airway Epithelium by Human and Avian Strains of Influenza A Virus." *Journal of Virology,* 2006, *80,* 8060–8068.

World Health Organization. *Cumulative Number of Confirmed Human Cases of Avian Influenza A/(H5N1) Reported to WHO.* Geneva, Switzerland: World Health Organization, 2008.

CHAPTER 20

HANTAVIRUS PULMONARY SYNDROME

LEARNING OBJECTIVES

- Define hantavirus pulmonary syndrome and hemorrhagic fever with renal syndrome
- Describe the viruses responsible for causing these illnesses
- Discuss modes of infection
- Discuss the host's response to infection
- Describe symptomatology and diagnosis
- Discuss methods of treatment
- Discuss methods of prevention

Major Concepts

Diseases and Symptoms

Hantaviruses cause two major types of disease in humans: hemorrhagic fever with renal syndrome (HFRS) and hantavirus pulmonary syndrome (HPS). Severe cases of HFRS result from infection with the Hantaan virus in Asia and Europe or the Dobrava virus in the Balkans. HFRS is characterized by the abrupt onset of high fever, severe abdominal or lower back pain, hemorrhagic symptoms, and renal dysfunction that severely diminishes the ability of the kidneys to produce urine. Fluid accumulates in the lungs, particularly if large volumes of water are consumed. The hemorrhagic manifestations include petechiae, severe hemorrhaging, and disseminated intravascular coagulation. The mortality rate is 5% to 15%, and between 40,000 and 100,000 persons are afflicted annually. HPS is caused by the Sin Nombre virus in North America and the Andes and the Laguna Negra, HU39694, Lechiguanas, Oran, and Juquitiba viruses in South America. Kidney involvement is limited, and hemorrhagic symptoms are uncommon. The early symptoms of this disease are fever, chills, fatigue, myalgia, headache, malaise, and dizziness, accompanied by gastrointestinal symptoms. The cardiorespiratory phase follows with leakage of high-protein-content fluid into the alveoli of the lungs and hypoxia, tachypnea, tachycardia, and mild hypotension. Later, respiratory symptoms such as coughing and shortness of breath develop in all patients. In many cases, death occurs rapidly after fluid enters the lungs and may be attributable to hypoxia or circulatory collapse due to low cardiac output and high systemic vascular resistance, hypotension, or shock. Overall mortality rate ranges from 20% to 40%.

Infection

Hantaviruses are spheroid to oval, enveloped negative-sense single-stranded RNA viruses of the Bunyaviridae family. They infect primarily endothelial cells. Other hantaviruses causing less severe HFRS-like pathology in humans are the Seoul virus (worldwide), the Puumala virus (Scandinavia), and the Bayou, Black Creek Canal, Monongahela, and New York viruses (North America). Hantaviruses are transmitted through dried, aerosolized excreta of rodents: Sin Nombre virus uses the deer mouse as its vector. A major outbreak of HPS occurred in 1993 due to increased deer mouse populations resulting from more plentiful food sources and mild weather produced by El Niño climatic conditions.

Immune Response

The immune system's response to hantavirus infection is often pathogenic. Atypical T lymphocytes induce capillary leakage during HPS. CD4$^+$ Th1 T helper cells secrete interferon-γ, activating macrophages that are present in high numbers in the alveoli of the lungs. These cells produce additional cytokines, stimulating inflammatory responses that accentuate lung pathology. IFN-α and IFN-β, by contrast, appear to play protective roles in HFRS. Differences occur in the immune responses to nonpathogenic versus pathogenic hantaviruses. The former induce expression of a number of interferon-stimulated genes that are not activated by the latter. The Hantaan virus, for its part, stimulates expression of some genes involved in the pathology of HFRS, including hematopoietic growth factors, chemokines, cell adhesion molecules, and the complement system.

Treatment and Prevention

Treatment for HPS is supportive and requires hospitalization to maintain fluid balance and blood oxygenation levels and to avoid hypoxia and shock. Preventive measures may be taken to decrease contact with infectious rodent excreta. Infrequently inhabited cabins or vacation homes should be carefully cleaned to avoid inhaling dried urine, feces, or saliva. Areas such as floors, walls, and shelving that contain rodent droppings should be sprayed or liberally wetted with disinfectants to kill viruses prior to sweeping or dusting. Gloves and a respiratory mask should be worn during this process. Persons working with rodents need to take special precautions during contact with rodents or their excretions.

Introduction

In the early 1990s, a highly pathogenic outbreak of respiratory illness began in portions of the southwestern United States. Its route of transmission was unknown, and it appeared to be caused by a novel infectious organism. This agent was soon discovered to be a close relative of the **Hantaan virus**, which causes a hemorrhagic disease with renal manifestations, primarily in Asia. By June 2002, a total of 318 cases of the new disease, designated as **hantavirus pulmonary syndrome (HPS)**, were confirmed, with a mortality rate of 37%. By tracing Native American legends, however, it appears that periodic outbreaks of this disease have occurred for a much longer period of time and are related to changes in rodent populations in response to climatic conditions. Native Americans were affected at a disproportionately high rate: 22% of infected individuals belonged to that group, while 76% were white Americans. At least 31 U.S. states, parts of western Canada, and a number of countries in South America have reported cases of this respiratory syndrome. Infection in the eastern United States is uncommon, particularly in the American South. The largest numbers have occurred in Arizona, New Mexico, California, and Washington. HPS is rare or absent in Mexico, Central America, and the Caribbean, despite the presence of infected sigmodontine rodents in the continental areas. (Many of the native rodents in the Caribbean have been displaced by Old World rats and mice.)

Some segments of the population are at higher risk of acquiring HPS than others. Fully 75% of the cases were reported in rural locales with increased exposure to the rodent reservoirs and vectors. Males tend to have a higher rate of infection than females, perhaps due to their increased exposure to infectious material in cabins or through agricultural pursuits.

FIGURE 20.1 Hantavirus pulmonary syndrome (HPS) cases, by reporting states

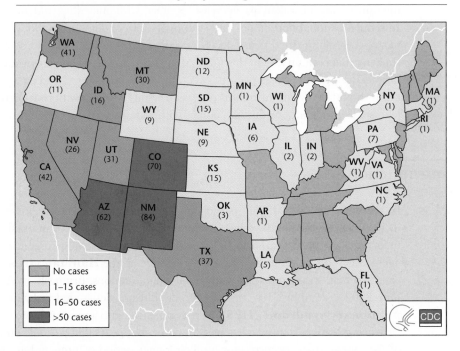

Note: Cumulative case counts as of July 1, 2010. Total cases: 545 in 32 states.
Source: CDC.

History

Hemorrhagic fever with renal syndrome was described by Soviets and Japanese in Manchuria near the Amur River; 12,000 Japanese troops stationed in the area were affected by this disease in the 1930s. Similar symptoms were described in a Chinese medical book written in A.D. 960. The disease was later noted in other areas of Asia as well in 1951 during the Korean War, when more than 3,200 United Nations troops came down with a hemorrhagic fever associated with greatly reduced urine production. This disease was found to be caused by infection with the Hantaan virus and is currently a major health threat in China and South Korea. Several other hantaviruses were later detected in various areas of the world, and some of these were associated with similar or differing illnesses.

Although several species of hantavirus were found in North America, these were not known to be pathogenic until 1993. At that time, an epidemic of adult respiratory distress syndrome began in the Navaho population of the American Southwest, particularly in the Four Corners area where the states of Colorado, Utah, New Mexico, and Arizona meet. The high numbers of Navahos in the initial outbreak led some observers to call this illness the "Navaho disease" and to avoid contact with Native Americans in that region. The affected persons were screened against a large panel of infectious agents and were eventually found to produce antibodies that were cross-reactive with the types of hantavirus occurring in Asia. The disease was subsequently named hantavirus pulmonary syndrome. The causative agent was initially dubbed the Muerto (Death) Canyon virus, but because it differed from previously identified hantaviruses, it was later designated the **Sin Nombre** ("without a name") **virus** (SNV). An earlier confirmed case of HPS in the United States was later backdated to 1959 in Utah.

Prior to 1993, two species of hantavirus were recognized in the Americas. The Prospect Hill virus from meadow voles caused no human illness in the United States, and the Seoul virus of Old World rats rarely caused disease in humans in the Western Hemisphere. The Seoul virus is found throughout the country, as well as on other continents, and is associated with hemorrhagic fever with renal syndrome in some locations.

The Diseases

Hantavirus infection leads to two distinct and serious illnesses. These diseases are caused by different species of virus and occur largely in different parts of the world, although some overlap exists in the ranges of the appropriate reservoir

Table 20.1 Distinguishing clinical characteristics for HFRS and HPS

Disease	Death Rate	Viruses	Hemorrhage	Distinguishing Characteristics				
				Azotemia/ Proteinuria	Pulmonary Capillary Leak	Myositis	Conjunctival Injection	Eye Pain/ Myopia
Hemorraghic fever with renal syndrome (moderate to severe)	1%–15%	Hantaan, Seoul, Dobrava-Belgrade	+++	+++/++++	+/++	+/++++	++/+++++	++/+++++
Hemorraghic fever with renal syndrome (mild)	<1%	Puumala	+	+/++++	–/+	+	+	+++/+++++
Hantavirus pulmonary syndrome (prototype)	>40%	Sin Nombre, New York	+	+	++++	–	–/+	–
Hantavirus pulmonary syndrome, renal variant	>40%	Bayou, Black Creek Canal, Andes	+	++/++++	+++/+++++	++/+++++	–/++	–

*Minimum/maximum occurrence of the characteristic; scale ranges from infrequent or mild manifestation (+) to frequent and severe manifestation (++++); (–) indicates that the characteristic is rarely reported.

Source: CDC.

and viral species. The bulk of this chapter is devoted to hantavirus pulmonary syndrome and its vectors, which are found in the Americas.

Hemorrhagic Fever with Renal Syndrome (HFRS)

Individuals with **hemorrhagic fever with renal syndrome (HFRS)**, also known as Korean hemorrhagic fever, experience an abrupt onset of high fever, severe abdominal or lower back pain, hemorrhagic symptoms, and renal dysfunction. The kidneys have greatly diminished ability to produce urine. Fluid accumulates in the lungs, a condition that may be worsened if the person consumes large volumes of water to stimulate urination. As its name suggests, HFRS induces hemorrhagic manifestations, such as petechiae, severe hemorrhaging, and disseminated intravascular coagulation. Cellular damage occurs in the kidneys, the anterior pituitary gland, and the right atrium of the heart. Symptoms may include hypotension and shock, headache, nausea, and vomiting. Other laboratory findings include thrombocytopenia and increased serum creatinine and blood urea nitrogen levels. Although the majority of patients recover in weeks or months, others are more severely affected, and the mortality rate is 1% to 15%.

HFRS is caused primarily by two hantaviruses, the Hantaan and Dobrava viruses. Approximately 40,000 to 100,000 cases of HFRS due to the Hantaan virus are reported annually in Asia, with greater than half that number from China. Several hundred cases due to the Dobrava virus are also reported in the Balkans each year. The Seoul virus may also cause HFRS. It thrives in rats in major cities throughout the world but is regularly linked to disease only in Asia. A generally milder disease called nephropathia epidemica results from infection with another hantavirus, the Puumala virus. This form of the disease occurs in most European countries, including the Balkans and Russia west of the Ural Mountains.

Hantavirus Pulmonary Syndrome (HPS)

The early symptoms of HPS include fever, chills, fatigue, muscle aches, headache, malaise, and dizziness, which typically last four to six days. These may be accompanied by gastrointestinal symptoms, including nausea, vomiting, and abdominal pain, but not by cough during the initial stages of infection. The later-occurring cardiorespiratory phase begins with the leakage of high-protein-content fluid into the alveoli (terminal air sacs) of the lungs, causing hypoxia (low blood oxygen levels), tachypnea (rapid breathing), tachycardia (rapid heart rate), and mild hypotension. Blood profiles include thrombocytopenia (low platelet levels) in almost all patients. Decreased platelet numbers generally inhibit the blood-clotting process, but hemorrhage is uncommon during HPS. These findings are often accompanied by hemoconcentration and an elevated hematocrit due to loss of fluid from the blood into the lungs and pleural cavity, resulting in pulmonary edema. Circulatory abnormalities include a "left shift"—the presence of immature white blood cells (myelocytes) in the circulation; circulating immunoblasts; hypoalbuminemia; and metabolic or lactic acidosis in the late stages of disease. Elevated levels of aspartate aminotransferase and lactate dehydrogenase are also frequently seen. Radiography of the chest is useful in diagnosis, and the disease progresses to frank bilateral alveolar edema (accumulation of fluid in the air sacs of the lungs). Late respiratory symptoms in all patients are coughing and shortness of breath. Unlike HFRS caused by a similar virus, HPS has a limited involvement of the kidneys, although proteinuria and abnormal urinary sediment are often found. The hemorrhagic manifestations of HFRS, such as overt bleeding or disseminated intravascular coagulation, are not common. The differential diagnosis needs to consider leptospirosis, rickettsial infection, American hemorrhagic fevers, and acute respiratory distress syndrome resulting from influenza A, mycoplasmosis, pneumonic plague, or pulmonary anthrax.

In many cases, progression to death occurs rapidly upon the entry of fluid into the lungs, often within 24 to 48 hours after hospital admission, and is generally attributable to hypoxia or circulatory collapse, commonly associated with low cardiac output and high systemic vascular resistance. Hypotension and shock may also occur. The mortality rate is high—in the 1993 outbreak, more than 50% of infected individuals died. The rate was 40% between 1994 and 1996 and

FIGURE 20.2   Bilateral pulmonary effusion during HPS

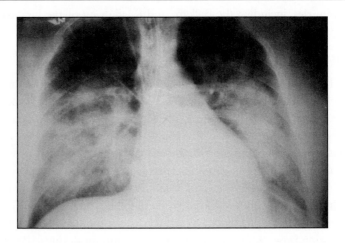

Source: CDC/D. Loren Ketai.

FIGURE 20.3   Interstitial pneumonitis and intra-alveolar edema

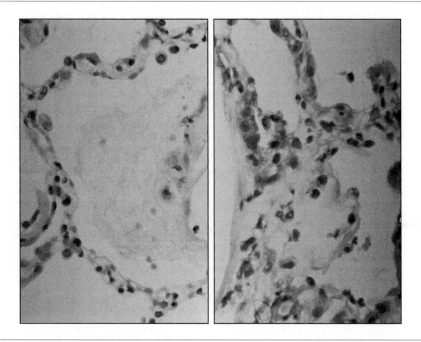

Source: CDC/Sherif R. Zaki.

20% in 1997. Mild disease is not the normal outcome of SNV infection; most infections progress to HPS. Young children are exceptions to this generalization, small numbers of them being infected with milder courses of disease.

The viruses themselves are not directly destructive to infected cells; rather, the damage appears to result from actions of the immune system. The lungs are a major entry site for microbes and therefore contain a large number of T lymphocytes, particularly the CD8$^+$ T killer cells that kill infected cells as well as uninfected cells in the vicinity. Pathogenesis is also due to the production of cytokines by CD4$^+$ T helper cells, activating further injury by other leukocytes (discussed later in this chapter).

The Causative Agents

Hantaviruses belong to the family **Bunyaviridae**, of which at least 20 species occur in the Americas. These are enveloped negative-sense single-stranded RNA viruses containing three RNA segments, large, medium, and small. They encode a number of viral proteins, such as RNA-dependent RNA transcriptase

Table 20.2   Pathogenic members of the genus *Hantavirus*, family Bunyaviridae

Species	Disease	Virus Distribution
Hantaan	HFRS	China, Russia, Korea
Dobrava-Belgrade	HFRS	Balkans
Seoul	HFRS	Worldwide
Puumala	HFRS	Europe, Russia, Scandinavia
Sin Nombre	HPS	United States, Canada, northern Mexico
New York	HPS	United States
Black Creek Canal	HPS	United States
Monongahela virus	HPS	Eastern United States
Bayou	HPS	United States
Laguna Negra virus	HPS	Paraguay and Bolivia
HU39694	HPS	Argentina
Lechiguanas virus	HPS	Central Argentina
Oran virus	HPS	Northwestern Argentina
Andes virus	HPS	Argentina and Chile
Juquitiba virus	HPS	Brazil

Source: CDC.

(responsible for transcription of RNA), the envelope glycoproteins, and the nucleocapsid protein. These viruses are spheroid to oval with a diameter of 95 to 110 nanometers. They primarily infect endothelial cells, which line the vasculature. Pathogenic, but not nonpathogenic, hantaviruses utilize the $\alpha v\beta 3$ integrin during entry into the cells. This integrin interacts with vascular endothelial growth factor receptor-2 (VEGFR-2). Alterations in vascular permeability occur in both HFRS and HPS.

Four groups of hantaviruses are defined on the basis of their vectors, several subfamilies of Muridae, Arvicolinae (voles), Murinae (Old World mice and rats), and Sigmodontinae (New World mice and rats).

Hantaan Virus and Other Hantaviruses Causing HFRS

The causative agent of HFRS was isolated in 1976 and named the Hantaan virus. It is present throughout Asia and sometimes in Europe. Its vector is the striped field mouse. The other hantavirus responsible for the severe form of HFRS is the **Dobrava virus** from the Balkans. Viruses associated with less serious pathology are the **Seoul virus** of brown and Norway rats, with worldwide distribution, and the **Puumala virus** of bank voles, found in Scandinavia. Other nonpathogenic hantaviruses are the Thailand, Khabarousk, Thottapalayam, and Tula viruses of Thailand, Russia, India, and Europe, respectively.

Sin Nombre Virus and Other Hantaviruses Causing HPS

The hantaviruses that cause HPS are found in rodents. They do not affect these animals' survival or reproductive fitness, although minor histological changes have been seen in the rodents' lungs and livers. Infection of these viral hosts is lifelong; however, hantaviruses do not persist in the circulating blood due to the presence of neutralizing IgA antibodies. It is not known how the viruses escape elimination from the rodents by either these antibodies or the hosts' CD8$^+$ T killer cells.

Sin Nombre virus (SNV) is responsible for the majority of the cases of HPS in North America and occurs in the United States and western Canada. The deer mouse (grassland form) serves as the disease reservoir and vector. In some areas and under certain conditions, the proportion of infected mice is quite high, while in other areas, it is much lower: on some of the Channel Islands off the coast of California, this number ranges from 58% to 71%, while on some of the other islands, no infected mice are found. The normal rate

FIGURE 20.4   Electron micrograph of the Sin Nombre virus

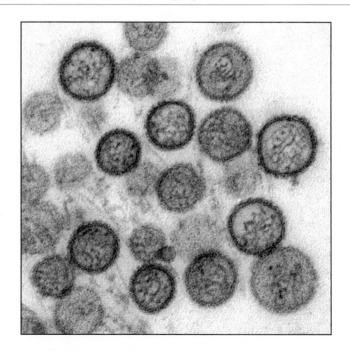

Source: CDC/Cynthia Goldsmith and Luanne Elliott.

of seroprevalance in the southwestern United States is 10%, but this number tripled in 1993 due to environmental factors causing crowded conditions in the mouse population.

Later investigations revealed that other hantaviruses may serve as disease agents in North America. These include the **Bayou virus** (southeastern United States), **Black Creek Canal virus** (primarily Dade County, Florida), **Monongahela virus** (eastern United States), and **New York virus** (eastern United States), all of which may lead to slightly different disease presentations with renal involvement including proteinuria and sometimes renal failure. The vectors for these viruses are the river rat found in moist to swampy grasslands, the cotton rat inhabiting grassland with scattered brush, the deer mouse (forest form), and the white-footed mouse, respectively. Other hantaviruses of sigmodontine rodents in North America that have not been associated with human disease are the Prospect Hill, Blue River, Muleshoe, and El Moro Canyon viruses. Many of these viruses are closely related and may differ by only 3% to 6% in amino acid sequence.

HPS is found throughout South America, with Argentina, Chile, and Brazil having the highest number of cases. The species of hantaviruses that are responsible for the disease in that region include the **Laguna Negra virus** (Paraguay and Bolivia), **HU39694** (Argentina), **Lechiguanas virus** (central Argentina), **Oran virus** (northwestern Argentina), **Andes virus** (Argentina and Chile), and **Juquitiba virus** (São Paulo, Brazil). The Oran and Lechiguanas viruses were known to be pathogenic prior to the 1993 outbreak in the United States but were not linked to HPS until 1994. Pathology induced by these viruses may differ slightly from SNV-caused HPS, including a higher rate of infection in

Table 20.3   Hantavirus pulmonary syndrome in the Americas, 1993–2004

Country	Cases	Deaths	% Fatal
Argentina	592	11	2
Bolivia	36	17	47
Brazil	321	71	22
Canada	88	0	0
Chile	331	124	37
Panama	35	3	9
Paraguay	99	13	13
Uruguay	48	13	27
United States	362	132	36
Total	1910	384	20

Source: Pan American Health Organization.

individuals under the age of 18 years. Similar hantaviruses in Central and South America that are not known to cause human disease include the Rio Segundo, Caño Delgadito, Rio Mamore, Maciel, and Pergamino viruses.

Viral Transmission

New World hantaviruses are transmitted to humans via dried and aerosolized excreta of **sigmodontine rodents**. Disease incidence occurs year round but is greatest in the spring and summer when the numbers of the rodent vectors peak. Environmental factors affect vector populations and disease transmission and occurrence. Pinyon juniper forests near the altitude of 1,980 meters in western portions of North America are hot zones, owing to the fact that deer mice eat nuts. This area is also home to many humans living in rural settings who may be at greater risk if rodent populations in that area increase. The outbreak of 1993 is believed to have resulted from the combination of a warm winter and mild spring and increased numbers of pinyon juniper nuts, leading to an explosion of the deer mouse population. The subsequent crowded conditions permitted rapid dissemination of Sin Nombre virus between mice. Such increases in rodent populations may occur following the excessive rains and mild winters present during El Niño years.

FIGURE 20.5   Deer mouse vector of the Sin Nombre virus

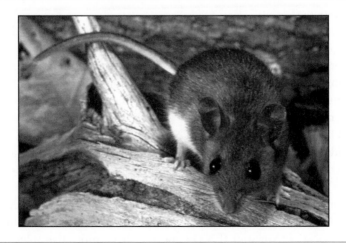

Source: CDC/James Gathany.

Sin Nombre virus is transmitted between mice by biting during combat. It is spread to humans via inhalation of infectious small particles present within aerosolized dried mouse excreta, such as saliva, urine, and feces, in human dwellings. Mice are believed to be most likely to transmit the virus early after infection due to the higher rate of shedding of infectious organisms in the urine and throat at that time. Risk factors for humans include living in rural areas in close contact with the environment or in areas with high numbers of infected vectors, as occurs in the Navaho population; having high numbers of rodents in or around the home; and cleaning rodent excreta from vacation homes, cabins, and outbuildings. In the United States, Europe, and Asia, no transmission has been demonstrated to occur directly between humans, including hospital personnel performing resuscitations. However, this means of transmission is strongly suspected to have occurred during an outbreak of the Andes virus infection in southern Argentina in 1996–1997 but not in a different outbreak of this virus in 1997 in Chile.

The Immune Response

The presence of immature phagocytes, myelocytes, and immunoblasts in the circulation of individuals with HPS suggests that the immune system is active and that the bone marrow is producing large numbers of new leukocytes. The causative agents of HFRS and HPS appear to do no direct damage to cells, and serious disease is not seen until after the development of an immune response.

The lungs are a major site of entry for infectious organisms via inhalation. As such, they produce a highly active immune response and harbor a particularly large number of $CD8^+$ T killer cells. These cells are among the most effective leukocytes during viral invasion, readily killing infected host cells but also inducing capillary leakage. In HPS, many of the T killer cells are classified as atypical lymphocytes. Other leukocytes are also involved in the response to hantaviruses. The cytokine interferon-γ (IFN-γ) secreted by $CD4^+$ Th1 T helper cells of the adaptive immune response activates macrophages of the innate immune system, which are also present in high numbers in the alveoli of the lungs. Macrophages in turn release additional cytokines, stimulating an inflammatory response and lung fibrosis and accentuating lung pathology. Alveolar macrophages may play a larger role in the pathology induced by the Andes virus than in that caused by SNV. IFN-α and IFN-β appear to have protective roles in HFRS, as mice without the corresponding receptors are more susceptible to infection by the Hantaan virus.

FIGURE 20.6   Activated immune system: lymph node
from an HPS patient

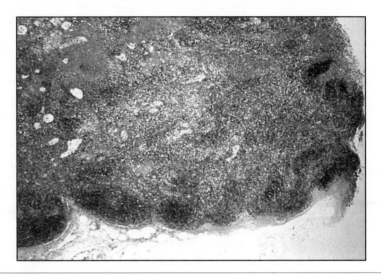

Source: CDC.

Diagnosis

Analysis of formalin-fixed samples by immunohistochemistry has been an important diagnostic tool that led to the recognition of HPS in many areas of South America. Other immunological tests, such as the immunofluorescence assay (IFA) and ELISA, are serological tests commonly used in the diagnosis of HPS. They permit a moderate degree of cross-reaction among the various hantaviruses, allowing the detection of previously unknown virus species. IFA is unreliable at low antibody titers and should be confirmed by other means. SNV antigens may be used in IgG and IgM antigen-capture ELISAs for all American hantaviruses of sigmodontine rodents. The latter type of ELISA uses the nucleocapsid protein and produces a very small number of false positive results. Western blot is used for rapid and specific diagnosis. Focus reduction and hemagglutination tests have been used to detect infection with other hantaviruses.

Molecular diagnostic assays for hantavirus infection include the reverse transcriptase polymerase chain reaction (RT-PCR). This test detects viral RNA in samples from rodents or the sera or blood clots of patients during their first seven to ten days of illness. It is too expensive and cumbersome for use in routine diagnosis, however.

RECENT DEVELOPMENTS

Infection of humans by different species of hantaviruses leads to either no disease, HFRS, or HPS. Recent studies have attempted to establish the differences that determine whether a given species is pathogenic or nonpathogenic. One approach has examined patterns of gene expression following infection of endothelial cells. The different types of hantaviruses induce or repress transcription and expression of different genes by their hosts. The IFNs are a group of cytokines that as part of the immune system generally protect the host from viral infections, in part by inducing transcription of a number of genes, the interferon-stimulated genes. Early after infection of cells, the Prospect Hill virus induces or represses expression of 67 host genes, including the protective IFN-β, while the Hantaan virus and the New York virus affect the expression of only three. The former is nonpathogenic to humans, whereas the latter two cause HFRS and HPS, respectively. Twenty-four interferon-stimulated genes in particular are induced early after infection by the nonpathogenic but not the pathogenic hantavirus species. In a separate study, induction of IFN-β transcription by the Prospect Hill virus correlated with activation of IFN regulatory factor 3. The New York virus, by contrast, repressed activity of the IFN-β promoter. Later after infection, however, the pathogenic viral species induced 13 genes that were not activated by the nonpathogenic Prospect Hill virus. Differences were seen between the viruses responsible for HFRS and HPS as well. The Hantaan virus induced expression of several genes suspected to be involved in the immune-mediated pathology of HFRS, such as hematopoietic growth factors, chemokines, cell adhesion molecules, and components of the complement system, including GM-CSF, G-CSF, IL-6, IL-8, GRO-β, GRO-γ, ICAM, and complement component 1 inhibitor. The New York virus stimulated transcription of β3 intergrin-linked potassium channels, which may be associated with vascular permeability in HPS. Further studies are needed to determine whether these findings can be generalized among all of the nonpathogenic and HFRS- or HPS-inducing hantaviruses. Together, these studies may allow the development of treatment options that target the genes altered by each group of virus.

Treatment

The most effective treatment for HPS has been the provision of circulatory and respiratory support in a hospital setting. This includes restoration of fluid balance and the management of hypoxia and shock. Blood oxygenation and inspiration

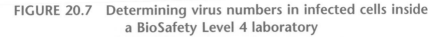

FIGURE 20.7   Determining virus numbers in infected cells inside a BioSafety Level 4 laboratory

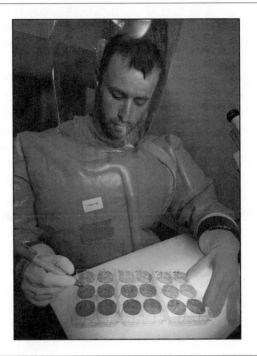

Source: CDC/Scott Smith.

of oxygen must be carefully monitored to avoid further fluid accumulation in the lungs and pleural cavity, worsening the pulmonary edema. Shock may be corrected by the use of ionotropic agents, maintenance of cardiac filling pressure, treatment of hypoxia, and administration of cardiostimulatory drugs.

Because several treatable respiratory diseases of bacterial origin must be included in the differential diagnosis, antibiotics such as doxycycline should be administered until the establishment of a definitive diagnosis. The antiviral compound ribavirin is effective in the treatment of HFRS and is active against SNV in vitro and in vivo in deer mice but not in human trials.

Prevention

Once rodentborne SNV was associated with the highly pathogenic HPS, the United States government began an intensive educational program concerning disease recognition and prevention. Education is particularly important for Native American populations of the southwestern United States and visitors, hunters, and campers in the affected areas, and it may be most effective if a multicultural approach is used. Because transmission of this virus to humans requires their exposure to infected dried rodent saliva, urine, or feces, limiting vsuch exposure decreases the incidence of HPS. Controlling rodent populations in nature is not practical, but steps may be taken to rodent-proof dwellings. Unfortunately, deer mice readily enter human residences and in some areas are trapped in homes more frequently than house mice. To avoid attracting rodents, food, water, and garbage should be kept in containers with tight-fitting lids. Food in bags should be kept in containers to which rodents cannot gain access, such as plastic storage bins. Pet food or water should not be left out at night. Food should be removed from dishes and cooking utensils soon after use, or such items should be placed in a dishwasher with the door closed. Care should also be exercised during agricultural practices, such as threshing.

Another means of preventing infection is to decrease the chance of inhaling infectious material. Sleeping on floors or outdoors increases the risk of infection by bringing a person closer to areas potentially contaminated with rodent excreta. Cabins or vacation homes that are infrequently inhabited may be used by rodents. Cleaning such areas is a risk factor because dried urine, feces, and saliva may become aerosolized and inhaled. To decrease such exposure, areas that are known or suspected to have been used by rodents, such as floors, walls, and shelving, may be sprayed or wetted liberally with disinfectants, such as Lysol, or bleach to kill the viruses by destroying their envelope. Rather than sweeping or dusting areas contaminated with rodent droppings, a wet mop or towels moistened with disinfectants should be used. Gloves and an approved respiratory mask should be worn during this process.

People who work with rodents need to take special precautions during contact with the animals or their excretions. Fortunately, fewer than 1% of biologists who handled large numbers of reservoir species were found to have antibodies to SNV, and only one individual had an illness suggestive of HPS. Nevertheless, biologists and animal support staff (especially those handling wild deer mice) need to be familiar with the symptoms of HPS and should seek medical attention if developing a fever followed by respiratory illness within 45 days of rodent exposure. To minimize contact, gloves and coveralls should be used when handling rodents or traps containing them. The CDC recommends wearing an appropriate respirator when in contact with rodents in an endemic area. Traps, equipment, gloves, and work areas may be cleaned with bleach or other disinfectants. Rodent carcasses or material contaminated with rodent excretions should be soaked in disinfectant and then placed in double bags and buried, autoclaved, or burned.

FIGURE 20.8   Examining samples suspected of involvement
in a hantavirus outbreak

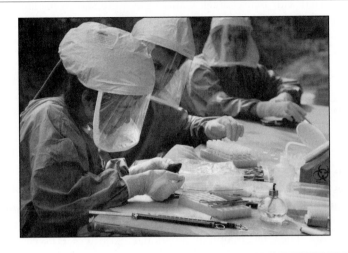

Source: CDC.

Vaccines would be useful to protect susceptible populations; however, their development has been complicated by difficulties in finding an appropriate animal model system for HFRS or HPS disease. Researchers have had limited success along these lines with HPS because the Andes virus does cause lethal disease in adult Syrian hamsters that is similar to the human illness, whereas SNV does not. Cynomolgus macaques also develop nephropathia epidemica upon infection with the Puumala virus. The effects of candidate vaccines on viral load may also be measured. Work is under way to develop vaccines reactive with the Hantaan and Seoul viruses. Because a number of viral agents induce either HFRS or HPS, development of a specific vaccine for each virus is impractical. Fortunately, these viruses have similar genetic composition, and antibodies are frequently cross-reactive. Accordingly, although the glycoprotein precursors of the Hantaan virus and the Seoul virus differ by 23% at the amino acid level, antibodies induced by either molecule neutralize both viruses. $CD8^+$ T killer cell responses may also be stimulated, and these are cross-reactive in vitro and in vivo. Vaccinia viral vectors containing hantavirus glycoprotein precursor similarly protect against infection with both of these viruses. Such cross-protection is not seen with the Hantaan and Puumala viruses, whose proteins differ by 46%. The hantaviruses of sigmodontine rodents in North and South America differ by a maximum of 27%, leading to the hope that cross-protective immunity among these species will be similar to that seen between and Hantaan and Seoul viruses. Neutralizing antibodies from convalescent serum of an individual infected with Black Creek Canal virus were shown to neutralize SNV as well. Syrian hamsters previously infected with different hantavirus (Hantaan, Seoul, Dobrava, Puumala, or SNV) survived challenge with lethal doses of Andes virus, demonstrating that cross-protection does occur in vivo.

Surveillance

The 1993 outbreak of HPS in the American Southwest led to the establishment of a special hotline to monitor the occurrence of this disease. During a period of six months, over 21,000 calls were placed and 280 samples from outside of the initial sites were submitted for analysis. Twenty-one of these samples were confirmed to be infected with the Bayou, Black Creek Canal, and New York viruses. The CDC maintains a national registrar of HPS cases. In Argentina and Brazil, surveillance of rodent and human sera, including that of animal caretakers, for reactivity with hantavirus antigens revealed high titers of neutralizing antibody. Surveillance for Argentine hemorrhagic fever detected many of the Lechiguanas-type cases of HPS. Future surveillance for hantavirus involvement in cases of renal failure may be indicated for individuals exposed to rodents in areas endemic for Bayou, Black Creek Canyon, or New York viruses and may indicate the presence of a mild form of HFRS induced by the Seoul virus, which is also present in the Americas.

Alert clinicians play a vital role in disease surveillance. They detected an outbreak of an unusual respiratory illness in Argentina in 1984 that was later recognized as HPS. Well-trained health care providers may allow rapid response to a potential outbreak by sending samples from persons suspected to have contracted HPS to a reference laboratory. Diagnosis may be made by ELISA and the specific virus involved determined by RT-PCR. Community surveillance and monitoring of patient contacts are especially critical in the case of Andes virus infection in light of the potential for human-to-human transmission.

Due to the association between HPS outbreaks and large surges in the populations of the corresponding rodent reservoir species, surveillance efforts might include monitoring rodent numbers and the factors associated with increases in their populations, including mild winters that may increase the rodent food supply. Such studies should also include determining the rate of infection in susceptible rodent populations. This infection rate is dependent on the animals' age, sex, rodent population density, the season, and the climate.

FIGURE 20.9   Donning protective wear prior to collecting
deer mice during a hantavirus field study

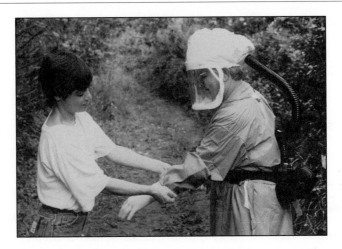

Source: CDC.

Summary

Diseases

• Hantavirus pulmonary syndrome   • Hemorrhagic fever with renal
syndrome   • Nephropathia epidemica

Causative Agents

• Primarily the Sin Nombre virus in North America and the Andes, Laguna
Negra, HU39694, Lechiguanas, Oran, and Juquitiba viruses in South
America   • Primarily the Hantaan and Dobrava viruses and also the Seoul
virus   • Puumala virus

Agent Type

• Hantavirus of the Bunyaviridae family

Genome

• Single-stranded, negative-sense RNA

Vectors

• Sigmodontine rodents, primarily deer mice   • Primarily striped field
mice   • Bank voles

Common Reservoirs

• Deer mice for SNV, other sigmodontine rodents for the other viral species

Mode of Transmission

• Airborne by inhalation of infectious dried rodent urine, feces, or urine

Geographical Distribution

• North and South America • Primarily Asia • Most of Europe

Year of Emergence

• 1993 • 1930s • Unknown

Key Terms

Andes virus Primary causative agent of hantavirus pulmonary syndrome in South America; responsible for outbreaks in Argentina and Chile

Bayou virus Pathogenic hantavirus found in the southeastern United States

Black Creek Canal virus Pathogenic hantavirus found in Dade County, Florida

Bunyaviridae Family to which hantaviruses belong; most members of this family instead cause arthropod-borne diseases, including Crimean-Congo hemorrhagic fever, Rift Valley fever, and California encephalitis

Dobrava virus Causative agent of hemorrhagic fever with renal syndrome in the Balkans

Hantaan virus Primary viral causative agent of hemorrhagic fever with renal syndrome

Hantavirus pulmonary syndrome (HPS) Highly pathogenic respiratory disease that may lead to adult respiratory distress syndrome; caused by various hantaviruses of sigmodontine rodents in the Americas

Hemorrhagic fever with renal syndrome (HFRS) Severe disease characterized by renal dysfunction, hemorrhagic manifestations, fever, and cardiovascular injury; caused by hantaviruses in Asia and parts of Europe

HU39694 Causative agent of hantavirus pulmonary syndrome in Argentina

Juquitiba virus Causative agent of hantavirus pulmonary syndrome in Brazil

Laguna Negra virus Causative agent of hantavirus pulmonary syndrome in Paraguay and Bolivia

Lechiguanas virus Causative agent of hantavirus pulmonary syndrome in central Argentina

Monongahela virus Pathogenic hantavirus found in the eastern United States

New York virus Pathogenic hantavirus found in the eastern United States

Oran virus Causative agent of hantavirus pulmonary syndrome in northwestern Argentina

Puumala virus European hantavirus associated with nephropathia epidemica

Seoul virus Cosmopolitan hantavirus associated with hemorrhagic fever with renal syndrome

Sigmodontine rodents Subfamily of New World mice and rats

Sin Nombre virus (SNV) Primary viral causative agent of hantavirus pulmonary syndrome in North America; distributed in the United States, Canada, and northern Mexico

Review Questions

1. What are the two diseases associated with infection by hantaviruses? What viruses cause each of these, and where are they found?
2. What are the primary symptoms associated with these two diseases? What antiviral compounds have been used successfully to treat each?
3. What cell types are infected by pathogenic hantaviruses? What cellular receptor is involved, and how might the use of this receptor lead to the viruses' effects on the vasculature?
4. What general types of animals serve as the vector for hantavirus-associated disease in the Americas? What methods might members of the general public use to protect themselves from infection?
5. Do the hantaviruses cause direct damage to host cells? If so, how do they do so? How does the immune system affect pathology?

Topics for Further Discussion

1. The Seoul virus and its reservoir species and vector are present in the Americas as well as Asia, but it is associated with disease only in Asia. Speculate as to possible reasons for this observation.
2. Hantaan virus–based vaccines provide cross-protection against infection of animals with the Seoul virus but not the Puumala virus. Why do current

vaccines based on Hantaan virus components not protect against the Puumala virus? How might this affect the development of vaccines against the various hantaviruses that cause HPS?

3. How might the associations between alterations in deer mouse populations in the American Southwest and western Canada with disease incidence and environmental conditions be used to protect humans from infection? Consider the roles of public education and surveillance and suggest which agencies and professionals might be involved in this effort.

4. In HPS as in other infectious diseases, the immune system plays a protective role as well as induces some of the pathology. How might this affect vaccine development? How might the immune-mediated protection be increased and the pathology decreased?

Resources

Alff, P. J., and others. "The Pathogenic NY-1 Hantavirus G1 Cytoplasmic Tail Inhibits RIG-I and TBK-1-Directed Interferon Responses." *Journal of Virology,* 2006, *80,* 9676–9686.

Chin, J. *Control of Communicable Diseases Manual* (17th ed.). Washington, D.C.: American Public Health Association, 2000.

Geimonen, E., and others. "Pathogenic and Nonpathogenic Hantaviruses Differentially Regulate Endothelial Cell Responses." *Proceedings of the National Academy of Sciences,* 2002, *99,* 13837–13842.

Hooper, J. W., Larsen, T., Custer, D. M., and Schmaljohn, C. S. "A Lethal Disease Model for Hantavirus Pulmonary Syndrome." *Virology,* 2001, *289,* 6–14.

Medina, R. A., Mirowsky-Garcia, C., Hutt, J., and Hjelle, B. "Ribavirin, Human Convalescent Plasma and Anti-b3 Integrin Antibody Inhibit Infection by Sin Nombre Virus in the Deer Mouse Model." *Journal of General Virology,* 2007, *88,* 493–505.

Peters, C. J. "Hantavirus Pulmonary Syndrome in the Americas." In *Emerging Infectious* (Vol. 2), ed. W. M. Scheld, W. A. Craig, and J. M. Hughes. Washington, D.C.: ASM Press, 1998.

Spiropoulou, C. F., Albarino, C. G., Ksiazek, T. G., and Rollin, P. E. "Andes and Prospect Hill Hantaviruses Differ in Early Induction of Interferon Although Both Can Downregulate Interferon Signaling." *Journal of Virology,* 2007, *81,* 2769–2776.

Terajima, M., Hayasaka, D., Maeda, K., and Ennis, F. A. "Immunopathogenesis of Hantavirus Pulmonary Syndrome and Hemorrhagic Fever with Renal Syndrome: Do CD8[+] T Cells Trigger Capillary Leakage in Viral Hemorrhagic Fevers?" *Immunology Letters,* 2007, *113,* 117–120.

Wichmann, D., and others. "Hantaan Virus Infection Causes an Acute Neurological Disease That Is Fatal in Adult Laboratory Mice." *Journal of Virology,* 2002, *76,* 8890–8899.

CHAPTER 21

SEVERE ACUTE RESPIRATORY SYNDROME

LEARNING OBJECTIVES

- Define severe acute respiratory syndrome

- Describe the coronavirus responsible for causing this illness and explain how it differs from the other, less pathogenic coronaviruses

- Discuss modes of infection

- Discuss the host's response to infection

- Describe symptomatology and diagnosis

- Discuss potential methods of treatment

- Discuss methods of prevention

Major Concepts

Outbreak

A previously unknown severe respiratory illness appeared toward the end of 2002. Before being brought under control the following spring, more than 8,000 cases and 774 deaths had occurred in 29 countries. It reemerged in December 2003 and January 2004, causing four cases of mild disease in humans. This disease, designated severe acute respiratory syndrome (SARS), is caused by a newly discovered coronavirus, SARS-CoV, which is able to infect cells of the lower respiratory tract and cause an atypical pneumonia. It differs from other coronaviruses, which infect the upper respiratory tract, causing the common cold, by being able to survive at human body temperature.

Transmission

SARS appears to have entered the human population following the mutation of a closely related animal virus of palm civets and other animals found in live-game markets in Asia. The mutated virus has an enhanced ability to bind to human ACE-2, its cellular receptor. Transmission of human SARS-CoV readily occurs between people through inhalation or mucosal exposure to infectious respiratory droplets or by contact with contaminated surfaces. The major outbreak in 2002–2003 was contained by a combination of strategies including quarantine, travel notices, surveillance of travelers, and institution of public and private hygienic measures.

Immune Response

The immune system appears to have both pathogenic and protective roles in SARS. Much of the lung injury results from inflammatory responses by Th1 cells and macrophages brought into the affected area. Immunosuppressive corticosteroids were therefore used to treat the disease. Other components of the immune response are beneficial, especially neutralizing antibodies. A number of vaccines using viral components are being developed to stimulate their production. These efforts should proceed with caution due to concerns that the antibodies induced may actually enhance infection.

Control of the Outbreak

Given the ease of transmission between humans and the severity of the disease, a massive collaborative effort was quickly undertaken to identify the causative agent, map its genome, determine the route of transmission to and between people, develop means of diagnosis, and monitor and reduce disease spread, with the result that the outbreak was contained within six months of its emergence in humans.

Introduction

Starting in late 2002, a new and deadly respiratory illness struck several locations in Asia and Canada as well as other countries throughout the world. Unlike past outbreaks of avian influenza in humans, this disease was easily transmitted from person to person by causal contact, similar to the common cold but much more serious. By the end of this outbreak in early 2003, there had been 8,096 reported cases of human infection with 774 deaths (9.6% fatality rate). An intensive research effort rapidly determined that the organism responsible for this outbreak was a coldlike virus, raising public and professional fears of a possible pandemic with a highly pathogenic, readily transmissible microbe. Unlike many respiratory diseases, including the common cold and influenza, relatively few children became infected, and those who did developed less severe disease manifestations. Individuals over the age of 65 years were at significantly higher risk of developing serious or fatal illness.

Massive efforts by biomedical researchers and the international health community led to the rapid accumulation of relevant information about the disease agent and its transmission, allowing the outbreak to be swiftly brought under control using both traditional and novel surveillance and protection strategies. The successes in dealing with this crisis may aid in the control of future epidemics or pandemics that pose serious health threats.

History

Severe acute respiratory syndrome (SARS) was first recognized in the Guangdong province of China in November 2002, although serological evidence from stored blood components later indicated that 1.8% of healthy members of the Hong Kong population had developed antibodies to the animal form of the virus by 2001. This treatment-resistant emerging infection spread rapidly to seven other Chinese provinces, including a large outbreak of atypical pneumonia in the provincial capital of Guangzhou. Many of the afflicted persons were health care workers. The disease was then disseminated by a physician traveling to Hong Kong who infected 16 guests staying on the same floor of his hotel (Hotel M). These people spread the disease elsewhere. SARS had become a global health threat by spring 2003, with clusters occurring in China, Hong Kong, Vietnam, Singapore, and parts of Canada, including Toronto. It ultimately affected 29 countries on five continents; only eight cases were confirmed in the United States, and these did not originate there but were imported by travelers from affected areas. On March 12, the World Health Organization issued a global health alert. The next month, due to fears of an outbreak with endogenous transmission in the United States, SARS was added to the U.S. list of **quarantinable communicable diseases**. This required a presidential order and an amendment to the CDC quarantine regulations. Diseases in this group include cholera, diphtheria, infectious tuberculosis, plague, smallpox, yellow fever, and viral hemorrhagic diseases. The CDC prevents introduction of disease into the United States from foreign countries by requiring the reporting of ill passengers on incoming vessels and airplanes and restricting imports with the potential to transmit disease to humans. The Food and Drug Administration then regulates interstate quarantine regulations. By the use of travel advisories, screening of international travelers, and quarantine of contacts of infected persons, the world public health community was able to contain SARS infections worldwide by July 2003. In September and December 2003 and February 2004, laboratory-acquired infections occurred in Singapore, Taiwan, and China, respectively. Community spread resulted during the last instance. Four mild cases occurred during a SARS reemergence in China in December 2003 and January 2004; two of these appear to have arisen through contact with live infected palm civets at a restaurant in which all six of the animals there were found to be infected with an isolate genetically similar to that found in the humans. Fortunately, no further outbreaks have been detected since then; however, given the ease and rapidity of transmission and the high mortality rate, health care workers have remained vigilant against a reemergence.

This outbreak of disease, like many others throughout history, had an associated societal impact, leading to fear of several groups of people and discrimination against them or their communities. Due to its geographical distribution, the SARS epidemic led to fear of contact with Asians and people from Toronto, resulting in economic losses of tens of billions of dollars to those areas. Other similar instances include the shunning of residents of the Chinatown community of San Francisco in 1900 after an outbreak of bubonic plague struck the city, imported by rats carried by ship from Hong Kong. The hantavirus outbreak in the American West in 1993 led to stigmatization of Navahos, whose communities were the first and hardest hit. Leprosy, epilepsy, and mental illnesses raised fears that led to discrimination and avoidance of segments of the population, as more recently occurred with respect to the gay community and Haitians during the initial phase of the AIDS epidemic.

Table 21.1 Summary of probable SARS cases, November 1, 2002–July 31, 2003

Areas	Number of Cases	Median Age (Range)	Number of Deaths	Mortality Rate (%)	Date of Probable First Case	Date of Probable Last Case
Australia	6	15 (1–45)	0	0	26-Feb-03	1-Apr-03
Canada	251	49 (1–98)	43	17	23-Feb-03	12-Jun-03
China	5,327	N.A.	349	7	16-Nov-02	3-Jun-03
France	7	49 (26–61)	1	14	21-Mar-03	3-May-03
Germany	9	44 (4–73)	0	0	9-Mar-03	6-May-03
Hong Kong (China)	1,755	40 (0–100)	299	17	15-Feb-03	31-May-03
India	3	25 (25–30)	0	0	25-Apr-03	6-May-03
Indonesia	2	56 (47–65)	0	0	6-Apr-03	17-Apr-03
Ireland	1	56	0	0	27-Feb-03	27-Feb-03
Italy	4	31 (25–54)	0	0	12-Mar-03	20-Apr-03
Kuwait	1	50	0	0	9-Apr-03	9-Apr-03
Macao (China)	1	28	0	0	5-May-03	5-May-03
Malaysia	5	30 (26–84)	2	40	14-Mar-03	22-Apr-03
Mongolia	9	32 (17–63)	0	0	31-Mar-03	6-May-03
New Zealand	1	67	0	0	20-Apr-03	20-Apr-03
Philippines	14	41 (29–73)	2	14	25-Feb-03	5-May-03
Romania	1	52	0	0	19-Mar-03	19-Mar-03
Russia	1	25	0	0	5-May-03	5-May-03
Singapore	238	35 (1–90)	33	14	25-Feb-03	5-May-03
South Africa	1	62	1	100	3-Apr-03	3-Apr-03
South Korea	3	40 (20–80)	0	0	25-Apr-03	10-May-03
Spain	1	33	0	0	26-Mar-03	26-Mar-03
Sweden	5	43 (33–55)	0	0	28-Mar-03	23-Apr-03
Switzerland	1	35	0	0	9-Mar-03	9-Mar-03
Taiwan	346	42 (0–93)	37	11	25-Feb-03	15-Jun-03
Thailand	9	42 (2–79)	2	22	11-Mar-03	27-May-03
United Kingdom	4	59 (28–74)	0	0	1-Mar-03	1-Apr-03
United States	27	36 (0–83)	0	0	24-Feb-03	13-Jul-03
Vietnam	63	43 (20–76)	5	8	23-Feb-03	14-Apr-03

Note: N.A. = not available.

Source: World Health Organization.

The Disease

SARS often develops into a serious lower respiratory tract infection, progressing to atypical pneumonia. Its incubation period is typically four to six days but may last up to two weeks. Asymptomatic infections are uncommon. In its initial stages, SARS is characterized by fever, chills, headache, malaise, and rigor. Respiratory symptoms of cough, sore throat, and dyspnea commence two to seven days later. The cough is productive in 25% of patients. Gastrointestinal symptoms, including nausea, vomiting, and watery diarrhea, are present in a similar number of people. Central nervous system and liver involvement may also occur. Associated hematological findings are discussed later in this chapter. Tachypnea, tachycardia, and hypoxia occur in 40% to 75% of patients admitted to hospitals. About 20% to 30% of all patients require intensive care, and many need mechanical ventilation. Radiographical evidence of pneumonia involving one or both lungs has been found in all individuals with SARS to date. Pneumomediastinum may occur later in the course of the disease. In patients with fatal outcome, the terminal events included severe respiratory or multiorgan failure, sepsis, and acute myocardial infarction. For those who die in the initial ten days of infection, autopsy findings include diffuse alveolar damage, inflammatory infiltrates, edema, desquamation of lung cells, and hyaline membrane formation, while those who die later during infection have organizing diffuse alveolar damage, squamous metaplasia, and multinucleate giant cells. The major factor underlying lung pathology appears to be direct viral damage of type 1 and type 2 pneumocytes.

Alterations in differential blood counts occur during SARS. Although the total number of leukocytes remains normal, 70% to 95% of infected individuals become lymphopenic. Lymphoid tissue of the lymph nodes and white pulp of the spleen become necrotic and atrophy, with decreased numbers of $CD4^+$ T helper cells and $CD8^+$ T killer cells, natural killer cells, and dendritic cells. Platelet numbers may also be slightly reduced. Due to the major roles of lymphocytes in adaptive immunity, including antibody production, and platelets in clotting, infected persons may be more susceptible to infections and bleeding disorders. Other hematological abnormalities include increased levels of alanine aminotransferase, creatine kinase, and lactic dehydrogenase.

Several factors influence the course and transmission of the illness. One of these is viral burden. A short duration of illness (less than 21 days) correlates with having a viral load of less than 1 million copies per gram of lung tissue. Transmission usually occurs after the fifth day of infection as the viral load in the upper respiratory tract and feces gradually increases. Age is also a factor. Attack rates are highest in persons between the ages of 20 and 39 years, and

FIGURE 21.1   Damage to the alveoli of the lungs caused by SARS

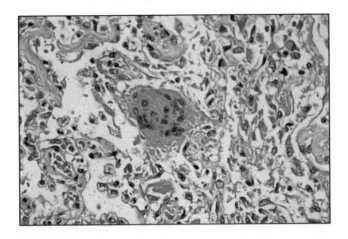

Source: CDC/Sherif Zaki.

only 1% of the infected were under the age of 10. Mortality rates are highest in individuals older than 65 years (52%) and decreased progressively in younger persons (45–64 years, 15%; 25–44 years, 6%; 0–24 years, 0%). The presence of comorbidities, extensive lung involvement, neutrophilia (high neutrophil count) at presentation, increased levels of lactic dehydrogenase, hyperuricemia, acute renal failure, and pregnancy are associated with a poor prognosis.

Pregnant women are particularly vulnerable to SARS. Infection with SARS-CoV increases the incidence of spontaneous abortion, premature birth, and need for emergency cesarean section. The development of disease during the second or third trimester of pregnancy is more likely to result in renal failure, secondary bacterial pneumonia, sepsis, adult respiratory distress syndrome, disseminated intravascular coagulation, and death than is the case for women who are not pregnant.

The Causative Agent

Intensive research rapidly determined that the disease epidemic resulted from infection with a new group 2b coronavirus, the **SARS-associated coronavirus (SARS-CoV)**, identified in March 2003 and found in the lungs of all patients with fatal disease. Mapping of the viral genome was completed on April 12 of that year. Other animals, including bats, macaques, ferrets, domestic and wild cats, pigs, and chickens, may be infected with SARS-CoV. Unlike the typical pattern for most epidemic-inducing agents, this virus is not amplified by passage through pigs or chickens after intravenous, intranasal, ocular, or oral inoculation, although it is detectable in their blood by polymerase chain reaction (PCR) or antibody detection.

Although *Rhinolophus* bats may be the principal reservoir species, SARS-CoV was believed to have entered the human population through contact with a very similar animal form of the virus in Himalayan palm civets or raccoon dogs because the first known cases of SARS occurred in animal vendors at live-game-animal markets or workers in restaurants serving civets. Severe respiratory disease does not occur in these animals. The humanized virus then spread rapidly from person to person via inhalation of large droplets of infectious respiratory secretions or through the conjunctival mucosal epithelium. Viruses are also present in feces, urine, and tears and remain viable for days on inanimate objects. Hospital equipment and procedures that generate aerosols, such as nebulizers and the use of suction, high-flow oxygen, and intubation devices, also facilitate transmission. Aerosolization of fecal material by a sewage system in the Amoy Gardens housing estate in Hong Kong, along with contact with contaminated surfaces (elevator buttons and door handles), may have contributed to infection of more than 300 residents. Transmission also occurred in an airliner, but it is not known whether this resulted from inhalation or contact with contaminated surfaces in areas such as the lavatory. A population of **"superspreaders"** appeared to have played a major role in viral transmission during the 2002–2003 epidemic. These persons tended to have more severe disease manifestations with a higher fatality rate, were older, and had a greater number of contacts with other persons.

Coronaviruses (in the *Coronaviridae* family) are enveloped single-stranded positive-sense RNA viruses with a large genome of 2,732 kilobases. Their surface bears projecting petal-shaped spike proteins, giving them a crownlike ("corona") appearance. Coronaviruses are spherical, with a diameter of 80 to 160 nanometers and have helical symmetry. More than 20 strains are known, and they generally infect the upper respiratory tract and cause a mild form of the common cold. Unlike other less pathogenic coronaviruses, SARS-CoV grows at 98.6°F (37°C), human internal body temperature. This enables it to invade the lower respiratory tract, leading to more serious symptoms, such as pneumonia. Typical coronaviruses grow at the lower temperatures present in the upper respiratory tract. SARS-CoV infecting humans during the later phases of the 2003 outbreak had a 29- or 415-base pair deletion in open reading frame 8 that is not present

FIGURE 21.2   SARS-CoV with projecting spike proteins

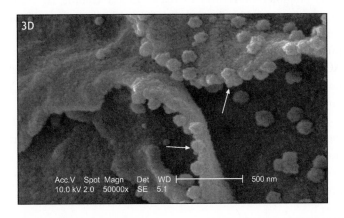

Source: CDC/Erskine Palmer.

in most SARS-CoV derived from animals. A number of new coronaviruses of animals and humans have been discovered since 2003. Research is needed to determine the potential of these or other yet unknown coronaviruses to infect humans and cause disease or outbreaks.

SARS-CoV from humans in the 2002–2003 outbreak uses its spike protein to bind **angiotensin-converting enzyme 2 (ACE-2)** on the surface of human and civet target cells in order to facilitate entry. The wild-type spike protein of civet SARS-CoV binds human ACE-2 poorly, but the mutation of two viral amino acids increased the binding 1,000-fold. The improved binding affinity may be an important determinant of pathology, for the 2003–2004 isolates from persons with mild disease were similar to those from civets but differed from those of the previous human strain in the binding area; these less pathogenic viruses bound ACE-2 only weakly. ACE-2 is expressed on smooth muscle cells and cells of the circulatory system, lung, kidney, and gastrointestinal tract. Viral RNA or viral particles have been found in lungs, kidney, intestines, liver, lymphocytes, lymph nodes, spleen, and skeletal muscle.

ACE-2 plays a vital role in human physiology raising blood pressure by two mechanisms. First, it aids renin in the production of angiotensin II, a hormonal vasoconstrictor that raises blood pressure. Second, it increases blood volume by reducing glomerular filtration rate and stimulating secretion of aldosterone by the adrenal cortex and antidiruretic hormone, encouraging salt and water reabsorption from the kidneys and decreasing fluid loss by reducing urine volume. Angiotensin II also increases blood volume by stimulating thirst. Due to its effects on blood pressure, ACE-2 is one target of medications used to treat hypertension. SARS-CoV binding to ACE-2, and thus its ability to infect human cells, is also blocked by several such medications, including soluble ACE-2 or anti-ACE-2 antibodies. ACE-2 also helps to defend against acute lung injury: by binding to this protective enzyme, SARS-CoV may aggravate lung damage.

Several other human cell surface molecules also bind SARS-CoV; these include DC-SIGN and L-SIGN. DC-SIGN may allow transport of viruses bound to dendritic cells of the innate immune system to new sites of infection. L-SIGN facilitates viral entry into cells but results in its degradation in the proteosome.

The Immune Response

The immune system may be both protective and pathogenic during SARS. Neutralizing antibodies to the outer spike protein (amino acids 441–700) produced by B lymphocytes during the adaptive immune response block viral replication. Many vaccine strategies under development attempt to stimulate the production of such beneficial antibodies. T cell responses play much smaller roles in host defense in this disease. The innate immune system may also provide protection. The mannose-binding lectin of the complement system binds and neutralizes SARS-CoV.

The immune response also contributes to the generation of disease during SARS. Some of the respiratory manifestations may be caused by inflammatory responses induced by the immune system, leading to the use of immunosuppressive corticosteroids in treatment regimens. Antibody titer rose earlier and to higher levels in persons with more severe disease course and higher mortality rate. Older individuals were more likely to be such "early responders." Strong Th1 T helper cell responses also were associated with poorer outcomes. Elevated levels of the proinflammatory cytokines IL-1, IL-6, and IL-12 and chemokines IL-8, CCL2, and CXCL10 may cause inflammation and stimulate macrophage migration into infected areas, potentially leading to tissue injury. The inheritance of certain forms of genes encoding elements of the immune response also affect disease susceptibility and severity. The major histocompatibility complex molecules HLA-B*4601 and HLA-B*0703 or low levels of mannose-binding lectin correlate with increased susceptibility.

RECENT DEVELOPMENTS

Both passive and active immunization strategies to prevent SARS are under development. **Passive immunization** by administration of humanized anti–spike protein antibodies to ferrets and mice decreased SARS-CoV replication in the lungs but was less effective in the nasopharnyx. **Active immunization** by vaccination is also being pursued. An attenuated parainfluenza virus type 3 vector was engineered to express viral spike, envelope, membrane, or nucleocapsid proteins that stimulated production of neutralizing antibody able to prevent experimental infection of hamsters and African green monkeys. Other viral vectors being used to express SARS-CoV spike protein include adenovirus, vaccinia, baculovirus, and vesicular stomatitis virus. DNA vaccines are also under development, including a spike protein DNA vaccine that protects mice by stimulating an antibody, rather than a T cell, response. A DNA vaccine consisting of nucleocapsid linked to the immune component calreticulin generates both T and B cell associated types of immunity and reduces viral replication in mice.

Several obstacles exist for SARS vaccine development. One obstacle is the fear of antibody-dependent enhancement of infection. Some vaccines based on the spike protein of isolates from the 2002–2003 outbreak increased infectiousness of the 2003–2004 human SARS-CoV isolate and the closely related civet SARS-CoV. Removal of the spike protein ACE-2-binding domain, however, appears to eliminate antibody-dependent enhancement while still inducing protective neutralizing antibodies. Another obstacle is the relative lack of a clear demand for a vaccine due to the disappearance of widespread or current infections. A vaccine may, however, be used to protect health care workers in regions with higher risk of infection or in the case of reemergence of SARS in the general population. Vaccines might also be useful for animals being raised in captivity for live-game-animal markets to prevent future transmission to humans.

Diagnosis

Due to massive efforts of researchers from 17 countries, the causative agent of SARS was discovered and its genome mapped within six months of the first known human case. Diagnostic tests were also rapidly developed. Virus may be cultured from respiratory secretions, feces, and urine.

Molecular and immunological detection techniques are more sensitive than viral culture. SARS RNA may be detected by molecular methods, such as

FIGURE 21.3   Processing samples from a SARS patient

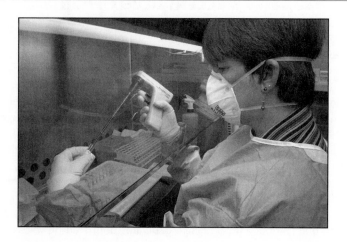

Source: CDC/Anthony Sanchez.

quantitative reverse transcriptase PCR (RT-PCR), in the stool or respiratory secretions by day 11 or 12. It may be detected more readily from samples obtained by endotracheal aspiration or bronchoalveolar lavage due to higher viral numbers. Real-time PCR now has a sensitivity rate of 80% early in infection. RT-PCR has sensitivity and specificity of approximately 100% in postmortem samples. Serological techniques, such as immunofluorescence or virus neutralization, are the gold standards for confirmation of SARS; however, other immunological assays, such as detection of SARS-CoV-specific antibodies by ELISA, are also useful. The production of antibodies by the adaptive immune response requires two weeks. ELISA has a sensitivity of 92% to 100% by day 28 of infection.

Treatment

Treatment for SARS may require respiratory support and intensive care. Care must be taken to prevent nosocomial spread. Antibiotics are not useful against agents like SARS-CoV, but several antiviral compounds are available that are effective in some viral diseases. Ribavirin is one such compound; however, it was not active against SARS-CoV in all cell types in vitro. During the outbreak, high doses of ribavirin were used initially in the hopes of in vivo efficacy, but this led to a high incidence of adverse effects. Medication dosage was decreased, and solo therapy was eventually abandoned. Other agents were more promising in vitro.

The **Type I interferons** (IFN-β-1a and IFN-α) halt viral replication, and the former eliminated 99.5% of virus after 24 hours in culture. These interferons bind to the IFN α/β receptor, setting into motion a pathway that activates the enzyme RNAse L that degrades viral RNA. The anticoagulant heparin inhibited infection of Vero (African green monkey kidney) cells in the laboratory. This agent may be beneficial in vivo as well, for it inhibits coagulation in the immediate vicinity of microbes, trapping them in a fluid phase inside the surrounding clot and thus allowing their destruction by antibodies and phagocytes within this enclosed area. Other compounds with activity against SARS-CoV include glycyrrhizin, baicalin, reserpine, niclosamide, the antimalarial compound chloroquine, and several HIV protease inhibitors. Research is being conducted on inhibitors of the viral helicase, protease, and spike proteins as well as analogues of the host ACE-2 protein.

When it was suggested that lung pathology during SARS might be immune-mediated, the immunosuppressive corticosteroid methylprednisolone was used in treatment. **Corticosteroids** reduce lymphocyte circulation and T cell functions by inhibiting the activity of NF-κB, a key participant in T cell activation and cytokine production. Corticosteroids also affect phagocytic cells, decreasing macrophage expression of the T cell activators, MHC class I and II complex molecules, inhibiting viral phagocytosis and killing by macrophages and neutrophils, and reducing release of the digestive lysosomal contents onto viruses found outside the cells. They also decrease chemotaxis. All of these factors combine to reduce inflammatory reactions, such as those occurring in the lungs of SARS patients. Corticosteroids should be used in combination with antiviral agents because when they are used alone, their immunosuppressive actions may worsen disease by increasing viral burden. Dual treatment with ribavirin and methylprednisolone did not lower viral load; however, when used together with alfacon-1 or protease inhibitors, methylprednisolone improved clinical outcomes in comparison with historical controls. Other immunomodulators explored for use in SARS therapy include pentaglobins, intravenous antibodies, antitumor necrosis factor antibodies, thymosin, and thalidomide. Given the current absence of new human infections, these agents have not been tested in controlled clinical trials but rely on testing in animal models. However, few animals—cynomolgus macaques, hamsters, marmosets, and ferrets—develop lesions upon experimental infection, and overt disease occurs only in ferrets.

Prevention

Individuals at the highest risk of becoming infected during the 2002–2003 outbreak were those in close proximity to SARS patients, such as medical personal. In Singapore and Toronto, health care workers accounted for 41% and 43% of the infected, respectively. Secondary infection due to close contact occurred less frequently, in 15% of all households and involving 8% of the household members of infected persons. Other risk factors were the presence of a chronic medical condition, visiting a fever clinic, eating out, and using taxi cabs frequently. Health care workers reduced their risk of infection by using respirators, gowns, gloves, and eye protection. Procedures that generate aerosols were minimized and preferably performed in negative-pressure isolation rooms. Members of the general population were advised to avoid situations under which

Table 21.2 Graded implementation of community containment measures

Level of Sars Activity	Response
No SARS-CoV transmission globally	Preparedness planning
SARS-CoV transmission in the world, but all cases locally either are imported or have an identifiable epidemiologic link to other cases at the time of initial evaluation	Passive or active surveillance/ monitoring of contacts
SARS activity in the area, with either a small number of cases in persons without an identifiable epidemiologic link at the time of initial evaluation or increased occurrence of SARS among known contacts	Quarantine of close contacts
SARS activity in the area, with a large number of cases in persons without an identifiable epidemiologic link at the time of initial evaluation; control measures are believed to be effective to increase social distance	Focused measures to increase social distance; consider community-level measures
SARS activity in the area, with a large number of cases in persons without an identifiable epidemiologic link at the time of initial evaluation; control measures are believed to be ineffective	Community-level measures to increase social distance; consider community-wide quarantine
Decreases in the number of new cases, unlinked (or "unexpected") cases, and generations of transmission	Quarantine of contacts
Transmission has been controlled/ eliminated; no new cases reported	Active monitoring in high-risk populations

Source: CDC.

they might be exposed to infected individuals, especially enclosed environments, such as restaurants, airplanes, and taxis. Other methods used in the 2002–2003 outbreak included those designed to "increase social distance" by canceling large gatherings and closing schools and theaters and requiring the use of face masks for persons using public transportation, working in restaurants, or entering hospitals. Disinfectants were applied to residences and vehicles of infected persons, to ambulance tires, and in pedestrian walking zones. The effectiveness of these strategies is unknown. To limit international spread, travel advisories were issued and travelers were educated by signs and videos, public address announcements, and the distribution of 31 million public health alert notices.

Surveillance

Due to the seriousness of human infection with the H5N1 avian influenza virus beginning in 1997, the world health community was watchful for clusters of cases of severe respiratory disease, especially in Asia, in 2002–2003. After detection of the SARS outbreak, rapid international responses identified the causative agent and its genetic structure, traced its transmission to and between humans, and halted the spread of infection.

During the outbreak, several unusual strategies were adapted to attempt to rapidly detect ill persons in order to isolate them and limit disease spread. Infrared thermal screening was one novel method used in some areas to attempt to identify persons with fever in public areas and at border crossings. Other methods included the recommendation that all persons in affected areas measure their temperature daily and the institution of fever telephone hotlines and evaluation clinics. Entry and exit screening of travelers included the use of questionnaires to determine the presence of symptoms or possible exposure and visual inspections. The utility of these strategies has been questioned.

Retrospective surveillance techniques were developed to identify and interrupt otherwise undetected chains of SARS transmission. A peptide-based ELISA for detection of anti-SARS-CoV IgG was used for a retrospective survey of healthy Taiwanese health care workers who had treated patients with SARS. Seroconversion among asymptomatic workers was found in two hospitals reporting nosocomial transmission. The assay had a sensitivity rate of 100% with seroconversion detected by the second week after the onset of fever. Individuals remained seropositive greater than 100 days. No cross-reaction was seen with other noncoronavirus respiratory illnesses. By contrast, RT-PCR is impractical for mass retrospective screening given the expense and the requirement for sophisticated equipment. Viral load also begins to rapidly decrease by day 9 or 10, decreasing the sensitivity of this technique.

In a number of countries, detection and isolation of infected individuals was combined with rapid identification and management of their contacts. These contacts were often placed in quarantine in their homes. Other people, such as travelers, the homeless, noncompliant persons, and those who feared exposure of their families were placed in residential facilities. Some people were temporarily excused from quarantine restrictions provided they wore masks, did not use public transportation, and avoided crowded public areas. Quarantine in the modern setting stresses the separation of symptomatic individuals from exposed contacts, isolating exposed persons for the minimal time period, closely monitoring them for disease symptoms, and rapidly providing medical assistance for those who do become ill. SARS was diagnosed in 0.2% to 6.3% of quarantined contacts.

Because SARS has a zoonotic origin (entering the human population via animals) and does not result in pathology in the animal hosts, inapparent infections as well as overt disease in animals sold in live-game markets and people exposed to these animals should be monitored to avoid future transmission to humans and to enable a rapid response should such transmission occur. This would involve cooperative efforts between public health workers, veterinarians, and those monitoring wild animal populations.

Summary

Disease

- Severe acute respiratory syndrome (SARS)

Causative Agent

- SARS-associated coronavirus (SARS-CoV)

Agent Type

- Virus in the Coronaviridae family

Genome

- Positive-sense, single-stranded RNA

Vector

- None

Common Reservoir

• Possibly bats

Modes of Transmission

• Primarily airborne by inhalation of large droplets of infected respiratory secretions or by their deposition on conjunctival mucosal epithelium

Geographical Distribution

• Highest incidence in parts of Asia and Canada

Year of Emergence

• 2002

Key Terms

Active immunization Induction of immunity by stimulating the recipient to generate an adaptive immune response

Angiotensin-converting enzyme 2 (ACE-2) Enzyme that raises blood pressure by converting angiotensin I to angiotensin II

Coronaviruses Group of spherical RNA viruses with a crown of projecting spike proteins

Corticosteroids Immunosuppressive compounds that decrease inflammatory reactions by inhibiting T lymphocyte and phagocyte responses

Passive immunization Induction of immunity by direct transfer of immune elements into a naive (never before exposed) recipient

Quarantinable communicable diseases Restricted group of highly communicable infectious diseases that require quarantine of infected individuals and often others with whom they are in direct contact

SARS-associated coronavirus (SARS-CoV) Novel member of the Coronaviridae family that was discovered to cause SARS in March 2003

Severe acute respiratory syndrome (SARS) Severe lower respiratory tract infection, often leading to atypical pneumonia, that emerged in China in November 2002

"Superspreaders" Individuals responsible for causing an unusually large number of secondary infections

Type I interferons Group of several cytokines that inhibit viral replication

Review Questions

1. When did SARS first emerge, and when did it reemerge? How did the severity and numbers of cases differ between the two outbreaks?
2. To what family of organisms does the causative agent of SARS belong? What disease is normally associated with this group? Why does the SARS agent cause a more severe disease?
3. What is the receptor on host cells to which the virus binds prior to entry? What viral molecule binds to this receptor? What is the normal role of the receptor in the human body?
4. What part of the immune system is protective in SARS? How does the immune system lead to lung pathology, and what cell types are involved? What drug may be used to decrease this type of injury?
5. What factors increased the risk of contracting SARS during the 2002–2003 outbreak? What protective measures were implemented at that time?

Topics for Further Discussion

1. What are some of the major novel surveillance and protective techniques used during the 2002–2003 outbreak? How effective were these in containing the spread of infection? What other disease situations may benefit from the use of these techniques?
2. Millions of people were screened for infection when entering or exiting countries. A relatively small number of travelers was determined to have SARS. Huge investments were made in extensive public education programs and in the quarantine of contacts of infected individuals. Considering the amount of money spent during this severe disease outbreak, the potential for widespread distribution, and the rapid end of this crisis, how do you think that international health funds should be allocated in the future? Factor into your answer other serious diseases that currently kill or sicken millions of people, such as tuberculosis, malaria, AIDS, measles, trypanosomiasis, schistosomiasis, infection with other parasitic worms, and diarrheal diseases.
3. Discuss the similarities and differences between SARS-CoV in humans and in palm civets. What measures might be taken to reduce the possibility of another jump of the civet virus into the human population in the future? What other serious human diseases originated by alterations that "humanized" animal viruses? How might the measures you cited be modified to prevent other human diseases from emerging in this fashion?

4. Quarantine procedures in the past differed from those used in the SARS outbreak and were often discriminatory. Compare and contrast the procedures used in the quarantine of individuals with smallpox in the early 1900s in the United States with those used in the 2003 SARS outbreak in Asia and Toronto, and discuss their relative effectiveness.

Resources

Bell, D. M., and World Health Organization Working Group on Prevention of International and Community Transmission of SARS. "Public Health Interventions and SARS Spread." *Emerging Infectious Diseases,* 2003, *10,* 1900–1906.

Chu, C.-M., and others. "Viral Load Distribution in SARS Outbreak." *Emerging Infectious Diseases,* 2005, *11,* 1882–1886.

Ho, M.-S., and others. "Neutralizing Antibody Response and SARS Severity." *Emerging Infectious Diseases,* 2005, *11,* 1730–1737.

Hsueh, P.-R., and others. "SARS Antibody Test for Serosurveillance." *Emerging Infectious Diseases,* 2004, *10,* 1558–1562.

Jiang, S., He, Y., and Liu, S. "SARS Vaccine Development. *Emerging Infectious Diseases,* 2005, *11,* 1016–1020.

Kindt, T. J., Goldsby, R. A., and Osbourne, B. A. *Kuby Immunology* (6th ed.). New York: Freeman, 2007.

Peiris, J. S. M., and others. "Severe Acute Respiratory Syndrome (SARS)." In W. M. Scheld, D. C. Hooper, and J. M. Hughes (eds.), *Emerging Infections* (Vol. 7). Washington, D.C.: ASM Press, 2007.

Saladin, K. S. *Anatomy and Physiology: The Unity of Form and Function* (4th ed.). New York: McGraw-Hill, 2007.

Wang, M., and others. "SARS-CoV Infection in a Restaurant from Palm Civet." *Emerging Infectious Diseases,* 2005, *11,* 1860–1865.

CHAPTER 22

WEST NILE DISEASE IN THE UNITED STATES

LEARNING OBJECTIVES

- Define and contrast the various diseases associated with infection by the West Nile virus

- Describe the flavivirus responsible for causing these illnesses

- Discuss modes of infection

- Discuss the host's response to infection

- Describe symptomatology and diagnosis

- Discuss methods of treatment

- Discuss methods of prevention

Major Concepts

Outbreaks

West Nile virus was first described in Uganda in 1937. For the next six decades, it caused mild infections in parts of Africa, the Middle East, Europe, Asia, and Australia. Severe disease became increasingly common in the 1990s. The virus entered the Western Hemisphere in 1999, carried by infected mosquitoes, most likely aboard a cargo ship that docked in New York Harbor. Despite large-scale spraying programs, West Nile established a firm foothold in the mosquito population of the northeastern United States and rapidly moved across North America. The greatest number of West Nile infections and severe disease in North America occurred in 2003, and incidence is currently declining.

Symptoms

Around 80% of infections with West Nile virus are asymptomatic. Most of the remaining cases take the form of West Nile fever, a mild condition characterized by fever and chills, severe frontal headache, ache in the eyes, pain in the chest and lumbar regions, fatigue, nausea and vomiting, swollen lymph nodes, or skin rash. Severe neurological illness results in fewer than 1% of infected individuals. Some develop West Nile meningitis, an inflammation of the covering of the brain and spinal cord, the outcome of which is usually favorable. West Nile encephalitis ranges in severity from a mild state of confusion to coma or death. Parkinson's-like symptoms or abnormal movement with gait impairment may persist following severe disease, and fatigue, headache, and cognitive dysfunction last for more than a year. West Nile poliomyelitis is due to inflammation of the spinal cord with symptoms similar to those induced by poliovirus, such as sudden weakness of the limbs or breathing muscles accompanied by great pain. Respiratory failure may occur due to paralysis of the diaphragm and intercostal muscles. This form of infection has a high morbidity and mortality rate, and survivors may require extended ventilatory support.

Infection

West Nile virus is a spherical, single-stranded RNA virus of the Flaviviridae family, which includes dengue and yellow fever viruses of humans and equine encephalitis viruses of horses. Some of the virus's closest relatives are the Saint Louis, Japanese, Rocio, and Murray Valley encephalitis viruses. Transmission usually occurs via the bite of a *Culex* mosquito vector. West Nile virus primarily infects birds (especially crows and blue jays), humans, and horses but may infect cats, dogs, squirrels, chipmunks, bats, skunks, bears, and domestic rabbits. Human-to-human transmission may occur following blood transfusion or organ transplantation.

Prevention

No effective drug has been developed for treatment of neuroinvasive West Nile disease. Risk of infection may be reduced by decreasing exposure to infected mosquitoes. Tight-fitting screens block insects from entering residences. Mosquito netting may be used to cover infant carriers. Light-colored long-sleeved shirts and long pants reduce skin exposure and aid in detecting mosquitoes that alight. Insect repellents containing DEET or picaridin reduce mosquito contact. Efforts may be undertaken to eliminate mosquito breeding grounds by removing bodies of standing water near residences. Larvacides and insecticides may be sprayed aerially to protect large areas.

Introduction

West Nile virus was first isolated in 1937 in the West Nile district of Uganda and was subsequently reported in other areas of Africa, the Middle East, Europe, South Asia, and Australia. For many decades, infections were generally mild and infrequent. This changed in the 1990s as severe disease became increasingly common and widespread. Cases of infection were first seen in the United States in 1999, and the virus began to overwinter in *Culex* mosquitoes in New York City in early 2000. It is now permanently established throughout North, South, and Central America.

Infection with West Nile virus is usually asymptomatic, but in approximately 20% of infected persons, a mild, self-limiting form of febrile illness ensues. A small number of those infected (less than 1%) develop severe neuroinvasive disease, which may be fatal. Some survivors have long-term or permanent neurological damage. The recent rapid geographical spread of the virus and the increase in both disease incidence and severity brought West Nile virus to the attention of both the health care community and the general public.

History

Infection with West Nile virus ordinarily resulted in occasional cases of mild febrile illness from its discovery in 1937 until 1957, when an outbreak produced severe neurological symptoms in residents of Israeli nursing homes. Serious disease manifestations remained uncommon until the mid-1990s. Large outbreaks of severe disease occurred in Algeria (1994), Romania (1996), Tunisia (1997), Russia (1999), the United States (1999–2005), Israel (2000), Sudan (2002), and Canada (2003–2004).

The virus is believed to have entered the United States toward the end of summer in 1999 from mosquitoes aboard cargo ships docked in New York Harbor. In August of that year, 62 cases of human West Nile disease, 59 of which were severe, resulting in hospitalization and seven deaths, and an **epizootic** outbreak in birds occurred in and around New York City, initially in the northern part of the borough of Queens. Genetic sequencing suggests that the strain (NY99) originated in the Middle East, with close similarity to that isolated from storks in Israel. Both isolates are unusual in their ability to cause a high mortality rate in birds. Prior to this flavivirus outbreak, most cases of viral meningitis were caused by an enterovirus and primarily involved children. Enteroviruses are transmitted by contact with contaminated fecal material. The persons involved in the 1999 outbreak did not know each other and had no common exposure history, but all reported spending time outdoors, particularly in the evenings. Serological testing of serum and cerebrospinal fluid samples indicated that the causative agent was antigenically similar to the Saint Louis encephalitis virus. West Nile virus was identified as the agent responsible for the human disease following its discovery during a large bird die-off involving thousands of animals in a simultaneous epizootic.

In 2000, there were 21 cases in humans, two of whom died, again occurring in New York, particularly on Staten Island. The epizootic in birds, however, had spread to 12 states, from Vermont to South Carolina, and the District of Columbia. That year also saw 63 cases of infection in horses in seven states, with a 39% fatality rate. In 2001, a total of 66 human cases and nine deaths were reported. In 2002, the number of cases increased to 4,156 with 284 deaths and the following year ballooned to 9,862 cases with 264 deaths. By 2004, the disease had appeared in almost all of the states in the continental United States. The state with the highest number of cases was California. The numbers of cases of human West Nile disease in the nation then dropped in 2004 and 2005 to less than one-third the number reported in 2003.

In recent years, the numbers of cases of West Nile diseases in the United States have fallen. From January 1 to December 16, 2008, a total of 1,370 cases of confirmed West Nile disease in the United States were reported to the CDC, of which 679 (49.6%) were West Nile fever, 640 (46.7%) were encephalitis or meningitis, 51 (3.7%) led to other clinical manifestations, and 37 (2.7%) were fatal. The state with the highest number of cases (411, with 13 deaths) was California; this accounted for 30% of the total number of cases in the country.

FIGURE 22.1 West Nile cases in the United States, 2000

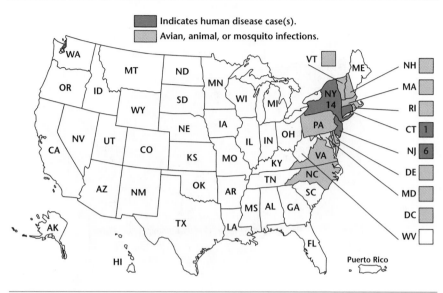

Source: CDC.

FIGURE 22.2 West Nile cases in the United States, 2003

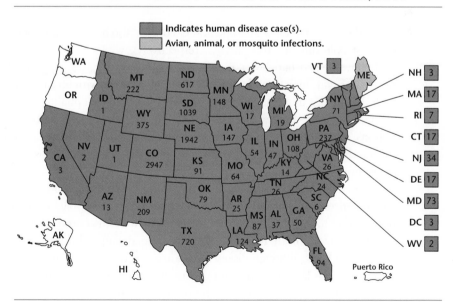

Source: CDC.

FIGURE 22.3 West Nile cases in the United States through December 15, 2008

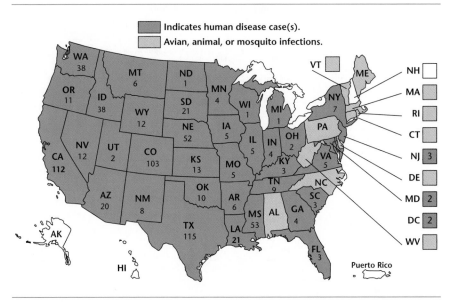

Source: CDC.

Two other western states, Arizona and Colorado, also had high numbers of cases of West Nile disease (109 and 95, respectively), while nearby Utah, Nevada, and New Mexico had lower numbers (26, 16, and 9 cases, respectively). The other state with high numbers of cases was Mississippi, with 99 cases. The states with the highest incidence rates of human West Nile encephalitis or meningitis in 2008 (highest number of cases per million population) were South Dakota, Kansas, and Nebraska. California, Arizona, and Nebraska also had the highest number of infected blood donors in 2008 (68, 26, and 13 positive donors, respectively).

West Nile disease appeared south of the United States in 2001 when a case of encephalitis occurred in the Cayman Islands. Surveillance of bird and horse blood found that antibodies to the virus were also present in Colombia, Cuba, the Dominican Republic, Jamaica, Guadeloupe, El Salvador, Mexico, and Puerto Rico, although disease incidence and death in animals and humans were rare. The lack of significant disease in these areas may indicate the presence of a less virulent strain or false-positive test results due to cross-reactivity to other flaviviruses.

West Nile disease among humans in Canada was first noted in 2002 as 426 people in Quebec and Ontario became ill and 20 died. As the number of cases in the United States peaked in 2003, a total of 1,494 cases with ten deaths occurred in Canada. As in the United States, disease incidence in Canada fell in subsequent years. West Nile disease during 2008 occurred in the southern portions of the Canadian provinces of Manitoba, Saskatchewan, and Ontario, and British Columbia and Alberta reported travel-related cases.

The Diseases

West Nile diseases occur in many areas of the world, including Africa, the Middle East, southwestern Asia, Europe, and North America. In temperate regions (latitudes 23.5° to 66.5°), they are most common during the late summer and fall in northern latitudes, in accordance with the biting habits of their mosquito vectors. In warmer climates, such as the American South, the diseases occur year round.

Mild West Nile Infection

Most infected individuals remain asymptomatic; no illness occurs in approximately 80% of those infected. **West Nile fever** is a mild illness arising in about 20% of those infected by West Nile virus and occurs in all age groups. It is characterized by fever and chills, severe frontal headache, ache in the eyes upon movement, pain in the chest and lumbar regions, tiredness, nausea and vomiting, swollen lymph nodes, and a nonitching skin rash. This condition may last from several days to several weeks. No permanent ill effects are associated with West Nile fever.

Neuroinvasive Disease

Serious disease symptoms occur in 0.75% of individuals infected with the West Nile virus; the fatality rate is 3% to 15%, and over half of patients with neuroinvasive illness develop long-term nervous system disorders. Most of the damage occurs in the brain stem, hippocampus, cerebellum, and anterior horn of the spinal cord. After a 3- to 14-day incubation period, a small percentage of infected individuals develop at least one of the following symptoms: severe headache, high fever, stiff neck, stupor, disorientation, confusion, coma, tremors, convulsions, muscle weakness, loss of vision, numbness, or paralysis. These may persist for several weeks with the possibility of becoming a long-term or permanent nervous system disorder. Neuroinvasive disease may be manifest in several forms.

West Nile Encephalitis and West Nile Meningitis

West Nile encephalitis and meningitis are inflammations of the brain and the meninges (coverings of the brain and spinal cord), respectively, following infection with the West Nile virus. West Nile meningoencephalitis may also occur. These conditions are found most commonly in individuals who are over the age of 50 years or are immunosuppressed, such as recipients of organ transplants, 40% of whom develop neuroinvasive disease. Half of the deaths in 2002 occurred in people older than 77 years. Meningitis is more common among younger persons, while encephalitis is more prevalent in older individuals. Severe disease manifestations are rare in children under the age of 1 year. Diabetes is a risk factor for death from West Nile virus infection.

The symptoms of **West Nile meningitis** are similar to those of other viral meningitis and include abrupt onset of fever, severe headache, Kernig's and Brudzinski's signs, and sensitivity to light and noise. Kernig's sign is the production of pain induced by flexion of the hip 90 degrees followed by extension of the knee. Brudzinski's sign is that flexion of the neck results in flexion of the hips and knees. Gastrointestinal upset may lead to dehydration. The outcome is usually favorable, although headache, fatigue, and muscle aches may persist in some persons. The fatality rate in the U.S. is approximately 2%.

West Nile encephalitis varies widely in severity and may manifest as a mild state of confusion or a severe form resulting in coma or death. A coarse tremor of the upper extremities is common and may be associated with movement. Parkinson's-like symptoms may also be seen, as well as abnormal movement or cerebellar ataxia with gait impairment. These generally resolve over time but may persist in patients with severe disease. Impaired movement appears to result from an attraction of the virus for the neurons in the brain areas involved in motor control, including the brain stem, the substantia nigra, and the cerebellum. Fatigue, headache, and cognitive dysfunction may continue for more than one year. Dysfunctions include difficulties in concentration, decreased attention span, apathy, and depression.

West Nile Poliomyelitis

West Nile poliomyelitis, also known as acute flaccid paralysis, results from inflammation of and damage to the spinal cord, especially the lower motor neurons, due to infection with the West Nile virus. It is manifested by sudden onset of weakness of the muscles of the limbs or the breathing muscles similar to that induced by the poliovirus. This weakness may be rapidly progressive and tends to affect one side of the body more than the other. Severe disease may lead to a more symmetrical dense quadriplegia. Weakness may also affect the facial muscles. Numbness or loss of sensation usually does not occur, but affected individuals may experience great pain. Respiratory failure may result from inflammation of the high cervical region of the spinal cord or the lower brain stem, paralyzing the diaphragm and intercostal muscles. This manifestation is associated with high morbidity and mortality, and survivors may require extended ventilatory support.

West Nile poliomyelitis was first widely observed in the United States in 2002. This condition occurs less commonly than encephalitis or meningitis and is seen in younger persons, with the peak incidence occurring between the ages of 35 and 65 years. Persons with this disease may recover limb strength completely or may not recover to any significant extent. Recovery of those experiencing quadriplegia or respiratory failure is slow and rarely complete.

Other Neuroinvasive Diseases Due to West Nile Virus

Another serious neuroinvasive manifestation of West Nile virus infection is the inflammation and demyelination of peripheral nerves, leading to a condition similar to Guillain-Barré syndrome. Affected persons experience fatigue and generalized weakness and sensory and autonomic dysfunction. The cerebrospinal fluid may contain elevated protein levels.

Table 22.1   West Nile disease in the United States, 2008

State	West Nile Encephalitis or Meningitis	West Nile Fever	Other Clinical or Unspecified Disease	Total	Fatalities
Alabama	11	10	0	21	0
Arizona	62	36	11	109	5
Arkansas	7	2	0	9	0
California	267	135	9	411	13
Colorado	17	78	0	95	1
Connecticut	5	2	1	8	0
Delaware	0	0	1	1	0
Florida	2	0	0	2	0
Georgia	4	3	1	8	0
Idaho	1	26	6	33	1
Illinois	11	4	4	19	1
Indiana	2	0	1	3	0
Iowa	5	1	4	10	1
Kansas	8	30	0	38	0

(Continued)

Table 22.1   West Nile disease in the United States, 2008 (Continued)

State	West Nile Encephalitis or Meningitis	West Nile Fever	Other Clinical or Unspecified Disease	Total	Fatalities
Kentucky	3	0	0	3	0
Louisiana	9	27	0	36	0
Maryland	7	6	1	14	0
Michigan	11	4	2	17	0
Minnesota	3	18	0	21	0
Mississippi	32	66	1	99	3
Missouri	12	7	0	19	1
Montana	0	3	2	5	0
Nebraska	5	44	0	49	0
Nevada	9	5	2	16	0
New Jersey	3	4	0	7	1
New Mexico	6	3	0	9	0
New York	31	13	0	44	6
North Dakota	2	41	0	43	0
Ohio	17	2	1	20	1
Oklahoma	2	5	0	7	0
Oregon	3	13	0	16	0
Pennsylvania	12	2	0	14	1
Rhode Island	1	0	0	1	0
South Dakota	11	28	0	39	0
Tennessee	10	7	0	17	0
Texas	38	24	0	62	1
Utah	6	18	2	26	0
Virginia	0	0	1	1	0
Washington	1	1	0	2	0
West Virginia	1	0	0	1	0
Wisconsin	3	3	1	7	1
Wyoming	0	8	0	8	0
Totals	640	679	51	1370	37

Source: CDC.

The Causative Agent

The Virus

West Nile virus is a member of the Flaviviridae family (genus **Flavivirus**). The dengue and yellow fever viruses are included in this family, as are the equine encephalitis viruses of horses. The West Nile virus belongs to the Japanese

FIGURE 22.4   Electron micrograph of West Nile Virus

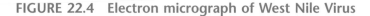

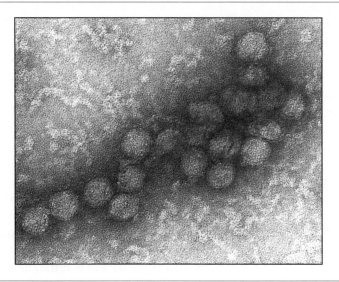

Source: CDC/P. E. Rollins.

encephalitis virus antigenic complex, which contains other viruses associated with neurological diseases, such as the Saint Louis, Japanese, Rocio, Kunjin, and Murray Valley encephalitis viruses. These viruses are spherical with a diameter of 40 nanometers and are surrounded by a lipoprotein envelope. Their genome is composed of single-stranded positive-sense RNA and is transcribed as one polyprotein that is subsequently cleaved to produce three structural and seven nonstructural proteins. The structural proteins are the capsid protein, which binds the RNA; the premembrane protein (prM), which prevents premature viral fusion; and the E protein, which functions in attachment, fusion, and assembly of the virus. A number of the nonstructural proteins (NSs) inhibit the host IFN response system. NS1 also impedes activation of the complement cascade by binding to factor H, a complement system regulatory protein. N-linked glycosylation of the E protein or NS1 increases viral virulence.

West Nile virus is cytolytic (it kills cells), and both NS3 and capsid proteins stimulate rapid, caspase-dependent apoptosis of infected neurons. Apoptosis is a form of cellular self-destruction and in the case of West Nile virus infection involves the host cell molecule caspase-3. Apoptosis is a common defense mechanism used by the body to limit viral spread by killing infected cells but may be pathogenic when nondividing cells, such as neurons, are eliminated as well.

West Nile virus is common in Africa, southern Asia, and the Middle East and is found throughout Europe, Australia, North America, and South America as well. Viral strains have been assigned to two lineages based on analysis of either the E protein gene sequence or the sequence of the complete genome. Human outbreaks are confined to lineage 1, while lineage 2 is maintained in **enzootic** cycles, primarily in Africa. The Kunjin virus in Australia has now been classified by a lineage 1 West Nile virus. The large outbreaks of severe neuroinvasive disease during the 1990s are believed to be due to the emergence of new, more virulent lineage 1 variants.

In addition to its mosquito vector, the West Nile virus infects birds, humans, and horses and may infect other animals as well, including domestic cats, dogs, squirrels, chipmunks, bats, skunks, bears, tigers, domestic rabbits, and alligators. Birds are the most important reservoir species. Horses usually recover after infection with West Nile virus; however, some become sick and die. A vaccine is currently available for use in horses. Experimentally infected cats developed a mild fever and were slightly lethargic for approximately one week; dogs remained asymptomatic. The low level of virus in the blood of these animals suggests that they may not be able to infect a mosquito and that they are therefore unlikely to serve as reservoirs for human infection.

Transmission

The vectors for the West Nile virus are mosquitoes, primarily of the genus *Culex*, which generally feed between dusk and dawn and are able to survive the winter in temperate areas such as New York. Fifty-eight species of infected mosquitoes have been identified in North America; the most important of these are *C. pipiens* and *C. restuans* (northeastern United States and Canada), *C. quinquefasciatus* (southern United States), *C. tarsalis* (western United States and Canada), and *C. nigripalpus* (Florida). Other species of infected mosquitoes include *Oclerotatus triseriatus*, *O. japonicas*, *O. vexans*, *Aedes albopictus*, and *C. salinarius*, which are more likely to bite humans. The primary route of infection occurs by the bite of a mosquito that previously fed on an infected bird. Birds circulate high levels of virus in their blood for several days. Over 280 species of birds in North America are able to host the virus, but birds of the Corvidae family, such as crows and blue jays, are the most susceptible. Once inside the mosquito, the virus travels to the salivary glands and is injected into the next host during a blood meal. The virus then enters the blood and crosses the blood-brain barrier to cause inflammation of the central or peripheral nervous systems. Fortunately, the infection rate among mosquitoes is generally low. In parts of Asia and Africa, the West Nile virus has been found in ticks; however, it is not known whether these insects play a role in transmission to humans.

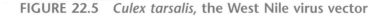

FIGURE 22.5   *Culex tarsalis*, the West Nile virus vector

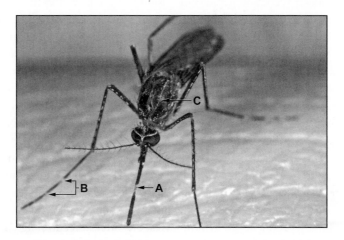

Source: CDC.

Human-to-human transmission occurs by several routes, including blood transfusion and organ transplantation. In 2003, two instances of transmission from contaminated blood were reported in the United States out of a total of 4.5 million transfusions. Both blood and organs are now screened for the virus by nucleic acid testing. Slightly over 1,000 viremic but asymptomatic blood donors were found. A very small number of infections have occurred through breast-feeding or transplacental transmission to the fetus, and transmission may have also occurred from use of a contaminated dialysis machine.

Infection with West Nile virus has not been found to result from casual contact with infected humans or other mammals. Contact with infected horses or living or dead birds has not been shown to cause viral transmission, nor has eating infected birds or other animals. Hunters dressing wild game birds, such as turkeys and ducks, may decrease their risk of infection by using gloves to prevent contacting the bird's blood.

The Immune Response

The immune system produces several types of IFN in response to viral infections. Virus replication is decreased in neurons pretreated with IFN-α or IFN-β in vitro, but after infection, these cytokines are less effective. IFN-γ is produced by several types of leukocytes, including CD4$^+$ Th1 helper cells and natural killer cells. It reduces early dissemination of the virus to the central nervous system. TLR3 and melanoma differentiation-associated gene 5 (MDA5) are pathogen recognition molecules found on cells of the innate immune system. Their engagement leads to the activation of transcription factors, including IFN regulatory factor 3 (IRF3) and IRF7 and the subsequent expression of IFN-stimulated genes. IRF3 is a major component in the host response to West Nile virus infection. TLR3 may also have detrimental effects, as it induces production of TNF-α, which allows viral dissemination (to be discussed shortly). One of the IFN-stimulated genes is 2-5-oligoadenylate synthase (OAS), which produces 2-5-linked oligoadenylates. These in turn activate RNAse L, an enzyme that cleaves viral RNA. Several of the West Nile NS proteins block production of IFN-β and activation of IRF3. Other components of the innate immune response, including the complement cascade, macrophages, and dendritic cells, are also important in host defense against the West Nile virus.

Adaptive immunity is vital in protection against the virus. Mice without antibody-producing B lymphocytes die after infection. IgM, in particular, is important, and the viral E protein and to a lesser extent the prM protein are targeted by host neutralizing antibodies. Antibodies to NS1 are also protective. CD4$^+$ T helper cells increase the production of antiviral antibodies, and their depletion increases mortality. CD8$^+$ T killer cells destroy lineage 1 West Nile viruses and reduce viral load in the brain.

The host immune response may also be subverted by the West Nile virus. The inflammatory cytokine TNF-α may induce alterations in endothelial cell permeability, allowing the virus to cross the blood-brain barrier. White blood cells that traffic into the brain may also serve as "Trojan horses" to transport virus into the CNS.

Diagnosis

Infection with West Nile virus may be determined by immunological means, such as an IgM capture or IgG ELISA of the blood or cerebrospinal fluid. IgM antibodies are produced early during infection, and this ELISA generally yields positive results using cerebrospinal fluid within eight days after the beginning of symptoms. IgG antibodies are typically produced later during infection. A plaque reduction neutralization test may be necessary if the person has been exposed to a similar virus, such as the Saint Louis encephalitis virus, which also occurs in the United States and has some antigenic similarities to the West Nile virus that may lead to a false positive result using ELISA. Antigenic cross-reactivity may also be observed following infection with the dengue virus or vaccination for the yellow fever virus.

RECENT DEVELOPMENTS

West Nile virus induces neurons to undergo a form of cellular self-destruction. CD8$^+$ T killer cells play a vital role in controlling West Nile virus in the central nervous system (CNS) by the secretion of perforin, an immune system molecule which produces pores in the virus membrane. To target the virus, T killer cells must first pass through the blood-brain barrier (BBB). This barrier prevents the passage of most immune cells, including T lymphocytes, into the CNS in order to prevent pathogenic inflammation such as occurs in multiple sclerosis. West Nile virus stimulates neurons to produce the chemokine CXCL10, which recruits CD8$^+$ T killer cells into the CNS after binding to CXCR3 on the T cell surface. Once they have entered the CNS, CD4$^+$ T helper cells help sustain antiviral CD8$^+$ T killer cell numbers in that location.

In addition to preventing immune-mediated damage to the brain, the BBB also inhibits elimination of viruses already present in that location. The chemokine CXCL12 and its receptor, CXCR4 on T cells, are found at the BBB. The interaction between these molecules serves to localize T cells to the perivascular spaces of the CNS microvasculature and restrict entry into the inner parenchyma, thus limiting their access to the virus. Recent studies have found that inhibition of CXCR4 enhances T cell entry into the CNS and increases viral clearance 1,000-fold. This subsequently improved survival of experimentally infected mice from 10% to 50% while reducing the development of a local pathologic immune response by activated astrocytes or microglia. Drugs which act as CXCR4 antagonists may therefore be beneficial in the treatment of West Nile virus infection.

Diagnosis may also employ virus isolation in a susceptible cell line followed by indirect immunofluorescent assay (indirect IFA) or nucleic acid sequence-based amplification confirmation. The Procleix WNV Assay on the Procleix TIGRIS system is a newly licensed automated nucleic acid test for West Nile virus. Reverse transcriptase polymerase chain reaction (RT-PCR) testing for viral RNA is less sensitive.

Treatment

No effective means of treatment is currently available for neuroinvasive West Nile diseases. Individuals with serious illness should be hospitalized. They may require supportive care, such as intravenous fluids and mechanical respiration. Care should be taken to prevent the development of secondary infections. The vast majority of infections are asymptomatic or mild manifestations, such as West Nile fever, and resolve spontaneously. Analgesic medication may reduce the symptoms of West Nile fever, such as head and body aches.

The antiviral compound ribavirin has in vitro activity against West Nile virus but has not been shown to be effective in experimental animal infections. It was not beneficial, and perhaps even increased pathology, in humans with neuroinvasive disease in Israel. Interferon, but not ribavirin, reduced disease in Syrian golden hamsters. Case reports in humans indicate potential clinical improvement in those treated with IFN-α2b. High-titer virus-specific gamma globulin (containing antiviral antibodies) appears to be useful for treatment in animal models of infection.

Prevention

Public education is a vital part of preventing disease, and New York City used a door-to-door campaign, a telephone hotline, and a Web site during the 1999 outbreak to inform city residents of protective strategies. The media also communicated valuable information to people in the affected area. Since the primary means of becoming infected with West Nile virus is by the bite of an infected mosquito, the best way to avoid the West Nile diseases is to avoid being bitten by these vectors. Windows and doors should be covered with tight-fitting, intact screens to avoid entry of the insects into residences. Mosquito netting may be used over infant carriers. During mosquito season and while outdoors in areas with large numbers of these vectors, light-colored long-sleeved shirts and long pants should be worn to reduce the amount of exposed skin and to aid in detecting mosquitoes that have alighted.

When outdoors, especially at times during which mosquitoes are more prone to bite humans, such as dawn and dusk, insect repellents should be used. Repellents do not kill insects but merely decrease the attractiveness of human skin. The Centers for Disease Control and Prevention consider repellents containing either DEET or picaridin (KBR 3023 or Bayrepel) to be the most effective. DEET may be applied to clothing and sparingly to exposed skin but not to the skin under clothing or to broken or irritated skin. To apply DEET-containing repellents to the face or to the skin of children, the repellent should be sprayed onto the hands and then rubbed onto the skin. Because repellents may irritate the mouth and eyes, they should not be applied to children's hands. Repellents should be removed from the skin with soap and water after returning indoors.

FIGURE 22.6   Application of DEET to clothing

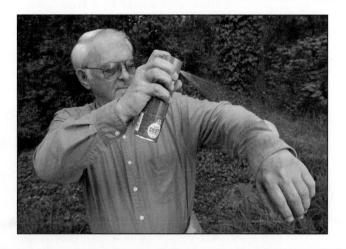

Source: CDC/PHPPO/DPDE/CAB/PhotoServices.

DEET has been shown to be safe for pregnant and breast-feeding women. These women are recommended to use insecticides because transmission may occur during pregnancy or breast-feeding even though infants rarely develop neuroinvasive diseases. DEET is not recommended for use in infants under the age of 2 months. It should also not be applied to dogs or cats because these animals lick their fur and would thus ingest the chemical. Insect repellents with DEET may be used at the same time as a sunscreen.

The percentage of DEET that should be used is dependent on the time to be spent outdoors. For example, 23.8% DEET provides protection for up to five hours; 20% DEET protects for four hours; 6.65%, for two hours; and 4.75%, for 90 minutes. Oil of lemon eucalyptus (containing p-methane 3,8-diol) is derived from a natural material and appears to provide the same degree of protection as repellents containing low concentrations of DEET but should not be used on children under the age of 3 years. Another long-lasting repellent produced from natural materials is IR3535 (3-[N-butyl-N-acetyl]-aminopropionic acid, ethyl ester). If the individual sweats or becomes wet, the repellent needs to be reapplied.

Insecticides, such as permethrin, kill adult insects. Permethrin may be used on clothing, footwear, bed nets, and camping gear but not the skin. Permethrin kills mosquitoes and ticks and may continue to be active after repeated laundering.

Other means of decreasing transmission of the virus from mosquitoes to humans or their pets includes the elimination of insect breeding grounds, which

FIGURE 22.7 Breeding grounds for *Culex* mosquitoes: irrigation ditch and water in a tree hole

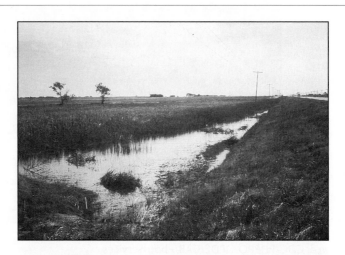

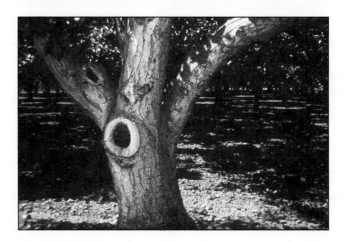

Source: CDC.

are areas of standing water such as may be found in flowerpots, buckets, wading pools, swimming pool covers, or clogged gutters. Holes may be drilled in tire swings to allow drainage. Water should be changed in outdoor pet bowls and birdbaths twice a week to eliminate the aquatic insect larvae. Communities may use biological larvicides or chemical insecticides to kill eggs, larvae, and adult mosquitoes. Larvicides are applied to the surface of water. Insecticides (such as malathion, resmethrin, and sumithrin) may be sprayed by hand or from trucks or airplanes. These compounds, which are regulated by the U.S. Environmental Protection Agency, were used in New York City during the emergence of the West Nile virus. They must be used repeatedly over a large geographical area to be effective.

Even though contact with live or dead infected birds has not been shown to lead to infection, dead birds should not be handled with bare hands. If dead birds are found, especially crows or blue jays that have died for no apparent reason, they should be reported to the local health department. If individuals are instructed to dispose of a dead bird, disposable gloves or an inverted plastic bag should be used to handle the bird, which should be sealed in double plastic bags before placement in a trash container.

Because transmission may also occur through contaminated blood or organs, the American Red Cross asks donors whether they are known to have had a past infection with West Nile virus and whether they have been at high risk for infection. Because the majority of West Nile infections are asymptomatic, the blood supply in the United States and Canada has since 2003 been screened for the virus using a nucleic acid amplification test. This procedure has detected more than 1,000 infected blood donors.

Currently, no vaccine is available for human use. Three effective vaccines have been developed for use in horses; however, they may not be safe for use in humans. The incidence of disease in horses fell after the first vaccine became available. Several human vaccine candidates are in clinical trials. Two of these are chimeric viruses in which West Nile virus genes are inserted into a live attenuated yellow fever virus or a dengue virus type 4 backbone.

Surveillance

The CDC is coordinating an electronic nationwide database (Arbonet Surveillance System) to allow states to rapidly share information concerning infection and diseases caused by the West Nile or similar viruses. Surveillance for West Nile virus should include infections of humans, mosquitoes, birds, horses, and other suitable hosts. When the virus is detected in an area, residents may be notified and educated about methods to reduce their risk of being bitten by a mosquito. During the 1999 New York City outbreak, both passive and active surveillance was implemented. Passive surveillance included weekly fax updates to the medical community and reminders to report suspected cases and provide samples for diagnostic analysis, which were then entered into a computerized database. Active surveillance included weekly phone calls to nine specialty areas (infection control, adult and pediatric general wards, and adult and pediatric infectious

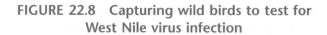

FIGURE 22.8   Capturing wild birds to test for West Nile virus infection

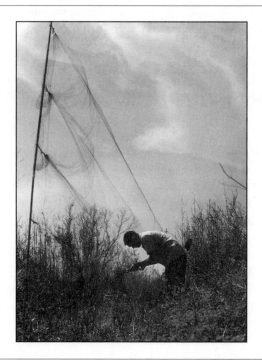

Source: CDC.

disease, neurology, and intensive care specialists) in 70 hospitals to ascertain the presence of new patients meeting the clinical criteria. A retrospective study of hospital discharge data was performed to determine the beginning of the outbreak. Suspect human cerebrospinal fluid samples were also screened by the CDC for antibodies to the virus. Surveillance of infection in birds has involved testing of dead birds and blood from live wild birds by the CDC in collaboration with the U.S. Geological Survey's national Wildlife Health Center.

Surveillance measures to detect the presence of West Nile virus in a given area have included the use of **sentinel animals**. This refers to the practice of keeping animals (usually chickens but also horses) in known locations and routinely sampling their blood for the presence of the virus (typically every 7 to 14 days). During the 1999 outbreak in New York City, the police department additionally used helicopters to detect unmaintained swimming pools that could host mosquito larvae, and the health department then sent sanitary workers to clean up the pools and apply larvicides.

Summary

Diseases
- West Nile fever • West Nile encephalitis • West Nile meningitis
- West Nile meningoencephalitis • West Nile poliomyelitis
- Inflammation of peripheral nerves

Causative Agent
- West Nile virus

Agent Type
- Flavivirus of the Japanese encephalitis virus serocomplex

Genome
- Single-stranded positive-sense RNA

Vector
- Mosquitoes, primarily *Culex* species

Common Reservoir
- Wild birds

Modes of Transmission
- Bite of an infected mosquito • Blood transfusion or organ donation • Mother-to-child transplacentally or during breast-feeding

Geographical Distribution
- Africa, the Middle East, Europe, South Asia, Australia, North America, Central America, South America

Year of Emergence
- 1999 (United States) • 1937 (Uganda)

Key Terms

Enzootic Endemic disease in animals

Epizootic Epidemic disease in animals

Flavivirus Genus of viruses that include the West Nile, Saint Louis, Japanese, Kunjin, and Murray Valley encephalitis viruses

Sentinel animals Animals deliberately placed in a particular environment to detect the presence of infectious agents

West Nile encephalitis Inflammation of the brain due to infection with the West Nile virus

West Nile fever Mild illness characterized by fever, headache, body ache, fatigue, nausea, vomiting, swollen lymph nodes, and skin rash following infection with the West Nile virus

West Nile meningitis Inflammation of the meninges due to infection with the West Nile virus

West Nile poliomyelitis Weakness of the muscles of the limbs or the breathing muscles resulting from inflammation of the spinal cord due to infection with the West Nile virus

Review Questions

1. What U.S. states have the highest number of cases of West Nile virus–related diseases? Where and when did the virus enter the United States?
2. What are the symptoms of the neuroinvasive diseases associated with West Nile virus infection?
3. To what family does the West Nile virus belong? What are other closely related viruses?
4. What are the most important vector and reservoir species for the West Nile virus in the United States?
5. How can infection with West Nile virus be avoided?

Topics for Further Discussion

1. West Nile disease was typically mild for approximately 60 years. In 1994, outbreaks of severe disease began to grow larger and more frequent. In 1999, West Nile virus entered North America and rapidly spread throughout the continent. By 2003, the number of infections peaked and began to decline. Discuss what factors may have led to the sudden increase in disease severity in the mid-1990s and why disease incidence in North America fell several years after West Nile entry into the region.
2. A number of severe diseases are transmitted by mosquitoes in various parts of the world today, and many other illnesses were more widespread in the past. What are the most problematic mosquito-borne illnesses in the world today, and where is each found? How were other such diseases eliminated from some parts of the world?

3. Most West Nile infections are asymptomatic, and the majority of the remainder result in mild illness. Speculate on what viral or human factors might lead a small percentage of infected individuals to develop severe disease.

4. Research the symptoms of diseases caused by other flaviviruses that infect humans. Where are these viruses located, and how many of them are newly emerging viruses?

Resources

Centers for Disease Control and Prevention. *Epidemic/Epizootic West Nile Virus in the United States: Guidelines for Surveillance, Prevention, and Control*. Atlanta, Ga.: CDC, 2003.

Centers for Disease Control and Prevention. *Interim Guidance for States Conducting Avian Mortality Surveillance for West Nile Virus (WNV) and/or Highly Pathogenic H5N1 Avian Influenza Virus*. Atlanta, Ga.: CDC, n.d.

Centers for Disease Control and Prevention, Division of Vector-Borne Diseases. "West Nile Virus Fact Sheet" http://www.cdc.gov/ncidod/dvbid/westnile, Dec. 2008.

McCandless, E. E., Zhang, B., Diamond, M. S., and Klein, R. S. "CXCR4 Antagonism Increases T Cell Trafficking in the Central Nervous System and Improves Survival from West Nile Virus Encephalitis." *Proceedings of the National Academy of Sciences*, 2008, *105*, 11270–11275.

Nash D., Cohen, N., and Layton, M. "West Nile Virus Infection in New York City: The Public Health Perspective." In W. M. Scheld, W. A. Craig, and J. M. Hughes (eds.), *Emerging Infections* (Vol. 5). Washington, D.C.: ASM Press, 2001.

Peterson, L. R. "West Nile Virus." In W. M. Scheld, D. C. Hooper, and J. M. Hughes (eds.), *Emerging Infections* (Vol. 7). Washington, D.C.: ASM Press, 2007.

Samuel, M. A., and Diamond, M. S. "Pathogenesis of West Nile Virus Infection: A Balance Between Virulence, Innate and Adaptive Immunity, and Viral Evasion." *Journal of Virology*, 2006, *80*, 9349–9360.

Samuel, M. A., Morrey, J. D., and Diamond, M. S. "Caspase 3-Dependent Cell Death of Neurons Contributes to the Pathogenesis of West Nile Virus Encephalitis." *Journal of Virology*, 2007, *81*, 2614–2623.

Shrestha, B., Samuel, M. A., and Diamond, M. S. "CD8$^+$ T Cells Require Perforin to Clear West Nile Virus from Infected Neurons." *Journal of Virology*, 2006, *80*, 119–129.

U.S. Food and Drug Administration. "FDA Approves First Fully Automated Test to Screen for West Nile Virus in Blood and Tissue Donors." Press release, Mar. 2, 2007.

CHAPTER 23

MONKEYPOX

LEARNING OBJECTIVES

- Describe monkeypox and compare and contrast it with smallpox
- Describe the orthopoxvirus responsible for causing this illness
- Discuss modes of infection
- Discuss the host's response to infection
- Describe symptomatology and diagnosis
- Discuss methods of treatment
- Discuss methods of prevention

Major Concepts

Outbreaks

Monkeypox is a zoonotic infection that occurs in several species of nonhuman primates and African rodents. Its natural reservoir is believed to be the rope squirrel. This disease was first noted in humans in 1970 in parts of Central Africa, particularly the Congo River basin, where it affected hundreds of people. It was later found to occur much less commonly in West Africa. In 2003, monkeypox entered the United States in a shipment containing infected West African rodents. The ill animals were housed in close proximity to prairie dogs, which became infected prior to their distribution as pets in several states in the Midwest. At least 37 persons became infected through contact with these animals and another 32 suspected cases were reported.

Symptoms

Monkeypox in humans is characterized by a smallpoxlike rash and lymphadenopathy. The causative agent is the monkeypox virus, an orthopoxvirus. The *Orthopoxvirus* genus is a group of large, double-stranded DNA viruses that include variola, vaccinia, cowpox virus, and buffalopox virus. Monkypox virus shares 85% DNA sequence homology with variola. Two distinctive forms of the disease have been reported. The first and more common form is found in humid lowland forests of Central Africa. This form generally has higher numbers of skin lesions than the second form. It has a case fatality rate of 10% to 16% and a moderate potential for transmission between humans, although at a rate lower than that seen for smallpox. The form of disease reported in West Africa and the United States is typically milder, with fewer lesions and a much lower mortality rate. It is also rarely transmitted through human-to-human contact. Genetic analysis of isolates of the monkeypox virus from Central Africa and the United States has led to their placement into two distinct clades.

Immune Response

Neutralizing antibodies play an important role in host defense against this illness. The monkeypox virus, in response, employs several mechanisms to evade both the adaptive and innate immune responses. These include the ability to block activation of $CD4^+$ T helper cells and $CD8^+$ T killer cells, blocking simulation of natural killer cells by producing a competitive inhibitor of the cell's activating receptor, and blocking binding of key cytokines involved in monocyte migration.

Diagnosis

Antigenic similarities between monkeypox virus and other more common poxviruses, such as varicella, make definitive diagnosis by serological means difficult. More sensitive and specific PCR and ELISA assays have recently been developed, however.

Protection

Treatment of monkeypox is often primarily supportive, although several antiviral compounds, including cidovir and ribavirin, are being developed or tested for use in humans with this disease. Prior immunization with vaccinia results in lower disease incidence and severity for those infected with the Central African–type virus. The risk of serious complications following vaccination, especially in regions with a high incidence of HIV-positive individuals, however, dictates against its routine use, even in endemic regions. Several promising vaccine candidates are being produced. These are highly attenuated vaccinia derivatives that provide rapid protection in nonhuman primate models and have good safety profiles in human testing.

Introduction

Smallpox (caused by the variola orthopoxvirus) was a dreaded disease throughout most of human history, resulting in great loss of life and often permanently disfiguring the survivors. Due to a heroic effort, this killer was eradicated from the natural world by an extensive campaign that concluded in the 1970s. One of the cornerstones of this campaign was large-scale immunization with vaccinia, another orthopoxvirus, which provided a high degree of cross-protection. Routine vaccination was then halted due to the high potential for development of serious complications, particularly in immunocompromised individuals.

After the elimination of smallpox and as a result of the heightened awareness of pox-forming diseases, human monkeypox infections were detected in parts of Central and occasionally West Africa in small villages located in the humid lowland areas. It was later determined that prior immunization with vaccinia protected humans against monkeypox virus infection and that vaccinated persons had less severe illness. As time has passed since vaccinia immunization ended and more and more people go unvaccinated, the incidence of human monkeypox cases has risen. In 2003, the importation of West African rodents into the United States led to the infection of prairie dogs housed in the same facility. Some of these animals subsequently infected humans in the Midwest. The clinical manifestations and transmission patterns of the Central African and West African and U.S. forms of monkeypox differ in several respects, leading to their separation into two separate clades that also differ genetically. The potential for serious disease and death from monkeypox, especially the Central African form, and the potential for its use in bioterrorism make surveillance for this disease a matter of great importance.

History

Monkeypox virus was first reported in 1958 as the causative agent of smallpox-type rash in cynomolgus macaques housed in a colony in Denmark. Nine instances of outbreaks of monkeypox were reported in similar colonies of nonhuman primates and in a zoo between 1958 and 1968. Six of the nine outbreaks occurred in the United States. A variety of species of monkeys and great apes were involved, including cynomolgus, rhesus, and pigtailed macaques; African green monkeys; squirrel monkeys; langurs; marmosets; orangutans; gibbons; gorillas; and chimpanzees. An anteater was also infected after close contact with an infected primate. The affected species of primates naturally occur in Africa, Asia,

FIGURE 23.1 Humans and nonhuman primates share living space in many countries in Africa and Asia

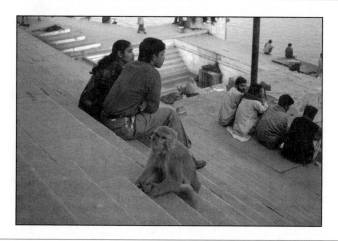

Source: CDC/Chris Zahniser.

and South America. The index animals in the outbreaks originated in Singapore, Malaysia, the Philippines, India, and Sierra Leone. Persons having close contact with the animals during these events, including their handlers, did not appear to contract the disease. No serological evidence of infection was detected at this time in other animals from Chad, India, Kenya, Mali, or Upper Volta.

Monkeypox was first recognized in humans in 1970, in the Democratic Republic of Congo (DRC; formerly Zaire) in Central Africa. Smallpox had once been widespread in the region but had been absent from the area for two years. Given the similarities in presentation between these two diseases, it is likely that human infections with monkeypox had been present in the area for some time and had been misdiagnosed as smallpox. Between 1970 and 1979, some 54 cases of monkeypox in humans were reported in tropical rain forest regions of seven countries in Central Africa, particularly the Congo River basin, and less commonly, in West Africa. The DRC had the overwhelming majority of these cases. Prior to 1980, studies of monkeypox were performed during the campaign to eradicate smallpox or to confirm the success of the eradication efforts. Vaccination against smallpox with vaccinia also produced a high degree of protection against monkeypox and decreased the severity of disease in individuals who did become infected. After the elimination of natural transmission of smallpox in 1980, monkeypox surveillance in the DRC was increased, resulting

FIGURE 23.2   Vaccination with vaccinia virus during the smallpox eradication program of the 1970s in West Africa

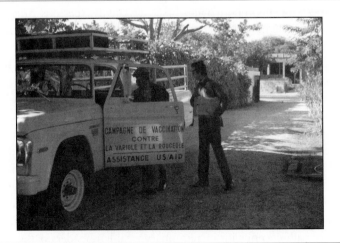

Source: CDC/Jean Roy.

in the detection of 350 human cases. Small numbers of infections were also reported in Cameroon, Central African Republic, Ivory Coast (Côte d'Ivoire), Liberia, Nigeria, Congo Republic, and Sierra Leone. Secondary transmission of the disease between humans was also reported in the DRC.

The number of reported cases of monkeypox dropped dramatically between 1987 and 1995 (14 cases total) and then rose after 1996, with several outbreaks involving over 500 suspected cases occurring over the next three or four years. One village was especially hard hit, with 12% of the population becoming ill. The war in DRC as well as the termination of routine smallpox vaccination may have been factors in the increased disease incidence, as the majority of infected individuals were under the age of 25 years and unvaccinated. Many cases in 1997 had serological evidence of recent or past exposure to varicella-zoster virus. Coinfection with HIV was not common.

In 1998 and 1999, several hundred suspected cases of monkeypox were reported. Definitive diagnosis was not made in the majority of these cases due to military battles, civil unrest, and security issues in the region, which is a major diamond-mining area. The cases during these outbreaks differed in several respects from the previously confirmed cases: the large number of cases, an increased incidence of secondary spread between humans (estimated at 88%), and decreased clinical severity with a lower mortality rate (1%). These differences suggest either misdiagnosis (confusion with chickenpox) or a change in the character of the circulating strains of the monkeypox virus. In cases for which a definite diagnosis was possible, 75% of the rashes resulted from monkeypox and the remaining 25% were chickenpox.

Monkeypox entered the United States in April 2003 in a shipment of six types of African rodents imported into Texas. Seventy-two persons (37 laboratory-confirmed cases and 35 meeting the case definition) were infected in Illinois, Indiana, Kansas, Missouri, Ohio, and Wisconsin. The origin of this outbreak was traced to close contact with black-tailed prairie dogs, including animals in a household day care facility. Increased length or extent of exposure to the prairie dogs was associated with greater risk of acquiring illness. Of the 11 persons initially infected, many had been scratched or bitten by the rodents. None of these individuals died, and in the majority (80% to 90%), the disease severity as ascertained by the number of rash lesions was minimal (1 to 50 lesions), even though more than half of the infected had no prior history of vaccinia vaccination including one child under the age of 5 years. In contrast to prior infections in Africa, vaccination did not appear to diminish disease severity, and few overall symptomatic differences were noted between pediatric and adult patients, although two children were admitted to intensive care units with encephalitis or retropharyngeal lymphadenopathy and abscess. Unlike the reports of infection in Africa, no human-to-human transmission of overt disease was reported in the U.S. outbreak, although subclinical illness may have occurred in three persons previously vaccinated.

The distributor of the infected prairie dogs in Illinois had housed an infected giant Gambian pouched rat from a shipment of animals originating in Ghana. Rope squirrels and African dormice from the shipment were also infected. The prairie dogs appear to have been the source of the human infections; virus was found in their skin, eyelids, tongues, respiratory systems, and mucosal secretions. Gambian rats have now gained a foothold in the Florida Keys. North American ground squirrels are also susceptible to infection. The viral strain involved in this outbreak bore genetic similarity to that previously found in primate colonies in West Africa and differed from strains originating in the DRC.

An outbreak involving 11 cases occurred in Congo Republic in Central Africa at the same time as the one in the United States, but the two outbreaks were quite different. One remarkable aspect of the infection in the Congo was that it resulted in seven rounds of human-to-human transmission, longer than previous instances in the DRC. The mortality rate was 10%, and disease was severe (more than 200 lesions) in a third of the cases. Most of the infected persons had an association with a hospital or lived in its vicinity.

The Disease

Monkeypox leads to a papulovesicular eruption in humans. Other infectious diseases characterized by this type of skin lesion include viral infections, such as smallpox (**variola virus**); chickenpox and shingles (**varicella-zoster virus**); hand, foot, and mouth disease (Coxsackie virus); atypical measles (rubella); eczema herpeticum (herpes simplex virus); and rickettsialpox (*Rickettsia akari*), as well as bacterial infections, such as yaws (*Treponema pallidum*) and impetigo (group A streptococci).

Initially, infection with the monkeypox virus (Central African type) results in microbial uptake by regional lymph nodes, followed by viral replication in lymphoid organs and viremia from 3 to 14 days postinfection. Early symptoms include fever, headache, backache, and fatigue. During the second week, skin eruptions begin to appear, evolving from macular (flat) to papular (palpable) to vesicular (fluid-filled) to pustular (pus-filled) lesions that crust and then scar during the 8 to 23 days following infection. These generalized skin lesions are in the same stage of development and have a **centrifugal distribution** (more concentrated on the extremities and head than the trunk). The illness is systemic, and lymphadenopathy is present in postauricular, submandibular, cervical, and inguinal regions in many patients. This Central African form of monkeypox is

FIGURE 23.3   Monkeypox skin lesions

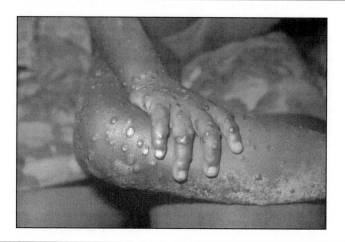

Source: CDC.

similar in many aspects to smallpox, which also has generalized papulovesicular lesions in the same stage of evolution with a centrifugal distribution pattern and is a systemic disease. Because of the similarities in the clinical disease seen during monkeypox and smallpox, the former has also been categorized as a category A select bioterrorism agent by the CDC. Smallpox, however, does not present with lymphadenopathy. Furthermore, cases of monkeypox generally occur in small villages in forests of Central Africa and occasionally West Africa, with the median age of infection being 4 years. Smallpox, by contrast, was cosmopolitan and struck unvaccinated persons of any age group. Monkeypox is transmitted fairly ineffectively between humans in comparison with smallpox (10% or less spread of clinical disease to family members for monkeypox versus 37% to 88% for smallpox); however, serological studies suggest that subclinical infection may occur in up to 28% of individuals who are in close contact with an infected person. Another difference between these two pox-producing illnesses is that monkeypox rarely passes through four rounds of transmission in humans, whereas smallpox, with no hosts other than humans, was passed on in this manner indefinitely.

Other closely related poxviruses may be differentiated from monkeypox by several characteristics. Cowpox and buffalopox are characterized by localized, pustular lesions. The lesions caused by varicella during chickenpox, by contrast, are smaller and more superficial, appear in successive waves ("crops"), and are more commonly located on the trunk. Varicella also causes less pronounced

FIGURE 23.4   Chickenpox rash on the chest

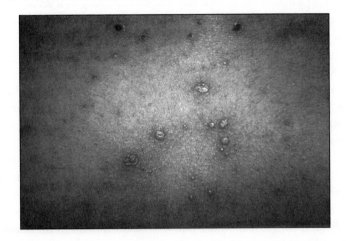

Source: CDC.

lymphadenopathy and is not often fatal. Other distinguishing characteristics of monkeypox virus include the production of small, opaque, hemorrhagic pocks when inoculated into chicken eggs; an upper growth temperature of 39°C (102°F); production of a generalized rash in monkeys; and a high lethality rate in mice and a lower rate for chick embryos. Atypical or severe chickenpox may pose diagnostic challenges in immunocompromised persons, including those with AIDS. HIV infection and AIDS are quite prevalent in parts of rural Africa where monkeypox and chickenpox also exist. Chickenpox has an increased fatality rate among such immunosuppressed people.

For the Central African type of infection, focal infection and necrotic cell death are found in the tonsils, lymph nodes, digestive tract, ovaries, testes, kidneys, liver (hepatocellular necrosis, portal inflammation), and lungs (pulmonary edema and hemorrhage). Necrosis also occurs in the epithelial tissues of the skin and mucous membranes. The overall fatality rate for this type of human monkeypox is 10% to 16%, similar to that of smallpox in the same geographical region. The form of infection found in West Africa is far milder, with fewer lesions, a lower fatality rate, and less human-to-human transmission. This type of infection is also characterized by sore throat, myalgia, sweating, cough, nausea, vomiting, nasal congestion, back pain, mouth sores, conjunctivitis, and gastrointestinal symptoms. Lymphadenopathy is less prominent. In the West African and U.S. form of disease, healing of skin lesions is sometimes accompanied by the presence of hemorrhagic crusts, which are not seen in the

Central African disease. This may be due to the inability of the West African strain to inhibit the complement system, leading to a greater tendency to bleed. Centrifugal distribution of skin lesions is less common as well (fewer than half of cases).

Monkeypox in Central Africa usually occurs in children under the age of 10 (80% of cases) and is most often found in males. This form is much less frequent and severe among vaccinia-vaccinated persons. Monkeypox in the United States is found approximately equally between the sexes and is not as skewed in age distribution. Prior vaccination does not appear to influence the rate or severity of infection.

Disease severity in nonhuman primates varies among species. Rhesus macaques, African green monkeys, baboons, and chimpanzees have only a mild form of infection, whereas orangutans develop severe disease with fatality rates of 3% to 40%. In these animals, illness is characterized by abrupt onset of fever, cough, listlessness, and decreased appetite. This is followed by generalized lymphadenopathy and eruptions after 7 to 11 days, with lesions especially numerous on the palms of the hands and soles of the feet. The evolution of lesions to the pustular form and crusting follows the same general course as seen in humans. Fatal disease corresponds to the development of a severe rash, dehydration, loss of weight, hypothermia (low body temperature), and collapse of the vascular system. Serological evidence of asymptomatic or subclinical infection is also seen in exposed primates in captivity and in rodents, large mammals, and some species of birds captured in Africa. It is assumed that monkeypox is a **zoonosis** acquired by humans from animals and that direct animal-to-human contact is required.

The Causative Agent

The monkeypox virus belongs to the ***Orthopoxvirus*** group, which includes variola virus (causative agent of smallpox), **vaccinia virus** (used to immunize against variola infection), cowpox virus, and buffalopox virus. Viruses isolated from humans are very similar to those derived from monkeys of the same geographical region. Tree squirrels, terrestrial rodents, and one domestic pig have been found to have monkeypox-specific antibodies. Disease incidence in Africa is greatest in regions with high mean annual precipitation and low elevation such as occurs in lowland evergreen rain forests.

The genome of the monkeypox virus consists of a single molecule of double-stranded DNA flanked by inverted terminal repeats. It consists of approximately 200 kilobases that code for about 200 proteins. Monkeypox virus and variola

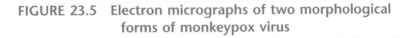

FIGURE 23.5   Electron micrographs of two morphological forms of monkeypox virus

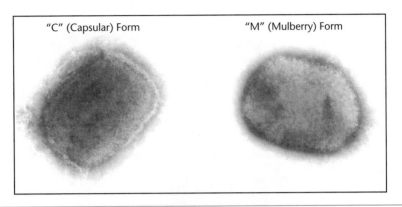

"C" (Capsular) Form   "M" (Mulberry) Form

Note: Depending on penetration of the stain, the surface of "M" (or "mulberry") virions are covered with short, whorled filaments, whereas "C" (or "capsular") virions present as a sharply defined, dense core surrounded by several laminated zones of differing densities.

Source: CDC/Cynthia S. Goldsmith, Inger K. Damon, and Sherif R. Zaki.

share approximately 85% homology at the DNA level. Virions are enveloped and are very large, approximately 250 by 200 nanometers (almost the size of small bacteria). Mature virions are produced by a complex process of acquiring and shedding lipid layers, which results in four forms of the virus (intracellular mature virus, intracellular enveloped virus, cell-associated enveloped virus, and extracellular enveloped virus), each with its own distinctive infectivity and immune evasion characteristics as well as associated proteins. Proteomic analysis of monkeypox virus and vaccinia revealed nine proteins that were specific to the former and eight to the latter. These proteins may be responsible for the differences in clinical severity of the two associated diseases. The monkeypox tumor necrosis factor receptor analogues were fragmented or truncated in vaccinia, suggesting an important role for this cytokine receptor in host avoidance of pathology.

Viral infection of experimental animals, including nonhuman primates, may be achieved by inhalation of aerosolized virus or by the intranasal or parenteral routes. In the case of infections in the United States from prairie dogs, transmission may have occurred via contact with infected urine or feces in an infected animal's bedding or by bites or scratches. Human-to-human transmission by contact with aerosolized droplets or body fluids is inefficient, and the virus is not often passed through more than three rounds of human-to-human transmission,

FIGURE 23.6　Electron micrographs of other orthopoxviruses that infect humans

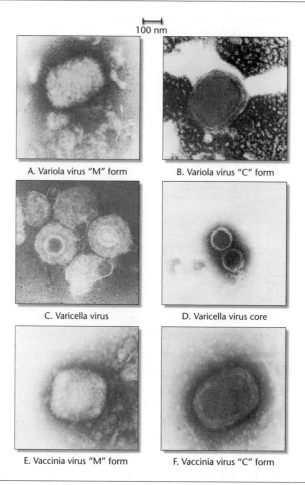

100 nm

A. Variola virus "M" form

B. Variola virus "C" form

C. Varicella virus

D. Varicella virus core

E. Vaccinia virus "M" form

F. Vaccinia virus "C" form

Source: CDC/James Nakano.

thus limiting the threat of large, uncontrollable outbreaks in human populations. The majority of human cases are therefore believed to have resulted from contact with an infected nonhuman primate, as frequently occurs in the small villages of the endemic area when monkeys raid crops of farmers, and from residents hunting these animals for food. Close contact may result from the monkeys attacking humans while being driven from the crops or from skinning or cooking the animals. Squirrels that live in the vicinity of oil palms near African villages may be the primary disease reservoir. Of 338 patients from the DRC from 1981 to 1986, 72% were infected by contact with an animal or animal tissue. In that study, young children were at highest risk for monkeypox—52% were aged 4 years or younger, and an additional 37% were 5 to 9 years old. Significantly, 96% of the infected children had not been immunized against smallpox, having been born after the termination of the eradication campaign or during its final stages.

Several varieties of the monkeypox virus may exist. The first of these predominates in the Central Africa Congo River basin countries of the DRC and Congo Republic and is characterized by relatively higher mortality rates and greater disease severity. More prolonged periods of viremia and a greater magnitude of infection have been reported. These isolates had a higher proclivity for human-to-human transmission, especially those originating in the recent outbreaks in Congo. Their strikingly high rate of interhuman transmission may be the result of genetic differences from DRC isolates or may reflect a recent trend in the evolution of this clade. Disease associated with isolates from the West African and U.S. clade is generally less severe and involves a lower level of viremia over a shorter time period. These isolates have decreased incidence of transmission between humans. The differences in the character of illness associated with these isolates could be due to genuine differences in the viruses or may reflect acquisition from different animal species or differences in the health care environment in these locales. Sequencing data support the former hypothesis, dividing the monkeypox species into two distinct clades, one containing isolates from the DRC and Congo and the other represented by isolates from the United States (imported from Ghana) and Liberia. Experimental infection of nonhuman primates with isolates from Central Africa results in more severe disease manifestations (earlier and more severe respiratory tract infection, higher viremia and viral load in the lungs, more severe depletion of clotting factors) and a higher fatality rate.

The Immune Response

$CD14^+$ monocytes are phagocytes of the innate immune system that serve as the primary host cells for monkeypox viruses in humans. Monkeypox-specific $CD4^+$ and $CD8^+$ T lymphocytes recognize monocytes infected with vaccinia virus, producing cytokines, such as IFN-γ and TNF-α. These T cells are not able to respond similarly to monocytes infected by the monkeypox virus in vitro, however. The monkeypox-infected cells prevent activation of lymphocytes via the T cell receptor but, unlike cowpox virus, do not affect expression of MHC class I molecules that are critical to $CD8^+$ T lymphocyte recognition

RECENT DEVELOPMENTS

Monkeypox virus has several mechanisms for evading the host defense system. One of these is the production of vCCI, a 35-kilodalton chemokine-binding protein secreted by virally infected cells. This suppressive molecule binds with high affinity to several chemokines, including migration inhibitory protein-1α (MIP-1α) from rhesus macaques, interfering with their ability to bind to their cellular receptors. In both in vitro and in vivo chemotaxic assays, vCCI completely inhibits trafficking of CD14$^+$ macrophages to sites of infection in response to this chemokine. While monkeypox virus may use vCCI to its own ends, the suppressive properties of this molecule may be used to the benefit of people suffering from diseases that involve exaggerated chemokine activity. One such disease is multiple sclerosis (MS). The vCCI protein is able to lessen the severity of the acute phase of this disease and completely abolish the relapsing phase of experimental allergic encephalomyelitis, an animal model for MS. Other autoimmune or neurodegenerative disorders that have the potential to benefit from therapy using vCCI include rheumatoid arthritis, type 1 diabetes, Grave's disease, Alzheimer's disease, Parkinson's disease, and HIV-associated dementia.

of monkeypox antigen. Expression of MHC class II molecules is similarly not reduced. Activation of both CD4$^+$ and CD8$^+$ T lymphocytes is inhibited by monkeypox, and this inhibition is generalized (decreased responses to other viruses as well as to monkeypox virus). The inhibition appears to be caused by a factor found on the infected cells. The generalized state of immunosuppression triggered by monkeypox viruses may allow for their escape from the host immune system. Interestingly, UV-inactivated monkeypox viruses are able to activate T lymphocytes, suggesting that alternative forms of antigen processing by the immune cells may still stimulate T cell responses. This type of processing may occur in vivo.

In addition to CD8$^+$ T killer cells, NK cells play a vital role in host defense against viral infections. The activity of these cells is stimulated by engagement of the **NKG2D activating receptor**. Monkeypox virus produces and secretes a protein that functions as a competitive antagonist of this NK receptor. The orthopoxvirus MHC class I–like protein is related to host MHC class I molecules. It binds to NKG2D with high affinity and blocks killing of the monkeypox virus by human NK cells. By inhibiting activation of both CD8$^+$ T killer cells and NK cells, monkeypox virus is able evade two of the most important cells used in defense against viral infection, increasing its ability to survive in the host and the likelihood of inducing pathological changes.

Diagnosis

Infection by the monkeypox virus may be determined using Western blot analysis for virus-specific IgG antibody. Other diagnostic tools include assays for plaque reduction neutralization and hemagglutination inhibition. The monkeypox virus displays antigenic and serological cross-reactivity with other orthopoxviruses, however, complicating the use of antibody-based tests in specific diagnosis. The use of monkeypox-specific monoclonal antibodies in IgM capture ELISAs or real-time polymerase chain reaction (PCR) directed against the monkeypox B21 protein appear to be more sensitive and specific diagnostic techniques. This approach has also shortened the time needed for data acquisition and allowed higher throughput of samples.

The ability to accurately diagnose monkeypox infection in individuals with clinically inapparent disease is difficult, particularly in those who were previously immunized with vaccinia. A recent diagnostic modification has proved useful: when samples are preadsorbed with vaccinia antigens prior to ELISA, the overall sensitivity for detecting monkeypox (including asymptomatic infection) is 86%, which increases to 100% for clinically apparent disease. The specificity appears to be 100%; however, cross-reaction with other orthopoxviruses, such as varicella, was not tested. A similar preadsorption approach to Western blot analysis was less sensitive.

FIGURE 23.7   Real-time PCR

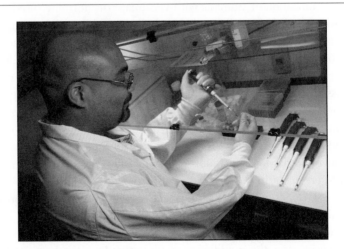

Source: CDC/Hsi Liu and James Gathany.

In light of the prevalence of chickenpox in the affected areas of the DRC and the high rate of coinfection with monkeypox, care needs to be taken not to confuse the two infections or to fail to recognize the presence of both in the case of coinfection. This is particularly true when the epidemiological evidence supports a less virulent infection with a lower fatality rate or in the face of increased levels of secondary transmission between humans.

Treatment

No specific treatment is recommended for monkeypox. A panel of 23 antiviral compounds was evaluated for their effectiveness against a variety of orthopoxviruses. Three of these were significantly effective against variola infection in tissue culture cells but had only moderate activity against monkeypox. Cidofovir and ribavirin are undergoing clinical testing in rodents and macaques.

Supportive care is used to prevent complications and decrease risk of death. Measures include hydration, proper nutrition, and the use of antibiotics for accompanying bacterial infections of the skin or respiratory tract.

Prevention

Immunization of humans with vaccinia virus (formerly used to protect humans from acquiring smallpox due to infection with variola virus) safeguards more than 85% of the recipients against monkeypox. Routine use of this vaccine is not recommended, even in areas where monkeypox is endemic, because the frequency of this disease is low and there is a high risk of serious complications associated with vaccinia administration, particularly for immunosuppressed individuals or those with eczema. Immunization with vaccinia is estimated to lead to one death and 20 serious complications per million vaccinations for the general public. Vaccination with the commercially licensed Dryvax vaccine poses a considerable risk for individuals with HIV infection or AIDS, since these conditions are prevalent in the affected regions.

The development of an effective killed vaccinia or monkeypox vaccine, a subunit vaccine, or a safer attenuated vaccinia vaccine may allow protection in endemic areas without the risk of developing vaccine-associated pathology. One such vaccine, the modified vaccinia virus *Ankara*, is being evaluated in animals

FIGURE 23.8 Dryvax vaccine used to prevent smallpox and monkeypox

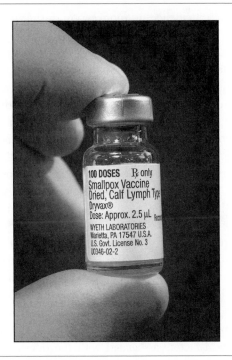

Source: CDC.

and humans. Priming and boosting efforts using this highly attenuated strain have induced humoral (neutralizing antibody) and cellular immunity ($CD8^+$ T lymphocyte and IFN-γ) that has proved protective for over two years in a monkeypox virus challenge model. Neutralizing antibodies are vital to protective immunity against monkeypox viruses. This vaccine also provides protection as early as four days following immunization. Protection is accomplished in a single round of vaccination and was shown to be safe in a trial of over 100,000 persons.

In the 2003 U.S. outbreak, implementation of personal protective measures appeared to have prevented development of infection and illness in medical personnel, even when compliance was less than optimal among a partially vaccinated group of health care workers. In a follow-up study, only 29% of the participants reported consistently strict adherence to measures such as the use of gloves and masks or N-95 respirators.

Surveillance

The increased incidence of monkeypox during the mid to late 1990s, as well as the uncertainty of the correct diagnosis for many of these cases, suggests that more vigorous surveillance and diagnostic measures are needed to accurately track the incidence and spread of monkeypox throughout Africa, with particular emphasis on the endemic regions of the DRC, and to ascertain whether the characteristics of infection are indeed changing with time (incidence of human-to-human spread, disease severity). A major factor in the increased prevalence of monkeypox is the halting of routine immunization with vaccinia after the successful eradication of naturally occurring smallpox. It may be advisable to consider surveillance measures for atypical chickenpox cases in the United States as well due to the presence of susceptible rodent species such as prairie dogs, ground squirrels, and the presence of giant Gambian pouched rats in Florida.

In 1999, the World Health Organization Monkeypox Technical Advisory Group prepared a list of recommendations for continuing surveillance efforts. Factors that interfere with the proper implementation of such surveillance studies include military action, civil unrest, poor public health infrastructure, confusion with chickenpox infection, and difficulty in serological differentiation of monkeypox and other orthopoxviruses. Further studies are needed to address these challenges and to establish the natural history of infection and the associated ecological and epidemiological factors associated with the disease and its geographical spread. Increased awareness of monkeypox among the health care community and public health workers, as well as education programs for the general public in endemic areas, are needed to identify and limit the spread of this disease. To accomplish these tasks, increased financial resources, training, and logistical support will be needed.

Summary

Disease

- Monkeypox

Causative Agent

- Monkeypox virus

Agent Type

- Orthopoxvirus

Genome

- Double-stranded DNA

Vector

- None

Common Reservoir

- Squirrels (most likely)

Modes of Transmission

- Inhalation • Contact with mucosal secretions or skin lesions
- Human-to-human transmission (limited)

Geographical Distribution

- Central and West Africa • United States

Year of Emergence

- 1970 • 2003

Key Terms

Centrifugal distribution Concentration of skin lesions on the extremities and head greater than those located on the trunk; occurs in smallpox and the Central African form of monkeypox

Monkeypox Illness similar to smallpox characterized by papulovesicular rash and lymphadenopathy; affects human and nonhuman primates and rodents

Monkeypox virus An orthopoxvirus; causative agent of monkeypox

NKG2D activating receptor Receptor on natural killer cells whose engagement activates these cells

Orthopoxvirus Viral group that includes the monkeypox, variola, vaccinia, and buffalopox viruses

Vaccinia virus Virus used for massive vaccination against variola

Varicella-zoster virus Causative agent of chickenpox and shingles

Variola virus Causative agent of smallpox

Zoonosis Disease that occurs primarily in animals but may be transmitted to humans

Review Questions

1. How do the forms of monkeypox from Central Africa differ from those found in West Africa and the United States?
2. To what viral group does the monkeypox virus belong? Name some other closely related poxviruses. What are several other diseases with similar rashes?
3. How is monkeypox transmitted from animals to humans? What animal species transmitted the disease to humans in the U.S. Midwest?
4. How might monkeypox infection be prevented? What are the possible risks involved?
5. What are the two most sensitive and specific means of diagnosing infection with monkeypox? Why have other serological assays had low specificity in the past?

Topics for Further Discussion

1. The Central African form of monkeypox results in a rash similar to that seen previously during outbreaks of smallpox. The mortality rate for this form of the disease is 10% to 16%. With the eradication of naturally occurring smallpox in the late 1970s, monkeypox became the most dangerous of the remaining orthopoxviruses that infect humans. For this reason, it is considered a potential bioweapon. What disease feature has stopped the development of large-scale outbreaks and prevented the use of the monkeypox virus as an agent of mass destruction in humans?
2. Should terrorists ever convert the monkeypox virus into a bioweapon or if they would acquire a vial of the remaining stocks of variola virus, what methods could be employed to prevent or halt large-scale loss of life? Would these methods be of practical use in areas with limited financial resources?
3. In regions where the more virulent form of monkeypox is currently endemic and where the incidence of HIV and AIDS is substantial, what methods might be undertaken to prevent human infection or to limit its spread should an outbreak occur? The cowpox virus, which induced a mild form of disease in milkmaids, was used by Edward Jenner to immunize people against the far more pathogenic but antigenically similar variola virus. Discuss the pros and cons of the possible use of the West African clade of monkeypox virus to prevent infection with viruses from the Central African clade.
4. More detailed surveillance for monkeypox occurrence and studies of its natural ecology and disease reservoirs in Central and West Africa would be

of great use in better understanding current trends in viral evolution and in predicting or detecting future outbreaks. Such studies are hampered by lack of available funds, trained personnel, proper education of health care workers and the general populace, and civil unrest or war in the affected regions. Discuss how these obstacles might be overcome, not only for monkeypox but also for other emerging diseases in this part of the world.

Resources

Bernard, S. M., and Anderson, S. A. "Qualitative Assessment of Risk for Monkeypox Associated with Domestic Trade in Certain Animal Species, United States." *Emerging Infectious Diseases,* 2006, *12,* 1827–1833.

Breman, J. G. "Monkeypox: An Emerging Infection for Humans?" In W. M. Scheld, W. A. Craig, and J. M. Hughes (eds.), *Emerging Infections* (Vol. 4). Washington, D.C.: ASM Press, 2000.

Campbell, J. A., Trossman, D. S., Yokoyama, W. M., and Carayannopoulos, L. M. "Zoonotic Orthopoxviruses Encode a High-Affinity Antagonist of NKG2D." *Journal of Experimental Medicine,* 2007, *204,* 1311–1317.

Damon, I. "Monkeypox Virus: Insights on Its Emergence in Human Populations." In W. M. Scheld, D. C. Hooper, and J. M. Hughes (eds.), *Emerging Infections* (Vol. 7). Washington, D.C.: ASM Press, 2007.

Dubois, M. E., and Slifka, M. K. "Retrospective Analysis of Monkeypox Infection." *Emerging Infectious Diseases,* 2008, *14,* 592–599.

Earl, P. E., and others. "Rapid Protection in a Monkeypox Model by a Single Injection of a Replication-Deficient Vaccinia Virus." *Proceedings of the National Academy of Sciences,* 2008, *105,* 10889–10894.

Hammarlund, E., and others. "Monkeypox Virus Evades Antiviral CD^+ and $CD8^+$ T Cell Responses by Suppressing Cognate T Cell Activation." *Proceedings of the National Academy of Sciences,* 2008, *105,* 14567–14572.

Jones, J. M., and others. "Monkeypox Virus Viral Chemokine Inhibitor (MPV vCCI), a Potent Inhibitor of Rhesus Macrophage Inflammatory Protein-1." *Cytokine,* 2008, *43,* 220–228.

Manes, N. P., and others. "Comparative Proteomics of Human Monkeypox and Vaccinia Intracellular Mature and Extracellular Enveloped Virions." *Journal of Proteome Research,* 2008, *7,* 960–968.

Sale, T. A., Melski, J. W., and Stratman, E. J. "Monkeypox: An Epidemiologic and Clinical Comparison of African and U.S. Disease." *Journal of the American Academy of Dermatologists,* 2006, *55,* 478–481.

Sbrana, E., Xiao, S.-Y., Newman, P. C., and Tesh, R. B. "Comparative Pathology of North American and Central African Strains of Monkeypox Virus in a Ground Squirrel Model of the Disease." *American Journal of Tropical Medicine and Hygiene,* 2007, *76,* 155–164.

PARASITIC INFECTIONS

CHAPTER 24

MALARIA: REEMERGENCE AND RECENT SUCCESSES

LEARNING OBJECTIVES

- Define and contrast the various forms of malaria

- Describe the Apicomplexan protozoa responsible for causing this illness

- Discuss modes of infection

- Discuss the host's response to infection

- Describe symptomatology and diagnosis

- Discuss methods of treatment

- Discuss methods of prevention

Major Concepts

Historical Incidence

Malaria has plagued humankind since antiquity. In the third century B.C., the conquests of Alexander the Great were cut short by this disease. Italy was long affected by the illness. A swampy area near ancient Rome, the Pontina, was noted for its high rate of infection. In the 1930s, the Italian dictator Benito Mussolini drained the swamps and greatly decreased disease incidence. Malaria was once common in parts of the United States, particularly the southern states but also in areas such as northern Ohio. In the early 1900s, construction of the Panama Canal required decreasing the incidence of mosquito-borne malaria and yellow fever by reducing vector numbers. Toward the end of that century, after several major battles in the war against malaria had been won, the tide began to turn and malaria began to reemerge in some areas of the world due to resistance and increased travel and migration to endemic areas.

Current Impact

At present, 350 to 500 million people are infected with the malaria parasites, and more than 1 million of them die each year, making malaria one of the major causes of death from infectious diseases today. Sub-Saharan Africa has been and remains one of the hardest-hit areas, with about 90% of the world's cases, the majority occurring in young children. In addition to the high death toll in the very young, infection of either expectant mother or fetus leads to premature birth, low birth weight, anemia, epilepsy, and learning difficulties in children. Countries in this region suffer huge economic losses resulting from ill workers, decreased tourism, and the unwillingness of companies to invest in high-risk areas.

Symptoms

Malaria is best known for its cyclical periods of severe high fever and chills, but nonspecific symptoms occur as well, including headache, fatigue, abdominal discomfort and vomiting, muscle and joint aches, loss of appetite, and malaise. The cycles last either 48 or 72 hours, depending on the species of parasite. These result from periodic rupture of infected erythrocytes, the release of large amounts of hemoglobin, and its conversion into the toxic compound bilirubin. Exposure to bilirubin may result in renal or heart failure. One of the more serious consequences of infection is cerebral malaria, characterized by progressive headache, very high fever, psychosis, convulsions, coma, and rapid death. Another very serious condition is blackwater fever, in which the kidneys are damaged by massive amounts of hemoglobin, producing black urine and death from renal failure. The mortality rate for cerebral malaria and blackwater fever is 20% to 50%. Other serious complications of malaria include severe anemia, metabolic acidosis, hypoglycemia, and acute pulmonary edema. Young children are most vulnerable to developing severe disease due to their lack of protective antibodies.

Infection

Four members of the *Plasmodium* genus of Apicomplexan protozoa cause human malaria. The most pathogenic of these is *P. falciparum*, which kills more erythrocytes than the other species because it infects red blood cells of any age. This species also has the highest rate of drug resistance. *P. vivax* is found more commonly in temperate zones and causes a milder form of the disease. It infects only immature erythrocytes. *P. malariae* infects older cells and has a longer cycle than the other species. *P. ovale* is the rarest of the malarial parasites. *Plasmodium* species have a complex life cycle involving two different hosts, the *Anopheles* mosquito and a human host. Sporozoites are injected into humans as female mosquitoes take a blood meal. They travel to the liver and infect hepatocytes, transforming into merozoites, which multiply asexually and subsequently burst the host cell to travel into the bloodstream and infect erythrocytes. Once inside these blood cells, asexual reproduction leads to the production of more merozoites. These rupture the infected cells and enter new erythrocytes to continue the cycle in humans. Other merozoites transform into male and female gametocytes that are ingested by a mosquito feeding on the infected person. Once inside the mosquito, the gametocytes produce micro- and macrogametes, similar to sperm and eggs. A microgamete fertilizes the macrogamete and produces a motile zygote, the ookinete, which penetrates the mosquito's stomach and transforms into an oocyst on the exterior of that organ. Asexual reproduction results in the formation of multiple sporozoites that travel to the mosquito's salivary glands in preparation for being transferred to the next human host.

Protection

Treatment for malaria has historically included drugs such as artemisinin from wormwood, quinine, and chloroquine. Drug resistance reduced the effectiveness of these and other more recently developed drugs, leading to a resurgence in disease incidence. The insecticide DDT was once very effective in reducing numbers of the mosquito vectors, but many regions either banned or severely restricted its use, and mosquitoes subsequently became resistant to this inexpensive and non-toxic insecticide. Several effective campaigns are currently under way to decrease malarial incidence, particularly in sub-Saharan Africa. These rely heavily on the use of DDT-treated bed nets and indoor residual insecticide use.

Introduction

In human beings, malaria is caused by four species of parasitic blood protozoa of the genus *Plasmodium*. Malaria is a huge health problem worldwide, with 350 to 500 million people infected and 1 to 2 million dying each year. Approximately 41% of the world's population is at risk for contracting disease, with 90% of the cases occurring in sub-Saharan Africa. Most of these are in children less than 5 years of age and are responsible for 20% of the childhood deaths in Africa. In addition to death, malarial infection induces premature birth, low birth weight, anemia, epilepsy, and learning difficulties in children. This decreases educational opportunities for children and may lead to permanent neurological damage. Malaria is estimated to cost Africa $12 billion per year in lost income as a result of illness in workers, decreased tourism, and an unwillingness of many companies to invest in high-risk areas. Together, these factors magnify malaria's toll on countries with high rates of infection.

Chemicals have been developed to kill either the malarial vector or the parasites themselves, leading many people to believe that malaria might be brought under control. However, the development of resistance has been problematic. Furthermore, some of the most effective agents have been cited as harmful environmental contaminants. New drugs and new strategies are raising cautious optimism in the health care community.

History

At one time, malarial infection was problematic throughout the world. In addition to areas currently affected, such as parts of Africa and Asia, southern Italy was particularly hard-hit. Many swamps were found in close proximity to ancient Rome, the Pontina, which had very high infection rates. "Bad air" (*mal aria*) from swamps was thought to be responsible. The Italian dictator Benito Mussolini drained these swamps and greatly decreased disease incidence in Italy during the 1930s. Malaria was also common in parts of the United States, particularly in the southern states but also was found as far north as Cleveland and Toledo, in northern Ohio, until the 1830s.

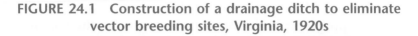

FIGURE 24.1   Construction of a drainage ditch to eliminate vector breeding sites, Virginia, 1920s

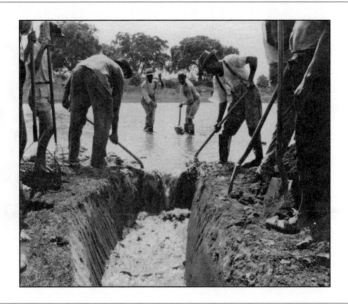

Source: CDC.

Controlling malaria and yellow fever by decreasing the numbers of their mosquito vectors was vital to the construction of the Panama Canal in the first decade of the 1900s. This was accomplished under the direction of W. C. Gorgas of the U.S. Army Medical Corps through a combination of drainage, cutting of brush and grasses, adding oil to standing water that served as habitat for larvae, and the use of quinine. Thanks to these efforts, death rates of canal workers decreased from 11.6 per 1,000 in 1906 to 1.2 per 1,000 in 1909, permitting completion of the canal that decreased the need for ships to make the dangerous passage around Cape Horn at the tip of South America, facilitating travel and trade between the Atlantic and Pacific Oceans

The decrease in numbers of mosquitoes of the *Anopheles* genus in affected areas was vital to freeing them from the burden of malaria, as was the development of effective drugs that killed the protozoa responsible for causing the disease. As mosquitoes and parasites developed resistance, however, the incidence of malaria rose greatly. In some areas of Africa, the infection rate of the population was 150% annually (virtually all members of the population became infected, many of them more than once a year). In the United States between 1957 and 2003, a total of 63 outbreaks were attributed to bites of locally occurring

FIGURE 24.2 One of the fruits of malaria reduction programs in the Western Hemisphere: the Panama Canal

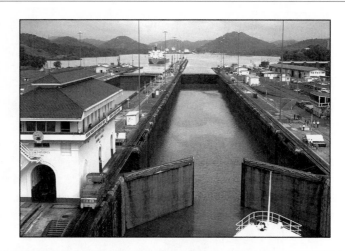

Source: CDC/Edwin P. Ewing Jr.

mosquitoes. Two mosquito species capable of malaria transmission remain common in the United States, allowing the possibility of reintroduction. Currently, however, most cases in North Americans do not occur in the traditional manner. Between 1963 and 1999, some 93 cases resulted from blood transfusion. In 2002, a total of 1,337 cases were reported, all but 5 of them imported from regions in which the disease is endemic.

The Disease

Malaria is best known for the development of alternating periods of fever and chills, but its initial symptoms are nonspecific and similar to mild viral infections. These symptoms include headache, fatigue, abdominal discomfort and vomiting, muscle and joint aches, loss of appetite, and malaise. A high body temperature is present during both fever and chill stages as the erythrocytes periodically rupture and release intracellular contents, such as hemoglobin and its toxic byproduct, **bilirubin**. Cycles occur every two to three days, depending on the parasite species. Individuals with most types of malaria often feel better between cycles. The fever and chills may be very intense and debilitating; the affected individual might shake hard enough to damage the bed. Anemia, sometimes severe, results from erythrocyte rupture. The person may experience severe nausea and continuous vomiting. Renal or heart failure may result from bilirubin exposure.

Several far more serious disease manifestations may occur. One such manifestation is **cerebral malaria**, resulting from parasite entry into the central nervous system. Cerebral malaria is characterized by a progressive headache, very high fever which may exceed 108°F (42°C), psychosis, convulsions, coma, and death within hours. This form of the disease has a mortality rate of 25% to 50% and is usually restricted to infection caused by *Plasmodium falciparum*. Another very serious condition associated primarily with *P. falciparum* is **blackwater fever**. During this manifestation, the kidneys are damaged by massive releases of hemoglobin from ruptured erythrocytes. The presence of this pigment produces black urine. Death usually results from renal failure. This condition is believed to have an autoimmune component, as antibodies aid in the erythrocyte lysis. Mortality rate is 20% to 50%. Other serious complications of malaria include metabolic acidosis, hypoglycemia, and acute pulmonary edema.

Malaria may be especially harmful to the very young. Infection raises the risk of low birth weight, childhood mortality, and neurological damage and is particularly problematic in areas where access to proper nutrition and health care is limited. Pregnant women are more susceptible to infection with the highly pathogenic *P. falciparum*.

After a person's initial infection, a state of partial immunity often occurs, reducing the individual's parasite burden and subsequent disease severity during future infections. In areas of the world with high and stable rates of infection, therefore, severe malaria is often restricted to the very young, travelers, or the immunocompromised, including HIV-positive individuals. In some areas, such as sub-Saharan Africa, incidence of both HIV and malaria is very high. In parts of the world with lower or fluctuating rates of infection, severe disease occurs in any age group and may result in epidemics. Travelers or immigrants from malaria-free areas entering endemic areas, including military personnel, are at higher risk of more severe disease due to their complete lack of protective immunity. Currently, no effective vaccine exists for malaria prevention despite enormous amounts of research having been conducted for decades.

The Causative Agents

In humans, four species of parasitic blood protozoa of the genus *Plasmodium* cause malaria. These parasites are members of the Apicomplexan class Sporozoa. Other species of the genus cause disease in animals.

Life Cycle

The life cycle of the *Plasmodium* species responsible for malaria is split between the human host and the vectors, *Anopheles* mosquitoes.

The portion of the cycle occurring in humans begins when **sporozoites** are injected into the human host from the salivary glands of an infected female mosquito during a blood meal. The sporozoites travel via the blood to the liver and there infect hepatocytes within 30 minutes. They then divide repeatedly asexually, forming **schizonts** containing 30,000 to 40,000 individual **merozoites**. The schizont ruptures, releasing merozoites that infect erythrocytes. In these cells, the merozoites first develop into the **ring form,** which resembles a signet ring, and then divide rapidly, each parasite producing 8 to 24 daughter cells. The cells lyse with a periodicity related to the parasite species, releasing the newly formed merozoites. For most malaria-inducing parasite species, cell rupture is synchronized, occurring in waves. Some merozoites infect new erythrocytes, continuing the blood cycle, while others develop into sexual stages of **male and female gametocytes**. Some of these are ingested by another feeding mosquito to start the next stage of the life cycle.

Once inside the female mosquito, gametocytes develop into the female **macrogamete**, similar to an egg, or multiple male **microgametes**, similar to sperm. The microgamete penetrates a macrogamete, and fertilization occurs inside the mosquito's stomach, producing an **ookinete**. This motile form of the parasite passes through the wall of the stomach to form an **oocyst** on its outer wall. The oocyst divides asexually to produce multiple sporozoites, which migrate to the mosquito's salivary glands and from there are passed to another human to continue the cycle in a new host.

Plasmodium falciparum

Plasmodium falciparum is responsible for the most pathogenic type of malaria, **malignant tertian malaria**. The **erythrocytic cycle** lasts 48 hours from the time of infection of the red blood cell to its rupture, and unlike infection with other *Plasmodium* species, the individual may not feel well between cycles. At one time cosmopolitan, distribution of the species is currently much more limited, often restricted to the tropical zones. These parasites infect erythrocytes of any age and so have a wide target range. Often more than one parasite will infect a given cell. As many as 65% of a person's erythrocytes may be infected; for individuals with an infection rate of greater than 25%, the disease is usually fatal. Even just two or three parasites per milliliter of blood may induce disease symptoms. *P. falciparum* may have led to the downfall of ancient Greek civilization

FIGURE 24.3 Malaria parasite life cycle

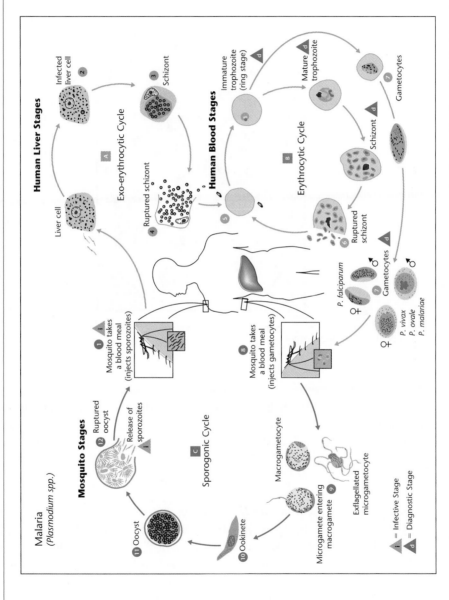

Source: CDC/Alexander J. da Silva.

FIGURE 24.4 Microgametocyte and macrogametocyte:
Plasmodium falciparum

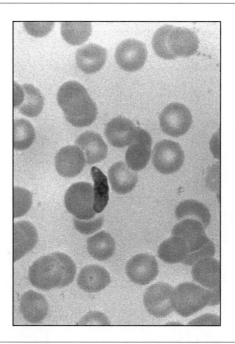

Source: CDC/Steven Glenn.

and is reputed to have halted the progress of Alexander the Great's army by killing its leader at the age of 32. In addition to causing the most severe malaria symptoms, *P. falciparum* has shown the greatest ability to develop drug resistance.

Plasmodium vivax

Disease induced by ***Plasmodium vivax*** is generally milder than that of *P. falciparum*. Similar to *P. falciparum,* the erythrocytic cycle lasts 48 hours and so is named **benign tertian malaria**. This form of disease may be lifelong because *P. vivax* may produce multiple rounds of hepatic infection in the liver, where it may remain hidden for decades. This parasite resides primarily in temperate zones. It has a more restricted range of target cells: it invades only reticulocytes (young erythrocytes). Accordingly, lower numbers of cells are infected, leading to less severe symptoms.

FIGURE 24.5   Erythrocytes infected by multiple
ring-stage *Plasmodium falciparum*

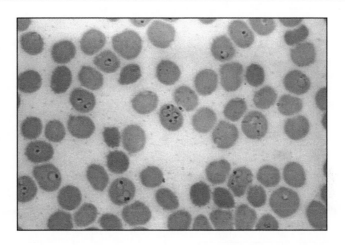

Source: CDC/Steven Glenn.

Plasmodium malariae

Plasmodium malariae causes **quartan malaria**, with a 72-hour erythro-cytic cycle. This parasite is less common than *P. falciparum* and *P. vivax*. It is able to induce relapses up to 53 years after the initial infection. It tends to infect older erythrocytes.

Plasmodium ovale

Mild tertian malaria, with a cycle of 48 hours, is produced by ***Plasmodium ovale***. It occurs primarily in tropical areas and is the least common form of human malaria.

The Immune Response

Individuals repeatedly exposed to *Plasmodium* often develop a fairly robust immune response to the parasite, which declines after removal from an endemic environment and reappears after reexposure. The humeral immune response is particularly stimulated, with persons developing high levels of antibodies. Despite this, many people are repeatedly infected, sometimes annually. Although this immune response is not completely protective, it is nevertheless beneficial in

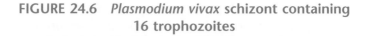

FIGURE 24.6 *Plasmodium vivax* schizont containing
16 trophozoites

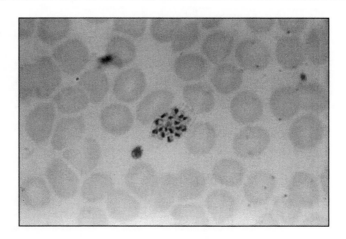

Source: CDC/Steven Glenn.

that individuals without previous immunity (children and persons from malaria-free areas) have higher mortality rates. CD8$^+$ T killer cells and interferon-γ are believed to be much more protective than antibodies.

Great effort has been expended unsuccessfully to develop a protective malaria vaccine for widespread use. Much research focused on sporozoite subunit vaccines, fueled by successful protection of mice inoculated with irradiated sporozoites in the 1960s. Obtaining a large number of sporozoites was very difficult, however, since this form of the parasite is found only in the salivary glands of mosquitoes and no method has yet been developed to grow them in culture. Vaccine efforts for many years concentrated on using sporozoite components instead, such as the circumsporozoite protein, since molecular biological techniques are able to easily produce large amounts of these proteins. The **circumsporozoite protein** was particularly attractive since its multiple sets of repeated amino acid sequences produced vigorous antibody production and protective immunity in some species of mice. The results of this work did not translate well into humans, however, perhaps due to the complexity of the parasite's life cycle—immunity to sporozoites is not cross-reactive with merozoites or gametocytes, thus any sporozoites that escaped killing shortly after infection quickly infected hepatocytes and produced the other forms of the parasite against which the host was not protected. Some people also respond better to certain sporozoite antigens than others due to individual genetic differences in the type of MHC antigens expressed by the person's cells: some persons were found to have little to no response to the parasite antigens used in some of the vaccine preparations. Subsequent efforts to combine antigens from more than one parasite developmental stage also met with very limited success. Other work concentrated on developing a vaccine using gametocyte antigens. Such a vaccine would not protect the person immunized but may instead block transmission of the sexual forms of the parasite to mosquitoes, thus preventing continuation of the malarial life cycle and hence transmission to other people. Some researchers now suggest returning to the use of whole-organism vaccines, employing new techniques to mass-produce sporozoites in mosquitoes. Such sporozoites are either irradiated or genetically altered before incorporation into a vaccine.

Diagnosis

Diagnosis is based on evidence of clinical and laboratory findings. The latter often involve detection and typing of parasites microscopically in blood smears, especially in areas with limited financial resources. Typing parasite species is based on unique characteristics of each of the four species, such as the size and number of signet-ring-stage parasites per erythrocyte and the age of the infected host cells. The full delineation of these characteristics is beyond the scope of this chapter. Microscopic determination requires skilled technicians. Another laboratory assay is the rapid diagnostic test. This test is more expensive and is vulnerable to high temperature and humidity, factors often encountered in regions with high incidence of malaria.

Treatment and Drug Resistance

Antimalarial Compounds

One of the oldest drugs used in the treatment of malaria was **artemisinin**, derived from the qinghao plant, wormwood (*Artemisia annua*). This material was used in China as early as the fourth century A.D. Another early drug was **quinine**, a derivative of cinchona tree bark. Records indicate that quinine was used in South America in the seventeenth century. It remains a major factor in the treatment of cerebral malaria. The cost of lifesaving treatment with this compound is approximately $2.68. **Chloroquine**, which acts by insertion into the parasite's DNA, was developed more recently and was highly effective and inexpensive, with a treatment cost of approximately 13 cents. It was particularly useful in the developing world,

FIGURE 24.7   Chemical structures of quinine (left) and chloroquine (right)

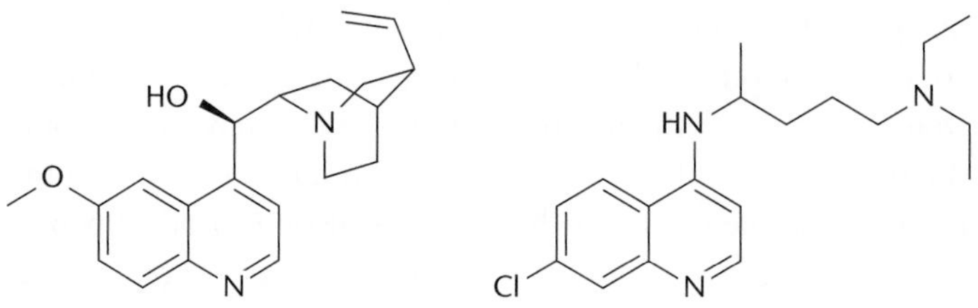

where the disease rate is high and resources are scarce. Unfortunately, resistance to this drug developed rapidly, especially in the most pathogenic species, *P. falciparum*, as the parasite began to produce pumps that export chloroquine through the plasma membrane. By 1998, 20% to 35% of this species were highly resistant to chloroquine. Chloroquine resistance remains widespread and is particularly problematic in East Africa. Resistance has also been noted in *P. vivax* in parts of Asia and the Brazilian Amazon. More than ten African countries have switched to sulfadoxine-pyrimethamine as their first-line drug, despite the rapid advent of *P. vivax* resistance to this agent.

Drug Resistance

Drug resistance is becoming increasingly worrisome for malaria as it is for bacterial diseases. Resistance to quinine required more than 250 years to develop. Chloroquine resistance was first noted around 50 years ago, just 12 years after its introduction. Such resistance has not only decreased the usefulness of a previously highly effective drug but has also reduced the options in a region of the world that is severely challenged economically. During the 1980s, resistance began to develop to sulfadoxine-pyrimethamine, the second least expensive drug, and to mefloquine in Thailand. These protozoan strains are multidrug-resistant (MDR). They are spreading rapidly, and affected areas now include portions of Brazil and East Africa. Changes in the *pfmdr1* gene allow resistance to chloroquine, mefloquine, quinine, and artemisinin. Other polymorphisms in *pfcrt* and in *dhfr/dhps* are associated with resistance to chloroquine and sulfadoxine-pyrimethamine, respectively.

Newer drugs under development include ones that stop electron transport in the mitochondria of the parasites but not those of humans. Derivatives

RECENT DEVELOPMENTS

Molecular biology is playing an increasing role in malaria research programs. Some current work focuses on sequencing *P. falciparum* and *Anopheles* DNA. Sequences of the parasite's genome and studies of differential expression of various genes and proteins during the different stages of the life cycle are being exploited to develop new drugs targeting metabolic pathways of the different parasitic developmental forms (genetic variation). Molecular monitoring of mosquito genomes allows detection and quantification of the prevalence of resistance to DDT and permethrin by monitoring expression of *kdr* resistance alleles in vector populations. This information, along with other DNA- and RNA-based strategies, is being used to develop potential vaccine candidates and drug targets.

Enhanced laboratory testing may lead to improved treatments. Such tests include in vitro drug susceptibility assays and determination of the presence of molecular markers of resistance in the parasite's DNA. The cost of these tests, like the cost of new malaria drugs, is a limiting factor in their broad application in regions where they would most benefit the population.

of artemisinin, including artemether, artemotil, artesunate, and dihydroartemisinin, are under consideration for treatment of cerebral malaria. The pairing of artemisinin-based therapy with compounds that have differing modes of action is becoming more common. This combination therapy is often effective against uncomplicated *P. falciparum* malaria and may involve the use of lumefantrine, tetracycline, clindamycin, chloroquine, mefloquine, sulfadoxine-pyrimethamine, amodiaquine, or other antimalarial compounds.

Prevention: Failures and Successes

The World Health Organization's Global Malaria Eradication Campaign was an optimistic attempt during the 1950s and 1960s to force malaria into extinction. Great effort and large amounts of resources were expended in the campaign that nevertheless resulted in an enormous failure to control the disease. Instead, the numbers of infected persons eventually exceeded those at the start of the campaign, and the rate of infection soared well beyond those numbers during the 1990s. Some high-risk areas, such as Africa, were not even included in this global campaign. Following the successful decline of both malaria and yellow fever in Panama, a similar strategy was employed during the attempt to eradicate malaria throughout the world. The insecticide DDT was widely used to spray the walls

FIGURE 24.8   Skin exposure during mixing
of the pesticide malathion

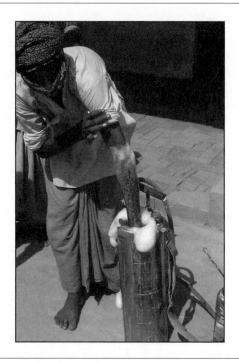

Source: CDC/Edward Baker Jr.

of houses in high-risk areas in order to decrease exposure of mosquito vectors to human hosts. Many of the vector species tend to feed on people indoors rather than outside their homes. DDT residues remain on indoor walls for months after application, providing some level of protection during that time. This strategy failed for several reasons. First, use of DDT was banned in large areas of the world, due largely to the book *Silent Spring* by Rachel Carson, which claimed that massive death of songbirds would result from the thinning of eggshells induced by the insecticide. Whether or not this claim had any merit, we now know that DDT is of fairly low toxicity to humans. Furthermore, decreasing mosquito contact with humans reduces the incidence of malaria and a number of other mosquito-borne illnesses, potentially saving many lives and increasing the quality of many more. Some parts of the world chose to continue using DDT but were unable to do so due to pressure to shut down production exerted by groups such as the International Pesticide Action Network on countries that were major manufacturers of the chemical, including the United States. Another problem

FIGURE 24.9   Female *Anopheles gambiae* laying eggs

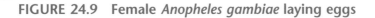

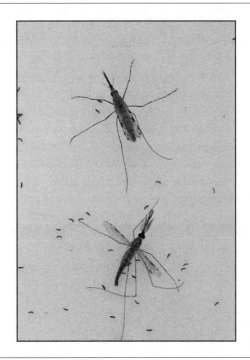

Source: CDC/Mary F. Adams.

with relying heavily on DDT as a key component in eradication attempts was the fairly rapid development of resistance in mosquito populations in some parts of the world. Unfortunately, the suggested DDT alternatives are less effective in controlling disease incidence and are much less affordable in developing countries where the need for such insecticides is greatest. For example, expenses associated with use of the alternative compound, malathione, are five times that of DDT, and the use of this pesticide on dishware or on skin may cause poisoning.

Another major international plan was the 1992 Global Malaria Control Strategy, emphasizing case detection and treatment and not vector control. Unfortunately, once treated, individuals often returned to sleep in homes in which infected vectors still resided and subsequently became reinfected. Such a cycle could be repeated several times because the vectors were not removed from the premises. In some areas where the eradication efforts of the 1960s had largely succeeded, such as the Peruvian Amazon, malaria incidence increased 50-fold between 1992 and 1997, with *P. falciparum* becoming the dominant species. Vector numbers similarly rose during that time.

In addition to the decreased use of DDT, several other factors contributed to malaria's reemergence in the 1970s. The spread of chloroquine-resistant parasites reduced the benefits derived from this previously effective and affordable drug. Resettlement and population movements resulting from civil war and unrest moved infected persons into previously disease-free zones and drove uninfected people into high-risk areas. Economic conditions also led to the relocation of large numbers of people. Especially problematic was movement from areas of high altitude, with low disease rates, to those of lower altitude, which are more supportive of disease transmission. New breeding grounds for mosquitoes were created by dams and irrigation projects. Economic pressures in the developing world reduced resources for drugs and other health care measures. High birth rates in many affected areas also provided a supply of young children at great risk for infection and severe disease. Moreover, some vector species changed their biting habits from indoors to outdoors, hampering prevention strategies emphasizing the spraying of home interiors.

A number of successful projects have begun more recently. One of the most prominent is the Roll Back Malaria Partnership, launched in 1998. This project is a major effort to substantially reduce malaria incidence by 2015. It is based on interactions between many agencies, including international health groups, such as the World Health Organization, the United Nations, the Red Cross, and the World Bank; the private sector, including BASF and ExxonMobil; foundations, including the Bill and Melinda Gates Foundation and the Clinton Foundation; pharmaceutical companies, including Bayer and Novartis; and researchers. One major focus has been the use of insecticide-treated bed nets. These are quite effective and are being widely distributed in affected areas. Formerly, conventionally treated nets were retreated annually. Newer, longer-lasting treated nets are effective for at least three years. Another major focus relies on indoor residual spraying and has been useful in many countries. DDT remains the insecticide of choice. If employed primarily for public health uses and not agriculturally, much smaller amounts are required and are restricted to a closed and protected setting (the house) to which it generally remains confined, as DDT is not readily soluble in water. Much of the spraying occurs in rural areas where homes are spread over large areas and all household members benefit. This strategy greatly reduces environment impact while protecting humans from a devastating disease. Other strategies include distribution of artemisinin-based combination therapy drugs and vaccine development.

A more recent program is the 2005 President's Malaria Initiative under direction of the U.S. Agency for International Development, the Departments of State and Health and Human Services, and the White House. The initiative uses methods similar to Roll Back Malaria and targets 15 African countries. At the end of its second year, 25 million people had been reached, with positive impacts in Tanzania, Zanzibar, Malawi, and Uganda.

Surveillance

The Pan American Health Organization has been monitoring malaria infections in the Western Hemisphere since 1959. Two reported parameters are the annual parasite index (number of blood slides testing positive for *Plasmodium* per 100,000 population) and the annual blood examination rate. When calculated in a manner that compensates for the number of slides examined in different years, malaria rates in Brazil were either stable or increased slightly from 1965 to the late 1970s. The annual parasite index increased fivefold, however, between 1978 and 1995. This was true for both *P. falciparum* and *P. vivax* malaria and was echoed in 18 other countries, including Peru and Guyana. Such surveillance may detect developing trends, which in this case could reflect decreased use of DDT to spray homes, as vector resistance to DDT was not widespread in South America at the time. In Ecuador, where DDT use increased, a large reduction in malaria rates occurred. Thus surveillance may highlight successes and failures among control strategies.

Sentinel sites throughout Africa monitor the spread and prevalence of drug resistance. A pan-African program to measure transmission intensity has used GPS technology to allow time-spatial mapping of malaria across the continent and potentially predict epidemics and monitor control measures.

Summary

Disease

- Drug-resistant malaria

Causative Agents

- *Plasmodium falciparum*, *P. vivax*, *P. ovale*, and *P. malariae*

Agent Type

- Parasitic members of the Apicomplexan class Sporozoa

Genome

- DNA

Vector

- *Anopheles* mosquitoes

Common Reservoir

- Humans

Mode of Transmission

- Mosquito bite

Geographical Distribution

- Primarily tropical regions of the world; *P. vivax* is found in temperate regions

Years of Emergence

- Resistance to chloroquine: 1950s–1960s • Resistance to sulfadoxine-pyrimethamine: 1980s

Key Terms

Artemisinin Wormwood derivative that was among the first drugs used to treat malaria

Benign tertian malaria Type of malaria caused by *Plasmodium vivax* whose erythrocytic cycle has a 48-hour periodicity

Bilirubin Toxic by-product of hemoglobin released in large quantities during the rupture of erythrocytes in malaria

Blackwater fever Severe manifestation of infection by *P. falciparum* in which the kidneys are damaged by massive release of hemoglobin from ruptured erythrocytes

Cerebral malaria Severe manifestation of infection by *P. falciparum* after parasites enter the central nervous system; characterized by progressive headache, very high fever, psychosis, convulsions, coma, and death within hours

Chloroquine Inexpensive contemporary drug used to treat malaria to which many strains of *P. falciparum* have developed resistance

Circumsporozoite protein Component of *Plasmodium* sporozoites that contain multiple sets of repeated amino acid sequences; produces vigorous antibody production and +protective immunity in some species of mice

Erythrocytic cycle Time from the infection of the red blood cell to its rupture

Macrogamete Large female gamete of *Plasmodium* species; similar to an egg

Malaria Disease characterized by alternating cycles of debilitating fever and chills, anemia, and more severe manifestations such as cerebral malaria and renal failure during blackwater fever

Male and female gametocyte Stage of malaria parasite that produces either multiple microgametes or a single macrogamete

Malignant tertian malaria Severe type of malaria caused by *Plasmodium falciparum* whose erythrocytic cycle has a 48-hour periodicity

Merozoites Form of malaria parasite within infected liver or red blood cells; produced by multiple rounds of asexual reproduction of sprozoites

Microgametes Small male gametes of *Plasmodium* species; similar to sperm

Mild tertian malaria Rare type of malaria caused by *Plasmodium ovale* whose erythrocytic cycle has a 48-hour periodicity

Oocyst Stage of *Plasmodium* species' life cycle which follows encystment of the ookinete on the outer wall of the mosquito's stomach; undergoes many rounds of reproduction to produce multiple sporozoites

Ookinete Motile zygote of *Plasmodium* species that is produced by fertilization of a macrogamete by a microgamete

Plasmodium falciparum Species of parasite causing the deadliest form of malaria in humans; also has the highest rate of drug resistance

Plasmodium malariae Species of human malaria parasite that causes quartan malaria

Plasmodium ovale Least common of the parasites that cause malaria in humans

Plasmodium vivax Species of parasite most often responsible for malaria in the temperate zones

Quartan malaria Type of malaria caused by *Plasmodium malariae* whose erythrocytic cycle has a 72-hour periodicity

Quinine One of the earlier drugs used to treat malaria, to which many strains of *Plasmodium* have developed resistance

Ring form Early stage of merozoite in *Plasmodium*-infected erythrocytes; resembles a signet ring

Schizonts Stage of *Plasmodium* species life cycle in which the infected cell is filled with multiple merozoites produced by asexual reproduction

Sporozoite Stage of the life cycle in *Plasmodium* species that infects the mammalian host via a mosquito bite

Review Questions

1. What are the four malarial parasites? How do they differ biologically, and how may these differences affect the resulting clinical conditions?
2. Describe the life cycle of *Plasmodium* species in humans and mosquitoes.
3. What are the major disease manifestations of malaria?
4. What antimalarial drugs were widely used in the past? Name some newer treatments.
5. What approaches are currently most effective in the prevention of malarial infection?

Topics for Further Discussion

1. Convalescent serum, involving elements of blood taken from patients who have previously recovered from an infection, is occasionally used in treating serious diseases that do not respond to other means of treatment, such as Ebola and Marburg hemorrhagic fevers. These diseases occur in areas with a high incidence of malaria and HIV infection, both transmissible via serum. When do the benefits of this treatment option outweigh the risks of developing other serious diseases?
2. What is the incidence of coinfection with malaria and HIV in various parts of the developing world? What effects does coinfection have on the immune response and pathology?
3. In addition to malaria and yellow fever, what other serious diseases are transmitted by mosquitoes? What is the most effective, affordable, and environmentally safe way of eliminating these vectors?
4. What is the relationship between rates and severity of malaria infection and economic development? Recognizing that medications are costly, raising an area's economic status could increase the health of the workforce. How might businesses be initially attracted into malaria-prone areas where many of the workers are stricken with debilitating illness for parts of the year?

Resources

De Santana Filho, F. S., and others. "Chloroquine-Resistant *Plasmodium vivax*, Brazilian Amazon." *Emerging Infectious Diseases*, 2007, *13*, 1125–1126.

Guarda, J. A., Asayag, C. R., and Witzig, R. "Malaria Reemergence in the Peruvian Amazon Region." *Emerging Infectious Diseases*, 1999, *5*, 209–215.

Himeidan, Y. E., and others. "Permethrin and DDT Resistance in the Malaria Vector *Anopheles arabiensis* from Eastern Sudan." *American Journal of Tropical Medicine and Hygiene,* 2007, *77,* 1066–1068.

Nchinda, T. C. "Malaria: A Reemerging Disease in Africa." *Emerging Infectious Diseases,* 1998, *4,* 398–403.

Ntoumi, F., and others. "New Interventions for Malaria: Mining the Human and Parasite Genomes." *American Journal of Tropical Medicine and Hygiene,* 2007, *77,* 270–275.

Pinzon-Charry, A., and Good, M. F. "Malaria Vaccines: The Case for a Whole-Organism Approach." *Expert Opinions in Biological Therapy,* 2008, *8,* 441–448.

Roberts, D. R., Laughlin, L. L., Hsheih, P., and Legters, L. J. "DDT, Global Strategies, and a Malaria Control Crisis in South America." *Emerging Infectious Diseases,* 1997, *3,* 295–302.

Salyers, A. A., and Whitt, D. D. *Revenge of the Microbes: How Bacterial Resistance Is Undermining the Antibiotic Miracle.* Washington, D.C.: ASM Press, 2005.

Wongsrichanaiai, C., Pickard, A. L., Wernsdorfer, W. H., and Mechnick, S. R. "Epidemiology of Drug-Resistant Malaria." *Lancet Infectious Diseases,* 2002, *2,* 209–218.

CHAPTER 25

BABESIOSIS

LEARNING OBJECTIVES

- Define babesiosis and compare and contrast it to malaria

- Describe the Apicomplexan protozoa responsible for causing the illness

- Discuss modes of infection

- Discuss the host's response to infection

- Describe symptomatology and diagnosis

- Discuss potential methods of treatment

- Discuss methods of prevention

Major Concepts

Symptoms

Babesiosis is an emerging infectious disease among people living in temperate areas of the world. Though often asymptomatic in younger healthy individuals, this illness may be very serious or fatal in immunocompromised persons. People at high risk for severe disease include those who lack a spleen, are over the age of 50 years, or are immunosuppressed. Illness in these persons may lead to development of high fever, pulmonary edema, hemolytic anemia, hemoglobin in the urine, renal failure, disseminated intravascular coagulation, adult respiratory distress syndrome, and multiorgan failure.

Infection

Most cases of babesiosis result from infection with *Babesia divergens* (in Europe), *B. microti* (in the northeastern United States), or *Babesia* isolate type WA-1 (in the western United States). Infection with *B. divergens* leads to the most severe pathology. *Babesia* species are parasitic protozoa belonging to the phylum Apicomplexa. Several species produce lethal infections in animals, including cattle, horses, and dogs. Apicomplexa includes several other genera of closely related human and animal pathogens such as *Theileria* (in cattle), *Plasmodium* (which causes malaria in humans and animals), and *Eimeria* (in birds). These parasites have significant negative effects on the economy and agriculture of affected regions. *Babesia* protozoa are transmitted to humans by deer ticks, and pathology is magnified by coinfection with *Borrelia burgdorferi* (the causative agent of Lyme disease), which is transmitted by the same species of tick. In addition to the domestic animals listed, several mammals in the wild (white-footed mice, mule deer, bighorn sheep, voles, and shrews) serve as hosts and potential reservoir species.

Immune Response

Several elements of the host immune response are protective, including IgG antibodies, NK cells, macrophages, and CD4$^+$ Th1 helper lymphocytes. These last, however, may interfere with defense against Lyme disease, which relies on a Th2 lymphocyte response. Other elements of the immune system such as IgM antibody and complement may in fact worsen babesiosis.

Protection

Preventive measures for babesiosis are similar to those used for erhlichiosis and Lyme disease. They involve decreasing host contact with infected ticks or tick removal prior to the introduction of the infective form of the parasite to the vertebrate host.

Introduction

Babesiosis (also known as piroplasmosis) is a potentially serious illness resulting from infection of erythrocytes with a parasitic protozoan belonging to one of several species of **Babesia**. These intracellular parasites are similar to the causative agents of malaria in humans, and the disease induced by *Babesia* is usually similar to a mild case of malaria. Among individuals with decreased immune responses, however, the illness is much more severe and may even prove fatal. Hundreds of cases of babesiosis have been identified since it was first reported in humans in the late 1950s; in New Jersey alone, 189 cases were noted between 1989 and 2004, and in New York, 560 cases were recorded between 1986 and 2001. This illness is found in scattered locations around the world, including portions of the United States that are home to deer ticks, one of the disease vectors. Some areas of the country in which the parasite is endemic include islands off of the Atlantic Coast (Nantucket, Block Island, and Shelter Island), eastern Long Island, Maine, upstate New York, southern Connecticut, Massachusetts, Rhode Island, New Jersey, Wisconsin, Minnesota, Missouri, California, and Washington. Mexico has reported cases of infection, as have European countries, including France, Ireland, Scotland, Spain, Switzerland, Sweden, Russia, and Yugoslavia. Infection with various *Babesia* species has also occurred in China, Taiwan, Japan, Korea, Egypt, South Africa, Mozambique, and the Canary Islands.

Babesiosis is one of the most common infections of free-living animals worldwide and is problematic for agriculture. *Babesia bovis* causes a severe disease in cattle known as Texas cattle fever (redwater fever). The effects of this and similar diseases on livestock severely diminish food availability and economic health in some regions of the world. Other species of *Babesia* cause serious disease in horses and dogs (discussed later in this chapter). The freed lioness Elsa, featured in the film *Born Free*, succumbed to *Babesia* infection.

History

Babesia species were first described by the Romanian scientist Viktor Babeş in 1888, who found them in the erythrocytes of cattle. Babesiosis may, however, have been noted much earlier as the plague of the Egyptian cattle described in Exodus. Infection of humans with *Babesia divergens* was first noted in 1957 in a 33-year old asplenic (lacking a spleen) farmer in Yugoslavia who had grazed his herd of infected cattle in a tick-infested field. A number of cases were detected over the next 20 years in Russia. Most individuals with symptomatic infection have lost their spleens. In these people, disease is severe and symptoms include fever, hemolytic anemia, and hemoglobin in the urine and renal failure resembling malarial blackwater fever. In the United States, human babesiosis was first recognized in California, and later, a separate species, *Babesia microti*, was found to cause human illness on Nantucket, off the coast of Massachusetts (Nantucket fever) in the mid-1960s and 1970s. Some areas not known to be endemic were found on closer examination to have widespread infection that is mounting over time due to a combination of increased tick prevalence and range, better surveillance and reporting of infection, and greater awareness of the disease. These areas include south and central New Jersey, where 2 cases were reported in 1994 and 48 in 2004. A third species, *Babesia* isolate type WA-1, was discovered to be the cause of an acute malaria-like disease in Washington in 1991. In 1991 and 1993, isolate type CA-1 was found in California. This isolate is closely related to, but distinct from, type WA-1. Isolate type MO-1 caused a fatal disease in a 73-year-old splenectomized man in Missouri in 1992. Type MO-1 is similar to *B. divergens* in Europe, although this individual had never traveled outside of the United States and rarely left his home state.

The Disease

Babesiosis is an arthropod-borne disease caused by infection of erythrocytes with one of three species of *Babesia* (piroplasms). Given the cellular location and the appearance of the parasites, babesiosis may be mistaken for malaria. Some 25% of infections in adults and 50% of those in children are asymptomatic or resolve without treatment. Nevertheless, babesiosis is a potentially severe or even fatal condition. In the United States, the mortality rate is about 5%, but in Europe, 42% of the infected become comatose and die. Babesiosis in the United States and in Europe are caused by different species of parasite. Furthermore, most of the European cases occur in asplenic individuals, who may be at greater risk in that the spleen is a major organ of the immune system in which many B lymphocytes, which produce antibodies, and phagocytic macrophages reside. Its removal thus results in immunosuppression.

The incubation period ranges from 1 to 8 weeks. The symptoms of babesiosis include persistent fever as high as 41°C (105.8°F), intense sweating, shaking chills, malaise, depression, sensitivity to light, stiffness of the neck, cough, shortness of breath, pulmonary edema, nausea, vomiting, abdominal pain, bone pain, rigors, myalgia, headache, fatigue, hypotension, and hepatosplenomegaly. Laboratory findings may include thrombocytopenia and high levels of serum transaminase, alkaline phosphatases, unconjugated bilirubin, and lactic dehydrogenase. Jaundice may result from hemolytic anemia, which lasts from days to several months. Severe renal symptoms include hemoglobin in the urine (released from lysed red blood cells) and renal failure. Other extremely serious disease manifestations include disseminated intravascular coagulation, adult respiratory distress syndrome, and multiorgan failure.

In individuals without clinical signs of infection, parasitemia (presence of parasites dividing in the blood) persists for months or years. Symptoms may resume after a year of an asymptomatic parasitemia. Although serious disease manifestations can occur in previously healthy persons, immunocompromised individuals, including those without a spleen (particularly true for infection with *B. divergens*), older individuals (over the age of 50 years), and those receiving immunosuppressive drugs during chemotherapy for cancer or to prevent rejection of transplanted organs, are at increased risk of developing severe symptoms after infection. In areas with large or rising numbers of HIV-infected persons, this infection may become more problematic as persons with inapparent infections with *Babesia* lose immune functions during the course of HIV disease progression. The increase in the elderly population may also affect the numbers of susceptible individuals. Other conditions that weaken the immune response, such as diabetes, have also been associated with higher risk for symptomatic babesiosis.

Coinfection of a person with another tickborne microbe, *Borrelia burgdorferi*, may occur. This bacterial spirochete causes Lyme disease, and dual infection increases the severity of both conditions. Infection with *Borrelia* persists longer in coinfected persons, and they are more likely to develop persistent postinfection fatigue. Surveys of deer ticks in endemic areas often detect the presence of both microbes in individual ticks. In the United States, 20% of humans with *Babesia* infection are coinfected with *Borrelia*. *Ehrlichia* species and *Anaplasma* species are also transmitted by deer ticks in the United States. The former infect white blood cells, as is the case for *Theileria* species. These tickborne infections are discussed in other chapters.

In addition to humans, *Babesia* species cause serious illness in animals, including some domestic livestock of agricultural importance and some species of birds. Dogs, cattle, and horses may develop disease. Among dogs, *B. canis* and *B. gibsoni* are the most common disease-causing species. Racing greyhounds and pitbulls are particularly affected by these species. Illness in canines may be acute, hyperacute, or chronic. During the acute form, dogs may develop fever, jaundice,

Table 25.1 Tickborne diseases of humans

Disease	Microbe	Tick
Babesiosis	*Babesia divergens, B. microti*	Deer tick (*Ixodes scapularis, I. ricinus*)
Ehrlichiosis	*Ehrlichia chaffeensis, E. ewinigii*	Lone star tick (*Amblyomma americanum*)
Anaplasmosis	*Anaplasma phagocytophilum*	Deer tick (*I. scapularis*), western black-legged tick (*I. pacificus*)
Lyme disease	*Borrelia burgdorferi*	Lone star tick (*A. americanum*)
Southern tick-associated rash illness	*Borrelia lonestari*	Lone star tick (*A. americanum*)
Rocky Mountain spotted fever	*Rickettsia rickettsii*	American dog tick (*Dermacentor variabilis*), Rocky Mountain wood tick (*D. andersoni*)
Tularemia	*Francisella tularensis*	Dog tick (*D. variabilis*), Rocky Mountain wood tick (*D. andersoni*), Lone star tick (*A. americanum*)
Tickborne relapsing fever	*Borrelia parkeri, Borrelia hermsii*	Soft ticks (*Ornithodoros parkeri, Ornithodoros hermsii*)
Colorado tick fever	Colorado tick fever virus	Wood ticks (*D. andersoni*)

hemoglobinuria, anemia, or death. Infection may be transmitted between dogs by biting. *Theileria equi* (*Babesia equi*) and *B. caballi* are the species found in horses, while *B. bovis, B. divergens, B. bigemina,* and *B. major* infect cattle. In horses, *T. equi* may cause acute tickborne hemolytic anemia that progresses into a chronic carrier state. This illness leads to reduced oxygen-carrying capacity and poor performance of racehorses. *B. bigemina,* the cattle pathogen, may have the most impact on the economy of Europe and other major cattle-producing countries. In the infected cattle, 30% to 45% of the erythrocytes may be parasitized and then destroyed. In addition to the symptoms seen in humans, infected cattle may be unable to rise and may experience severe dehydration, diarrhea that is followed by constipation, lower than normal body temperature, and reduced levels of oxygen in the brain, leading to behavioral changes. They have very rapid heart rates with extremely loud cardiac sounds that can be heard even from a distance of several feet. Toxemic shock may subsequently result in death. In addition to domestic animals, this protozoan may also parasitize water buffalo and wild ruminants, such as reindeer, in other regions of the world.

Table 25.2 *Babesia* species and their hosts

Babesia Species	Animals Infected
B. divergens, B. microti, Type WA-1, Type CA-1, Type MO-1	Humans
B. canis, B. gibsoni	Dogs
Thileria equi (B. equi), B. caballi	Horses
B. bovis, B. major	Cattle
B. bigemina	Cattle, water buffalo, reindeer

The Causative Agent

The Parasites

Members of the *Babesia* genus are parasitic protozoa that infect erythrocytes of humans and animals, including some domestic animals. They may be grouped into either small or large species. The small species measure 1.5 to 3 micrometers in diameter, and the large species measure 3 to 5 micrometers. After division in the erythrocytes, the small forms produce four daughter parasites (a tetrad), while the large produce two (a pair).

These protozoa belong to the phylum Apicomplexa (Sporozoa), class Aconoidasida (Piroplasmea), order Piroplasmida, whose name reflects the pear shape of these organisms within the erythrocytes. This order includes another genus of parasites of cattle blood, *Theileria. Theileria parva* causes East Coast fever, while *T. annulata* causes tropical theileriosis. These infections both result in severe lymphoproliferative diseases because the life cycle of *Theileria* species includes a stage that invades white blood cells. Other Apicomplexan parasites include *Plasmodium* species (which cause malaria) and *Eimeria* species (which cause lethal infections of birds). *Babesia* protozoa differ from the more common *Plasmodium* species in that they divide by binary fission, develop in the erythrocyte cytoplasm, and neither invade liver cells nor form the pigment hemozoin. *Plasmodium* species, by contrast, divide by schizogony to produce multiple merozoites, develop inside parasitophorous vacuoles within the erythrocytes, and induce hemozoin production.

Although more than 100 species of *Babesia* are known, three are responsible for most of the disease in humans: *B. microti* is most common in the eastern and midwestern United States, *Babesia* isolate type WA-1 predominates along the U.S. West Coast, and *B. divergens* occurs in Europe. These are small forms of *Babesia* that produce "Maltese cross" tetrads in which the four parasites are joined at

FIGURE 25.1 *Babesia* protozoa in the tetrad conformation

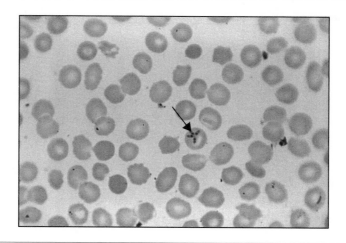

Source: CDC/Steven Glenn.

their pointed ends. *Babesia* isolate type MO-1, first reported in Missouri, and type CA-1, found in California, have also been identified as disease agents.

The relationship between piroplasma genera and among the various human and animal species is uncertain. Whereas *Theileria* species have not been reported in humans, *Babesia* type WA-1 has many features in common with *Theileria*, and the distinction between the two groups is unclear. Furthermore, based on sequencing data, type WA-1 may be more closely related to the small *Babesia* from dogs and wildlife (*B. gibsoni*) in California than to *B. microti*. Type MO-1 in the United States appears to be closely related to *B. divergens* from Europe. PB-1 is a *B. microti*–like species found in baboons, infecting up 40% of animals in colonies. Given the similarities between baboons and humans, concern has been raised that cross-species transmission of PB-1 might occur. *B. divergens*, a member of the small group, is more closely related to members of the large group of the genus based on small subunit ribosomal DNA (ssrDNA) sequencing. Another small *Babesia* (*B. microti*), however, appears to be a sister to the *Theileria* species on the basis of ssrDNA phylogeny.

Babesia parasites are transmitted to humans and other animals via the bite of an infected hard tick such as the deer tick, *Ixodes scapularis* (formerly *I. dammini*) in the United States and *I. ricinus* in Europe. The geographical area affected by *Babesia* species is increasing in the United States as the range of this tick vector expands. The adults of this tick feed primarily on deer, and increased numbers of these hosts has led to a corresponding rise in the tick population and in babesiosis. This situation is similar to that occurring with ehrlichiosis, Lyme disease, and a new species of *Bartonella*, who share *I. scapularis* and *I. ricinus* as vectors and also infect white-footed mice.

Life Cycle

The life cycle of *B. microti* requires two hosts, a rodent reservoir species, usually the white-footed mouse or a meadow vole in the northeastern United States, and a hard tick. *B. divergens* uses cattle as a reservoir host, and type WA-1 may reside in mule deer and bighorn sheep. Surveys have reported infection rates of up to 60% among white-footed mice. Infection has also been reported among other rodents, such as the southern redbacked vole, the masked shrew, and the northern short-tail shrew. In the American South, the tick vectors frequently feed on lizards, which do not appear to support *Babesia* infection. *Babesia*, like other parasitic protozoa, has several stages in its life cycle, and due to their close relationship, these are similar to those occurring in *Theileria* and *Plasmodium*.

While feeding in the spring, a *Babesia*-infected nymphal deer tick introduces sporozoites into an uninfected rodent, which serves as an **intermediate host** (host in which asexual reproduction occurs). Up to 40% of the nymphs are infected in some areas, such as Nantucket. The sporozoites enter erythrocytes through invagination of the cell's plasma membrane and are initially enclosed

FIGURE 25.2   *Babesia* ring-form trophozoites

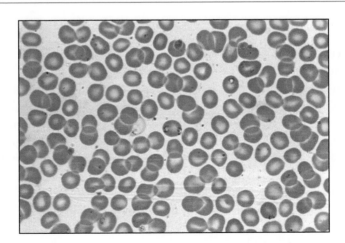

Source: CDC/Mae Melvin.

within a parasitophorous vacuole. The vacuole membrane then disintegrates, leaving only a single plasma membrane around the parasite. Sporozoites then transform into the **trophozoite** (feeding) stage resembling a signet ring (ring form) and undergo one or two rounds of asexual reproduction by binary fission to produce two to four merozoites (daughter parasites).

As the erythrocyte fills with parasites, it bursts, releasing the merozoites and hemoglobin from the erythrocyte into the blood. Some of the merozoites infect and multiply in additional erythrocytes to continue the cycle in the rodent, while others differentiate into **gametocytes**, which produce the sexual stages. During a blood meal, the gametocytes are ingested by a larval deer tick during August or September, which serves as the **definitive host** (the host in which sexual reproduction occurs). Within the tick, the gametocytes develop into gametes with an arrowhead-shaped organelle at their anterior end (**Strahlenkörper**, or **ray bodies**). Two of these gametes unite to form a mobile **kinete** (zygote), and the organelle is then used during the entry of the zygote into epithelial cells of the tick gut. The parasite subsequently enters the insect's hemolymph and travels to other tissues, such as the salivary glands, where it undergoes one or two rounds of asexual reproduction to form a multinucleate **sporoblast**. The sporoblast in turn buds from its surface 5,000 to 10,000 haploid sporozoites (the infective form for rodents), which are transmitted to a new mammalian host as the tick develops into the nymphal stage the following year to continue the life cycle. The life cycle of some species of *Babesia* may also include invasion of lymphocytes, a type of white blood cell, similar to the events occurring during *Theieria*'s life cycle.

Transmission to Humans

Transmission of sporozoites to humans is generally a dead-end for the *Babesia* parasite and usually occurs via a nymphal tick that has previously been infected through feeding on an infected rodent. The infected nymph feeds on humans or other larger animals and transmits the protozoan sporozoites by its bite. This primarily happens between May and September when humans are most likely to encounter ticks of this stage while walking, hiking, camping, or playing in an area containing deer ticks. Deer are one of the most important hosts for the adult ticks; they do not develop an illness, although some other mammals and birds do.

Other modes of parasite transmission are also known to occur, including infection of blood recipients following transfusion. In addition to transfusion of packed red blood cells, infection has also resulted from the use of frozen deglycerolized red cell and platelet units. As of 2003, more than 40 such transfusion-related cases had been recorded in the United States. Asymptomatic blood donors have remained infectious for at least a year. One 54-year-old heart transplant patient with an intact spleen was infected with *Babesia* by blood transfusion. He developed severe disease with fever, hemolytic anemia, acute renal failure, and adult respiratory distress syndrome. Transplant recipients are particularly vulnerable to babesiosis due to the immunosuppressants they receive to prevent rejection. Several cases of babesiosis have been identified in which mothers transmitted the parasite to their infants transplacentally.

The Immune Response

The immune response is involved in controlling the extent of infection by *Babesia* species. Early during infection, IgG produced by B lymphocytes of the adaptive immune system may inhibit the initial sporozoite invasion of erythrocytes. NK cells and macrophages of the innate immune system later limit parasitemia caused by whatever sporozoites succeeded in evading the antibodies and infecting erythrocytes. The NK cells may function by the production of IFN-γ, while the macrophages may contribute TNF-α, nitric oxide, and reactive oxygen species. In the mouse model, the infection begins to resolve after ten days, due to degradation of the parasites within host erythrocytes and their removal by the spleen. Parasite destruction is due to the action of $CD4^+$ Th1 helper lymphocytes, which also secrete IFN-γ. $CD8^+$ T killer cells do not appear to be protective during babesiosis.

In addition to its protective role during babesiosis, the immune system may contribute to the pathology. It recognizes infected erythrocytes and kills these cells. If the rate of infection of red blood cells is high, this may lead to the development of anemia. The release of hemoglobin from erythrocytes destroyed by the immune system or lysed by the parasites and the resulting production of bilirubin (a toxic by-product of hemoglobin breakdown) may result in the production of dark urine or jaundice. IgM and the complement system may actually aid in the infection of erythrocytes and prevent their phagocytosis by macrophages, respectively. TNF-α and IFN-γ appear to act synergistically in the development of pulmonary edema.

The increased severity of disease in hosts that are coinfected with *Babesia* and *Borrelia* may be due to immune alterations. *Babesia* (protozoa) infection tends to engender a Th1-like immune response, while *Borrelia* (bacteria) responds most favorable to Th2 responses. Because these two types of T helper cell responses are generally mutually antagonistic, the Th1 responses to *Babesia* would then lower the protective Th2 responses to *Borrelia*.

Diagnosis

Infection of humans or animals with a *Babesia* species may be determined by viewing parasite-infected erythrocytes in thin or thick blood smears by light microscopy. The ring form of the parasite is typically viewed in the host erythrocytes. This procedure is inexpensive but requires a trained technician who is able to differentiate this parasite from similar stages of *Plasmodium* species in erythrocytes, particularly if the patient has visited or resided in an area endemic for malaria or has received a blood transfusion. In contrast to infection by *P. falciparum*, *Babesia*-infected cells lack the pigment hemozoin and so have a pale cytoplasm. Care must be taken in the examination of the blood smears because thin smears may fail to identify parasites if the level of parasitemia is low, while thick smears may not allow detection of smaller species of the parasite.

Diagnosis may be confirmed by the detection of parasite-specific antibodies in the blood by indirect immunofluorescence analysis or parasite DNA by polymerase chain reaction (PCR). Immunofluorescent techniques may be misleading because they can cross-react with other similar parasitic protozoa. Under investigation is an immunoblot test that detects the presence of parasite-specific IgG antibody in an infected person's blood: this test has a sensitivity of 96% and a specificity of 99%. Alternatively, *Babesia* from a blood sample may be amplified and grown in a susceptible laboratory animal (hamsters for *B. microti* and type WA-1 and splenectomized calves or gerbils for *B. divergens*) prior to analysis. Hamsters and mice infected with type WA-1 develop much more serious illness than those inoculated with *B. microti*, which may aid in differentiation of these two species, both found in the United States. The sensitivity and usefulness of growing parasites in hamsters is offset by the time required (seven to ten days) and the expense.

Treatment

Given the similarities between *Babesia* and *Plasmodium* species, some of the drugs that successfully treat malaria are used in combination with other medications to treat babesiosis. Combined therapy with clindamycin and quinine is usually effective for the treatment of babesiosis but may result in serious side effects such as hearing loss, tinnitus (ringing in the ears), hypotension, and gastrointestinal distress. Clindamycin is best known as an agent that inhibits protein synthesis of anaerobic bacteria, and quinine is active against infection of malarial parasites. Another antimalarial drug, chloroquine, is not clinically useful in the treatment of babesiosis.

FIGURE 25.3   The chemical structure of clindamycin

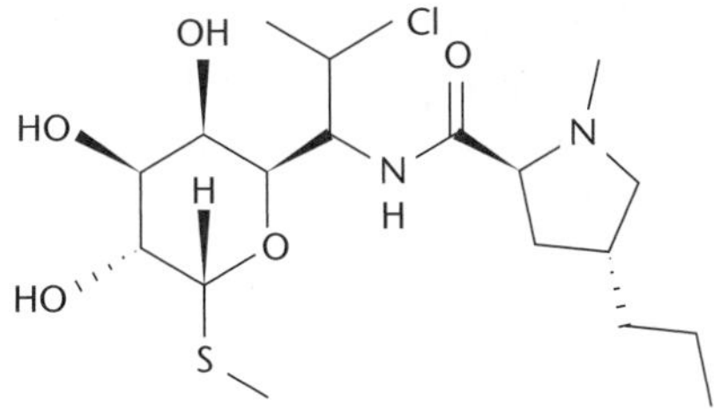

Other combinations that are effective in either some human cases or experimental animal models are azithromycin plus quinine or atovaquone, clindamycin plus doxycline, or pentamidine plus trimethoprim-sulfamethoxazole (TMP-SMX, Bactrim). Azithromycin is a macrolide antibiotic used to kill sexually transmitted bacteria. Doxycline inhibits protein synthesis by distorting the small ribosomal subunit, inhibiting the interaction of tRNA and mRNA. Pentamidine blocks DNA synthesis in *Pneumoncystis jiroveci* (*P. carinii*), a fungus that causes pneumonia in HIV-positive persons, and *Trypanosoma*, protozoan parasites (both discussed

RECENT DEVELOPMENTS

Two cholesterol-lowering drugs, lovastatin and simvastatin, block the development of *B. divergens* in human erythrocytes in the laboratory. This parasite, and its Apicomplexan relative *P. falciparum,* are unable to synthesize fatty acids or cholesterol for themselves but must derive these substances from their hosts. Phospholipids from human high-density lipoproteins are transported to *Babesia* within the erythrocytes. Cholesterol is produced by the isoprenoid pathway; this is required for a number of vital cellular functions, including mitochondrial electron transport, tRNA synthesis, cell growth regulation, and glycosylation of proteins. The isoprenoid pathway uses the enzyme 3-hydroxy-3-methylglutaryl coenzyme A reductase, and its inhibitors, such as lovastatin and simvastatin, decrease cholesterol production. These drugs target the protozoan's reliance on the import of fatty acids and cholesterol from the host's plasma by lowering available plasma cholesterol levels. In vitro tests demonstrated their ability to reduce *B. divergens* growth. A more recent report studied the effects of the cholesterol depletion agent methyl-β-cyclodextrin on *B. bovis*. This agent decreased the amount of cholesterol in the erythrocytic membrane and also reduced the parasite's ability to invade erythrocytes and to divide.

in other chapters). Atovaquone and TMP-SMX are naphthalenes used to treat malaria, pneumonocystis pneumonia, and toxoplasmosis (a severe illness of the nervous system of immunosuppressed individuals resulting from infection with *Toxoplasma gondii*, a related protozoan). In additional to drugs, blood exchange transfusion may be necessary if the percentage of parasitized erythrocytes is high. Dialysis may be needed in the case of renal failure.

Prevention

Preventive measures for babesiosis are similar to those for several other diseases (Lyme disease and ehrlichiosis) transmitted by the bite of infected deer ticks. These measures include decreasing the risk of tick bites by avoiding tick habitat (woody or grassy areas), using proper tick repellents (those containing 10% to 35% DEET), dressing in light-colored clothing that cover one's arms and legs, and careful examination of persons and their dogs after exposure to ticks and the prompt removal of the insects in an approved manner (discussed in Chapter Four).

It usually requires 24 hours for human infection to occur after tick attachment. To prevent human exposure to the ticks, rodent numbers in the vicinity of human dwellings may be reduced by not allowing scrub, weedy vegetation, or wood to be close to homes. To kill the ticks, acaricides may be applied to nests of rodent hosts or the coats of other reservoirs, such as cattle. Thinning deer populations near residential areas also reduces the availability of hosts for the adult form of the deer ticks.

Cases of babesiosis should be reported to local health authorities, particularly if occurring outside a known risk area. Due to the lack of transmission by casual or intimate association with infected persons, contacts do not require testing unless exposed to the same risk factor as the infected individual. In such a case, contacts should be tested for infection and monitored for signs of a fever.

No vaccine is currently available or in the process of large-scale development for human babesiosis due to the relatively low numbers of severe infections in people. Work is under way to develop a preventive vaccine for babesiosis in cattle in light of this disease's economic significance in agricultural areas.

Surveillance

Areas known to be endemic for other tickborne infections, such as Lyme disease and ehrlichiosis, are also at risk for human babesiosis. In one such locale with a very high incidence of Lyme disease in western New Jersey, 100 deer ticks were surveyed by PCR for the prevalence of infection with *B. microti* and the causative agents of the other two diseases. This is a rapidly developing region and many of the homes are located in wooded areas where contact between humans, ticks, deer, and infected rodents may easily occur. Five of the ticks were infected with *B. microti;* two were coinfected with *B. burgdorferi;* and two others with the human granulocytic ehrlichiosis agent. A previous study indicated an infection rate of 9% in deer ticks on Nantucket. The discovery of more than one tickborne pathogen in individual ticks is a matter of concern because a person bitten by such a tick may become infected with both agents simultaneously. At least in the case of *B. burgdorferi* and *B. microti,* the two microbes together induce more severe pathology than either alone. Given the differences in the categories of the infecting microbes (spirochete bacteria and protozoa), treatment may be complicated in the case of dual infection.

Although babesiosis is not a nationally reportable disease in the United States, its reporting is required in some states. Reporting data are therefore incomplete, so other means of surveillance and risk assessment must also be employed. Several studies have compared the abundance of nymphal ticks in an area, determined by the number of nymphs collected per hour, with the presence of human disease. A threshold of more than 20 nymphs per hour in an area was determined to be the most likely to support parasite maintenance in nature with a potential for causing human disease. In Rhode Island, where the study was conducted in an area of the state undergoing development, numbers of nymphal ticks are at or above this threshold number. Approximately 13% of the state's population lives in locations that are at risk for acquiring infection with *Babesia.* This supports the recent trend of increasing reports of human disease in locations where deer and deer tick numbers have been rising due to increasing conservation measures, decreases in the populations of deer predators, and the shift from farmland to forested, semiurban areas.

Summary

Disease

- Babesiosis

Causative Agents

- *B. microti* • *Babesia* isolate type WA-1 • *B. divergens* • Isolate types CA-1 and MO-1

Agent Type

- Apicomplexan protozoan

Genome

- DNA

Vector

- Deer ticks: Ixodes scapularis, Ixodes ricinus

Common Reservoir

Rodents • Cattle • Possibly mule deer or bighorn sheep

Modes of Transmission

- Bite of infected hard-tick nymph • Blood transfusion
- Transplacental transmission

Geographical Distribution

- Scattered areas worldwide, particularly temperate areas of Europe and the northeastern, Great Lakes region, and West Coast of the United State

Year of Emergence

- 1888 in cattle • 1957 in humans

Key Terms

Babesia Several species of parasitic protozoa that infect red blood cells and cause babesiosis in humans and animals; close relatives of *Plasmodium* species (causative agents of malaria)

Babesiosis Serious to fatal infection of erythrocytes with a *Babesia* species

Definitive host Host species in which sexual reproduction occurs

Gametocyte Stage of the life cycle of several parasitic species, including *Plasmodium* and *Babesia*, that produces gametes

Intermediate host Host species in which asexual reproduction occurs

Kinete Motile zygote formed by the union of gametes in Apicomplexan parasites

Sporoblast Undifferentiated, multinucleated form of *Babesia* parasite in salivary glands; buds from its surface 5,000 to 10,000 sporozoites

Strahlenkörper (ray body) Gamete of *Babesia* parasites that contain an arrowhead-shaped organelle

Trophozoite Feeding stage in the life cycle of protozoan parasites

Review Questions

1. What parasite species cause human babesiosis? Where are each located, and what species of tick serves as its vector?
2. What symptoms of a severe case of babesiosis might occur in an asplenic individual? Are asymptomatic persons able to transmit *Babesia* by blood donation?
3. How do the mortality rates of human babesiosis in the United States compare with those in Europe? What may account for this difference? What groups of persons are most susceptible to the development of serious babesiosis?
4. What is the detailed life cycle of *B. microti*?
5. What are the protective actions of the immune system during babesiosis?

Topics for Further Discussion

1. *Ixodes* ticks, including the deer tick, are vectors for a number of important infectious diseases in temperate regions, including several emerging infections. Discuss the pathogens transmitted by these ticks in the United States and Europe and the role of their interactions in augmenting disease severity. What are the roles in the emergence of these diseases of increased deer numbers, conservation efforts, and greater use of natural areas by humans, and how might public health care agencies decrease their incidence without negatively affecting the natural environment?
2. Besides those discussed in this chapter, what are other Apicomplexan parasites of humans and with which diseases are they associated? What structures are unique to this phylum, and how might they be targeted to kill the parasites or inhibit their ability to infect people?
3. Discuss the impacts of *Babesia* species on agriculture and animal husbandry. What are possible economic implications of these impacts, and how might this affect the global economy and the worldwide availability of food?
4. *Babesia* infections are often asymptomatic but are particularly severe in immunosuppressed persons. Discuss the possible effects of the parallel increases in the numbers of immunocompromised individuals (HIV-positive persons, those receiving cancer chemotherapy, organ transplant recipients, the elderly) and those with inapparent babesiosis. How might the latter affect the safety of the blood supply, and what measures might be taken to counter this?

Resources

Chin, J. *Control of Communicable Diseases Manual* (17th ed.). Washington, D.C.: American Public Health Association, 2000.

Grellier, P., and others. "3-Hydroxy-3-Methylglutaryl Coenzyme A Reductase Inhibitors Lovastatin and Simvastatin Inhibit In Vitro Development of *Plasmodium falciparum* and *Babesia divergens* in Human Erythrocytes." *Antimicrobial Agents and Chemotherapy*, 1994, *38*, 1144–1148.

Herwaldt, B. L., and others. "Endemic Babesiosis in Another Eastern State: New Jersey." *Emerging Infectious Diseases*, 2003, *9*, 184–188.

Homer, M. J., and others. "Babesiosis." *Clinical Microbiology Reviews*, 2000, *13*, 451–469.

Lux, J. Z., and others. "Transfusion-Associated Babesiosis After Heart Transplant." *Emerging Infectious Diseases*, 2003, *9*, 116–119.

Manson-Bahr, P.E.C., and Apted, F.I.C. *Manson's Tropical Diseases*. Philadelphia: Baillière Tindall, 1982.

Rodgers, S. E., and Mather, T. N. "Human *Babesia microti* Incidence and *Ixodes scapularis* Distribution, Rhode Island, 1998–2004." *Emerging Infectious Diseases*, 2007, *13*, 633–635.

Schuster, F. L. "Cultivation of *Babesia* and *Babesia*-like Blood Parasites: Agents of an Emerging Zoonotic Disease." *Clinical Microbiology Reviews*, 2002, *15*, 365–373.

Varde, S., Beckley, J., and Schwartz, I. "Prevalence of Tickborne Pathogens in *Ixodes scapularis* in a Rural New Jersey County." *Emerging Infectious Diseases*, 1998, *4*, 97–99.

Zintl, A., and others. "*Babesia divergens*, a Bovine Blood Parasite of Veterinary and Zoonotic Importance." *Clinical Microbiology Reviews*, 2003, *16*, 622–636.

CHAPTER 26

CRYPTOSPORIDIOSIS

LEARNING OBJECTIVES

- Define cryptosporidiosis

- Describe the Apicomplexan protozoa responsible for causing this illness

- Discuss modes of infection

- Discuss the host's response to infection

- Describe symptomatology and diagnosis

- Discuss potential methods of treatment

- Discuss methods of prevention

Major Concepts

Incidence

The first known *Cryptosporidium* species was discovered in mice in 1907, but these parasitic protozoa were not detected in humans until 1976. Very few human infections were noted over the next few years until the organisms were linked to a serious diarrheal condition in HIV-positive men during the early 1980s. Since then, *Cryptosporidium* species have caused disease in diverse populations, including very young children, the elderly, persons in developing regions, campers and backpackers, people coming into contact with farm animals, and immunosuppressed individuals. Infection in this last group is often chronic, severe, and potentially life-threatening. Immunocompetent people may become ill as well. Several large outbreaks have occurred in industrialized nations, including the United States and Canada, due to waterborne transmission. The largest outbreak occurred in 1993 in Milwaukee and affected more than 400,000 people.

Symptoms

Most *Cryptosporidium* species that infect humans cause diarrhea. One species, however, causes fever, generalized malaise, nausea and vomiting, malnutrition, significant weight loss, and delayed growth. Infection of the intestine leads to blunting of villi and increased levels of transitional epithelium. This may result in malnutrition, altered absorption and secretion of sodium and chloride ions, and dehydration due to the loss of large amounts of water in the stools.

Infection

Cryptosporidiosis is caused primarily by either *C. hominis* or *C. parvum*, which closely resemble each other morphologically but differ genetically, in clinical presentation, and in host range. Infection with *C. hominis* is mainly restricted to humans and may cause serious disease. This parasite is most likely to be involved in large outbreaks due to contamination of either drinking or recreational water sources. *C. parvum* infects humans, calves, sheep, goats, and deer and may cause isolated cases by zoonotic transmission. It generally causes a milder form of disease than *C. hominis*. Both species are members of the Apicomplexa protozoan phylum. They have several life stages, including hardy oocysts released into the feces, motile sporozoites and merozoites, and sexual forms.

Immune Response

Cryptosporidium infection stimulates the production of chemokines, which attract cells of the innate and adaptive immune systems to the intestinal lamina propria. Cytokines such as TNF-α, IFN-γ, IL-4, and IL-10 are released into the area. Th1 CD4$^+$ T helper cells, IgG, and IgM are particularly important in resolving infection. Long-lasting immunity is not produced, however, and individuals are often reinfected.

Protection

Many drugs have been tested for the treatment of *Cryptosporidium* infection, without much success due to difficulty in accessing parasites located under the mucosal epithelium or within dense attachment complexes. Nitazoxanide is currently recommended to treat cryptosporidiosis in healthy persons over the age of 12 months, but it does not completely eliminate infection in all persons. Antiviral therapy given to HIV-positive individuals increases CD4$^+$ T cell numbers and helps resolve infection. Oral or intravenous rehydration therapy is useful to counteract water loss. Prevention involves decreasing ingestion of viable oocysts from fecal material. Oocysts are highly resistant to chlorination and pass through many filters. Persons with diarrhea should avoid using recreational water and preparing food. Fruits and vegetables that will not be cooked should be washed thoroughly with soap and clean water. Travelers, campers, and backpackers need to ensure the safety of their water supplies.

Introduction

Since the advent of the AIDS epidemic, a number of organisms have been identified that are responsible for serious or life-threatening infections in immunosuppressed persons. These include agents that cause respiratory illnesses, diarrheal disease, and unusual cancers. Some of these agents were later found to be pathogenic in immunocompetent individuals as well, particularly young children. Organisms that cause severe diarrhea in humans include *Cyclospora*, *Giardia*, and *Cryptosporidium* species. Several groups of the protozoan genus *Cryptosporidium* infect humans, the two major species being *C. hominis* and *C. parvum*. Infection with the former primarily occurs in humans and may result in severe illness, including fever, vomiting, dehydration, malnutrition, and growth deficiency. *C. parvum* infects a number of ruminants, including calves, sheep, and goats, in addition to humans and may be acquired via **zoonotic transmission** (transmission from animals to humans). Infection with this protozoan typically leads only to diarrhea.

Inhabitants of developing nations are far more likely to acquire infection than those living in developed regions. Children in developing areas are usually infected very early in life. Infection causes alterations of cells in the intestinal wall that interfere with the absorption of nutrients. Infected children may suffer long-term consequences, such as stunted growth, from the resulting malnutrition. Immunosuppressed individuals, especially those with low $CD4^+$ T helper cell numbers, often develop chronic, life-threatening disease. They should take particular care to avoid infection. Transmission may occur in a variety of manners, including via contaminated drinking water or recreational water, such as lakes, swimming pools, water slides, and hot tubs. *Cryptosporidium* parasites are highly resistant to chlorine, and their small size presents difficulties in removing them from drinking supplies by filtration. A major epidemic occurred in Milwaukee, Wisconsin, that sickened more than 400,000 persons and was particularly dangerous to HIV-positive individuals. Other outbreaks in industrialized nations, including the United States and Canada, have involved imported foods.

History

Cryptosporidium muris was discovered in the gastric glands of asymptomatic mice in 1907 by Edward Tyzzer, who later identified *C. parvum* in the small intestine of these rodents in 1912. Infection by various other *Cryptosporidium* species was linked to diarrheal disease in poultry, calves, and several other animals since the 1950s. In 1976, a 3-year-old child was found to be infected with *Cryptosporidium;* seven more human cases were reported over the next six years, five of which occurred in immunocompromised persons. These organisms were not widely recognized as human pathogens, however, until the advent of the AIDS epidemic starting around 1982. In 2002, the genus was divided into two primary species infecting humans, ***Cryptosporidium parvum*** and ***Cryptosporidium hominis***. These enteric (gut-associated) pathogens are two of several protozoa found to cause severe, persistent diarrhea that is life-threatening in HIV-positive individuals. The genus was subsequently discovered to lead to endemic persistent diarrhea in normal, healthy adults residing in tropical regions as well.

A large outbreak involving drinking water occurred in Milwaukee in 1993 and a smaller one in Las Vegas in 1996. The Milwaukee outbreak was unusually severe and involved 403,000 people. It was the largest waterborne infection in U.S. history and is believed to have cost $96.2 million: $31.7 million in medical costs and $64.6 million in lost productivity. The Las Vegas outbreak occurred in spite of a state-of-the-art water treatment facility and was detected only because *Cryptosporidium* infection is a reportable illness in Nevada. In 2007, more than

1,900 cases of cryptosporidiosis were reported in Utah. This outbreak was linked to recreational water use in pools, water parks, and interactive fountains. Children under the age of 5 years were particularly affected.

The Disease

Infection with *Cryptosporidium* may result in severe, persistent diarrhea by disrupting the epithelial lining of the intestinal tract. It may be accompanied by cramping abdominal pain and less commonly by fever, generalized malaise, nausea, or vomiting. This disease may be life-threatening in immunosuppressed persons, especially those who are HIV-positive. Besides causing diarrhea directly, infection predisposes young children to increased diarrheal burdens and malnutrition for months afterward. This protozoan may also infect and cause diarrhea in healthy adults who are not immunocompromised, especially those living in the tropics. It poses a potential threat to people residing in temperate areas as well, including northern portions of the United States. Developing regions have a higher incidence of infection than developed regions: the infection rate in developing countries is 1.5% among the general population and 6% in individuals with diarrhea, compared to 0.2% in the healthy and 2% in those with diarrhea in developed areas. The infection rate is even higher among HIV-positive individuals with diarrhea: 24% in developing areas and 14% in developed regions. Approximately 20% of young adults in the United States show evidence of a past infection with *Cryptosporidium,* and more than 90% of those in some developing countries had been infected during their early childhood.

Infection with *Cryptosporidium* results in watery diarrhea that may last two weeks or more, even in immunocompetent hosts. Significant weight loss or dehydration may occur. In the Milwaukee outbreak, infected persons were generally ill for 4 to 12 days, with 8 to 19 bowel movements a day, and lost 4.5 kilograms (10 pounds). Low-grade fever was noted in 36% to 57% of the infected. Other persons developed an upper gastrointestinal tract infection characterized by vomiting, indicating possible infection of the stomach by this parasite. Persons experiencing vomiting appear to represent a subgroup in which disease is universally fatal. Approximately 20% to 40% of the infected persons had a recurrence of watery diarrhea after three days of normal stools. The disease was particularly severe in HIV-positive persons with low $CD4^+$ T helper cell numbers. The elderly accounted for 36% of patients with cryptosporidiosis.

Disease in healthy persons is typically self-limiting and resolves within 30 days, while that occurring in immunocompromised individuals is most often chronic and life-threatening. Responses to infection, however, may be more complex. One or more relapses of diarrhea occurred in 45% of healthy persons who were voluntarily reinfected with the parasite, and 20% reported two to five relapses. Studies from Brazil indicate that normal children who are initially infected before the age of 1 year experience longer periods of diarrhea than those initially infected later in life and are much more likely to have multiple diarrheal episodes due to other gut pathogens. Infection of children in Africa and Peru had prolonged effects on their weight and height and also led to delayed mortality in which infected persons may not die until two years after infection. Diarrhea in children may be preceded by vomiting and anorexia. Among immunocompromised HIV-positive persons, the lower the $CD4^+$ T helper cell number, the greater the risk of developing protracted diarrhea. Those with 150 or more $CD4^+$ T cells per cubic millimeter of blood are usually able to clear the infection. Clinical responses in this group are nevertheless variable. While about one-third of the AIDS patients with low $CD4^+$ cell levels have cholera-type disease requiring intravenous rehydration, 15% have only transient diarrhea, defined as more than two bowel movements per day, controllable with antimotility agents or spontaneously resolving. It is not known whether the variability in disease course is due to individual differences in host responses, to the presence of copathogens such as cytomegalovirus, or to differences in virulence of the infecting protozoan strain.

The Causative Agents

C. parvum and *C. hominis* are protozoa belonging to the phylum Apicomplexa, which also includes other human and animal pathogens such as *Plasmodium* (malaria) and *Babesia* (discussed in other chapters). The latter infects erythrocytes, resulting in hemolytic anemia, renal failure, severe multiorgan failure, and other serious disease manifestations. The *Cryptosporidium* genus is a member of the order Eucoccidiida, suborder Eimeriina, which includes other pathogens, such as *Isospora*, *Cyclospora*, and *Toxoplasma*. *Cyclospora* species are enteric pathogens similar to *C. parvum*, and *Toxoplasma* infection may lead to severe disease in infants born to infected mothers. Both of these protozoa cause serious illness in HIV-positive persons as well. *Sarcocystis* species are other Apicomplexans whose oocysts may easily be mistaken for *Cryptosporidium*. In addition to humans, *Cryptosporidium* species infect at least 45 vertebrate species, including fish, reptiles, birds, small mammals (rodents, dogs, cats), and large mammals (cattle, sheep, goats, and deer). The genus name means "underground" or "hidden spore."

Cryptosporidia are small organisms, 3 to 6 micrometers in length, with a hardy, acid-fast, ovoid to spheroidal oocyst form. They are unable to replicate

Table 26.1 Several Apicomplexan parasites of humans

Genus	System Affected	Prominent Symptoms
Cryptosporidium	Gut	Diarrhea, acute gastroenteritis
Sarcocystis	Gut	Diarrhea
Cyclospora	Gut	Prolonged diarrhea
Isospora	Gut	Watery diarrhea
Plasmodium	Blood	Hemolytic anemia, renal failure, cerebral manifestations
Babesia	Blood	Hemolytic anemia, renal failure
Toxoplasma	Nervous system	Acute meningoencephalitis, seizures

outside of the host. Sequence analysis of small subunit rRNA suggests that there is a *Cryptosporidium* group that infects humans and that other isolates from monkeys, calves, and sheep are closely related to each other genetically and are slightly more distantly related to *C. felis* from cats. *C. felis*, however, may also be identified by rRNA analysis in stools of AIDS patients. *C. meleagridis* from turkeys, *C. canis* from dogs, *C. muris* from mice, the *Cryptosporidium* cervine genotype from deer, and the pig genotype I are occasionally found in humans as well. The *Cryptosporidium* group infecting humans has a great degree of molecular heterogeneity, enabling the protozoa to be placed into two major species. *C. hominis* (formerly genotype 1, the H genotype) infects primarily humans and monkeys but not calves, rodents, cats, or dogs. The Milwaukee outbreak, as well as the majority of other outbreaks, involved this genotype. Only 10% of the cases of cryptosporidiosis in the United States are attributable to outbreaks. The other major species of *Cryptosporidium* affecting humans, *C. parvum* (formerly genotype 2, the C genotype), infects neonatal ruminants (calves, sheep, goats, and deer), mice, and humans. It is further divided into several families, of which family IIc is acquired from other humans and family IIa is typically a zoonotic infection.

C. hominis was the predominant species isolated in studies of children from widespread geographical locations such as Malawi, Kenya, India, Haiti, and Brazil; in children and elderly persons from South Africa; and in hospitalized HIV-infected children from South Africa and Uganda. *C. parvum* may be more common in Europe. Coinfection with several *Cryptosporidium* species may also occur. A study of mucosal biopsy material from 13 AIDS patients found that all patients contained DNA of the *C. parvum* variety, while 60% also contained *C. hominis* variety DNA at the same site. Isolates of *C. parvum* have variable virulence in humans and differ up to 100-fold in infectious dose. The TAMU strain is most virulent, with an attack rate of 85% and diarrheal duration of 94 hours. As few as nine oocysts are able to infect 50% of the humans inoculated.

The UCP strain, by contrast, has an attack rate of only 59%, shorter disease duration (82 hours), and requires over 1,000 oocysts to infect 50% of inoculated volunteers. The two primary species of *Cryptosporidium* infecting humans differ in clinical manifestations. Infection with *C. hominis* is associated with diarrhea, nausea, vomiting, general malaise, and delayed growth, with increased intensity and duration of oocyst shedding and higher levels of fecal lactoferrin, an iron-binding protein produced by phagocytic white blood cells. *C. hominis* produces more serious disease in HIV-positive persons as well. In contrast, infection with *C. parvum, C. meleagridis, C. canis,* or *C. felis* is associated only with diarrhea. *C. hominis* is separated into several families (Ia, Ib, Id, and Ie), all of which are associated with diarrhea. Family Ib is also associated with nausea, vomiting, and general malaise and is more pathogenic than other *C. hominis* families in children. It is also the most common family found in epidemics of waterborne infection in industrialized nations. Family Id, however, is more virulent in HIV-positive persons.

The life cycle of cryptosporidia, like other Apicomplexan parasites, includes several stages involving both asexual and sexual reproductive forms. **Oocysts** are hardy, rounded, cyst-like protozoa that resist adverse environmental conditions, such as desiccation. They are the infectious stage for humans and animals. Each cryptosporidium oocyst releases four motile sporozoites, which invade and establish infection immediately below the luminal cell layer of the intestinal epithelial mucosa. The ileum is the preferred site of infection, but the protozoa may also be found in the colon. Sporozoites replicate asexually by **schizogony** (multiple fission) to produce eight mobile Type I merozoites. These may infect new epithelial cells to produce additional Type I merozoites or may form four Type II merozoites. The latter may produce 16 microgametes or a single macrogamete, the male and female sexual forms of the parasite. These fuse to produce a zygote, the thick-walled oocyst, that divides to produce four sporozoites. The oocyst is then released externally in the feces and may survive for prolonged periods of time (two to six months in moist environments) before being ingested by the next host.

After establishing an intestinal base, cryptosporidia may disseminate to the biliary (liver and gallbladder) or respiratory tracts, stomach, or pancreas. Cholecystitis-like symptoms (inflammation of the gallbladder) may occur in individuals with biliary infection. In the intestine, villi (projections that increase surface area to increase absorption of nutrients) may be blunted and fused, crypts may undergo hyperplasia, and epithelial barrier function may be disrupted. These alterations may involve inflammatory host molecules such as TNF-α and prostaglandins from macrophages. Levels of "transitional" epithelium that are dependent on glutamine for energy may also increase. Nearly two-thirds of the tip of the villi and surface area may be lost, linked to a 50% decrease in

FIGURE 26.1   Life cycle of *Cryptosporidium*

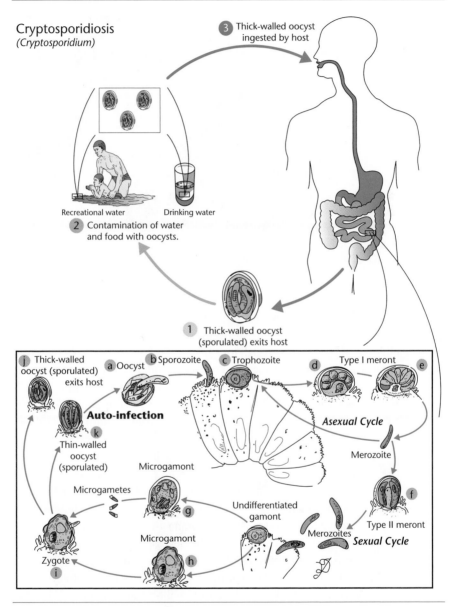

Cryptosporidiosis
(Cryptosporidium)

3 Thick-walled oocyst
    ingested by host

Recreational water   Drinking water

2 Contamination of water
   and food with oocysts.

1 Thick-walled oocyst
   (sporulated) exits host

j Thick-walled
   oocyst (sporulated)
   exits host

a Oocyst

b Sporozoite

c Trophozoite

d

e Type I meront

Auto-infection

k Thin-walled
   oocyst
   (sporulated)

Asexual Cycle

Merozoite

Microgamont

Microgametes

g

Undifferentiated
gamont

f Type II meront

Merozoites

Sexual Cycle

Microgamont

h

Zygote

i

Source: CDC/Alexander J. da Silva and Melanie Moser.

FIGURE 26.2   *Cryptosporidium* in the gallbladder

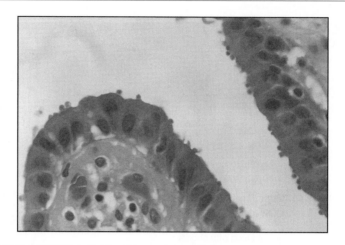

Source: CDC/Edwin P. Ewing Jr.

glucose-coupled sodium cotransport. The loss of absorptive surfaces due to villus blunting may cause malnutrition, which affects subsequent growth in young children; this effect on growth may be permanent. Even children with supposedly asymptomatic infection may experience blunted growth, indicating that cryptosporidial infection may be an underlying cause of malnutrition even in persons not experiencing overt diarrhea. Furthermore, disruption of epithelial barrier function may increase the susceptibility of young children to other diarrheal illnesses for many additional months.

Parasite adherence to and invasion of the intestinal epithelial cell lining induces the activation of several host cell enzymes (phosphatidylinositol-3-phosphate kinase, myosin light-chain kinase, and tyrosine kinases) and the transcription factor NF-κB, which aid in the production of a dense attachment zone between the protozoa and the host cells containing the cellular cytoskeleton component actin. This protected area in which the developmental forms mature is known as the intracellular but extracytoplasmic location. The kinases affect ion transport through cell membranes by inhibiting sodium absorption and stimulating chloride secretion out of the cell. The kinases also alter the functioning of tight junctions that join the epithelial cells together and form a tight barrier to the passage of material out of the intestinal lumen and into the interior of the body. This disruption of epithelial barrier function may allow infection by other gut pathogens, as described earlier. Infection of epithelial cells by the parasite also stimulates new protein synthesis, resulting in increased levels of the proinflammatory cytokines

TNF-α and chemokines, such as IL-8, which attracts neutrophils into the lamina propria, and the IFN-γ-inducible protein 10, which attracts leukocytes that produce IFN-γ. Infection also leads to the release of prostaglandins E2 and I2 from cells, perhaps triggered by the high levels of TNF-α. Prostaglandins themselves stimulate chloride secretion and further stimulate the enteric nervous system (involuntary branch of the nervous system that controls the digestive tract) to encourage this secretion. Levels of the neuropeptide substance P are increased in intestinal tissues of persons with cryptosporidiosis, being released by intraepithelial or lamina propria lymphocytes or monocytes. Substance P has several roles: it is involved in pain perception, helps stimulate production of cytokines, such as IFN-γ and TNF-α, and induces chloride secretion by human gastrointestinal cells. Because the removal of sodium from the intestinal lumen is inhibited and the secretion of chloride is promoted, increased levels of sodium chloride (table salt) are present in the gut, which increases the water content, leading to the production of watery diarrhea and possibly dehydration. Some infected cells also undergo apoptosis induced by activation of caspase 3.

Infection with *Cryptosporidium* is spread by oral-fecal transmission and may occur by four routes: waterborne, person-to-person, foodborne, and zoonotic. Waterborne transmission leads to epidemics and may occur through drinking water or recreational water, including that found in lakes, ponds, rivers, hot tubs, or fountains. Person-to-person spread, in contrast, causes endemic disease and may occur in settings such as day care centers. Foodborne infection may result from consumption of contaminated foods, such as raspberries irrigated or rinsed with infected water, or by beverages, such as unpasteurized apple cider or raw milk. Infected animals, such as calves or poultry, may also transmit cryptosporidia to humans. This route of infection may be particularly problematic for those inhabiting rural, pastoral settings. Soil coming into contact with infected animal feces is also contaminated. Cryptosporidial infection in the U.S. Upper Midwest appears to be primarily via the zoonotic route. Wisconsin had the highest incidence of cryptosporidiosis each year from 1999 to 2002. Persons at particular risk for becoming infected by all four routes are children under the age of 2 years; travelers; animal handlers; men who have sex with men; close contacts of infected individuals, such as family members and health care or day care workers; backpackers and campers drinking unfiltered, untreated water; persons drinking from shallow, untreated wells; and swimmers who swallow contaminated water. Immunosuppressed individuals, including HIV-positive persons, those with cancer or viral infections such as measles, recipients of transplants, the malnourished, individuals on immunosuppressive drugs, and persons with inherited immunodeficiency conditions, such as hyper-IgM syndrome, are at risk for developing serious disease. If the underlying cause of immunosuppression can be removed, the diarrheal disease often resolves.

Cryptosporidium oocysts are extremely resistant to chlorine and survive the amounts added to municipal drinking water, swimming pools, and waterslides. Over one-fourth of the tested chlorinated water samples meeting U.S. and Canadian turbidity standards were found to contain oocysts in 1991. In a 1994 outbreak among HIV-positive persons in Clark County, Nevada, the **nephelometry turbidity units (NTUs)** were below 0.17, well beneath the EPA maximum of 0.5 NTU, and in the Milwaukee outbreak, levels were between 0.45 and 1.7 NTU. High turbidity levels are an indicator of possible water contamination, but their absence does not guarantee water safety. The combination of great chlorine resistance and low infectious dose (as few as nine 10 oocysts) place *Cryptosporidium* among the most infectious of enteric pathogens. This is evidenced by their rapid spread through members of a household; their tendency to cause numerous outbreaks in day care centers and in chlorinated swimming pools and wave pools during the late summer, the ease of nosocomial infection, and their transmission through acidic apple cider.

The Immune Response

CD4$^+$ T helper cells and CD8$^+$ T killer cells play a role in resolving infection with *Cryptosporidium*. The intraepithelial region of the immune system, IL-12, and Th1-type immunity are important to this process, partially by inducing production of the Th1 cytokine IFN-γ. IFN-γ is vital to prevent acute disease in mice, and HIV-negative humans lacking IFN-γ develop severe disease. Th2 cytokines, such as IL-4, are protective as well. Amounts of the Treg cytokines IL-10 and TGF-β rise after resolution of symptoms. These cytokines may decrease inflammation and be involved in intestinal healing. Despite the role of these cytokines in eliminating infection, a single infection with cryptosporidia

Table 26.2 Immune system components activated by *Cryptosporidium* infection

Cell types involved	Th1 and Th2 lymphocytes
	B lymphocytes
	Macrophages
	Neutrophils
Immune mediators	Th1 cytokines (IL-12, IFN-γ)
	Th2 cytokines (IL-4)
	Treg cytokines (IL-10, TGF-β)
	Inflammatory cytokines (TNF-α)
	Chemokines (IL-8)
Antibody classes	IgA, IgG, IgM

is not likely to induce long-lasting protective immunity, and repeated infections are highly likely to occur. These reinfections often produce disease again with the same incidence as the first infection (70% symptomatic infection for the first and second infection). During the second infection, however, disease symptoms are less severe and fewer oocysts are released in the stool. Humoral immunity appears to be at least partially effective, however, for volunteers with anti-*Cryptosporidium* IgG antibody require a 20-fold higher inoculum to become infected and release lower numbers of oocysts. IgM and IgG may, however, function better in protection against illness rather than in protection against infection. Levels of antiprotozoan IgA are elevated in the mucosa and in stools.

Innate immune responses may have a role in eliminating cryptosporidial infection. Toll-like receptors (TLRs) of the innate immune system are important in providing resistance to infection by protozoa. TLRs are pathogen pattern recognition receptors that allow various groups of microbes to be recognized by the immune system on the basis of molecules unique to that group; many of these receptors rely on the recruitment of the adaptor protein myeloid differentiation protein 88 (MyD88) for signaling. Infection of cells by *Cryptosporidium* increases expression of TLRs 2 and 4, followed by the recruitment of MyD88. This in turn activates a kinase enzymatic cascade, resulting in the activation of transcription factors, such as NF-κB and c-Jun, and the production of inflammatory cytokines. NF-κB activation leads to production of the antiapoptotic molecule Bcl-2 in an attempt to compensate for the proapoptotic signals induced by the protozoan and to prolong survival of infected cells. MyD88-mediated innate immunity acts in concert with IFN-γ in the control of infection. Precise regulation of these pathways is critical, as inflammatory responses may either mediate resistance to infection or contribute to disease pathogenesis. IL-15 may also regulate the anticryptosporidial innate immune response by activating NK cells to eliminate infected intestinal cells.

Phagocytic cells travel to sites of cryptosporidial infection. Intestinal macrophages secrete the inflammatory cytokine TNF-α, which may induce prostaglandin-dependent secretion of chloride by chloride channels in intestinal crypts or by inhibition of sodium-hydrogen exchangers in the transitional epithelium. Increased production of the chemokine IL-8 attracts neutrophils into the area as well, contributing to the inflammatory milieu.

Diagnosis

The most efficient and effective means of diagnosis appear to be acid-fast stain or safranin-methylene blue stain of fecal material for oocysts and immunofluorescent microscopy without concentration. A fluorescein-labeled antibody is

FIGURE 26.3   Stool sample containing *Cryptosporidium*

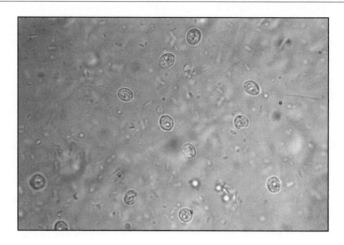

Source: CDC/Peter Drotman.

available for detecting oocysts in stool or environmental samples. Without proper staining, the small size of the oocysts may lead to their being mistaken for yeast. Multiple stool samples may be required to maximize detection (53% versus 73%, respectively). Endoscopy with mucosal biopsy of the terminal ileum (third portion of the small intestine) is much more sensitive, however (91%). The presence of merozoites in biopsy samples may also indicate infection.

Diagnostic techniques may also include polymerase chain reaction (PCR) and ELISA. Morphological and antibody-based diagnostic techniques are not able to differentiate between *C. hominis* and *C. parvum;* however, PCR-based techniques may do so by identifying genetic differences. One new technique uses amplification of the microsatellite locus, microsatellite-2 region, followed by hybridization with probes detecting a single nucleotide difference between *C. hominis* and *C. parvum* DNA sequences. The probes are then covalently bound to fluorescent microspheres and analyzed by flow cytometry. This technique may be performed in five hours, is less expensive than traditional PCR, and is 100% specific.

Treatment

Many antimicrobial and antiparasitic agents have been tested for the treatment of cryptosporidiosis; however, none has been effective at eliminating the parasites from 100% of the infected people, particularly immunosuppressed persons. The difficulty in finding useful drugs is due in part to the parasites' residing beneath the gel-like mucous layer of the epithelium or in intracellular but extracytoplasmic locales. The antiparasitic agent nitazoxanide is recommended by the U.S. Food and Drug Administration for the treatment of cryptosporidiosis in healthy persons over the age of 1 year. After five days, diarrheal disease resolves in 72% to 88% of those using this drug, and 60% to 75% of users have no detectable oocysts in their stools. Infection with *Cryptosporidium* is also partly treatable with paromomycin, reducing parasite load and bowel movement frequency, especially when administered early during infection. Paromomycin is beneficial for up to two-thirds of HIV-positive persons and AIDS patients but not those with low CD4 numbers. Combined treatment with paromomycin and azithromycin may be useful. HAART helps resolve diarrheal disease in AIDS patients due to increased CD4$^+$ T helper cell numbers and improved immune responsiveness. AIDS patients receiving clarithromycin or rifabutin for *Mycobacterium avium* infection noted decreased rates of infection with *Cryptosporidium* as well.

RECENT DEVELOPMENTS

DNA and RNA are composed of pyrimidine (cytosine, thymine, and uracil) and purine (guanine and adenine) nucelotide bases. These must be synthesized de novo or recycled from other bases (salvaged). *Cryptosporidium* lacks all of the enzymes required for the de novo synthesis of pyrimidines and therefore relies completely on salvaging these bases from its vertebrate host. The protozoa depend on three salvage enzymes to supply them with these DNA and RNA bases: uracil phosphoribosyltransferase (UPRT), a bifunctional uridine kinase UPRT (UK-UPRT), and thymidine kinase (TK). Protozoan UPRT salvages uracil by a mechanism that is not employed by mammalian cells. Analogues of uracil might be developed that are processed specifically by the parasite into toxic metabolites that would not be formed in host cells. Cytosine-arabinoside (Ara-C) is a drug commonly used in cancer chemotherapy. It is activated to a toxic form by *Cryptosporidium*'s UK. Other currently available drugs target TK, which *Cryptosporidium* appears to have derived from a bacterium.

Cryptosporidia obtain their purines solely from the salvage of adenosine. A key enzyme in the salvage pathway is inosine 5'-monophosphage dehydrogenase (IMPDH). This enzyme is inhibited by the drug ribavirin, currently in use as an antiviral agent. Ribavirin inhibits cryptosporidia in cultured cells. Evidence suggests that the IMPDH from *Cryptosporidium* is of bacterial origin and has different properties from that found in humans, a fact that might be exploited to specifically target the protozoa.

Considering that glutamine-coupled sodium absorption does not appear to be adversely affected by cryptosporidial infection, glutamine-based oral rehydration and nutrition therapies show promise in rehydrating infected persons and aiding in the repair of disrupted intestinal wall functioning. In milder cases, increasing fluid consumption may aid in countering dehydration. Another hopeful approach lies in attacking a parasite transporter protein found in the dense attachment zone. This member of the ATP-binding cassette protein family of transporters may be blocked by analogues of the drug cyclosporin.

Prevention

Removing viable *Cryptosporidium* from drinking water supplies is problematic due to its extreme resistance to chlorine and iodine. Its small size presents further difficulties with removal by filtration, unless the filters are able to remove particles smaller than 1 micrometer in diameter. "Reverse osmosis" and "cyst removal" filters are protective as well. Pasteurization of milk and fruit juices and bringing water to a rolling boil for at least one minute are effective means of killing these protozoa; however, boiling water tends to concentrate any pollutants that may be present. This may present problems in areas of the world with high levels of chemical contaminants, including nitrates from fertilizers. Other approaches using electronics or radiation may be useful in the removal of cryptosporidia and other infectious agents in the future. Ultimately, separation of water supplies used for drinking purposes from water serving other needs may prove to be advantageous, at least in some parts of the world.

Preventive interventions may include public education concerning proper hygiene, sanitary disposal of human and animal feces, and hand-washing for people coming into contact with animals with diarrhea, particularly calves. Persons with diarrhea should not prepare food that will not be subsequently cooked. Children with diarrhea should be excluded from day care centers and swimming pools while symptomatic. To prevent contamination of recreational water, people should wash with soap prior to entering these facilities. People should keep their mouths closed when in the water. Articles soiled with feces may be disinfected by heating for 5 to 20 minutes at 45°C (113°F) or for two minutes at 60°C (140°F). Chemical disinfection of such articles using 10% formalin or 5% ammonia is also effective.

Seeing that temperate areas and developed nations import seasonal food products from developing countries in tropical regions, it may be in the best interests of the developing nations to reduce contamination of the water used to irrigate or wash food. Fruits and vegetables that are eaten raw should be thoroughly cleaned in uncontaminated water. Travelers to regions with unsafe water supplies should avoid drinking water, using ice, or brushing their teeth with tap water. Hot tea and hot coffee are generally safe.

Safer sex practices may decrease risk of infection with *Cryptosporidium* and other organisms, such as hepatitis A and *Giardia*. Sexual practices that involve contact with feces should be avoided, including those in which oral-anal contact occurs. Condoms should be disposed of following anal contact. Because fecal material may also be present on the genitals, barrier methods should be used in instances of oral-genital contact.

Immunosuppressed persons need to use special care to prevent infection. They should avoid contact with fecal material from pets, especially puppies and kittens under the age of 6 months, and stray animals. After visiting a farm or petting zoo, these individuals should wash their hands thoroughly with soap and water and have an immunocompetent person clean their shoes. Special care must be paid to food and water sources, especially when traveling.

Surveillance

Drinking water is a potential source of diarrheal epidemics such as those that occurred in the 1990s in Milwaukee and Las Vegas. Filtration sampling of large water volumes may detect the presence of oocysts. In 1991, a study of 66 water treatment plants in 14 U.S. states revealed that 87% of inflow water contained *Cryptosporidium* oocysts and that they persisted in 27% of the treated, finished water samples. About 7% of oocysts detected visually in drinking water were found to be viable cryptosporidia.

Among immunocompetent children in Peru, community-based studies revealed that 30% of those infected experienced diarrhea. In a study of 533 Peruvian children, the rate of infection with *C. hominis* was four times that of *C. parvum*. Another four-year study of immunocompetent children without severe malnutrition was conducted in Brazilian slums. These children typically became infected prior to their first birthday. Infection was linked with both acute and persistent diarrhea. Relapsing *Cryptosporidium*-related diarrhea occurred in about a third of these children. Other studies found that number of days of diarrhea before the age of 2 years is associated with decreased physical fitness and cognitive defects four to seven years later. Given the important short- and long-term consequences of infection of the very young, surveillance of this population is key to early intervention.

In a 1998–1999 survey of 669 beef cows from 39 farms within 10 counties of Ontario, 18.4% of the animals were infected with *C. parvum* and 90%

of the farms had positive cattle. Infection appeared to be due to oocysts in the bedding and pen floor and was highest during calving season. Surveillance studies performed in dairy farms in Quebec yielded a three times higher incidence rate, perhaps reflecting greater indoor confinement of diary calves. Infected calves and cows may shed oocysts for weeks, so restricting their access to surface water may reduce contamination of watersheds, thereby decreasing transmission.

Summary

Disease

- Cryptosporidiosis, characterized by severe, persistent diarrhea, dehydration, and malnutrition with or without fever, nausea, vomiting, and weight loss

Causative Agents

- *Cryptosporidium parvum* • *Cryptosporidium hominis*

Agent Type

- Parasite of the phylum Apicomplexa, order Eucoccidiida, suborder Eimeriina

Genome

- Double-stranded DNA

Vector

- None

Common Reservoirs

- Humans • Cattle • Other domestic animals

Modes of Transmission

- Waterborne, person-to-person, foodborne, or zoonotic transmission

Geographical Distribution

- Worldwide (over 50 countries on six continents), but primarily tropical areas • Infection may occur in temperate zones, including the northern United States and Canada

Years of Emergence

- 1976 (first reports of human disease) • 1982 (life-threatening infection of HIV-positive persons)

Key Terms

Cryptosporidium hominis Apicomplexan parasite infecting humans, resulting in persistent diarrhea, nausea, vomiting, malaise, and delayed growth; life-threatening to HIV-positive persons

Cryptosporidium parvum Apicomplexan parasite infecting humans and other animals, resulting in persistent, watery diarrhea that may be life-threatening in HIV-positive persons

Nephelometry turbidity unit (NTU) A measure of water turbidity that estimates the risk of harmful microbial contamination; the EPA standard for safe water is less than 0.5 NTU

Oocyst Hardy, cyst-like stage of the Amplicomplexan parasite life cycle that is highly resistant to adverse environmental conditions

Schizogony Asexual form of reproduction involving multiple round of fission

Zoonotic transmission Transmission of disease from animals to humans

Review Questions

1. What species of *Cryptosporidium* infect humans? What other animal species do they infect?
2. What are the symptoms of infection with the two major species of *Cryptosporidium* infecting humans?
3. To what group of parasites do *Cryptosporidium* species belong? What are other pathogenic members of this group?
4. What are the four major routes of transmission of *Cryptosporidium* species?
5. How might infection via water be prevented or reduced?

Topics for Further Discussion

1. Cryptosporidial species cause chronic, life-threatening illness in immunosuppressed persons, including those who are HIV-positive. Disease is particularly serious if those in the latter group have low numbers of CD4$^+$ T helper cells. Th1 immune responses, particularly IFN-γ, are critical to resolving infection. Explore means by which physicians might boost Th1 immunity in infected immunosuppressed individuals.
2. Research other enteric pathogens of humans, particularly those that threaten immunocompromised persons. In what ways are these organisms similar to *Cryptosporidium,* and in what ways do they differ?

3. How common is coinfection with *Cryptosporidium* and other pathogens in immunosuppressed persons? What organisms are involved? What are the effects of such coinfection?

4. *C. parvum* is commonly found in dairy and beef cattle, especially in calves. This protozoan may be transmitted to humans. What effects does infection with *C. parvum* have on milk and meat production in developed and developing regions of the world? What efforts might be undertaken to protect farm animals, and subsequently humans, from infection?

Resources

Bandyopadhyay, K., and others. "Rapid Microsphere Assay for Identification of *Cryptosporidium hominis* and *Cryptosporidium parvum* in Stool and Environmental Samples." *Journal of Clinical Microbiology,* 2007, *45,* 2835–2840.

Cama, V. A., and others. "Cryptosporidium Species and Subtypes and Clinical Manifestations in Children, Peru." *Emerging Infectious Diseases,* 2008, *14,* 1567–1574.

Chin, J. *Control of Communicable Diseases Manual* (17th ed.). Washington, D.C.: American Public Health Association, 2000.

Guerrant, R. W., and Thielman, N. M. "Emerging Enteric Protozoa: *Cryptosporidium, Cyclospora,* and *Microsporidia.*" In W. M. Scheld, D. Armstrong, and J. M. Hughes (eds.), *Emerging Infections* (Vol. 1). Washington, D.C.: ASM Press, 1998.

Hyde, J. E. "Targeting Purine and Pyrimidine Metabolism in Human Apicomplexan Parasites." *Current Drug Targets,* 2007, *8,* 31–47.

McAllister, T. A., and others. "Prevalence of *Giardia* and *Cryptosporidium* in Beef Cows in Southern Ontario and in Beef Calves in Southern British Columbia." *Canadian Veterinary Journal,* 2005, *46,* 47–55.

Pantenburg, B., and others. "Intestinal Immune Response to Human *Cryptosporidium* spp. Infection." *Infection and Immunity,* 2008, *76,* 23–29.

Rogers, K. A., and others. "MyD88-Dependent Pathways Mediate Resistance to *Cryptosporidium parvum* Infection in Mice." *Infection and Immunity,* 2006, *74,* 549–556.

Sears, C. L. "*Cryptosporidium parvum*: Miniscule but Mighty." In W. M. Scheld, W. A. Craig, and J. M. Hughes (eds.), *Emerging Infections* (Vol. 4). Washington, D.C.: ASM Press, 2000.

CHAPTER 27

CHAGAS' DISEASE AND ITS EMERGENCE IN THE UNITED STATES

LEARNING OBJECTIVES

- Define Chagas' disease and its recent emergence in the United States

- Describe the Zoomastigopheran protozoan responsible for causing this illness

- Discuss modes of infection

- Discuss the host's response to infection

- Describe symptomatology and diagnosis

- Discuss methods of treatment

- Discuss methods of prevention

Major Concepts

Symptoms

Chagas' disease is a severe, debilitating, and sometimes fatal disease found throughout impoverished areas of Latin America, and imported as well as endemic cases of this illness are increasingly turning up in the southern United States. The disease course involves an often asymptomatic acute phase, a 20- to 30-year latent phase, and a pathogenic chronic phase. The chronic phase is characterized by either damage to the heart or by enlargement of the esophagus and colon. Heart pathology includes cardiomyopathy with or without congestive heart failure, arrhythmia, right bundle blockage, and sudden cardiac death. Enlargement of the esophagus and colon leads to difficulty in swallowing, malnutrition, constipation, and abdominal pain.

Infection

Chagas' disease is caused by the parasitic protozoan *Trypanosoma cruzi* and is transmitted to humans via the feces of infected triatomine bugs, blood transfusions, organ transplants, or transplacentally. *T. cruzi* and its close relatives, the causative agents of African sleeping sickness and leishmaniasis, have complex life cycles involving several life stages and insect as well as human hosts. The infective form of the parasite for humans is the blood-dwelling metacyclic trypomastigote, and the replicative form is the amastigote, which divides inside cells, such as macrophages. The infective form of the parasite for the insect host is the bloodstream trypomastigote, and the replicative form is the epimastigote.

Immune Response

Parasite-induced immunosuppression occurs during the acute phase of Chagas' disease, with decreased production of cytokines and expression of cell surface molecules. Lymphocyte growth is also inhibited. Suppressive molecules produced by the parasite may induce production of regulatory cytokines. Numbers of CD8$^+$ killer cells are increased during Chagas' disease, possibly augmenting heart pathology. Autoimmune responses may also play a role in heart damage.

Protection

Few compounds are currently used to treat Chagas' disease. These are most effective if administered during the acute phase of the disease and are not often curative. Prevention may be the best protective strategy and primarily involves decreasing human contact with infected insects by improving building construction materials or spraying insecticides in dwellings or structures housing domestic animals. Screening the blood supply for contamination could also decrease infection via transfusion. These strategies are often expensive, however, and may be impractical for the poverty-stricken areas most affected by this disease.

Introduction

An estimated 20 million people in the Western Hemisphere are infected with ***Trypanosoma cruzi***, the causative agent of **Chagas' disease**, and many additional millions may be at risk. Some 50,000 to 200,000 new infections occur each year. During the chronic phase of illness, infected individuals suffer progressive debilitating damage to the heart or digestive system that is often lethal. As a result of reduced productivity, disability, and death, Chagas' disease is responsible for the loss of 670,000 disability-adjusted life years annually. It is a neglected illness arising out of poverty and in turn leads to even greater poverty in the endemic regions in a vicious circle.

Originally believed to be restricted to tropical and subtropical regions of South and Central America and Mexico and to persons originating in or visiting those areas, increasing numbers of reports have now confirmed the presence of *T. cruzi* in invertebrate and vertebrate hosts, including wild and domestic animals, in the southern United States. As a result of immigration and travel of vacationing and military persons to high-risk areas in Latin America, about 500,000 persons in the United States are believed to be infected. These individuals may infect others through blood or organ donation or may transmit the disease to their offspring transplacentally. Endemic transmission of Chagas' disease involving infected insects and mammalian reservoir species in the United States is becoming an increasing concern as well. Because American physicians are generally not familiar with Chagas' disease, many cases of this serious illness remain undetected and are attributed to other causes of cardiac disease.

History

The Brazilian physician Carlos Chagas discovered the causative agent of the disease that now bears his name in its invertebrate host and then in domestic animals (dogs and cats) and humans. He dubbed it *Schizotrypanum cruzi* (later *T. cruzi*) in honor of his mentor, Oswaldo Cruz, and described the disease it caused, found hosts among wild animal populations, and traced the parasite's life cycle. Chagas first noted the infection in a 2-year old girl, Berenice, in 1909. At age 53, Berenice remained infected but displayed no symptoms of chronic infection, such as cardiac or digestive manifestations. She died at age 73, apparently of heart disease.

The noted biologist Charles Darwin is thought to have acquired Chagas' disease during his historic journey on the H.M.S. *Beagle*. He recorded in March 1835 having being bitten by the disease vector, which he had previously studied: "At night I experienced an attack (for it deserves no less name) of the Benchuca, a species of Reduvius, the great black bug of the Pampas. It is most disgusting to feel soft wingless insects about one inch long crawling over one's body. Before sucking, they are quite thin but afterwards they become round and bloated with blood, and in this state they are easily crushed."

From several years thereafter, Darwin may have been in the latent phase of disease, but for the following 25 years, he wrote of heart palpitations, lassitude, extreme fatigue, and occasional trembling, flatulence, and vomiting. Darwin's health later improved until early 1882, when he experienced the first of four heart attacks in the last four months of his life. Whether Darwin's mysterious illness was indeed Chagas' disease remains a matter of speculation; however, it is similar to that seen in Berenice.

The Disease

The Phases of Chagas' Disease

Chagas' disease (American trypanosomiasis), in its chronic form, is a highly pathogenic and often fatal illness for which no effective treatment is currently available. The disease may be divided into three phases—acute, latent, and chronic—which are not universal among infected individuals. The development of chronic-phase symptoms frequently signals that death will follow within one year. Disease incidence is greatest among individuals over the age of 35 years and is equally distributed among males and females. Frequency of infection is increasing in both the southern and northern parts of the Western Hemisphere.

The acute phase occurs early after infection and is often inapparent, manifesting itself most frequently among children. Most infected persons do not seek medical attention during this stage. It presents itself as either an indurated skin lesion (**chagoma**) or a unilateral edema of the eyelid, conjunctivitis, and an enlarged satellite lymph node (**Romaña's sign**). **Parasitemia** (the presence of demonstrable parasites in the blood) may be present during this time, diminishing within two to three months. Fever, hepatosplenomegaly, lymph-adenopathy, lymphocytosis, electrocardiograph abnormalities, heart failure, and meningoencephalitis may occur at this time. Infants and very young children are most susceptible to development of meningoencephalitis, which may be fatal. The mortality rate in the acute stage is 5% to 10% among individuals aged 4 years or younger who are untreated (90% of those infected in some regions). In most individuals, however, the acute phase symptoms resolve spontaneously after four to eight weeks.

The length of the latent phase of the disease is variable and may last 20 to 30 years. For approximately 30% of infected persons, this is followed by the more severe chronic phase in which the majority of the pathology is seen. During this phase, damage occurs to the cardiovascular system, in the form of myocarditis or congestive heart failure, or to the digestive system, as **megaesophagus** or **megacolon** (megaviscera), in which the initial or terminal sections of the digestive system greatly enlarge and become dysfunctional, inhibiting the passage of

FIGURE 27.1   Romaña's sign: edema above the right eye

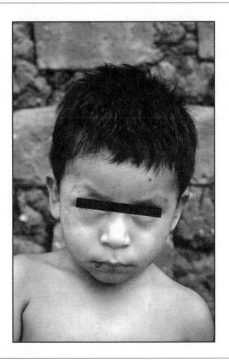

Source: CDC/Mae Melvin.

food through the gut. These changes are secondary to injury to nervous tissue innervating the heart and digestive musculature. The muscles lose tone and become flabby, and the associated structures enlarge and lose functional capacity. Among persons who progress to the chronic phase, average life expectancy is reduced by nine years. In some regions of South and Central America, 10% of the deaths among adults may result from chronic Chagas' disease.

In chronic Chagas' disease, it is estimated that 4% will develop cardiomyopathy with heart failure; 18%, cardiomyopathy without heart failure; and 3%, megaviscera. Symptoms of cardiovascular disease in the chronic phase include tachycardia and arrhythmia. This progresses to cardiomyopathy with or without congestive heart failure, right bundle branch blockage, apical aneurysm, and thromboembolism, followed by death within two to three years. The first symptom of the digestive form of the chronic phase may be difficulty in swallowing, which may lead to decreased food intake and malnutrition. This is followed by the development of megaesophagus and megacolon as the musculature weakens and the lumens enlarge. Megaesophagus may be responsible for the difficulty in swallowing, while megacolon may lead to constipation and abdominal pain. This manifestation occurs primarily in southern Brazil and Argentina.

Inflammation and apoptosis, a self-destructive form of cellular death, may underlie some of the pathology found in Chagas' disease. Parasite molecules attach to a toll-like receptor (TLR) on macrophages. TLRs serve as phagocyte receptors for recognition of molecular patterns of pathogens. Triggering of TLR2 stimulates macrophages to first secrete proinflammatory mediators, such as IL-12, TNF-α, and nitric oxide, and later induces a state of tolerance that may aid in long-term parasite persistence in the host. Cardiac damage may also occur at least in part from parasite-induced apoptosis of cardiomyocytes in inflammatory heart infiltrates during experimental Chagas' disease. Lymphocyte apoptosis also increases replication of *T. cruzi* in macrophages in the vicinity, and blocking apoptosis reduces the number of parasites in the blood.

Trypanosoma cruzi and Chagas' Disease in the United States

T. cruzi has been reported in appropriate insect vectors in several locations in the United States, including Alabama, Florida, Georgia, and Tennessee. Dogs and wild mammals, such as opossums and raccoons, are infected with *T. cruzi* in areas such as Texas, Oklahoma, Florida, Georgia, South Carolina, Virginia, California, and Louisiana. Infected dogs have abnormal electrocardiograms, arrhythmias, and signs of right-sided cardiac disease; half of those identified survive less than six months. In one study, 3.6% of the dogs were infected with the parasite. Veterinarians need to be aware of the possibility of canine Chagas' disease among domestic animals. Infection of wild animals in the southern United States must also monitored because these animals may serve as reservoirs for the infection of humans and their pets. The infection rate among wild opossums in some areas was 37% and up to 61% for raccoons.

Human infection with *T. cruzi* or development of Chagas' disease is being detected with ever greater frequency in the United States in California, Georgia, North Carolina, Tennessee, and Florida. In Los Angeles County, California, the proportion of infected blood samples containing antibodies to the parasite increased from 102 per 100,000 in 1996 to 185 per 100,000 in 1998. To assess the risk of transmission through blood transfusion in that region, donated blood was screened for antibodies to the parasite. Donors of infected blood were found to be 3.6 times more likely to have resided in Central America or Mexico and 8.7 times more likely to have previously donated blood. Infected organs donated for transplantation have been detected in California but not in a study of organs in the American Midwest.

In some cases, Americans who have no risk factors (travel to known endemic areas, blood transfusion, and drug usage) have developed Chagas' disease. Animals in the vicinity of these individuals were found to be infected, suggesting that this disease may also be endemic to parts of the southern United States. Analysis of enzyme profiles of *T. cruzi* isolated from wild animals in the United States suggests that this parasite in indigenous to the country and has not entered the country in the recent past.

The Causative Agent

The Protozoan

Chagas' disease is caused by the bloodborne parasite *Trypanosoma cruzi*. *T. cruzi* is a hemoflagellated protozoan of the class Zoomastigophera, order Kinetoplastida, family Trypanosomatidae, section **Stercoraria**. This section of protozoa develops in the posterior portions of the insect gut and is transmitted through fecal material expelled as the insect feeds. *T. cruzi* has been subdivided into zymodemes based on isoenzyme analysis. The Z1 zymodeme occurs in opossums and in domestic and peridomestic animals; Z2 is found in cats, dogs, domestic rodents, and guinea pigs; and Z3 is found primarily in opossums, with human infections uncommon. *Trypanosoma brucei gambesea* and *T. b. rhodesiensence* are relatives of *T. cruzi* that also cause human disease—African trypanosomiasis (African sleeping sickness). These parasites are from the section **Salivaria** and develop in the anterior gut with transmission via the saliva of tsetse bugs during biting. Other human pathogens related to *T. cruzi* include the *Leishmania* species, which cause cutaneous, mucocutaneous, and visceral leishmaniasis. The latter two conditions are extremely serious and often fatal.

T. cruzi assumes several morphologically and antigenically distinct forms throughout its life cycle. The **metacyclic trypomastigote** is the infectious form for humans. It is elongate and laterally flattened with the **flagellum** running along most of the length of its body, attached to the posterior end of the trypomastigote by an undulating membrane and extending beyond the parasite at its anterior end as a free flagellum. Members of the Trypanosomatidae family contain two distinct, dark-staining round bodies, the elongated central nucleus and the smaller **kinetoplast**. The latter is in close proximity to the origin of the flagellum in the basal body. It is posterior to the nucleus in the trypomastigote form, and its position relative the anterior of the parasite determines the length of the flagellum. The kinetoplast is a capsular extension of the single, large mitochondrion found in these parasites. It contains a high concentration of mitochondrial DNA existing in both linear and circular forms. A similar stage of the parasite found in the human bloodstream is the **bloodstream trypomastigote**, which looks much like the metacyclic trypomastigote, with a large round subterminal kinetoplast, but is more slender. It is the infectious form for the insect host. The bloodstream trypomastigote of *T. cruzi* typically assumes a "C" or "S" shape in stained blood smears. Both trypomastigote forms move through the blood using a distinctive undulating movement. One other form

FIGURE 27.2   *T. cruzi* bloodstream trypomastigote (center)

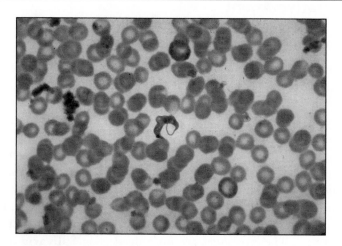

Source: CDC/Mae Melvin.

FIGURE 27.3 Cluster of *T. cruzi* amastigotes inside heart cells (center)

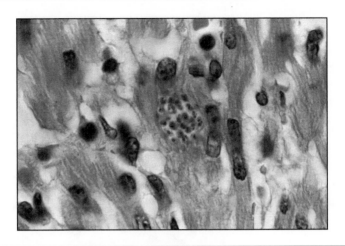

Source: CDC/L. L. Moore Jr.

exists in humans: the rounded **amastigote** that dwells inside macrophages and, as its name ("without a whip") implies, has only a rudimentary flagellum. This is the replicative form in humans. Two other life stages occur in the insect host, the **epimastigote** and the **sphaeromastigote**. The epimastigote has a shortened flagellum because its kinetoplast is anterior to the nucleus. It is the replicative form in the insect. The sphaeromastigote is a rounded form with a short undulating membrane and a free flagellum; it eventually transforms into the metacyclic trypomastigote, capable of infecting humans as noted earlier.

Life Cycle

As is true of the vast majority of parasites living within their hosts' bodies, the life cycle of *T. cruzi* is complex, involving not only several distinct life forms but also several host organisms. It requires transmission between an invertebrate host of the blood-sucking insect family Reduviidae, subfamily **Triatominae ("kissing bugs")**, and a vertebrate mammalian host. Several species of triatomine bugs of three genera (*Triatoma*, *Rhodnius*, and *Panstrongylus*) host the parasite. The most important of these insect vectors for humans are those that reside in human dwellings and are nocturnal feeders. A wide range of mammals—perhaps all mammals—may serve as the vertebrate host, including humans,

FIGURE 27.4 *Triatoma infestans,* a "kissing bug" vector of Chagas' disease

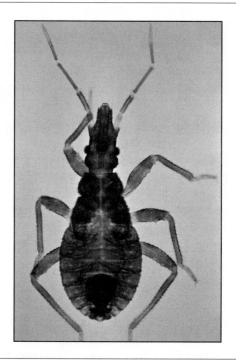

Source: CDC/World Health Organization.

domestic animals, rodents, and sylvatic (wild) mammals, which may serve as reservoirs of disease. The common opossum may be the most frequently infected and most important reservoir species. Opossums are nocturnal and frequently visit inhabited areas to search for food. Amphibians and birds are refractory to infection by this parasite.

The mammalian hosts are infected by metacyclic trypomastigotes found in feces of the insect vector. The triatomine bugs bite mammals at night, often near the mucous membranes of the mouth or eyes, in the vicinity of saliva and tears. Unlike other similar insects whose bite is painful (the "assassin bugs"), the vectors of *T. cruzi* do not inflict pain as they bite the mammals' faces and have therefore been nicknamed "kissing bugs." As they feed, the triatomine bugs produce liquid fecal material. This may cause an itchy sensation in the mammal, leading to scratching and the rubbing of the contaminated feces into the mucosa of the eyes or mouth or the abrasions of the bite site. Infection may also occur from infected mothers to their offspring during pregnancy or delivery, by blood transfusion or organ transplant, or by handling corpses of infected animals or eating uncooked food contaminated with feces from an infected insect vector. Mother-to-child transmission is responsible for 10% of the cases and, if transplacental, may result in spontaneous abortion or premature birth. The risk of infection by organ transplantation is augmented by immunosuppressants used to prevent rejection. Transmission through the milk of infected women is very rare.

After entry into the bloodstream of the mammalian host, the metacyclic trypomastigote enters a nearby host cell, usually muscular tissue (skeletal, cardiac, or smooth muscle), macrophages (phagocytic cells of the innate immune system), fibroblasts, or neuroglia of the peripheral or central nervous system. In macrophages, they initially enter a lysosome-like vacuole whose acidic pH activates TcTox, a pore-forming molecule that acts together with the trans-sialidase enzyme to allow parasite escape from the hostile lysosomal environment into the host cell's cytoplasm. Once in this safer location, metacyclic trypomastigotes transform into amastigotes, which then multiply repeatedly by binary fission in the host cell, forming a packed bunch of daughter cells, the **pseudocyst** ("false cyst"). These cysts form epimastigotes and then bloodstream trypomastigotes, eventually filling the cell, leading to its rupture and parasite release into the blood. In humans in the acute phase of disease, these trypomastigotes are numerous enough to permit their detection by examination of the blood, but such detection is very uncommon during the latent and chronic phases. The bloodstream trypomastigotes may then enter new host cells and replicate as before in the amastigote form or be ingested by an insect host during its blood meal.

Once trypomastigotes enter the insect, they transform into epimastigotes in the host's anterior midgut. The epimastigotes move to the insect's hindgut, attaching to the anterior glandular region of the rectum wall, dividing rapidly, and transforming into sphaeromastigotes and then metacyclic trypomastigotes. The infectious metacyclic trypomastigotes and the other two noninfectious forms are then expelled from the insect in its feces during a meal, allowing entry into mammals and continuation of the parasite's life cycle. Interestingly, amastigotes may also be found in the insects' guts, either singly or fused into an agglomerate, but their purpose is not known. Infection of the triatomine bugs is lifelong.

The Immune Response

During the acute phase of infection, *T. cruzi* escapes the immune response by inducing a state of immunosuppression, which resolves during the latent

FIGURE 27.5 Life cycle of *Trypanosoma cruzi*

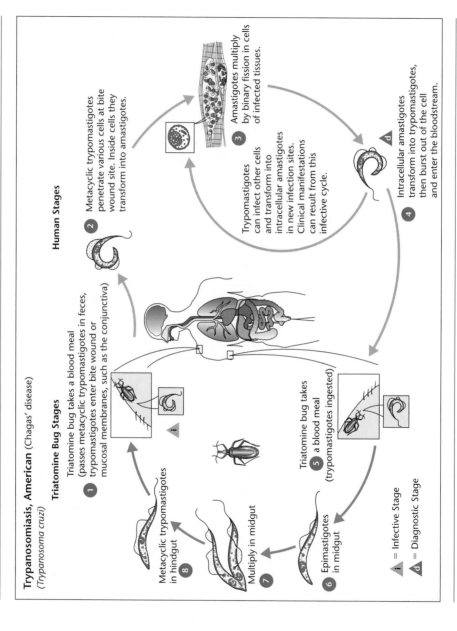

Trypanosomiasis, American (Chagas' disease)
(*Trypanosoma cruzi*)

Triatomine Bug Stages

Human Stages

① Triatomine bug takes a blood meal (passes metacyclic trypomastigotes in feces, trypomastigotes enter bite wound or mucosal membranes, such as the conjunctiva)

② Metacyclic trypomastigotes penetrate various cells at bite wound site. Inside cells they transform into amastigotes.

③ Amastigotes multiply by binary fission in cells of infected tissues.

Trypomastigotes can infect other cells and transform into intracellular amastigotes in new infection sites. Clinical manifestations can result from this infective cycle.

④ Intracellular amastigotes transform into trypomastigotes, then burst out of the cell and enter the bloodstream.

⑤ Triatomine bug takes a blood meal (trypomastigotes ingested)

⑥ Epimastigotes in midgut

⑦ Multiply in midgut

⑧ Metacyclic trypomastigotes in hindgut

△i = Infective Stage
△d = Diagnostic Stage

Source: CDC/Alexander J. da Silva and Melanie Moser.

and chronic phases. Similar to the immunosuppression associated with HIV infection, infected persons have an increase in the numbers of CD8$^+$ T killer cells and a decrease in CD4$^+$ T helper cells. B and T lymphocytes from acutely infected mice have blunted growth responses to nonspecific stimuli or to parasite antigens. B lymphocytes produce lower amounts of antibodies, especially IgG1 and IgG3. T lymphocytes from these infected mice produce lower amounts of the T cell growth factor IL-2, and the addition of IL-2 to cultures of these cells may restore their ability to grow. Many of these findings have been replicated by the addition of trypomastigotes or epimastigotes to normal human lymphocytes derived from uninfected persons. Exposure to these forms of *T. cruzi*, but not the intracellular amastigotes, decreases normal human T cell growth and production of the Th1 cytokines IL-2 and IFN-γ. Expression of α and β chains of the IL-2 receptor and the receptor's high-affinity binding of IL-2 also decreases, which may underlie decreased T lymphocyte growth. In vitro exposure to trypomastigotes reduces cell surface expression of other molecules essential to T lymphocyte function, including the transferrin receptor, CD4, and CD8. Several immunosuppressive factors appear to be secreted by trypomastigotes. One of these, cruzipain, induces production of the regulatory cytokines IL-10 and TGF-β by macrophages. Defective T lymphocyte activation may also result from the parasite's ability to inhibit expression of T cell costimulatory molecules (CD40, CD86, and MCH II) by dendritic cells.

The immune response later during the course of infection may be either protective or pathogenic, depending on the balance between various immune cell types in infected individuals. Those developing heart failure have increased numbers of CD8$^+$ T killer cells and decreased numbers of CD4$^+$ T helper cells, similar to the situation occurring in AIDS patients. It is unclear whether the T killer cells induce cardiac pathology or are recruited to reduce damage by killing parasites in the area. During the latent phase of disease, high numbers of CD4$^+$CD25^{hi} Treg cells and NKT cells are found in the blood, and the monocytes are primarily modulatory, secreting the regulatory cytokine IL-10. Increased numbers of activated CD8$^+$ T killer cells and proinflammatory monocytes are found in patients with severe cardiac damage in the chronic phase. It is believed that the regulatory and modulatory cell types associated with latent disease prevent the pathology induced by the activated T killer cells and inflammatory monocytes and that loss of the regulatory and modulatory cells may allow disease progression. It is possible that strategies that boost regulatory immune cell activity may induce a lifelong latent phase and thus be protective against chronic-phase tissue damage. Alternatively, the actions of these cells may result in parasite persistence.

Induction of autoimmune reactions has been suggested to play a pathogenic role in chagasic heart injury. T and B cell responses have both been implicated in this damage because cross-reactive immunity may be generated to *T. cruzi* antigens and host cell components such as cardiac myosin, acetylcholine receptors of neuromuscular junctions necessary for contraction of the heart, and β1 adrenergic receptors. Stimulation of the latter by these cross-reactive antibodies induces cardiac arrhythmia.

Diagnosis

Chronic Chagas' disease may be suspected for persons residing in or visiting endemic high-risk areas who develop cardiac symptoms confirmed by an abnormal ECG or thoracic X-ray. Tests are then indicated to confirm the diagnosis. During the chronic phase of infection, however, *T. cruzi* is difficult to detect in blood smears. One method of amplifying the low numbers of parasites present in the circulating blood during this phase is **xenodiagnosis**. In this procedure, a container of triatomine bugs is strapped to the arm of an individual suspected to be infected. The insects are allowed to feed and then divide. The insects are later dissected and gut contents examined for the presence of epimastigotes. Alternatively, the patient's blood may be inoculated into susceptible animal hosts, including mice and rats.

T. cruzi must be differentiated from its close, but nonpathogenic, relative *T. rangeli* because both infect several species of wild mammals and humans. This may be accomplished by isoenzyme analysis and morphological differences (more prominent undulating membrane, more central kinetoplast, lack of "C" shape in stained preparations).

No single serological assay has sufficient sensitivity and specificity for solo use, but a combination of tests is recommended to confirm diagnosis. Such tests include an IgG ELISA, immunofluorescent assay, or indirect hemagglutination. A commercial test for the large-scale screening of donated blood was developed in 2005 by Ortho-Clinical Diagnostics. It is an ELISA that uses antigens from epimastigote lysates to detect the presence of antibodies to *T. cruzi* in the serum or plasma. In clinical trials, blood samples scored as positive were retested twice. Those that remained positive upon retest were further subjected to a radioimmunoprecipitation assay, and those found to contain antibodies to the parasite in both assays were then considered positive. The U.S. Food and Drug Administration licensed this test in December 2006 for the screening of donated blood, cell and tissue donors, and live organ donors but not for general diagnostic purposes, and it went into use in many U.S. blood banks on January 29, 2007.

Treatment

Drug treatment options for Chagas' disease are currently limited and are most effective if administered during the acute phase. Recently, evidence has accumulated suggesting that treating persons during the chronic phase may cause the disappearance of antibodies to the parasite and may halt progression of cardiac manifestations. Treatment of infected women of childbearing age may reduce the risk of congenital transmission to their children. Antitrypanosomal medications in the United States are presently available only through the CDC. No drugs are highly effective in treating the chronic phase of Chagas' disease. Once an individual enters this phase, care is primarily supportive or based on management of symptoms.

Two drugs are used to treat Chagas' disease: nifurtimox (lampit) and benznidazole. Both are associated with toxic side effects that worsen as individuals age. These frequently include anorexia (loss of appetite and weight), nausea, abdominal pain, and problems with the hands and feet. Less frequently, difficulty sleeping, skin rash, dizziness and headaches, neuropathy (nerve pain), memory loss, difficulty concentrating, and sexual impotence are seen. The drugs are most effective when administered early during infection, require a 90-day treatment regimen, and at best cure less than half of the patients treated. Benznidazole blocks apoptotic death of $CD8^+$ T killer cells and decreases parasite load in the blood.

RECENT DEVELOPMENTS

Research is in progress to discover an effective drug for the treatment of Chagas' disease. Some of the recent work has focused on metabolism of polyamines, such as putrescine, spermidine, and spermine, which are essential for cell growth and division. In most organisms, putrescine is synthesized from L-ornithine by the enzyme ornithine decarboxylase (ODC). *T. cruzi* lacks this enzyme and must derive putrescine from its surroundings by an influx system. *S*-adenosylmethionine (AdoMet) is a part of the polyamine metabolic pathway as well and via transsulfuration is converted into cysteine, an essential amino acid, and glutathione. In *T. cruzi*, the glutathione conjugates with spermidine to form trypanothione, a key protective molecule that helps defend the parasite from oxidative molecules produced by the host's immune system. In the absence of environmental putrescine, *T. cruzi*'s stores of trypanothione are depleted, and the parasite is killed by reactive oxygen species from human macrophages. Drugs able to block putrescine uptake or target the production of AdoMet from L-methionine could selectively inhibit parasite growth or allow killing of the parasites by the innate immune system. Testing of the utility of polyamine analogues and polyamine biosynthesis inhibitors in the treatment of Chagas' disease has begun.

Prevention

One risk factor for Chagas' disease is residence in South or Central America, especially in impoverished areas where huts are composed of thatch, mud, or adobe, which provide dwelling places for triatomine bugs; another is blood transfusion from an infected individual. Prevention of transmission via the insect vector may include the use of insecticides and the construction of human dwellings that are not suitable for insect residence. The expenses associated with the latter may be prohibitive, especially in poverty-stricken areas in the interior of South America. The Southern Cone Initiative, however, has significantly reduced transmission by *Triatoma infestans* in Uruguay, Chile, and Brazil by spraying houses with insecticides. This insect vector has not yet been eliminated in the high-risk area of northern Argentina, Paraguay, and Bolivia, and further complications exist in other regions where a number of other vector species exist with distinct feeding and infestation behaviors. Because homes are frequently reinfested with the insects, they must be sprayed repeatedly, which may promote resistance to insecticides. Other strategies under exploration include the use of insecticide-treated bed nets and dog collars.

Preventing transmission by transfusion may involve screening of the blood supply and questioning potential donors. In 1991, a screening questionnaire was introduced by the American Red Cross for administration to potential blood donors. Most blood banks in the United States began to directly test donated blood for infection with *T. cruzi* in 2007, but this may not be practical in developing countries where many low-income donors from endemic areas may donate blood for payment in more affluent areas, thus increasing the range of the disease. Family members of infected blood donors who are at risk of infection (children of infected mothers and others with a history of similar exposure to the disease vectors) should also be tested. Although the blood supply in the United States and Canada is generally quite safe, seven cases of Chagas' disease in these two countries since 1988 have been associated with blood transfusions. In areas of Latin America that are not able to routinely screen blood products, killing parasites present in blood products may greatly decrease this mode of transmission, believed to result in thousands of infections per year. Gentian violet has been used to kill trypanosomes in the blood since the 1950s; however, it is unpopular due to the resulting bluish cast of recipients' skin. Combination treatment of plasma and platelet preparations with long-wavelength UVA light and psoralen (amotosalen hydrochloride) decreases parasite numbers to undetectable levels without affecting platelet functions. This combination also inactivates bacteria and viruses in the preparations.

Many cases of Chagas' disease in the United States are believed to be misdiagnosed due to lack of familiarity with the illness among American physicians and the general public. An educational program might raise the level of awareness of means of preventing infection by parasites residing in family pets and might allow rapid response after infection occurs to both treat the affected individual and to reduce the possibility of transmission to offspring or through blood or organ donation.

Surveillance

In many parts of Latin America, Chagas' disease is a reportable infectious illness. Health care agencies in high-risk areas undertake both active and passive surveillance for the acute and chronic phases of Chagas' disease. In many areas, local health inspectors examine residences regularly for the presence of insect vectors and collect and examine those that are found. Buildings for domestic animals, such as barns and chicken coops, and outhouses may also house insect vectors in close proximity to human habitations, especially because these insects feed on animal blood in addition to human blood. The percentage of insect-infested structures, the number and types of triatomine bugs in infested dwellings, and the percentage of insects that are infected are recorded. Epidemiological studies also note the types of construction materials used in human dwellings in the area. Blood of family members living in the same residence as infected persons is examined for infection.

Due to the presence of *T. cruzi*–infected insects and mammals throughout the American South and increasing reports of Chagas' disease among immigrants, travelers, and U.S.-born citizens, donated blood is being examined for the presence of the parasite in order to protect the blood supply. The American Red Cross undertook a screening of nearly 150,000 blood samples from three blood-collecting centers in the United States (Los Angeles and Oakland, California, and Tucson, Arizona) from August 2006 to January 2007. Of these, 32 units (215 per million) contained antibodies reactive with *T. cruzi*. At-risk populations in the United States are also being monitored. In a survey of blood from Hispanic and Haitian migrant farmworkers in North Carolina in the early 1990s, 2% of the laborers were found to be infected with the parasite. Health care providers treating migrant workers need to be aware of possible infection of this segment of the population with unusual microbes, including *T. cruzi*, *Plasmodium* species (causative agents of malaria), *Babesia*, and other organisms, so as to treat patients appropriately and effectively and to safeguard the general public. A study of *T. cruzi* in the blood of pregnant women from Houston, Texas, found a prevalence rate of 0.4% among Hispanic women and 0.1% among non-Hispanic women, indicating the potential for transplacental transmission and the possible utility of screening for infection during pregnancy to allow early intervention.

Summary

Disease

- Chagas' disease (American trypanosomiasis)

Causative Agent

- *Trypanosoma cruzi*

Agent Type

- Parasitic protozoan, class Zoomastigophera, order Kinetoplastida, family Trypanosomatidae, section Stercoraria

Genome

- Double-stranded DNA; microchromosomes

Vector

- Triatomine ("kissing") bugs

Common Reservoirs

- 150 possible reservoir species, primarily the common opossum

Modes of Transmissions

- Infectious insect feces rubbed into bite wound or mucosa   •   Blood or organ donation   •   Transplacentally

Geographical Distribution

- Primarily South and Central America and Mexico; emerging elsewhere in North America

Year of Emergence

- 1909

Key Terms

Amastigote Replicative form of *T. cruzi* in mammalian macrophages

Bloodstream trypomastigote Form of *T. cruzi* infective for macrophages and the insect host

Chagas' disease Parasitic disease characterized by damage to the heart or digestive tract, resulting in cardiomyopathy, arrhythmia, and sudden cardiac death or enlargement of the lumens of the esophagus and colon

Chagoma Indurated skin lesion present in the acute stage of Chagas' disease

Epimastigote Replicative form of *T. cruzi* in the midgut of its insect host

Flagellum Whiplike structure that allows motility; the names of the different stages in the life cycle of *T. cruzi* refer to the relative length of this structure

Kinetoplast Rounded structure found in members of the order Kinetoplastida, a capsular extension of the single large mitochondrion in close proximity to the origin of the flagellum

Megacolon Enlarged colon whose flabby musculature inhibits the passage of food

Megaesophagus Enlarged esophagus whose flabby musculature inhibits the swallowing of food

Metacyclic trypomastigote Form of *T. cruzi* that is infective for its mammalian host

Parasitemia Demonstrable presence of parasites in the blood

Pseudocyst "False cyst" of intracellular mammalian forms of *T. cruzi* daughter cells

Romaña's sign Unilateral edema of the eyelid, conjunctivitis, and enlarged satellite lymph node resulting from acute infection with *T. cruzi*

Salivaria Group of trypanosomes that develop in the anterior gut of the insect vector; transmitted via saliva during insect bites

Sphaeromastigote Rounded form of *T. cruzi* that has a short undulating membrane and a free flagellum; eventually transforms into a metacyclic trypomastigote

Stercoraria Group of trypanosomes that develops in the posterior portions of the insect gut; transmitted through fecal material expelled from the insect during feeding

Triatominae ("kissing bugs") Group of blood-sucking insects that include the vectors for Chagas' disease

Trypanosoma cruzi Hemoflagellated parasitic protozoan that causes Chagas' disease

Xenodiagnosis Diagnostic procedure for *T. cruzi* in which triatomine bugs are allowed to feed on the blood of a potentially infected individual to amplify the low numbers of parasites found in humans during the chronic stage of Chagas' disease

Review Questions

1. What protozoan is the causative agent of Chagas' disease? What are the names of two parasitic protozoa that are its close relatives, and what diseases do they cause? To what class and order do these parasites belong?

2. What are the three phases of Chagas' disease, and what are the symptoms of each? What percentage of individuals progress to the final phase of the illness? How many individuals have Chagas' disease in Latin America and in the United States?

3. What is the life cycle of the causative agent of Chagas' disease? Include in your description the modes of transmission to humans and the names of the life forms of the parasite in each host.

4. What drugs are currently being used to treat Chagas' disease, and what are their side effects? During which phase of infection are they most effective? What are some newer treatment strategies under development?

5. How might communities and individuals protect themselves from acquiring Chagas' disease?

Topics for Further Discussion

1. Structures that are peculiar to a group of microbes, such as cell walls in some types of bacteria, have been successfully targeted by drugs that attack organisms bearing that structure while not affecting the human host. Members of the order Kinetoplastida have several unique structures. What are these structures, and how might they be exploited for therapeutic purposes for Chagas' disease and African sleeping sickness?

2. Chagas' disease is primarily a neglected disease of the poor. Disability and death due to this illness result in loss of economic vitality in affected regions, leading to decreased availability of plentiful and nutritious food, modern housing, and adequate health care. These factors in turn lead to greater susceptibility to other illnesses. Several of the most useful preventive strategies for Chagas' disease—housing that is free of the insect vector and screening of the blood supply—are not financially practical in impoverished areas of Latin America. Suggest mechanisms by which the regional and world communities might interrupt this vicious circle of poverty and disease, thereby increasing the population's health and general standards of living. What positive effects could this intervention have on the global community and on other countries in the Western Hemisphere?

3. Imported and endemic cases of Chagas' disease in the United States in both humans and dogs are increasing, yet most physicians and members of the general public are ignorant of this illness. Suggest means by which this trend might be halted or reversed and the impact of greater public awareness on Chagas' disease in the United States.

4. Discuss the roles of the various components of the immune system in either protecting the host or inducing pathology during Chagas' disease. What implications does this have for vaccine development?

Resources

Adler S. "Darwin's Illness." Nature, 1959, *184*, 1102.

Barnabé, C., and others. "*Trypanosoma cruzi*: A Considerable Phylogenetic Divergence Indicates That the Agent of Chagas' Disease Is Indigenous to the Native Fauna of the United States." *Experimental Parasitology*, 2001, *99*, 73–79.

Beltz, L. A., Kierszenbaum, F., and Sztein, M. B. "Selective Suppressive Effects of *Trypanosoma cruzi* on Activated Human Lymphocytes." *Infection and Immunity*, 1989, *57*, 2301–2305.

Beltz, L. A., Sztein, M. B., and Kierszenbaum, F. "Novel Mechanism for *Trypanosoma cruzi*–Induced Suppression of Human Lymphocytes: Inhibition of Interleukin 2 Receptor Expression." *Journal of Immunology*, 1988, *141*, 289–294.

Denkers, E. Y., and Butcher, B. A. "Sabotage and Exploitation in Macrophages Parasitized by Intracellular Protozoans." *Trends in Parasitology*, 2005, *21*, 35–41.

Di Pentima, M. C., and others. "Prevalence of Antibody to *Trypanosoma cruzi* in Pregnant Hispanic Women in Houston." *Clinical Infectious Diseases*, 1999, *28*, 1281–1285.

Dos Reis, G. A., and others. "The Importance of Aberrant T-Cell Responses in Chagas' Disease." *Trends in Parasitology*, 2005, *21*, 237–243.

Herwaldt, B. L., and others. "Use of Polymerase Chain Reaction to Diagnose the Fifth Reported U.S. Case of Autochthonous Transmission of *Trypanosoma cruzi*, in Tennessee, 1998." *Journal of Infectious Diseases*, 2000, *181*, 395–398.

Minter, D. M. "Trypanosomes." In P.E.C. Manson-Bahr and F.I.C. Apted (eds.), *Manson's Tropical Diseases* (18th ed.). Philadelphia: Baillière Tindall, 1982.

Pung, O. J., and others "*Trypanosoma cruzi* in Wild Raccoons, Opossums, and Triatomine Bugs in Southeast Georgia, U.S.A." *Journal of Parasitology*, 1995, *81*, 324–326.

Reguera, R. M., Tekwani, B. L., and Balana-Fouce, R. "Polyamine Transport in Parasites: A Potential Target for New Antiparasitic Drug Development." *Comparative Biochemistry and Physiology*, 2005, *140*, 151–164.

Tarleton, R. L., and others. "The Challenges of Chagas' Disease: Grim Outlook or Glimmer of Hope?" *PLoS Medicine*, 2007, *4*, 1852–1857.

Van Voorhis, W. C., and others. "*Trypanosoma cruzi* Inactivation in Human Platelet Concentrates and Plasma by a Psoralen (Amotosalen HCl) and Long-Wavelength UV." *Antimicrobial Agents and Chemotherapy*, 2003, *47*, 475–479.

Vitelli-Avelar, D. M., Sathler-Avelar, R., and Massara, R. L. "Are Increased Frequency of Macrophage-Like and Natural Killer (NK) Cells, Together with High Levels of NKT and CD4[+]CD25[high] T Cells Balancing Activated CD8+ T Cells, the Key to Control Chagas' Disease Morbidity?" *Clinical and Experimental Immunology*, 2006, *145*, 81–92.

INFECTIOUS
PROTEINS

CHAPTER 28

CREUTZFELDT-JAKOB DISEASE AND OTHER TRANSMISSIBLE SPONGIFORM ENCEPHALOPATHIES

LEARNING OBJECTIVES

- Define and contrast the various prion diseases
- Describe the agent responsible for causing these illnesses and contrast it with all other forms of infectious organisms
- Discuss modes of infection
- Discuss the host's response to infection
- Describe symptomatology and diagnosis
- Discuss methods of prevention

Major Concepts

Diseases

Prions, self-replicating, infectious proteins, are responsible for transmissible spongiform encephalopathies (TSEs) in humans and animals. The human forms include several types of Creutzfeldt-Jakob disease (CJD), Gerstmann-Straussler-Scheinker syndrome (GSS), fatal familial insomnia, Alper's syndrome, and Huntington disease–like syndrome 1. Increased pathology may occur during Wilson disease and primary progressive aphasia. Prion diseases may be acquired by inherited mutations of the prion gene, PRNP, or by infection by malformed prions, PrPsc. The latter are transmitted by consumption of cattle or human prions or by medical procedures involving infected instruments or blood, meninges, corneas, or pituitary-derived human growth factor. Prion diseases of animals include bovine spongiform encephalopathy (BSE) (in cattle), scrapie (in sheep), chronic wasting syndrome (in deer, moose, and elk), transmissible mink encephalopathy (in mink), and feline spongiform encephalopathy (in domestic cats). Other than the BSE agent, none of the animal TSE agents appears to directly cause disease in humans.

Symptoms

Prion diseases are uniformly fatal and are accompanied by ataxia, paralysis, emotional disturbances, loss of cognition, and dementia due to the deposition of amyloid fibrils and spongiform degeneration of gray areas of the central nervous system. The cerebrum, cerebellum, basal ganglia, and thalamus may be affected.

Infection

The human prion protein exists in two forms. The normal form, PrPc, is found on the surface of neurons, glial cells, platelets, and various leukocytes; is protease-sensitive; and contains large amounts of α-helical secondary protein structure. The abnormal form, PrPsc, may be found in lysosomes within infected cells, is protease-resistant, and is aberrantly folded, containing large amounts of β-pleated sheets in its secondary structure. PrPsc is formed by interacting with PrPc and refolding the normal protein into PrPsc, with more β-pleated sheet content. Prions are thus able to replicate themselves without containing or using nucleic acids. The exact function of the normal PrPc is not known. Mice lacking this protein appear to be grossly normal but have alterations in circadian rhythms, sleep patterns, synaptic conduction, seizure thresholds, and hippocampus morphology. PrPc may be involved in copper transport, immune cell functioning, and inhibition of the processing of the Aβ amyloid protein found in Alzheimer's disease. In addition to mammalian prions, six prions have been found in fungi.

Immune Response

The immune system is activated during prion diseases because infection stimulates the release of T cell–tropic chemokines followed by the entry of $CD4^+$ T helper cells and $CD8^+$ T killer cells into the brain tissue. These cells do not appear to mount a protective response, however, and the disease proceeds until death. B lymphocytes appear to play a contributory role in disease progression. Leukocytes in the intestinal wall, as well as the cytokines TNF-α and TNF-β, may be required for infection by the oral route.

Protection

No treatment has thus far been able to stop the fatal progression of prion diseases in humans, although several drugs may slow the course of disease in animal models. Research is continuing to uncover new drugs that cure neuronal cells in culture, but delivery of these agents in vivo is complicated by the blood-brain barrier. Several efforts have been able to reduce or prevent transmission. Since humans may be infected by eating beef or other meat from BSE-infected cattle, a number of ruminant feed bans have been put into effect that have greatly reduced the incidence of BSE in cattle and the resultant variant Creutzfeldt-Jakob disease in humans. Kuru, another form of CJD, has been almost eliminated by halting funeral rites that involved consumption of human brains. Incidence of iatrogenic CJD is reduced by disposing of infected medical instruments and refusing blood from at-risk donors, such as those who have received a meningeal or corneal transplant, are receiving pituitary-derived human growth hormone, or have lived for more than six months in regions with a high incidence of BSE.

Introduction

Almost all infectious agents fall into several well-defined categories, including bacteria, viruses, fungi, and protozoan (unicellular) or metazoan (multicellular) parasites. All of these agents are considered by at least some authorities as alive (although others do not classify viruses as such), and all use a nucleic acid,

Table 28.1   Infectious agents of humans

Infectious Agent	Type	Number of Cells	Source of Hereditary Information
Bacterium	Prokaryote	1	DNA
Virus	Virus	1	DNA or RNA
Fungus	Eukaryote	1	DNA
Protozoan parasite	Eukaryote	1	DNA
Metazoan parasite	Eukaryote	2 or more	DNA
Prion	Protein	N.A.	Shape

Note: N.A. = not applicable.

either DNA or RNA, as their hereditary information. Prions are different from any other known infectious agent: they are not living and are composed solely of a single protein without any nucleic acid. Prion hereditary information used during reproduction appears to be contained in the shape of the protein. These agents may pass from one individual to another via an infectious route or may be transmitted to offspring through an inherited mutation in the gene that encodes a normal cellular form of the protein.

Prion proteins are found primarily on the surface of neurons but are also present on glial cells, platelets, and some leukocytes, including hematopoietic stem cells. The exact function of the normal protein is not clear, but it may function in copper ion transport, in blocking the formation of amyloid plaques associated with Alzheimer's disease, during T lymphocyte activation, during blood cell production, or in synaptic transmission. These unusual infectious agents cause several universally fatal diseases of the central nervous system, characterized by loss of coordination, inability to move, emotional disturbances, dementia, and finally death. "Mad cow disease" is one of these transmissible spongiform encephalopathies that infects cattle but may be transmitted to humans by consuming infected beef. Because prions are not inactivated by extremely high or low temperatures, normal cooking or freezing procedures do not block transmission. Iatrogenic transmission may also occur because normal decontamination procedures, including autoclaving, do not inactivate these hardy infectious agents.

History

Scrapie, a **transmissible spongiform encephalopathy (TSE)** of sheep, was reported in 1730 in Europe, and in 1936 it was found to be transmissible between sheep. The first of the human TSEs was identified by Hans Gerhard

Creutzfeldt and Alfons Maria Jakob in the 1920s and was named **Creutzfeldt-Jakob disease (CJD)**. Daniel Carleton Gajdusek described **kuru** among the cannibalistic Fore tribesmen of Papua New Guinea in 1957. Gajdusek received a Nobel Prize in 1976 for his work, which proved that the prions that caused kuru and CJD were transmissible. In 1966, Tikvah Alper found that the scrapie agent was extremely resistant to inactivation by ultraviolet light and questioned whether it could replicate without nucleic acids. **Prions**, the self-replicating, infectious proteins responsible for TSEs in humans and animals, were purified in 1982 by Stanley Prusiner, who received the Nobel Prize in Medicine in 1997 for this work.

Variant Creutzfeldt-Jakob disease (vCJD), the human form of "mad cow disease," was initially noted when ten persons with an atypical form of CJD were diagnosed between February 1994 and October 1995 in widely dispersed areas of the United Kingdom. This disease is linked to human consumption of beef originating in cattle from the United Kingdom that had **bovine spongiform encephalopathy (BSE)**. During the 1970s, changes were made in the methods for rendering sheep offal used in cattle feed by abandoning the use of organic solvents. Some of the sheep offal was derived from animals with scrapie, a spongiform encephalopathy of sheep that does not directly infect humans. Meat and bone meal from BSE-infected cattle was also included in the feed, amplifying the epidemic. By 1988, more than 168,000 cases of BSE had been reported in the United Kingdom, and the number of vCJD cases in humans was also rising. In an attempt to halt the outbreak, a ban on feeding ruminant-derived protein to other ruminants went into effect in July 1988. Between November 1989 and January 1990, this ban was expanded to preclude the use of cattle brain, spinal cord, tonsil, thymus, spleen, and lower intestine from animals over the age of 6 months in human foods; beginning in September of that year, the ban was extended to include feed for all animals and birds. "Beef on the bone" was later banned as well. Milk and milk products, however, are considered safe for human consumption. The outbreak in cattle is decreasing due in part to these measures: whereas 1,000 new cases were reported per week in 1993, the number had been reduced to 300 per week in 1996.

The Diseases

Prions are responsible for causing TSEs, fatal diseases in which areas of spongiform (spongelike, full of small holes) degeneration develop in gray areas of the brain and spinal cord. Vacuolation of the neuropil and astrocytosis (increased numbers of the astrocyte type of glial cell) may be present. Disorders of the pancreas may also occur. TSEs may be transmitted to laboratory animals by injecting material derived from affected brains. In addition to humans, TSEs have been reported to affect cattle, sheep, goats, mice, mink, deer, and cats.

Creutzfeldt-Jakob Disease (CJD)

Persons suffering from this group of uniformly fatal diseases demonstrate loss of motor control, including rapid jerky movements, progressive dementia, paralysis, wasting, and death typically within 3 to 12 months. The cerebellum, basal ganglia, and lower motor neurons are often affected.

Sporadic CJD Approximately 85% of the cases of CJD are sporadic, in which the means of disease acquisition is unknown. The incidence of sporadic CJD is one case per million persons per year. It primarily affects people between the ages of 50 and 75 years. This form of CJD has cerebral involvement associated with rapidly progressive dementia.

Familial CJD Familial CJD accounts for 10% to 15% of the cases of CJD. Disease is linked to a hereditary mutation of the gene encoding the prion protein. It is inherited as an autosomal dominant trait, meaning that only one mutated copy of the gene is required to cause disease. Familial clusters have been reported in Slovakia, Israel, and Chile.

Iatrogenic CJD Fewer than 5% of the cases of CJD are believed to be of iatrogenic origin (associated with medical procedures). Transmission of this form of disease occurs through contaminated surgical instruments, such as scalpels and cortical electrodes, via transplantation of brain meninges or corneas, or by the use of human growth hormone derived from human pituitaries. Prion transmission by blood transfusion or organ donation may also occur. Accordingly, the American Red Cross restricts blood donation by individuals who have been recipients of meningeal transplants, pituitary-derived human growth hormone, or non-U.S. licensed bovine insulin as well as those who have spent extended periods of time in the United Kingdom, due to the risk of consuming contained beef by persons in the latter group.

Kuru Kuru, also known as "laughing disease," was found only among women and children of the Fore Highlander tribe of Papua New Guinea. It was acquired by handling, preparing, or ingesting contaminated human brains. Fore

Highlanders formerly honored their dead relatives by eating their brains. After this practice was halted, kuru almost disappeared and is now found in fewer than ten persons per year.

Variant CJD Variant CJD (vCJD; formerly new variant CJD) is the human form of bovine spongiform encephalopathy and appears to be acquired by ingestion of contaminated beef. This form of CJD affects younger people than does sporadic CJD; the average age of onset is 27 years. The duration of illness is also longer for vCJD than for other forms of CJD (14 months versus 4½ months). Most cases of vCJD have been acquired in the United Kingdom or Ireland; a lower number were acquired in France and other parts of Europe. The incidence of vCJD has been decreasing as infected or potentially infected cattle are prevented from entering the human food chain.

Several differences exist between the clinical presentation of sporadic CJD and vCJD: patients with the former have more prominent dementia and early onset of neurological signs, whereas those with the latter have more delayed neurological signs, painful dysesthesias, prominent psychiatric symptoms such as depression or psychosis, and memory impairment. Later during the course of the disease, early ataxia (unsteadiness and loss of coordination) and involuntary movements appear; prior to death, affected individuals become completely immobile and mute. The disease is accompanied by extensive deposition of prion proteins (PrP) and amyloid plaques in the cerebellum (the region of the brain controlling balance, posture, and coordination of fine movements). Numerous "florid plaques" and the "pulvinar sign" are often present in vCJD as well. A florid plaque consists of a central area that stains with the red dye eosin and is surrounded by a region of spongiform degeneration, while the pulvinar sign is the presence of a high intensity signal from the pulvinar region of the thalamus that is detected by magnetic resonance imaging. Findings in electroencephalograms also differ between sporadic and variant CJD: the former often has periodic sharp waves that the latter typically lacks. In vCJD but not sporadic CJD, prions are typically detected in lymphoid organs. In vCJD, the spongiform changes are most evident in the brain's basal ganglia and thalamus. The basal ganglia regulate voluntary motor activity, while the thalamus serves as the major integrating and relay station for sensory impulses. Prions accumulate in high density in the cerebellum.

Variant CJD is caused by human infection with the BSE ("mad cow") agent. The causative agent of vCJD contains a molecular marker that is absent in other human CJDs but is present in BSE. Its transmission characteristics are almost identical to those of BSE. Evidence from animal models also supports the

Table 28.2   Differences between sporadic and variant CJD

Characteristic	Sporadic Cjd	Variant Cjd
Median age at death	68 years	28 years
Median duration of illness	4 to 5 months	13 to 14 months
Clinical signs and symptoms	Dementia; early neurological signs	Prominent psychiatric and behavioral symptoms; painful dyesthesiasis; delayed neurological signs
Periodic sharp waves on electroencephalogram	Often present	Often absent
"Pulvinar sign" on MRI	Not reported	Present in more than 75% of cases
Presence of "florid plaques" on neuropathology	Rare or absent	Present in large numbers
Immunohistochemical analysis of brain tissue	Variable accumulation of protease-resistant prions	Marked accumulation of protease-resistant prions
Presence of prion in lymphoid tissue	Not readily detected	Readily detected

Source: CDC

linkage between vCJD and BSE. Transgenic mice containing human genes are susceptible to BSE. Rhesus macaques injected with BSE material also develop a disease similar to vCJD in humans.

Gerstmann-Straussler-Scheinker Syndrome

Gerstmann-Straussler-Scheinker syndrome (GSS), like familial CJD, is caused by an inherited autosomal dominant mutation to the prion gene but may rarely occur spontaneously as well. It generally affects persons in their forties or fifties. GSS leads to cerebellar ataxia; dementia is seen less commonly than in CJD. Multicentric amyloid plaques are common. This condition typically persists for several years before terminating in death.

Fatal Familial Insomnia

Fatal familial insomnia (FFI) is a form of human TSE that involves the autonomic nervous system. It is characterized by progressive disturbances of sleep, blood pressure, body temperature, and appetite due to severe atrophy of the thalamus of the brain. Little involvement of the neuropil occurs during FFI. This disease is usually diagnosed among persons between 40 and 60 years of age, who generally live 7 to 18 months postdiagnosis.

FFI is associated with a mutation of codon 178 of the prion protein gene, which substitutes the amino acid aspartic acid for asparagine: this mutation is also seen in sporadic CJD. Which disease results appears to be dependent on codon 129: the amino acid methionine is present in FFI, while valine is often found in sporadic CJD.

Alper's Syndrome

Alper's syndrome is a prion disease of infants. It was named after Tikvah Alper, who discovered infectious material that lacked nucleic acid in the brains of infants with the disease.

Huntington Disease–Like Syndrome

Four types of **Huntington disease–like syndromes** are known, numbered HDL1 through HDL4. These are rare progressive brain disorders with symptoms resembling those found in Huntington disease. Persons with HDL syndromes, however, do not have a mutation in HD gene. Symptoms of HDL1, HDL2, and HDL4 typically appear during early to mid adulthood. Initial signs include irritability, emotional problems, small involuntary movements, loss of coordination, difficulty learning new information or making decisions, and chorea (involuntary twitching movements), which become more pronounced with time. Individuals may experience difficulty walking, speaking, and swallowing and may undergo changes in personality and a decreased ability to think or reason. Affected persons may survive for several years to more than a decade after diagnosis. HDL3 has an earlier onset, typically around the age of 3 or 4 years, and has an atypical presentation.

HDL1 has been described in just a single family. The condition is due to an inherited autosomal dominant mutation of the PRNP gene. The mutation involves an octapeptide repeat (a repeated segment of DNA encoding eight amino acids). This repeat normally occurs 5 times in the PRNP gene but is repeated around 11 times in those with HDL1, resulting in an abnormally long protein.

Other Disorders Associated with the PRNP Gene

Wilson Disease In **Wilson disease**, excessive levels of copper accumulate in the body. This disorder results from a mutation of the ATP7B gene but is modified by an abnormality in the PRNP gene. The PrP protein may also be involved in copper transport. In the normal PRNP gene, the amino acid valine is encoded by codon 129, but some persons with Wilson disease have methionine at that position instead, as also occurs in FFI. Persons with Wilson disease who also have the methionine substitution in PRNP develop disease several years later and appear to have more nervous system symptoms, especially tremors.

Primary Progressive Aphasia **Primary progressive aphasia** is a form of dementia characterized by a gradual loss of language function (reading, writing, and speaking) beginning in midlife. Other brain functions are affected later during the course of the disease. This disease is associated with the presence of methionine at codon 129 of the PRNP gene. Young healthy adults with methionine at this position have greater difficulty performing long-term memory tasks than those with valine.

Transmissible Spongiform Encephalopathies (TSEs) in Animals

Bovine Spongiform Encephalopathy (BSE) BSE occurs in cattle and is commonly known as "mad cow disease." Although both sexes of animal may be affected, dairy cows are affected at a higher rate. The median age of onset is 4 to 4½ years of age, and during most of its development, there is no obvious sign of infection. Symptomatic cattle become uncoordinated, highly sensitive to tactile or visual stimuli, very apprehensive, and prone to losing weight. They have difficulty maintaining posture and moving their hind limbs; a creeping paralysis may occur later during the disease course. Similar to TSE in humans, the brain and spinal cord of affected cattle develop spongiform changes that are visible under a light microscope. This disease is uniformly fatal within weeks to months after diagnosis. The causative agent of BSE is a prion of cattle that may be acquired by humans consuming infected meat, leading to the development of vCJD. The BSE agent is heat-stable, withstanding not only normal cooking temperatures and pasteurization but also the extremely high temperatures used during autoclaving; the prion cannot therefore be inactivated by heating food. It is also resistant to freezing, drying, and low pH, such as exists in the stomach.

BSE affects primarily cattle in the United Kingdom or that originated there. A substantial number of cases have occurred in other countries that imported cattle or cattle feed from the United Kingdom, including Ireland, France, Portugal, Poland, Switzerland, and Germany, and a smaller number of cases appeared in the Netherlands, Italy, Austria, Belgium, Denmark, Luxemburg,

FIGURE 28.1   Unsteadiness of a BSE-affected cow

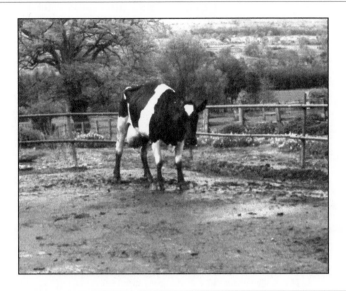

Source: U.S. Department of Agriculture/Animal and Plant Health Inspection Service.

Slovakia, Slovenia, Sweden, Canada, Oman, and the Falkland Islands. Due to the link between vCJD, BSE, and British cattle, the United States has banned importation of these cattle or their meat. Several cases of BSE have nevertheless been found in the United States; one of these is believed to have originated in a Canadian herd.

BSE may also occur in similar ruminants, such as the greater kudu and the oryx, and in domestic cats and members of the cat family in zoos (pumas and cheetahs) that had been fed material containing contaminated bovine offal.

Scrapie Scrapie is a TSE of sheep. Affected sheep lose coordination and eventually are unable to stand. The animals are irritable, extremely sensitive to sound and touch, lose coordination of their hind limbs, and develop severe itching that may lead them to scratch themselves against objects such as fences, often scraping off some of their fleece. Scrapie may be transmitted among the sheep herd either vertically or horizontally. Vertical transmission is believed to be the primary means of propagating the disease within a herd as infected ewes transmit the prions to their young in utero or soon after birth. Placentas and

FIGURE 28.2 **BSE cases in North America, by year and country of death, 1993 and 2003–2010**

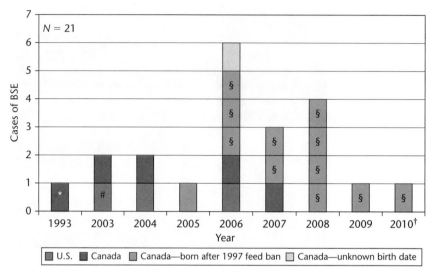

* Imported from UK into Canada. # Imported from Canada into U.S. § Born after March 1, 1999.
†Through March 12, 2010.

Source: CDC.

amniotic fluids are infective and may contaminate pens or pastures where lambing occurs.

Other TSEs TSEs have also been found in minks (transmissible mink encephalopathy), household cats (feline spongiform encephalopathy), and mule deer, white-tailed deer, elk, and moose (**chronic wasting syndrome**). This last affects many elk and deer in the United States, both in the wild and in captivity. States that have reported ill animals include Wyoming, Colorado, Utah, Nebraska, Illinois, New York, West Virginia, and Wisconsin. Hunters and other persons consuming infected meat have never been conclusively shown to develop a TSE. This may be due to a species barrier, which generally prevents transmission of prions between species including passage of the scrapie prion to humans. This barrier is not absolute, however, for sheep prions may infect cattle, undergo changes in the new host species, and then infect humans.

FIGURE 28.3   Areas reporting chronic wasting syndrome in wild deer, elk, and moose, as of March 2010

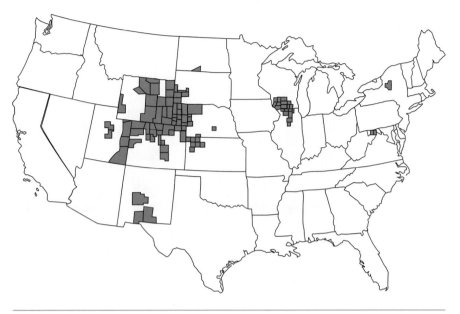

Source: CDC.

The Causative Agents

TSEs are caused by prions. These self-replicating proteins are classified as "small proteinaceous infectious particles that resist inactivation by procedures that modify nucleic acids" but are susceptible to agents that inactivate or unfold proteins. Unlike viruses and the even simpler viriods, both being infectious agents that contain either DNA or RNA, prions are extremely resistant to heat (including autoclaving), ultraviolet and ionizing radiation, and almost all chemical disinfectants. Prions are nonliving infectious agents that do not contain DNA, RNA, or any other nucleic acids; they consist entirely of a single malformed protein. They may undergo denaturation and then regain their former shape without a loss of function. The "hereditary" information that allows prions to replicate is encoded solely by the shape of the protein.

The protein capable of forming human prions exists in two forms, the normal cellular protein, PrPc, which is encoded by the chromosomal DNA gene PRNP, and the alternatively folded prion form, PrPsc. The PRNP gene is on the

FIGURE 28.4 Normal cellular form of the prion protein (left) versus the scrapie form (right)

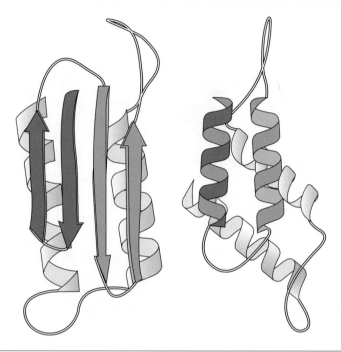

Source: Government of Alberta, Department of Agricultural and Rural Development.

short arm of human chromosome 20 (CD230 antigen). Both PrPc and PrPsc are 33- to 35-kilodalton proteins composed of 208 amino acids. They are found in neurons, glial cells, platelets, and leukocytes, where the PrPc form is normally anchored to lipid rafts in the plasma membrane by a phosphatidylinositol-glycolipid tail. PrPc is water-soluble and protease-sensitive (able to be degraded by protease enzymes). The precise functions of PrPc are unknown but may involve transportation of copper ions into cells, cell signal conduction, or regulation of β-secretase cleavage of the Alzheimer amyloid precursor protein or the immune response. Mice engineered to lack this protein appear to be grossly normal with the exception of some alterations in their circadian rhythms, sleep patterns, seizure thresholds, synaptic transmissions, and hippocampus morphology, indicating that while TSEs are not caused by the absence of the protein, PrPc does nevertheless play some role in normal brain functioning. Interestingly, mice lacking PrPc are not able to be infected by PrPsc, nor do they develop disease if exposed to prions.

The PrPsc form of the protein is protease-resistant (is not degraded by enzymes such as proteinase K) and resides in cytoplasmic vesicles. PrPsc may form thread-like aggregates known as fibrils. Many persons who have inherited spongiform encephalopathies (such as GSS) have a point mutation at position 102 in the PRNP gene, which leads to a substitution of the amino acid leucine for proline in the resulting protein. A substitution of methionine for valine occurs at codon 129 in prions of persons with vCJD. Mutations have also been found to concentrate in at least 16 other regions of PRNP. Mice with such mutant genes develop TSE. Excessive amounts of the normal PrPc form of the protein may also lead to neurodegeneration and the destruction of nerves and muscles.

Because prions do not contain DNA or RNA, they do not replicate in the same manner as other infectious agents or any known form of life. Most living organisms store hereditary information in the form of DNA. DNA is able to be transcribed into various forms of RNA, including mRNA, which is then

RECENT DEVELOPMENTS

The addition of partially purified PrPsc to either cultured neuronal cell lines or to neurons derived from the cerebral cortex increases levels of total cholesterol in cells as well as free cholesterol in the plasma membrane while reducing levels of cholesterol esters. PrPc does not have this effect. The increase in free cholesterol is not due to elevated cholesterol synthesis but may rather be due to its increased solubilization. Cholesterol is an important component of plasma membranes, and increasing its levels may alter membrane fluidity and endocytosis of material into cells. Free cholesterol is also involved in the formation and functioning of neural synapses. Alterations in cholesterol balance have been suggested to play roles in the pathology of Alzheimer's and Parkinson's diseases.

Cholesterol levels are particularly high in structures known as lipid rafts. A number of important molecules are located in the lipid rafts of neurons, including sphingolipids and gangliosides, the folate and p75 neurotrophin receptors, receptors for several neurotransmitters, and components of signaling pathways, such as the phospholipase A_2 (PLA_2) enzyme. The presence of PrPsc increases activation of PLA_2, and these molecules colocalize in lipid rafts. Interestingly, PLA_2 has been implicated in mediating prion-associated neurotoxicity. One of the products of PLA_2 is prostaglandin E_2, whose levels are increased in animals with scrapie and in the cerebrospinal fluid of persons with CJD. Further work is required to determine the outcome of the interactions between PrPsc, cholesterol, and lipid rafts and to ascertain the roles of activated PLA_2 and its products, such as prostaglandin E_2, in TSE pathology.

translated into all of the known proteins. The PRNP gene produces PrPc or the inherited forms of PrPsc by this route. The infectious forms of PrPsc are formed as the misfolded PrPsc protein interacts with PrPc, inducing it to refold and be converted into more PrPsc. PrPc is thus required for the reproduction of infectious PrPsc, explaining why mice that lack PrPc do not develop TSE. Moreover, mice with only one functional copy of the mouse version of the PRNP gene have longer incubation periods and slower disease progression than mice with two functional copies after infection by PrPsc. During the pathogenic refolding process, some of the alpha helical regions of secondary protein structure (spiral areas) of PrPc are converted into beta-pleated sheets in which the protein backbone is more fully extended. This refolded protein is then PrPsc. Some of the mutations in the prion gene that occur in the inherited forms of human TSE (familial CJD and GSS) make the resulting protein more susceptible to changing shape.

The exact mechanism by which PrPsc causes damage to the brain is not clear; however, the alternatively folded forms accumulate in lysosomes in the neurons. If these organelles become too full, they may break, releasing their powerful digestive enzymes into the cytoplasm of the cell. These enzymes, together with the acidic pH of the lysosomes, may damage the intracellular components of the cells, leading to their death.

A species barrier apparently prevents most prions from one animal species from infecting other species. For example, injecting hamster PrPsc into normal mice does not result in disease in the mice. If the mice are engineered to express the hamster form of PrPc, however, disease in the mice will then occur. This species barrier may be breached if the PrPc are very similar. Sheep and cattle PrPc differ by only seven amino acids, and scrapie in sheep may be transmitted to cattle. Cattle and human PrPc vary by 30 amino acids, and BSE may be transmitted to humans, resulting in vCJD.

When meat or lymphoid tissue of infected cattle is consumed by humans, the prions appear to be transported across the gastrointestinal tract wall. From there, the infectious proteins gain access to the enteric or sympathetic branches of the peripheral autonomic nervous system. Retrograde axonal transmission may then carry the prions to the brain and spinal cord of the central nervous system. Prions also accumulate in the spleen, tonsils, and other lymphoid tissue, perhaps entering the lymphatic system via Peyer's patches, small areas of lymphatic tissue scattered throughout the gut wall.

Interestingly, Alzheimer's and Parkinson's diseases are associated with neuronal death and the presence of abnormal, tangled proteins in the brains of affected persons. This has led some researchers to suggest that prions may be involved in causing these neurodegenerative diseases. Both Alzheimer's and

TSEs are characterized by the formation of amyloid fibers, highly organized protease-resistant protein aggregates with a filamentous morphology and a content of high beta-pleated sheet secondary structure. Thus far, however, of the more than 20 human amyloid proteins, only PrPsc is known to be infectious. During Alzheimer's disease, senile plaques are formed whose major component are amyloid β (Aβ) peptides, derived by enzymatic processing of the amyloid precursor protein (APP). The first step in this processing is cleavage of APP by the enzyme β-secretase. Normal PrPc inhibits the action of β-secretase, thus decreasing the formation of Aβ and senile plaques. PrPc needs to be located in lipid rafts in order to have this inhibitory effect. Mutant prions derived from persons with familial prion diseases are not able to inhibit β-secretase and consequently have increased levels of Aβ. The presence of mutated prions may therefore be linked to increased production of the type of senile plaques found in Alzheimer's disease. APP and PrPc may be structurally related as well, as both are processed by at least three of the same cellular enzymes. Furthermore, persons with the amino acid methionine rather than valine at position 129 of the prion protein have increased risk of developing early-onset Alzheimer's disease.

In addition to prions that cause TSEs, six prions have been identified in fungi; four of these are self-propagating amyloids, and two are enzymes necessary to activate their inactive precursors. [URE3] and [PSI+] are prions of the yeast *Saccharomyces cerevisiae*. The [URE3] prion results in inappropriate transcription of a number of genes into RNA, and the [PSI+] prion inhibits the recognition of the signals that end translation of proteins. [PIN+], by contrast, is a self-replicating amyloid protein. [Het-s], the first known prion of fungi, was described in 1952 as a nonchromosomal, non-Mendelian gene of the filamentous fungus *Podospora anserina*. The [β] prion in *S. cerevisiae* is a self-activating enzyme, vacuolar protease B, required for yeast meiosis, and the [C] prion of *P. anserina* serves as self-activating enzyme of the mitogen-activating protein kinase cascade.

The Immune Response

Given the lack of an effective immune response against prions, several studies have examined whether any immune response is engendered by prion infection. CD4$^+$ T helper cells and CD8$^+$ T killer lymphocytes were found to be present in the brains of mice after experimental infection with scrapie and also in the central nervous systems of patients with CJD. These cells did not appear to mount a functional immune response, however, such as the production of IFN-γ or TNF-α or the destruction of target cells. Elevated levels of several chemokines did occur, such as MIP-1β, IFN-γ-inducible factor, and RANTES, all of which attract T lymphocytes to the site of infection. Expression of MHC class I and II molecules were also increased. Activation of brain microglia also occurs during prion infections. None of these immune activities is sufficient to halt the uniformly fatal course of the disease.

Some components of the immune system, however, seem to amplify prions and to be necessary for disease dissemination; for instance, mice lacking B lymphocytes lack prions in the spleen and do not contract scrapie. Animals with lower numbers of Peyer's patches do not readily develop disease after oral infection with prions. M cells in the intestines appear to be important in the infection process. TNF-α and TFN-β are also important for infection by this route. Because the BSE agent may infect humans via consumption of contaminated beef or may infect cattle through infected feed, infection by the oral route may be of great importance for the spread of disease in humans and other animals. In addition to the gut-associated lymphoid tissue, ganglia of the enteric branch of the autonomic nervous system are infected prior to the central nervous system.

Recent work suggests that PrPc may have a role in normal immune system functioning. PrPc is found on the surface of lymphocytes, NK cells, monocytes, and dendritic cells, as well as hematopoietic stem cells. In the stem cells, PrPc may be involved in cell self-renewal, one of the key characteristics of stem cells. Levels of PrPc are higher on T cells than on B cells and higher on memory cells than on naive cells. In human T lymphocytes, PrPc expression is increased during aging and is up-regulated during T cell activation. Cross-linking of PrPc on the surface of T lymphocytes modulates the cells' activation, leading to rearrangements of lipid raft constituents and increased phosphorylation of signaling proteins in the rafts. Greater understanding of the normal physiological role of PrPc in the immune system and elsewhere is important to allow the development of effective therapies against PrPsc that do not prevent normal PrPc functions.

Diagnosis

Definitive diagnosis has traditionally required pathological examination of brains of the deceased. Such exams reveal the presence of plaques that are visible as microscopic aggregates encircled by holes, loss of neurons, and gliosis (increased numbers of glial cells). MRI has also been used in diagnosis. Diffusion-weighted imaging of persons with TSEs indicates the presence of high-intensity signals in the striatum and linear lesions. Individuals with vCJD show high-intensity signals in the posterior thalamus in this test.

Researchers at the National Prion Disease Pathology Surveillance Center at Case Western Reserve University perform assays of brain tissue for microscopic evidence of the disease by the presence of the protease-resistant PrPsc protein. They also search for the presence of elevated levels of the 14-3-3 protein in the cerebrospinal fluid (CSF). The 14-3-3 protein is involved in normal cellular division, differentiation, and signal transduction, and it regulates neurotransmitter production. This protein serves as a marker for some of the prion diseases, including CJD, after the exclusion of neurodegenerative diseases. Its levels are also elevated in individuals with encephalitis and cerebral infarction. Levels of neuron-specific enolase, the microtubule-associated protein tau, and S-100 protein are also elevated in the CSF, but sensitivity using these markers is lower than that seen using 14-3-3. Interestingly, abnormal deposits of hyperphosphorylated tau are also seen in persons with Alzheimer's disease. Tests for these proteins in the CSF may allow preliminary diagnosis of TSE while the person is still alive.

Several other diagnostic assays are also used. In one of these, DNA may be extracted from blood, brain, or other tissues to assay for the presence of mutations in the PRNP gene, particularly in codon 129. Western blotting of the prion protein following protease digestion may be used to identify the strain of PrPsc involved. Brain tissue extracts may be also tested for the presence of prions by ELISA or by immunohistochemistry. Diagnostic testing based on the presence of prions in tonsils has also been explored. Such a test would greatly aid in early detection of disease.

Treatment

Treatment of prion diseases is difficult because few agents are able to cross the blood-brain barrier. Chlorpromazine is able to inhibit PrPsc accumulation in cultured cells but does not alter disease course in infected humans, despite its ability to permeate the blood-brain barrier. Monoclonal antibodies against PrPsc cure neuronal cell lines of infection. These antibodies bind to the cell surface and internalize PrPsc. They act without removing normal PrPc from cells. Many other compounds have also been tested, primarily in vitro, but none has been found to be effective at halting disease in affected humans. No cure is therefore currently available, and death is the universal result among symptomatic individuals. Polyanions, such as dextran sulfate, pentosan sulfate, and Congo red, may block the conversion of PrPc into PrPsc in vitro. Congo red appears to be active against sheep and hamster prions but not mouse or human prions.

Very few treatments have shown any promise in slowing disease progression in vivo. One with activity in humans is the intraventricular infusion of pentosan polysulfate for the treatment of vCJD. Another promising treatment is guanabenz, which has slightly but significantly slowed disease progression in mice infected with the scrapie agent. This drug is an agonist of α2-adrenergic receptors that has been used for years to treat hypertension.

Prevention

Because prions are not alive, they cannot be killed, but they may perhaps be inactivated using extraordinary measures. To prevent iatrogenic transmission, equipment and instruments coming into contact with infected material must be properly decontaminated or disposed of and never reused. Surgical instruments cannot be reliably decontaminated by autoclaving. Chemical agents such as 5% sodium hypochlorite (the active agent in bleach) and 1N sodium hydroxide and aldehydes (formaldehyde, glutaraldehyde) are not completely effectively.

Meat infected with the BSE agent cannot be rendered safe for consumption by humans or other animals by any known means, including cooking at any temperature, freezing, or irradiation. Prions are not inactivated by passage through the acid environment of the stomach. Bile salts, which decrease infection by enveloped viruses, instead enhance the uptake of prions through the epithelium lining the intestinal walls. To prevent BSE and vCJD, prion-contaminated meat must not be allowed to enter the food supply. This has been accomplished by various bans on ruminant feeds, as noted earlier.

Surveillance

Active surveillance for BSE continues throughout the world. Between July and December 2008, the countries with active disease were the United Kingdom, Ireland, Canada, Portugal, Spain, Italy, and France. Germany and Poland reported infection but no clinical disease. By the end of 2008, more than 184,500 cases of BSE had been identified in about 35,000 herds in the United Kingdom, an increase of less than 20,000 cases in 20 years, fueling hope that the feed bans are effectively decreasing disease incidence.

Canada reported 17 cases of BSE from 1993 through June 2009; the last of these was a cow confirmed with the disease on May 15, 2009. Eleven of the 17 infected cattle were born after the implementation of the Canadian feed ban. The United States has had three cases during that time frame, two of which were in animals born in the country; the last of these occurred in March 2006. The two cases of BSE in U.S.-born cattle are classified as atypical BSE, which is believed to arise spontaneously rather than as a result of consuming infected feed.

Summary

Diseases

- Creutzfeldt-Jakob disease • Gerstmann-Straussler-Scheinker syndrome • Fatal familial insomnia • Alper's syndrome

Causative Agent

- PrPsc

Agent Type

- Prions, infectious proteinaceous material

Genome

- No DNA or RNA

Vector

- None

Common Reservoirs

- Humans • Cattle

Modes of Transmission

- Inherited • Consumption of contaminated human brains • Consumption of infected cattle products • Contact with infected surgical instruments, medical equipment, blood, or organs

Geographical Distribution

- Worldwide

Years of Emergence

- 1730s (scrapie) • 1920s (human spongiform encephalopathies)
- 1957 (kuru) • 1996 (vCJD)

Key Terms

Alper's syndrome Prion disease of infants

Bovine spongiform encephalopathy (BSE) "Mad cow disease," a fatal disease of cattle in which gray areas of the central nervous system undergo sponge-like degeneration

Chronic wasting syndrome Transmissible spongiform encephalopathy of mule deer and elk

Creutzfeldt-Jakob disease (CJD) Transmissible spongiform encephalopathy characterized by loss of motor control, dementia, paralysis, and wasting; death usually occurs within a year of diagnosis

Fatal familial insomnia Human transmissible spongiform encephalopathy characterized by progressive disturbances of sleep, blood pressure, and appetite due to severe atrophy of the thalamus

Gerstmann-Straussler-Scheinker syndrome (GSS) Form of fatal human transmissible spongiform encephalopathy due to an inherited autosomal dominant mutation of the prion gene; leads to ataxia

Huntington disease–like syndrome Progressive brain disorder due to a mutation of the PRPN gene, characterized by involuntary jerking movements; difficulty walking, speaking, and swallowing; changes in personality; and decreased ability to think or reason

Kuru "Laughing disease," a fatal human transmissible spongiform encephalopathy caused by ingestion of human brains containing the prion protein

Primary progressive aphasia Form of dementia characterized by gradual loss of language function

Prions Proteinaceous infectious particles; self-replicating proteins

Scrapie Transmissible spongiform encephalopathy of sheep

Transmissible spongiform encephalopathy Disease characterized by sponge-like degeneration of gray areas of the brain and spinal cord

Variant Creutzfeldt-Jakob disease (vCJD) Human transmissible spongiform encephalopathy obtained by eating material from cattle with "mad cow disease"

Wilson disease Accumulation of excessive levels of copper in the body due to a mutation of the ATP7B gene and modified by an abnormality in the PRCP gene

Review Questions

1. What are the five types of Creutzfeldt-Jakob disease? What populations are affected with each, and what are the mechanisms of transmission?
2. What is a prion? Which gene encodes human prions? How do they reproduce?

3. What is believed to have led to the huge increase in numbers of bovine spongiform encephalopathy in cattle and vCJD in humans? How was this epidemic stopped?
4. What is the connection between prions and Alzheimer's disease?
5. How can prion-contaminated surgical instruments be disinfected?

Topics for Further Discussion

1. Mice that lack PrPc are unable to develop prion diseases upon infection. Furthermore, mice without the gene encoding this protein appear to develop normally. These findings have led some investigators to attempt to find ways to eliminate PrPc production in the hope of preventing TSEs. Other research has hinted at roles for PrPc in preventing production of Aβ, found in plaques of Alzheimer's disease patients and in normal immune system functioning. Discuss the possible problems with therapy that eliminates production of PrPc in humans and how these problems might be minimalized or eliminated.
2. Because prions do not contain nucleic acids, they are not susceptible to many of the conventional disinfection agents. They are also resistant to the action of many proteases. Research methods that are currently being used to inactivate proteins, and suggest alternative means of inactivating prions that contaminate surgical instruments. Could these methods be used to inactivate prions in vivo?
3. What other diseases are associated with abnormally folded proteins or protein tangles?
4. For many decades, humans have been consuming meat from scrapie-infected sheep or from deer or elk with chronic wasting syndrome, yet no disease transmission from the animals to humans is believed to have ever occurred. Discuss reasons for the potential differences of these diseases in comparison with the documented transmission of bovine spongiform encephalopathy to humans.

Resources

Bate, C., Tayebi, M., and Williams, A. "Sequestration of Free Cholesterol in Cell Membranes by Prions Correlates with Cytoplasmic Phospholipase A2 Activation." *BMC Biology*, 2008, *6*, 8–17.

Chin, J. *Control of Communicable Diseases Manual* (17th ed.). Washington, D.C.: American Public Health Association, 2000.

Hope, J. "Transmissible Spongiform Encephalopathies of Man and Animals." In R. M. Krause (ed.), *Emerging Infections*. San Diego, Calif.: Academic Press, 1998.

Isaacs, J. D., Jackson, G. S., and Altmann, D. M. "The Role of the Cellular Prion Protein in the Immune System." *Clinical and Experimental Immunology*, 2006, *146*, 1–8.

Lewicki, H., and others. "T Cells Infiltrate the Brain in Murine and Human Transmissible Spongiform Encephalopathies." *Journal of Virology*, 2003, *77*, 3799–3808.

Pankiewicz, J., and others. "Clearance and Prevention of Prion Infection in Cell Culture by Anti-PrP Antibodies." *European Journal of Neuroscience*, 2006, *23*, 2635–2647.

Parkin, E. T., and others. "Cellular Prion Protein Regulates β-Secretase Cleavage of the Alzheimer's Amyloid Precursor Protein." *Proceedings of the National Academy of Sciences*, 2007, *104*, 11062–11067.

Prinz, M., and others. "Oral Prion Infection Requires Normal Numbers of Peyer's Patches but Not of Enteric Lymphocytes." *American Journal of Pathology*, 2003, *162*, 1103–1111.

Tribouillard-Tanvier, D., and others. "Antihypertensive Drug Guanabenz Is Active In Vivo Against Both Yeast and Mammalian Prion." *PLoS ONE*, 2008, *3*, 1–9.

Wickner, R. B., Edskes, H. K., Shewmaker, F., and Nakayashiki, T. "Prions of Fungi: Inherited Structures and Biological Roles." *Nature Reviews of Microbiology*, 2007, *5*, 611–618.

PART VI

SPECIAL ISSUES IN INFECTIOUS DISEASES

CHAPTER 29

THE EMERGING IMPORTANCE OF INFECTIOUS DISEASES IN THE IMMUNOSUPPRESSED

LEARNING OBJECTIVES

- Describe populations of immunosuppressed persons and explain why these populations are increasing

- Describe the causes of immunosuppression

- Describe the bacterial, viral, fungal, and parasitic infections of concern to immunosuppressed persons

Major Concepts

The Populations

Persons with compromised immune systems fall into various groups. Some of the causes of immunosuppression are transient, and the immune systems of these people return to a normal functional state with time. Such populations include infants, pregnant women, individuals receiving chemotherapy, and persons with a short-lived viral infection. Others are immunosuppressed for lengthy or indefinite periods of time, including those with metabolic disorders, with congenital immune deficiencies, on long-term immunosuppressive drug treatments, or with certain chronic viral infections. The number of immunocompromised persons is currently increasing, especially in developed areas of the world where those in a weakened state of health are surviving for longer periods of time.

Causes of Immunosuppression

A number of factors may induce a state of reduced immunity. Some of these factors relate to a person's age (fetuses, infants, and the elderly), special circumstance (pregnancy), genetic background (inherited immune deficiency disorders), or lack of immune system organs. Other immunosuppressive elements are acquired during one's lifetime, such as immunosuppressive bacterial or viral infections, including AIDS. Medical interventions may compromise a person's immune response. Immunosuppressive drugs may be administered during the treatment of several diseases, including cancer and inflammatory conditions. Chemotherapy drugs and dialysis also decrease immune responsiveness. Compounds naturally produced by the human body (some hormones and cytokines) may also inhibit activity of various parts of the immune system.

Diseases

Immunosuppressed persons are particularly vulnerable to diseases caused by some bacteria, viruses, fungi, protozoa, and helminths. Some of the most troublesome of these microbes are *Clostridium difficile*, agents that cause respiratory and diarrheal diseases, cytomegalovirus, rotavirus, *Toxoplasma gondii*, and *Cryptosporidium*. The pathogenic role of many fungi in immunosuppressed populations is becoming increasingly well known. Coinfection with HIV and other organisms, including *Mycobacterium tuberculosis*, *Trypanosoma cruzi*, and *Leishmania* species, is especially problematic.

Introduction

This book describes a number of infectious diseases that are presently emerging as novel threats to human health as well as infections that for a variety of reasons are reemerging to endanger new segments of humanity or have escaped the mechanisms that humans have carefully created over decades for our protection (antibiotics, vaccines). One of the large categories of emerging infectious diseases encompasses diseases that strike persons whose immune system is compromised, leaving them vulnerable to infection with one or more groups of microbes. Many of the diseases described in other chapters are either only pathogenic in immunosuppressed individuals or cause much more serious or life-threatening diseases in these people. Given the large increase in numbers of persons with dysfunctional immune responses, many people currently entering the health care or public health fields will find themselves addressing some unique forms of microbial infection as well as special needs of persons harboring the responsible microbes. This chapter describes specific populations of persons at high risk of developing these infections and the microbes involved in disease causation.

Immunosuppressed Populations

Several groups of people have compromised immune systems that leave them more susceptible to malignancies and infections than the general population. Immunocompromised persons are at greater risk for developing opportunistic infections by microbes that typically are a part of the normal flora or even some that under other circumstances act in a manner that benefits both host and microbe. In other cases, infections that usually result in mild or self-limiting infections in immunocompetent persons may engender chronic or severe and life-threatening infections in immunosuppressed individuals. The number of such persons is increasing in developed nations as the population ages, as organ transplantation becomes more common, as more individuals become obese and thus more prone to developing type 2 diabetes or requiring dialysis, and as persons with previously fatal medical conditions live for an extended number of years.

Immunocompromised individuals may be divided into several groups. The first group includes specific segments of the population, such as infants, the elderly, and pregnant women. The second group consists of persons whose immune system is affected by medical procedures. This group would include recipients of cancer chemotherapy, diabetics and hemodialysis patients, transplant recipients, and persons receiving anti-inflammatory therapy for the treatment of autoimmune, inflammatory, or allergic disorders. The third group encompasses individuals with other disease conditions or disorders. Persons in this category include those with congenital immune deficiency diseases; those with immunosuppressive bacterial or viral infections, including HIV-positive persons; those who are malnourished, debilitated, or depressed; diabetics; individuals without a spleen; those in burn units; and those with congenital diseases such as β-thalassemia, Down syndrome, or cystic fibrosis.

Selected Causes of Immunosuppression

A variety of factors may compromise an individual's defense systems. The immune system is not fully developed until well after birth and later in life loses functionality during the aging process. Several types of congenital immune system diseases affect various components of the immune system, whereas other immunosuppressive conditions are acquired.

Age- or Pregnancy-Related Defects in Immune System Functioning

Immune Alteration During Pregnancy A state of induced immunosuppression occurs during pregnancy to prevent rejection of the fetus, whose cells contain foreign MHC class I molecules from the father. Several changes occur in antibody production and T lymphocyte numbers and activity. While some of these alterations decrease autoimmune conditions, they nevertheless make the mother more susceptible to microbial infections, as demonstrated by the relatively high number of pregnant women becoming severely ill or dying during the 2009–2010 H1N1 flu season.

Estrogen levels increase during pregnancy. Estrogens, female sex hormones, trigger an increase in antibody production, and some of these antibodies are transported across the placenta to protect the fetus. The incidence of some autoimmune disorders, such as systemic lupus erythematosus and diabetes, increase during pregnancy and decrease immediately postpartum as estrogen levels fall.

The activity of Th1 cells is reduced during pregnancy and restored postpartum, partly due to alterations in estrogen levels as this hormone decreases Th1 immune responses. The decrease in Th1 activity during the third trimester reduces the relapse rate in individuals with multiple sclerosis; the rate increases again by three months after birth. Treg cells play a vital role in decreasing Th1 and NK activity during pregnancy to prevent immunological rejection of the fetus. Treg numbers rise early during pregnancy in response to increased estrogen levels. Treg cells have on their surface the immune-inhibitory molecule cytotoxic T-lymphocyte-associated antigen 4 (CTLA-4), which up-regulates the expression of another immunosuppressive molecule, indoleamine 2,3-dioxygenase (IDO), on cells that normally aid in T helper cell stimulation, including monocytes and macrophages; instead of stimulating T helper cells, IDO-expressing monocytes and macrophages instead block T cell activation.

Immune Defects in the Very Young Newborns, infants, and young children have low levels of immunity until their immune system develops, leaving them more susceptible to infections. Both antibody and T cell activities are affected. Young children have high numbers of naive T cells, but these do not generally respond well to microbes.

Fetal antibody production begins approximately 20 weeks after birth, and adult antibody levels are not attained for five years. During fetal development, maternal antibodies protect against infection. IgG antibodies from the mother are able to pass through the placenta to the fetus during the last ten weeks of pregnancy. After birth, IgA antibodies are obtained by infant through the mother's milk and play an important role in preventing lung and gastrointestinal infections. Infants who are bottle-fed are 60 times more likely to develop pneumonia during the first three months of life than those receiving maternal IgA through breast-feeding. Some children develop transient **hypogammaglobinemia** (low antibody levels), especially IgG2, during their first year of life due to a delay in maturation of antibody synthesis.

Premature infants are particularly prone to infections because they receive less of the IgG normally transported to the fetus during late gestation. They also have reduced complement activity: complement produces large pores in bacteria, which lyse the microbes. Premature infants also have more respiratory infections because the production of lung surfactant begins late during gestation. Surfactant contains **collectins**, defense proteins that bind sugars on microbial surfaces and aid in the killing of these invaders by phagocytes or the complement system.

Decreased Immunity in the Elderly During the aging process, many components of the immune system diminish in number, reaching very low levels in the elderly and leaving this population much more susceptible to infection. Because both innate and adaptive immune responses are affected, the elderly are prone to infection by many different types of microbes.

Production of neutrophils, monocytes, and macrophages is decreased in the elderly due to low levels of a key hematopoietic growth factor that stimulates the synthesis of the appropriate progenitor cells in the bone marrow. Macrophages' ability to kill microbes is diminished as well because their production of antimicrobial hydrogen peroxide and nitric oxide is reduced. Macrophages are activated by IFN-γ, and T cell production of that cytokine is also reduced.

Increases in prostaglandin synthesis may contribute to the decrease in T cell functions. Numbers of mature T lymphocytes are decreased during aging due to the loss of thymic tissue. The thymus is an immune system organ that is primarily responsible for the selection and maturation of T cells. Decreased activity of this organ during aging reduces the body's ability to replace T lymphocytes. During aging, T cells themselves are less able to divide in response to microbes and produce lower amounts of cytokines such as IL-2, IFN-γ, and IL-4. Loss of IL-2 impairs T and B lymphocyte division and activation. Decreased levels of IFN-γ reduce protection against viruses and impair macrophage activity. Reduced production of IL-4 impairs synthesis of some Th2 cytokines.

Genetic Defects in the Immune System

A number of inherited conditions reduce antimicrobial activity of the immune system by either decreasing numbers of leukocytes or leading to loss of functioning. These genetic immunodeficiency disorders (**primary immunodeficiencies**) may be divided into three categories: those that affect neutrophils and monocytes, lymphocytes, or the complement system. The first category of immunodeficiency diseases includes **congenital neutropenia** (decreased neutrophil numbers resulting from reduced levels of a growth factor, G-CSF, which normally triggers bone marrow stem cells to produce these cells) and **leukocyte adhesion deficiency** (defective expression of cell surface molecules that normally allow neutrophils and monocytes to adhere to and pass through the endothelial cells of the blood vessels, inhibiting passage of these cells to sites of infection). The second category of primary immunodeficiency diseases includes **common variable immunodeficiency** (reduced numbers of antibody-producing cells) and several types of **severe combined immunodeficiency syndrome** (lack of mature T and B lymphocytes). The third category of primary immunodeficiency disorders leads to defective killing of microbes by the complement system due to decreased levels of several components of the complement cascade or its regulatory molecules.

Immunosuppression Resulting from Bacterial or Viral Infections

Infection with several bacteria and viruses may lead to a generalized state of immunosuppression that worsens the effects of diseases caused by other pathogens or permits the development of severe disease by typically benign opportunistic microbes. *Anaplasma phagocytophilum* (discussed in Chapter Four) is one such bacterium that infects neutrophils and impairs their activity, increasing the host's susceptibility to opportunistic diseases caused by fungi or viruses. Several viruses may also impair the immune response. HIV (discussed in Chapter Sixteen) affects functions of many immune cells, including T helper cells, which it infects and kills. Infection with either the measles or Epstein-Barr virus induces a generalized state of immunosuppression as well.

Drugs That Suppress Immune Responses

Immunosuppressive antirejection drugs must be administered to recipients of solid organ or bone marrow transplants to prevent immune-induced graft rejection. Anti-inflammatory drugs, used in the treatment of conditions such as rheumatoid arthritis, psoriasis, and Crohn's disease, also suppress T cell activity in order to block excessive pathogenic immune activation. Antirejection and anti-inflammatory drugs include corticosteroids such as prednisolone, tacrolimus, mycophenolate mofetil, cyclosporine A, and azathioprine. Monoclonal antibodies directed against immune cells (anti-CD3 and anti-CD4 antibodies to eliminate T lymphocytes) or against cytokines (anti-TNF-α antibody) also decrease graft rejection. These drugs all greatly increase the risk of microbial infections.

Cancer patients, especially those with hematological malignancies such as leukemia or lymphoma, are debilitated and hence more susceptible to microbial infection. Chemotherapeutic medications increase cancer patient vulnerability. This is particularly true of drugs used to treat leukemia and lymphoma because the cancer cells being targeted are immune cells, and many nonmalignant white blood cells and bone marrow stem cells are killed as well.

Other drugs may also affect susceptibility to microbial infection. Alcohol and illicit drugs decrease nutritional status, leading to debilitation and decreased immune responsiveness.

Immunosuppressive Hormones and Cytokines

Corticosteroids, such as cortisol, are hormones produced by the adrenal cortex. These stress hormones inhibit T cell activity, and persons living with chronic stress are at higher risk for developing infections than nonstressed persons who produce less of these hormones.

Treg cells, a subset of CD4$^+$ T lymphocytes, down-regulate Th1 and Th2 immune responses. These cells act via the production of the regulatory cytokines IL-10 and TGF-β.

Table 29.1   Some factors that inhibit immune system functioning

Age-related conditions	Fetuses, infants, the elderly
Health conditions	Pregnancy, diabetes, dialysis, depression, Down syndrome, cystic fibrosis, β-thalassemia, surgery, malnutrition, debilitating conditions
Primary immunodeficiencies	Deficiencies in monocytes and neutrophils, lymphocytes, complement system
Immunosuppressive infectious agents	Some bacteria, some viruses
Drug therapy	Antirejection drugs, anti-inflammatory drugs, chemotherapeutic drugs
Lack of immune system organs	Lack of thymus, loss of spleen

Lack of Immune System Organs

The absence of immune system organs impairs defense against several types of microbes. In **DiGeorge syndrome**, children are born with a developmental defect that leads to the absence of a thymus, among other effects. Such children lack mature T lymphocytes. The spleen is an immune organ that may be severely damaged by trauma and removed surgically, often following a motorcycle accident. The spleen houses many B lymphocytes and macrophages.

Infectious Diseases of the Immunosuppressed

In a 2008 report, 199 pediatric kidney transplant recipients were followed for three years. A total of 64 episodes of diarrhea occurred during this period, 38 of them resulting from microbial infections: viruses in 16 patients, bacteria in 10, yeast in 4 (*Candida albicans*), and parasites in 8 (*Giardia lamblia* in one patient and *Cryptosporidium* in the others). The viral infections were as follows: cytomegalovirus (CMV; nine cases), rotavirus (five), and adenovirus (two). Of the bacterial infections, *Clostridium difficile* was found in four persons, especially within the first 30 days of transplant; *Helicobacter pylori* in three; and *Escherichia coli*, *Campylobacter jejuni*, and *Salmonella enteritidis* in one person each. In a 2007 study of kidney and liver transplant recipients, 33 episodes of diarrhea occurred due to infection by viruses—CMV (six cases) and rotavirus (one); bacteria—*C. difficile* (three), *C. jejuni* (two), *Shigella sonnei* (two), and *S. enteritidis* (one); parasites—*G. lamblia* (nine), *Cryptosporidium* (seven), *Entamoeba histolytica* (one); and a fungus—*Blastocystis hominis* (one). *C. difficile* again predominated early after transplant, while CMV was the most common microbial agent between months 1 and 6.

Bacterial Infections

Respiratory Tract Infections Immunocompromised persons are particularly vulnerable to severe respiratory tract infections as a result of infection by different groups of bacteria. Several of these bacteria are discussed elsewhere in this book (*Legionella pneumophila* in Chapter Nine, *Pneumocystis jiroveci* (*carinii*) in Chapter Sixteen, and *Mycobacterium tuberculosis* in Chapter Ten). Other species of the *Mycobacterium* group also cause disease in immunocompromised persons, including HIV-positive persons, children, alcoholics, and those with chronic lung disease. Infections with members of the *M. avium* complex, *M. kansasii, M. malmoense,* and *M. xenopi* are particularly likely to result in respiratory tract disease. *Pseudomonas aeruginosa* infection is common among persons with cystic fibrosis and may result in serious illness, while infection with *Burkholderia cepacia* is particularly dangerous.

Nocardia species are gram-positive, branched filamentous bacteria. Infection with members of this group is common among transplant recipients but not immunosuppressed cancer patients.

Mycoplasma pneumoniae is a member of an unusual group of very small bacteria that lack a cell wall. They are the primary agents responsible for

FIGURE 29.1   *Pseudomonas aeruginosa*

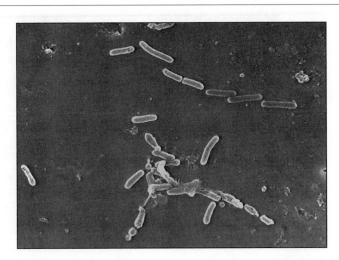

Source: CDC.

"walking pneumonia" and may also induce tracheobronchitis and bronchiolitis along with upper respiratory tract symptoms. Infection may also exacerbate asthma. Other nonpulmonary manifestations of infection include arthritis, gastro-intestinal disorders (nausea, vomiting, and diarrhea), muscle ache, kidney damage, and skin rash. Some persons with primary immunodeficiency disease are more likely to develop joint and respiratory disease, brain abscesses, and subcutaneous skin nodules or abscesses. Renal manifestations are found in persons with AIDS.

Digestive Tract Infections *Clostridium difficile* is particularly problematic in immunocompromised individuals. This bacterium is a normal inhabitant of the human intestine and a frequent cause of colitis in immunosuppressed persons. A ten-year study of transplant recipients in Minneapolis found an overall incidence of *C. difficile*–associated colitis of 8%, 16% in pediatric kidney recipients, 15.5% in kidney-pancreas recipients, and 3.5% in adult kidney recipients. The children generally became infected much sooner than the adults (33 days for pediatric kidney transplants versus 15 months for adult kidney transplants). Following general surgery, the incidence of *C. difficile* colitis is 1% to 4% and is partly linked to prior antibiotic use and length of hospitalization.

Other Bacterial Infections Several other groups of bacteria covered elsewhere in this text cause more serious infections in immunocompromised persons than

FIGURE 29.2 *Clostridium difficile*

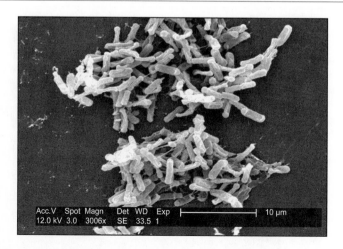

Source: CDC.

in members of the general population. *Ehrlichia chaffeensis* and *Anaplasma phagocytophila*, the causative agents of human monocytotropic ehrlichiosis and human granulocytotropic anaplamosis, respectively, are discussed in Chapter Four. *Bartonella henselae* and *B. quintana* (Chapter Five) cause bacillary angiomatosis and bacillary pelosis hapatis during late-stage AIDS and in cancer patients receiving chemotherapy.

Probiotic organisms, such as those found in yogurt, may be administered orally to outcompete other typically pathogenic organisms. These probiotic microbes occasionally also cause disease in individuals without a fully competent immune system. One such case involved a person with **Sjögren's syndrome**, an autoimmune condition characterized by decreased production of tears and saliva. The patient was treated with immunosuppressive agents to control her inappropriate immune response and subsequently developed a recalcitrant infection with *C. difficile* in addition to *Staphylococcus aureus* pneumonia and *S. pneumoniae* septicemia. After a prolonged course of several broad-spectrum antibiotics failed to contain these bacteria, "biotherapy" with yogurt was instituted. Yogurt contains the probiotic bacterium *Lactobacillus rhamnosus*, a gram-positive bacillus that rarely causes opportunistic infections. The *C. difficile* infection subsequently

SEVERAL BACTERIA THAT ARE PROBLEMATIC FOR IMMUNOSUPPRESSED PERSONS

Legionella pneumophila

Pneumocystis jiroveci (carinii)

Mycobacterium species

Pseudomonas aeruginosa

Burkholderia cepacia

Nocardia species

Mycoplasma pneumoniae

Clostridium difficile

Ehrlichia chaffeensis

Anaplasma phagocytophila

Bartonella species

Probiotic bacteria

Treponema pallidum

resolved; however, *L. rhamnosus* caused vancomycin-resistant septicemia with respiratory and cardiovascular dysfunction as well as very high fever. These conditions, as well as *S. pneumoniae* pneumonia, led to the person's death. More than 50 other cases of pathological *L. rhamnosus* infection have been reported in persons with cancer, organ transplant recipients, diabetics, or persons having had recent surgery. The mortality rate is 14%. These cases demonstrate that generally benign and beneficial microbes such as *L. rhamnosus* that are prescribed to counter *C. difficile* diarrhea may themselves cause life-threatening infections in debilitated persons receiving immunosuppressive drug therapy.

Treponema pallidum is the causative agent of syphilis. *T. pallidum*–induced disease is altered by coinfection with HIV, which accelerate the course of infection and increases the risk of developing neurosyphilis. Neurosyphilis is a progressive destruction of the brain and spinal cord characterized by an unsteady gait, incontinence, seizures, shaking, paralysis, dementia, mood disorders, personality changes, and psychosis.

Viral Infections

Respiratory and Digestive Tract Infections Influenza is often more severe in young children and the elderly than in most segments of the population. Pregnant women are also more likely to develop dangerous infections with influenza virus. During the H1N1 pandemic of 2009–2010, a disproportionally high number of fatalities occurred in pregnant women. Treg activity is increased during pregnancy, with the subsequent suppression of T lymphocyte and NK cell activity. These cells are normally our primary protection against viral infections, including influenza.

Cytomegalovirus (CMV) is another organism of concern for immuno-suppressed individuals. A Taiwanese study of 341 bone marrow recipients found that 20% developed diffuse pulmonary infiltrates, with a mortality rate of 50%. CMV pneumonitis was responsible for 20% of these cases and was often associated with hepatitis infection. Such infections often develop at least two weeks after transplant and are more common in persons with a history of prior infection. CMV also affects the digestive tract of transplant recipients, leading to nausea, vomiting, abdominal pain, and diarrhea and increasing the risk of graft rejection. This virus is also a major cause of blindness during AIDS.

Adenovirus infection commonly occurs within the first 100 days after transplant. It is found in 3% to 29% of bone marrow transplant recipients and in 5% to 10% of individuals receiving a solid organ. The commonly reported pathologies include hemorrhagic cystitis, renal failure, upper respiratory tract infection, interstitial pneumonia, pneumonitis, enteritis, hepatitis, confusion, seizures, encephalitis, and disseminated disease, including multiorgan failure. The overall mortality rate for infected bone marrow recipients is 26% to 54%, with higher rates occurring in those with pneumonia or disseminated disease (50% to 80%). Infection also increases the risk of graft rejection and coinfection with fungi.

Skin Infections Several viral infections originating in the skin are serious and potentially fatal in immunocompromised persons. Infection with varicella-zoster viruses may be reactivated during immunosuppression, as occurs during aging. This leads to **shingles**, in which the virus, formerly residing in a latent form in the nerves, travels to the skin, resulting in a vesicular rash on the waist, chest, back, or face. It is a very painful condition, and the pain may persist for months, even after the infection is brought under control. Among immunocompromised individuals, the mortality rate may reach 17%.

Infection with the measles virus may be fatal in the young, leading to a mortality rate of 15% to 25% among children in the developing world, who often are unvaccinated. A similar virus, rubella, causes German measles. Whereas it remains a mild, self-limiting illness in immunocompetent persons, it leads to a severe congenital disease in developing fetuses. Human herpesvirus-8 induces a severe and often fatal visceral form of Kaposi's sarcoma in HIV-positive homosexual men (discussed in Chapter Seventeen).

FIGURE 29.3 Shingles due to varicella-zoster virus in a person with a history of leukemia

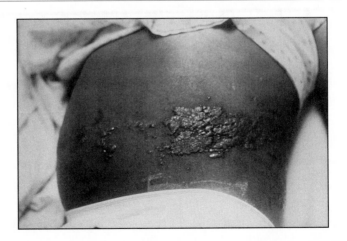

Source: CDC.

Other Viral Infections Hemophagocytic lymphohistiocytosis (HLH) results from the overproduction of several cytokines in response to a variety of microbial infections. These molecules include Th1-like cytokines (IL-12 and IFN-γ), inflammatory mediators (TNF-α and IL-6), and regulatory cytokines (IL-10), leading to the accumulation of T lymphocytes and macrophages in lymphocytic organs, such as the liver, spleen and bone marrow. Impairment of the host defense system as a result of primary immunodeficiency, hematological malignancy, or secondary to an infection may trigger HLH. Epstein-Barr virus, CMV, parvovirus, and HIV are the most common viruses associated with secondary HLH in immunocompromised persons. Other infectious causes of HLH include *Bartonella* species, *M. tuberculosis,* hepatitis C virus, and *T. gondii.*

Fungal Infections

Solid organ transplant recipients are at risk for a variety of fungal infections, usually within the first two to six months posttransplant. Liver transplant recipients are prone to early infection with *Candida* species. Half of all individuals who receive livers develop a fungal infection. Persons undergoing chronic rejection are more likely to develop later infections with *Aspergillus* or endemic fungi such as *Cryptococcus.* Lung and heart-lung transplant recipients are more apt to be infected by *Aspergillus* or other filamentous fungi due to exposure of the transplanted organ to the external environment. Factors associated with the

---

SEVERAL VIRUSES THAT ARE PROBLEMATIC FOR IMMUNOSUPPRESSED PERSONS

Influenza

Cytomegalovirus

Adenovirus

Varicella-zoster

Rubella

Human herpesvirus-8

Epstein-Barr

Parvovirus

Human immunodeficiency virus (HIV)

Hepatitis C virus

development of fungal infections following transplantation include preoperative steroid and antibiotic treatment, administration of broad-spectrum antibiotics, length of antibiotic use, steroid dose, central venous catheters, bacterial infections, systemic CMV infection, long initial transplant operation time, urgent status, prolonged operation time, blood transfusion during an operation, transfusion of a high number of red blood cell units posttransplant, vascular complications, renal insufficiency and hemodialysis, and use of antirejection drugs, including OKT3 monoclonal antibody to kill T lymphocytes.

Pneumonias of fungal origin were studied in immunosuppressed cancer patients from the relatively moist, temperate climates of the south central and southeastern United States. The fungi in this study were usually either *Candida* or *Aspergillus* species and, less commonly, members of the Mucorales order or the *Cryptococcus* or *Histoplasma* genus. Infection with *Aspirgillus* or Mucorales fungi results in rounded pneumonia (spherical area of consolidated lung infection) and hemorrhagic pulmonary infarctions. These fungi are acquired by inhalation. *Candida* caused nonspecific bronchopneumonia as a result of disseminated infection. These fungal infections typically occur at the height of chemotherapy-related leukopenia and are associated with hematological malignancies and use of broad-spectrum antibiotics.

Cryptococcus **and** ***Histoplasma*** *Cryptococcus neoformans* is a yeastlike fungus (unicellular) and *Histoplasma capsulatum* is a dimorphic fungus (may exist as either yeast or mold); both are endemic to soil and dust containing bird or bat excreta and may be aerosolized by construction or other activity that disturbs the soil. Areas under blackbird roosts, chicken coops, and caves may be heavily contaminated with the fungi. Humans are generally infected by inhaling the airborne fungal spores. *C. neoformans* is found thorough the world; *H. capsulatum* is present in the Ohio and Mississippi valleys of the United States, Central America, portions of South America, and Africa. *H. capsulatum* var. *capsulatum* (North and Central America) and *H. capsulatum* var. *duboisii* (Africa) are pathogenic to humans. Approximately 80% of young adults in the endemic areas of the United States have been infected by the former.

Primary lung infection is usually asymptomatic or results in a self-limiting, flulike illness. CD4$^+$ T helper cells control these fungal infections, but foci continue to persist if disseminated and may be reactivated if T cell function is compromised. Disseminated cryptococcosis and histoplasmosis may be reactivated in immunocompromised individuals, including those with AIDS, leukemia, or lymphoma; in infants and the elderly; or following organ transplantation or use of immunosuppressive drugs. Disseminated histoplasmosis is found in 5% to

FIGURE 29.4   *Histoplasma capsulatum*

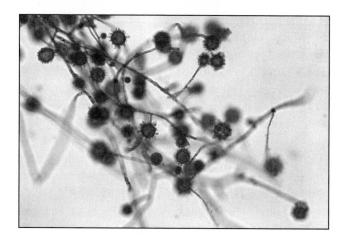

Source: CDC.

25% of AIDS patients in the Ohio and Mississippi valleys. Intense fungal multiplication begins in the lungs and moves to extrapulmonary sites, including the bone marrow, kidneys, brain and meninges, liver, skin, and rarely, the intestines. Disease manifestation include sepsis syndrome with hypotension, disseminated intravascular coagulation, renal failure, acute respiratory distress, meningitis, lesions of the mucous membranes, endocarditis, and ulceration, strictures, and perforations of the small intestine. Disseminated infection may be lethal if not appropriately treated.

Cutaneous manifestation of cryptococcosis and histoplasmosis are fairly uncommon but may signify the presence of underlying disseminated infection. Cutaneous *C. neoformans* and *H. capsulatum* may present as panniculus in immunocompromised persons—painless or painful subcutaneous nodules, ulcers, pustules, granulomas, localized cellulitis, or papules mimicking molluscum contagiosum (a viral infection). This condition may also result from infection with several gram-positive or gram-negative bacteria, *M. tuberculosis,* actinomyces, *Nocardia,* and *Candida albicans.*

Aspirgillus species   *Aspirgillus* species are filamentous fungi. Following transplantation, the incidence of invasive aspirgillosis ranges from 0.7% (kidney transplant) to 8.4% (lung), and mortality rates range from 55% (lung transplant) to 92% to 100% (bone marrow and pancreas transplants). Consequences of infection include bronchitis, ulcerative tracheobronchitis, aspergilloma, invasive pulmonary infection, empyema, and retroperitoneal abscess. *Aspergillus* is also the most common fungal cause of brain abscesses, although *Candida* and Mucorales species have also been implicated in this disease manifestation. Fungal brain abscess generally occurs early after transplant (median of 24 days), while nonfungal abscess due to *T. gondii* or *Nocardia* occurs much later (mean time of 264 days). Risk factors for infection in lung transplant patients are ongoing infection with CMV, single lung transplantation, smoking, immunosuppression with the OKT3 monoclonal antibody to kill T lymphocytes, poor allograft function, renal failure, and fulminant hepatitis. Aspirgillosis is also common in persons with cystic fibrosis, a genetic disorder in which thickened mucus inhibits the clearance of microbes from the respiratory tract.

Candida **species** Endogenous or nosocomially acquired *Candida* species are the fourth leading cause of bloodstream infection in critical care units. These fungi may lead to brain abscesses, pneumonia, and thrush or may induce lesions in the kidney, gastrointestinal tract, spleen, or eye. *C. albicans* is most commonly involved, but the rate of invasive infection by several other *Candida* species is on the rise. These emerging threats include *C. glabrata, C. tropicalis, C. parapsilosis, C. krusei, C. lusitaniae, C. tropicalis,* and *C. rugosa.* Many of these are resistant to the azoles and others to amphotericin B, 5-fluorocytosine, or nystatin.

Zygomycetes The class **Zygomycetes** contains filamentous fungi that grow at temperatures higher than that of the human body. They are inhabitants of soil,

FIGURE 29.5 Pneumonia resulting from *Candida* infection

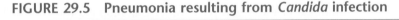

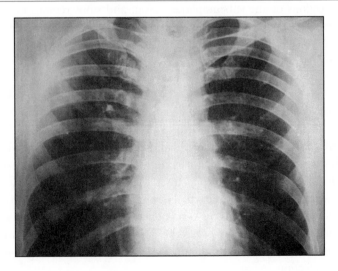

Source: CDC.

decaying organic matter, and foods, including bread. The class is divided into two orders. Members of the order Mucorales tend to invade blood vessels and cause thrombosis (blood clotting) and tissue death. They target persons with type 1 and type 2 diabetes mellitus, those with hematological malignancies, and transplant recipients but may also affect young children in high-risk nurseries, postoperative patients, and persons in trauma or burn wards. Mucorales fungi cause several forms of disease in humans. The craniofacial form is often encountered during poorly controlled diabetes and results in infection and necrosis of the sinuses around the nasal cavity, followed by destruction of the tissue of the nose, hard palate of the mouth, orbital cavity, cheeks, and brain. Fungi of the *Rhizopus* genus are typically the responsible agents. The pulmonary form of infection leads to thrombosis of pulmonary vessels, necrosis of lung tissue, or airway obstruction. Persons receiving immunosuppressive drugs and those with acute leukemia are most likely to develop these two forms of disease. In the cutaneous form, infection begins in or the under the skin and may extend into the adjacent fat, muscle, and bone tissue, resulting in necrotizing fasciitis with skin inflammation, ulceration, and necrosis. The gastrointestinal form of disease has a high mortality rate and is found primarily in premature infants and malnourished individuals. This form is characterized by ulceration and rupture of the abdominal wall, leading to peritonitis or thrombosis and gangrene of the stomach or intestinal lining. The pulmonary, cutaneous, and gastrointestinal forms usually involve infection with *Mucor, Rhizomucor, Rhizus,* or *Cunninghamella* species of Mucorales fungi.

Members of the Zygomycetes order Entomophthorales normally cause mild infections of the subcutaneous, nasal, and sinus regions of immunocompetent persons. They may, however, also engender dangerous, invasive infections in immunosuppressed persons. The Entomophthorales species that infect humans belong to the *Conidiobolusi* and *Basidiobolus* genera.

Coccidioides immitis *C. immitis* is a dimorphic fungus that produces a saprophytic mold in soil and a spherical endospore-forming parasite in tissues. Primary infection occurs only in the arid and semiarid regions of the Western Hemisphere. It has become increasingly common in California in the past two decades. Beginning as a respiratory tract infection, the fungi may later disseminate, causing lung lesions and abscesses in other regions of the body, especially the skin or subcutaneous tissues, bone, and central nervous system, leading to meningitis. The course of the disease is progressive and frequently fatal. Immunocompromised individuals are susceptible to reactivation and dissemination of infection.

FIGURE 29.6   *Coccidioides immitis* infection of the skin

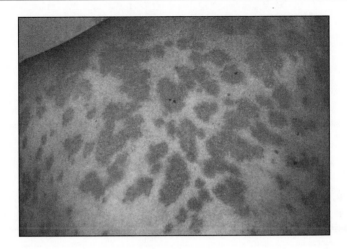

Source: CDC.

Dematiaceous Fungi **Dematiaceous fungi** are dark-pigmented fungi that are emerging infectious agents in transplant patients. They include *Cladosporium, Cladophialophora, Dactylaria, Exserohilum, Scopulariopsis, Alternaria, Curvularia, Bipolaris,* and *Exophiala* species. Two patterns of infection occur. The prominent pattern results in skin and soft tissue or joint infections, usually due to *Exophiala* species infection after environmental exposure to soil or plant matter (more common among gardeners, florists, farmers, and landscapers). Mortality is approximately 7%. The other pattern is characterized by a systemic invasive infection, often leading to brain abscesses, with a mortality rate of 57%.

Saccharomyces cerevisiae *S. cerevisiae* is "baker's yeast" used in baking and brewing and as a probiotic.

During a single two-week period, three cases of invasive infection by *S. cerevisiae* were diagnosed in an intensive care unit in Spain. All three patients had taken the probiotic Ultralevura intranasally to treat *Clostridium difficile*–associated diarrhea. More than 50 additional cases have been reported, 60% of which occurred in intensive care units and 50% of which were linked to probiotic use. These patients had a variety of underlying conditions, including HIV infection, hematological and nonhematological cancers, surgery, trauma, burn, tuberculosis, chronic obstructive pulmonary disease (COPD), cystic fibrosis, ulcerative colitis, heart attack, acute respiratory failure, transplantation, cerebral embolism, stroke, and infancy. The common theme among these persons was a compromised immune response.

SEVERAL FUNGI THAT ARE PROBLEMATIC FOR IMMUNOSUPPRESSED PERSONS

Cryptococcus neoformans

Histoplasma capsulatum

Aspirgillus species

Candida species

Zygomycetes

Coccidioides immitis

Dematiaceous fungi

Saccharomyces cerevisiae

Blastocystis hominis

Sporothrix schenkii

Other Fungi *Blastocystis hominis* is an agent of prolonged, severe diarrhea in transplant recipients. *Sporothrix schenkii* causes ulcerating skin nodules late after transplant, during the period of chronic rejection.

Protozoan Parasites

HIV-positive persons usually have gastrointestinal disorders, particularly diarrhea. Such people are often coinfected by variety of parasitic protozoa that cause diarrhea. A study of enteric protozoa in HIV-infected individuals in India found that over 60% were infected with *Cryptosporidium*, 13% with *Giardia lamblia*, and smaller numbers with microsporidia or *Isospora belli*. Persons with chronic diarrhea were often infected with more than one protozoan and had a lower number of CD4$^+$ T helper cells (mean of 141 cells per milliliter) than those without diarrhea (mean of 390). Persons infected by a single protozoan had a higher CD4 cell count (161 cells per milliliter) than those infected by two (105/mL) or three protozoa (33/mL), demonstrating a linkage between decreased T helper cell number and infection with enteric protozoa.

Phylum Apicomplexa Several parasites of the **phylum Apicomplexa** cause much more severe infections in individuals who are immunocompromised than in the general population. Such protozoa include *Plasmodium* species (discussed in Chapter Twenty-Four) and *Babesia* species (discussed in Chapter Twenty-Five), the agents of malaria and similar diseases. Other Apicomplexans lead to opportunistic infections in the immunosuppressed population. *Isospora belli* is one such protozoan that seldom infects immunocompetent persons but is a major cause of watery diarrhea in AIDS patients. *Cyclospora cayetanesis* is a similar coccidian responsible for large epidemics throughout the world. Infection is characterized by episodes of prolonged, watery diarrhea in both immunocompetent and immunosuppressed individuals, especially those who are HIV-positive. It is accompanied by nausea, anorexia, weight loss, and abdominal cramping. *C. cayetanesis* has caused several large outbreaks in North America. During May and June of 1996, more than 1,400 cases of diarrhea in 20 U.S. states and two Canadian provinces were associated with imported Guatemalan raspberries. Another outbreak involving over 350 individuals occurred from imported berries the following year. *C. cayetanesis*, like *Cryptosporidium* (to be discussed shortly), is often transmitted by ingestion of fecally contaminated water and is resistant to killing by chlorine.

Cryptosporidium parvum   Infection with *C. parvum* leads to severe, chronic diarrhea with dangerous fluid loss and dehydration in immunocompromised individuals (described in Chapter Twenty-Six). In a 2006 study of 214 immunosuppressed patients in Iran, 8.7% of those with AIDS and 2.3% of those with hematological malignancy had chronic diarrhea due to cryptosporidial infection. The diarrhea lasted for weeks and ended in death in the AIDS patients but resolved after discontinuation of the chemotherapeutic medication in the leukemia patient. No cases of cryptosporidial diarrhea were found in 48 persons with nonhematological cancer, 44 persons with skin disease, and 37 transplant recipients. Separate studies have reported an infection rate of 23.8% among cancer patients and 37.7% and 91% in immunodeficient children and adults, respectively. The prevalence of cryptosporidial infection among transplant recipients is 18% to 35% in developing nations. In one study, all seven persons infected with *Cryptosporidium* following renal transplantation developed acute renal failure. Patients undergoing long-term hemodialysis are also at greater risk of infection with *Cryptosporidium* (11.5%) compared with healthy family members (4.4%) and the population as a whole (3.6%).

Toxoplasma gondii   *T. gondii* is the most common protozoan infecting immunocompromised persons, with 50% of the world's population playing host to this parasite. The resulting disease manifestations include acute meningoencephalitis, dysfunctional motor activity, disturbances of consciousness, seizures, and disseminated infection that may be fatal if not treated early. *T. gondii* is an obligate intracellular parasite able to infect and replicate in all human cells, with the exception of erythrocytes.

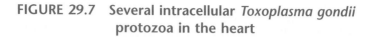

FIGURE 29.7   Several intracellular *Toxoplasma gondii*
protozoa in the heart

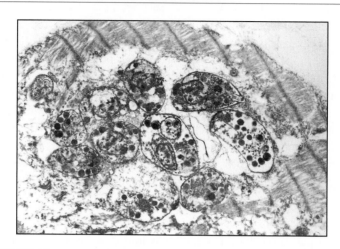

Source: CDC.

Oocysts are the infective form of *T. gondii* for humans and are transmitted via cat feces or from mother to child with up to five cases of congenital infection per 1,000 live births. During congenital infection, 5% to 24% of the affected neonatal children die, and many others develop severe neurological and visual sequelae requiring special education and costly care.

In immunocompetent hosts, *T. gondii* infection is usually asymptomatic or results in a mild, self-limiting illness. The parasite then persists in a slowly dividing stage as a cystlike form in the tissues throughout the person's lifetime. Parasite growth is kept in check during this chronic phase of infection by the host's immune system. CD4$^+$ T helper cells, CD8$^+$ T killer cells, and NK cells produce IL-2 or IFN-γ (or both) to contain the infection. IFN-γ activates macrophages to ingest and kill the parasite. The activated macrophages produce IL-12, which in turn augments a protective Th1 immune response. In tissues having limited interactions with lymphocytes, such as the central nervous system, parasite reproduction proceeds at a higher rate. The blood-brain barrier also impedes entry of antibodies and IFN-γ into the area. *T. gondii* may be reactivated by conditions that impair cell-mediated immunity.

Phylum Mastigophera Parasites of the **phylum Mastigophera** are protozoa that have one or more flagella. *Giardia duodenalis* (*lamblia*) is one such parasite found inhabiting waterways throughout the world, including the United States, and may be acquired by ingesting unfiltered water. The cysts are not killed by the levels of chlorine used in water treatment. *G. duodenalis* is a common cause of diarrhea in HIV-positive individuals and may be accompanied by abdominal cramping, bloating, fatigue, weight loss, and malabsorption of fats.

Trypanosoma cruzi Infection with *T. cruzi* (discussed in Chapter Twenty-Seven) leads to acute myocarditis and meningoencephalitis in immunosuppressed individuals, including those with AIDS, hematological malignancies, and transplanted organs, as a result of reactivation of latent parasites. This last group may actually become infected with *T. cruzi* from the transplant itself because persons with antibodies to the protozoan are not disqualified from organ donation in parts of South and Central America where infection is fairly common. Cardiac manifestations in the immunocompromised include enlargement of the heart, epicarditis, endocarditis, congestive heart failure, arrhythmia, and extensive pericardial hemorrhaging. Central nervous system involvement occurs in 75% to 80% of HIV and *T. cruzi* coinfected persons, resulting in generalized cerebral edema and hemorrhagic lesions in the cerebrum, cerebellum, and brainstem.

Leishmania **species** Members of the *Leishmania* genus are blood-dwelling protozoa that are endemic throughout tropical and subtropical regions of world. Several species infect humans, causing diseases with greatly differing degrees of severity. Infection of immunocompetent persons with several of these species, such as *L. braziliensis*, results in mild, self-resolving skin or mucous lesions.

Immunocompromised persons, however, develop often lethal mucocutaneous or visceral disease. Visceral leishmaniasis is characterized by fever, weight loss, and hepatosplenomegaly in 75% to 80% of the cases. Gastrointestinal tract involvement occurs in 30% of affected individuals, and the respiratory system may also be targeted.

Coinfection with *Leishmania* and HIV is reported most commonly in countries bordering the Mediterranean Sea and, to a lesser extent, equatorial Africa, Asia, and South America. HIV reactivates latent *Leishmania* infections, leading to widespread parasite dissemination, while *Leishmania* shortens the asymptomatic period of HIV infection. About 20% of HIV-positive patients die during their first episode of visceral leishmaniasis, and 70% die over the course of a year as additional relapses occur. Other diseases, such as activated tuberculosis and systemic mycoses, occur in HIV-*Leishmania* coinfected patients as well. *Leishmania*

FIGURE 29.8 Mild leishmanial lesion

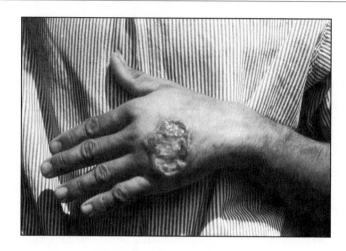

Source: CDC.

is often transmitted via contaminated syringes used by HIV-positive IV drug addicts. Severe leishmaniasis also occurs in renal transplant patients and persons with lymphocytic leukemia.

Phylum Microspora Members of the **phylum Microspora** are highly unusual protozoa that contain a membrane-bound nucleus but lack mitochondria and the Golgi apparatus. Two species cause disease in humans, almost exclusively in the immunosuppressed: *Enterocytozoon bieneusi* and *Encephalitozoon (Septata) intestinalis*. *E. bieneusi* is the more common pathogen, causing damage to the small intestine, malabsorption, and diarrhea. This microsporidium is detected in 7% to 39% of the cases of HIV-associated diarrhea. Several hundred cases of *E. bieneusi* infection have been reported in the HIV-positive population. A 2001 report also described disease in a woman five years after a liver transplant. She experienced chronic watery diarrhea, with 20 to 25 bowel movements per day, persisting for more than seven months. At that time, only five other cases of *E. bieneusi*–associated diarrhea had been found solid organ transplant recipients. In all cases, diarrhea began after at least 18 months on an immunosuppressive regimen. The diarrheal disease in transplant patients is less severe than that seen in HIV-positive individuals. *E. intestinalis* infection is less common but more systematic than that of *E. bieneusi*, and the microsporidium has been found in the urine and nasal mucosa.

SEVERAL PROTOZOA THAT ARE PROBLEMATIC FOR IMMUNOSUPPRESSED PERSONS

Phylum	Species
Apicomplexa	*Plasmodium* species, *Babesia* species, *Isospora belli*, *Cyclospora cayetanesis*, *Toxoplasma gondii*
Mastigophera	*Giardia duodenalis, Trypanosoma cruzi, Leishmania* species
Microspora	*Enterocytozoon bieneusi, Encephalitozoon intestinalis*

Helminth Parasites

In sub-Saharan Africa, the incidence of infection with both HIV and parasitic **helminths** (worms) is high. A 2005 study of 297 HIV-positive adults from urban Zambia found infection with at least one intestinal helminth in 25% of

FIGURE 29.9   *Ascaris lumbricoides*

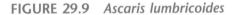

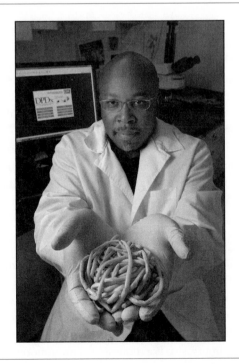

Source: CDC.

study participants. Over half of these persons had a low-intensity infection with the nematode *Ascaris lumbricoides* and 40% had hookworm (*Ancylostoma duodenale*).

The blood fluke *Schistosoma mansoni*, the nematode *Strongyloides stercoralis*, and the tapeworms *Hymenolepis nana* and *Taenia* species are helminths that were identified less frequently in HIV-positive persons. In addition to causing enteric disease, disseminated infection with *S. stercoralis* in immunocompromised persons may lead to cutaneous lesions, respiratory failure, neurological and musculoskeletal involvement, sepsis, and death in about a third of the cases in the United States. Dissemination of the worm throughout the body is caused by hyperinfection with the nematode resulting from autoinfection as larvae penetrate the gut wall. Disseminated *Strongyloides* infection also occurs in persons taking immunosuppressive therapy to control autoimmune disorders such as rheumatoid arthritis, sarcoidosis, and systemic lupus erythematous.

Helminth infection has a detrimental effect on the immune response and may result in malnutrition and blood loss. Helminths also affect the course of infection with HIV, shortening the time of disease progression. Elimination of intestinal helminths correlates with lower HIV plasma levels.

Summary

Immunosuppressed Populations

• Infants • the elderly • pregnant women • those receiving chemotherapy • diabetics • hemodialysis patients • transplant recipients • persons receiving anti-inflammatory therapy for the treatment of autoimmune, inflammatory, or allergic disorders • those with congenital immunodeficiency diseases • those with immunosuppressive bacterial or viral infections, including HIV$^+$ persons • those who are malnourished, debilitated, or depressed • those without a spleen • those in burn units • and those with congenital diseases such as β-thalassemia, Down syndrome, or cystic fibrosis

Causes of Immunosuppression

• Pregnancy-related changes in immune functioning • lack of fully developed immune system due to young age or prematurity • age-related decline in immune functioning • genetic immunodeficiency disorders • immunodeficiency resulting from bacterial or viral infection • anti-rejection drugs • anti-inflammatory drugs • chemotherapeutic drugs • alcohol • illicit drugs • immunosuppressive hormones • immunoregulatory cytokines • lack of a thymus or spleen • depression • congenital disease • surgery • malnutrition • debilitating conditions

Bacterial Infections of the Immunosuppressed

- *Legionella pneumophila* • *Pneumocystis jiroveci (carinii)* • *Mycobacterium tuberculosis* • *M. avium complex* • *M. kansasii* • *M. malmoense*
- *M. xenopi* • *Pseudomonas aeruginosa* • *Nocardia* species
- *Mycoplasma pneumoniae* • *Clostridium difficile* • *Ehrlichia chaffeensis* • *Anaplasma phagocytophila* • *Bartonella henselae*
- *B. quintana* • probiotic bacterium *Lactobacillus rhamnosus*
- *Treponema pallidum*

Viral Infections of the Immunosuppressed

- Influenza • cytomegalovirus • adenovirus • varicella-zoster • measles virus • rubella • human herpesvirus8 • Epstein-Barr virus • parvovirus • HIV

Fungal Infections of the Immunosuppressed

- *Cryptococcus neoformans* • *Histoplasma capsulatum* • *Aspergillus* species • *Candida albicans* • *C. glabrata* • *C. tropicalis* • *C. parapsilosis* • *C. krusei* • *C. lusitaniae* • *C. rugosa* • *Rhizopus* • *Mucor* • *Rhizomucor* • *Rhizus*
- *Cunninghamella* • *Conidiobolusi* • *Basidiobolus* • *Coccidioides immitis*
- *Cladosporium* • *Cladophialophora* • *Dactylaria* • *Exserohilum*
- *Scopulariopsis* • *Alternaria* • *Curvularia* • *Bipolaris* • *Exophiala*
- *Saccharomyces cerevisiae* • *Blastocystis hominis* • *Sporothrix schenkii*

Protozoan Infections of the Immunosuppressed

- Phylum Apicomplexa (*Plasmodium* species, *Babesia* species, *Isospora belli*, *Cyclospora cayetanesis*, *Cryptosporidium parvum*, *Toxoplasma gondii*) • Phylum Mastigophera (*Giardia duodenalis*, *Trypanosoma cruzi*, *Leishmania* species)
- Phylum Microspora (*Enterocytozoon bieneusi*, *Encephalitozoon intestinalis*)

Helminth Infections of the Immunosuppressed

- *Ascaris lumbricoides* • *Ancylostoma duodenale* • *Schistosoma mansoni*
- *Strongyloides stercoralis* • *Hymenolepis nana* • *Taenia*

Key Terms

Collectins Defense proteins that bind sugars on microbial surfaces and aid in their killing by phagocytes or complement

Common variable immunodeficiency Reduced numbers of antibody-producing cells

Congenital neutropenia Decreased neutrophil numbers resulting from reduced levels of the hematopoietic growth factor G-CSF

Corticosteroids Stress hormones produced by adrenal cortex that inhibit T cell activity

Dematiaceous fungi Dark-pigmented fungi which cause emerging infectious diseases in transplant patients, manifesting as either infection of skin, soft tissue, or joints or systemic invasive infection, often resulting in brain abscesses

DiGeorge Syndrome Developmental defect causing children to be born without a thymus, among other defects

Helminths Worms

Hypogammaglobinemia Low levels of antibody

Leukocyte adhesion deficiency Defective expression of the cell surface molecules that allow neutrophils and monocytes to adhere to and pass through endothelial cells

Phylum Apicomplexa Nonmotile protozoa containing a structure known as an apical complex

Phylum Mastigophera Protozoa possessing at least one flagellum

Phylum Microspora Highly unusual protozoa that contain a membrane-bound nucleus but lack mitochondria and the Golgi apparatus

Primary immunodeficiencies Inherited immunodeficiency diseases that inhibit activity of neutrophils or monocytes, lymphocytes, or the complement system

Severe combined immunodeficiency syndrome Lack of mature T and B lymphocytes

Shingles Reactivation of varicella-zoster which results in a vesicular rash on the waist, chest, back, or face

Sjögren's syndrome Autoimmune condition characterized by decreased production of tears and saliva

Zygomycetes Filamentous fungi that grow at temperatures greater than 37°C (98.6°F) and are divided into two orders: Mucorales and Entomophthorales

Review Questions

1. Why are the very young and the elderly more susceptible to infectious diseases?
2. Which causes of immunosuppression are temporary?
3. What types of medical interventions may result in immunosuppression?

4. What bacteria are responsible for many of the respiratory diseases in immunosuppressed persons?
5. What protozoa are responsible for digestive system diseases in immunosuppressed populations?

Topics for Further Discussion

1. Discuss possible reasons for the recent rise in numbers of immunosuppressed persons. Research whether this increase is found in developed countries and developing regions and whether the types of immunosuppressed persons differ between these areas.
2. Discuss methods of successfully treating drug-resistant bacterial and viral infections in immunosuppressed populations. Will these methods work for all groups of immunosuppressed persons or are different strategies needed for different groups?
3. Explore the public health implications of coinfection with HIV and tuberculosis or HIV and leishmaniasis in regions and populations where both diseases are common.
4. Many of the diseases of immunocompromised persons result from fungal infections. Discuss possible reasons why fungal infections are so common in this group.

Resources

Arslan, H., and others. "Etiologic Agents of Diarrhea in Solid Organ Recipients." *Transplantation and Infectious Diseases*, 2007, *9*, 270–275.

Bandin, F., and others. "Cryptosporidiosis in Paediatric Renal Transplantation." *Pediatric Nephrology*, 2009, *24*, 2245–2255.

Basile, A., and others. "Disseminated *Strongyloides stercoralis*: Hyperinfection During Medical Immunosuppression." *Journal of the American Academy of Dermatologists*, 2010, *63*, 896–902.

Bhowmik, D., and others. "Fungal Panniculitis in Renal Transplant Recipients." *Transplantation and Infectious Diseases*, 2008, *10*, 286–289.

Chin, J. *Control of Communicable Diseases Manual* (17th ed.). Washington, D.C.: American Public Health Association, 2000.

Dwivedi, K. K., and others. "Enteric Opportunistic Parasites Among HIV-Infected Individuals: Associated Risk Factors and Immune Status." *Japanese Journal of Infectious Diseases*, 2007, *60*, 76–81.

Ferreira, M. S., and Borges, A. S. "Some Aspects of Protozoan Infections in Immunocompromised Patients: A Review." *Memoirs of the Institute of Oswaldo Cruz,* 2002, *97,* 443–457.

Gonzalez, C. E., Antachopoulos, C., Shoham, S., and Walsh, T. J. "Zygomycosis." In W. M. Scheld, D. C. Hooper, and J. M. Hughes (eds.), *Emerging Infections* (Vol. 7). Washington, D.C.: ASM Press, 2007.

Guerrant, R. L., and Theilman, N. M. "Emerging Enteric Protozoa: *Cryptosporidium, Cyclospora,* and Microsporidia." In W. M. Scheld, D. Armstrong, and J. M. Hughes (eds.), *Emerging Infections* (Vol. 1). Washington, D.C.: ASM Press, 1998.

Ison, M. G., and Fishman, J. A. "Changing Patterns of Respiratory Viral Infections in Transplant Recipients." In W. M. Scheld, D. C. Hooper, and J. M. Hughes (eds.), *Emerging Infections* (Vol. 7). Washington, D.C.: ASM Press, 2007.

Kauffman, C. A. "Histoplasmosis: A Clinical and Laboratory Update." *Clinical Microbiology Reviews,* 2007, *20,* 115–132.

Kiehn, T. E., and White, M. H. "The Changing Nature of Nontuberculous Mycobacteriology." In W. M. Scheld, D. Armstrong, and J. M. Hughes (eds.), *Emerging Infections* (Vol. 1). Washington, D.C.: ASM Press, 1998.

Lo, M. M., Mo, J. Q., Dixon, B. P., and Czech, K. A. "Disseminated Histoplasmosis Associated with Hemophagocytic Lymphohistiocytosis in Kidney Transplant Recipients." *American Journal of Transplantation,* 2010, *10,* 687–691.

MacGregor, G., Smith, A. J., Thakker, B., and Kinsella, J. "Yoghurt Biotherapy: Contraindicated in Immunosuppressed Patients?" *Postgraduate Medical Journal,* 2002, *78,* 366–367.

Modjarrad, K., and others. "Prevalence and Predictors of Intestinal Helminth Infections Among Human Immunodeficiency Virus Type 1–Infected Adults in an Urban African Setting." *American Journal of Tropical Medicine and Hygiene,* 2005, *73,* 777–782.

Muñoz, P., and others. "*Saccharomyces cerevisiae* Fungemia: An Emerging Infectious Disease." *Clinical Infectious Diseases,* 2005, *40,* 1625–1634.

Nahrevanian, H., and Assmar, M. "Cryptosporidiosis in Immunocompromised Patients in the Islamic Republic of Iran." *Journal of Microbiology, Immunology and Infection,* 2008, *41,* 74–77.

Pagani, J. J., and Libshitz, H. I. "Opportunistic Fungal Pneumonias in Cancer Patients." *American Journal of Roentgens,* 1981, *137,* 1034–1039.

Patterson, J. E. "Epidemiology of Fungal Infections in Solid Organ Transplant Patients." *Transplantation and Infectious Diseases,* 1999, *1,* 229–236.

Seyrafian, S., and others. "Prevalence Rate of *Cryptosporidium* Infection in Hemodialysis Patients in Iran." *Hemodialysis International,* 2006, *10,* 375–379.

Sing, A., Tybus, K., and Heesemann, J. "Molecular Diagnosis of an *Enterocytozoon bieneusi* Human Genotype C Infection in a Moderately Immunosuppressed Human Immunodeficiency Virus–Seronegative Liver Transplant Recipient with Severe Chronic Diarrhea." *Journal of Clinical Microbiology,* 2001, *39,* 2371–2372.

Talkington, D. F., Waites, K. B., Schwartz, S. B., and Besser, R. E. "Emerging from Obscurity: Understanding Pulmonary and Extrapulmonary Syndromes, Pathogenesis, and Epidemiology of Human *Mycoplasma pneumoniae* Infections." In W. M. Scheld,

W. A. Craig, and J. M. Hughes (eds.), *Emerging Infections* (Vol. 5). Washington, D.C.: ASM Press, 2001.

Trofe, J., and others. "Human Granulocytic Ehrlichiosis in Pancreas Transplant Recipients." *Transplantation and Infectious Disease*, 2001, *3*, 34–39.

Wang, J.-Y., and others. "Diffuse Pulmonary Infiltrates After Bone Marrow Transplantation: The Role of Open Lung Biopsy." *Annals of Thoracic Surgery*, 2004, *78*, 267–272.

West, M., and others. "*Clostridium difficile* Colitis After Kidney and Kidney-Pancreas Transplantation." *Clinical Transplantation*, 1999, *13*, 318–323.

CHAPTER 30

THE EMERGING THREAT OF BIOWEAPONS

LEARNING OBJECTIVES

- Describe the bacterial and viral agents believed to be of potential use to bioterrorist groups and the diseases caused by each

- Describe bacterially derived toxins of potential use to bioterrorists

- Describe some of the actions that might be taken to respond to, detect, and prevent mass casualties in the event of the release of a bioweapon

Major Concepts

History

Infectious disease agents have been harnessed for centuries as weapons to neutralize armies, decrease the size of enemy populations, and create a state of terror that destabilizes societies. Such biological weapons research continued in many "civilized" nations until very recently, and clandestine work may be ongoing despite being banned by international treaty. Even though many known stocks of bioweapons have "disappeared," government groups around the world continue to prepare for attacks that hopefully will never occur.

Potential Bioweapon Agents and Diseases

Several species of bacteria and viruses and some bacterial toxins are perceived to be of potential use by bioterrorist groups. The agents believed to pose the greatest threat to humans are *Bacillus anthracis* (anthrax), *Yersinia pestis* (plague), *Francisella tularensis* (tularemia), *Variola major* (smallpox), hemorrhagic fever viruses, and *Clostridium botulinum* toxin (botulism). Many of these agents have been released intentionally. Other bacteria and viruses have also been the subject of research as agents of biological warfare. In addition to microbes that target humans, agents that kill animals have been studied for use in crippling a region's food supply or economy.

Preparation for an Attack

Governmental and public health organizations have ongoing plans for the early detection of and response to biological attacks. Researchers continue to prepare stocks of protective vaccines and antibiotics. Terrorist groups, however, have engineered bacteria and viruses in ways that increase their pathogenicity and allow them to circumvent the actions of current antibiotics and vaccines. The need to maintain active surveillance programs and to develop novel means of protection against genetically altered organisms consumes resources that might otherwise be used for more productive and beneficial projects.

Introduction

A number of biological agents have been judged to pose serious risks to human populations if used in a biological attack. Such agents possess several of the following characteristics:

- High morbidity and mortality rates

- Potential for person-to-person transmission

- Low infective dose

- High infectivity following aerosol dissemination by long-range missiles

- Ability to cause large outbreaks

- Lack of an effective vaccine (either not yet developed or available in limited quantities)

- Potential to cause public and health care worker anxiety and disrupt social stability

- Terrorist group access to the microbe or toxin

- Feasibility of large-scale production

- Stability in storage and in the environment

- Prior research and development as a weapons agent

Particular microbes or toxins are further favored if their release is difficult to detect (silent, invisible, odorless, tasteless), if they induce diseases that are difficult to diagnose, and if they have been engineered to contain pathogenic elements of several agents or to be resistant to currently used vaccines and antibiotics. Agents whose production requires the use of skilled workers or specialized equipment and those with a high risk of infecting production workers or the population of the surrounding region are less useful.

The agents have been divided into three categories, A, B, and C, with category A agents deemed to pose the greatest threat. Category A agents are those that are easily disseminated or transmitted from person to person, have a high mortality rate with the potential for major public health impact, would cause public panic and social disruption, and require special actions for public health preparedness. Category B agents are those that are moderately easy to disseminate, are associated

TABLE 30.1   Categories of potential biological weapons agents

Biological Agent	Disease	Infective Dose
Category A		
Bacillus anthracis	Anthrax	8,000–50,000 organisms
Yersinia pestis	Plague	100–500
Francisella tularensis	Tularemia	10–50
Variola major	Smallpox	10–100
Hemorrhagic fever viruses	Hemorrhagic fever	1–10
Clostridium botulinum toxin	Botulism	0.001 µg/kg body weight (via intravenous, subcutaneous, or intraperitoneal inoculation); 0.003 µg/kg body weight (via inhalation)
Category B		
Brucella species	Brucellosis	10–100 bacteria
Burkholderia mallei	Glanders	Low
Coxiella burnetii	Q fever	1–10
Encephalomyelitis viruses	Viral encephalomyelitis	1–100
Ricinus communis toxin	Ricin intoxication	1 molecule per cell
Category C		
Multidrug-resistant *Mycobacterium tuberculosi*	Tuberculosis	N.D.
Other encephalomyelitis viruses	Viral encephalomyelitis	N.D.

Note: N.D. = not yet determined.

with a moderate morbidity and a low mortality rate, and require specific enhancement of diagnostic capacity and enhanced disease surveillance. Category C includes emerging infectious agents with potential to be engineered for mass dissemination in the future due to their availability, ease of production and dissemination, potential for high morbidity and mortality, and major impact on health.

History

The Black Death (bubonic plague), which killed approximately one-third of the world's population, is believed to have originated in China in the 1330s and to have entered Europe in 1346 during a battle for the seaport city of Caffa on the Crimean Sea (currently part of Ukraine). Tartar forces catapulted plague victims into the city to spread the disease. Genoese merchants escaped Caffa in ships that later docked in Genoa, Italy, and spread the disease to Mediterranean ports through infected rats that escaped the ships. Plague then disseminated rapidly throughout Europe, claiming large numbers of victims and eventually destroying the feudal system in western Europe due to the fact that so many of the peasants who had formerly worked the land had died. Outbreaks continued to sweep the region from the fifteenth to eighteenth centuries.

Bubonic plague continued to be exploited as a bioweapon for centuries. During the battle of Carolstein in 1422 and the battle of Reval in 1710, Lithuanian and Russian forces also catapulted bodies of plague victims into the ranks of enemy troops. *Variola major* was much later rumored to have been used in the eighteenth century by the British, who gave clothing contaminated by smallpox scabs to Native Americans in order to initiate epidemics that would weaken the tribes to allow expansion of British colonies. During World War II, the Japanese attempted to develop smallpox for use in Mongolia and China.

A number of nations have performed basic research on and production of bioweapons in the recent past. These activities may be ongoing in some regions of the world. The U.S. offensive biological weapons program was officially ended in 1969–1970 by executive order of President Richard Nixon. The British program had ended much earlier, during the 1950s. The 1973 worldwide Biological and Toxin Weapons Convention banned development, production, stockpiling, and acquisition of biological weapons and was supposedly implemented in 1975. No effective international mechanism was set in place, however, for challenging development of these weapons. The number of countries engaged in such endeavors reportedly doubled over the course of the following decade.

In the Soviet Union, the bioweapons research and development program actually grew in size and scope from 1972 to 1987 under the auspices of several secret groups, including the Fifteenth Main Directorate of the Ministry of Defense and the "civilian" pharmaceutical complex Bioprepara. Microbial agents were genetically engineered for greater pathogenicity, to escape protective effects of the vaccines in use at the time, or to be resistant to antibiotics. Large stockpiles of plague and smallpox were prepared for delivery to large population centers using intercontinental ballistic missiles. Iraq also continued to run an active bioweapons production program.

Bioterrorism Agents and Diseases

Bacterial Diseases

Pneumonic Plague and *Yersinia pestis* *Yersinia pestis* is a nonmotile gram-negative coccobacillus that serves as the causative agents of the three forms of plague in humans: bubonic, septicemic, and pneumonic. *Y. pestis* typically infects

FIGURE 30.1   Skin lesions due to bubonic plague

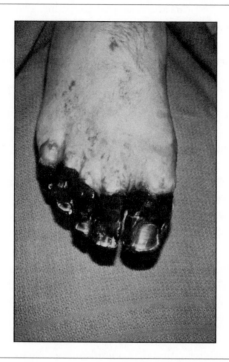

Source: CDC.

humans through the bite of an infected rat flea. Plague is an enzootic infection of rats, ground squirrels, prairie dogs, and other rodents in most continents, including North America, where it is found in the southwestern United States. The reservoir hosts often experience a large population die-off prior to an outbreak in humans. Most of the persons infected develop **bubonic plague**, with a sudden onset of fever, chills, and weakness and production of **buboes**— swollen, reddened, extremely tender lymph nodes in the groin, axillae, or neck.

Some persons develop primary **septicemic plague** in which septicemia (blood infection) occurs directly after the flea bite in the absence of buboes. Secondary septicemia may also appear following bubonic plague. Septicemic plague is characterized by disseminated intravascular coagulation, necrosis of small vessels, purpuric skin lesions, and gangrene in the digits or nose during advanced disease. Neither bubonic nor septicemic plague is transmitted via direct person-to-person contact.

Symptoms of **pneumonic plague** include severe bronchopneumonia, chest pain, dyspnea, cough, and bloody sputum. It may develop as a secondary illness in a small number of patients with bubonic plague as bacilli spread from the blood into the lungs or as a primary infection. During primary pneumonic

FIGURE 30.2   Rat flea, the vector of *Yersinia pestis,*
causative agent of bubonic plague

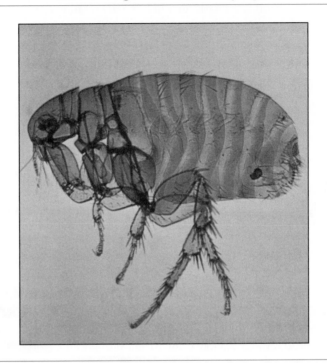

Source: CDC.

plague, pneumonic symptoms are accompanied by gastrointestinal symptoms such as nausea, vomiting, abdominal pain, and diarrhea. Pneumonic plague may be spread between people via inhalation of respiratory droplets, leading to primary pneumonic plague. Of the 390 cases of plague reported in the United States from 1947 to 1996, 84% were bubonic, 13% were septicemic, and 2% were pneumonic, with fatality rates of 14%, 22%, and 57%, respectively.

Pneumonic plague has received much attention for use in biological warfare. During World War II on at least three occasions, Unit 731 of the Japanese army is believed to have delivered a mixture of rice, wheat, and plague-infected fleas (*Pulex irritans*) to populated areas of China, leading to outbreaks of plague. In a twist of fate, cases of plague occurred in Japanese soldiers following a biological attack on Changde in 1941, resulting in 1,700 Japanese deaths.

The United States and the Soviet Union spent years perfecting this weapon by aerosolizing plague directly. A 1970 WHO study concluded that in a worst-case scenario, 50 kilograms of *Y. pestis* released as an aerosol over a city of 5 million could produce up to 150,000 cases of pneumonic plague and 36,000 deaths. Such an attack would differ from naturally occurring plague in that inhalation of aerosolized *Y. pestis* would cause rapidly progressive primary pneumonic plague one to six days from the time of exposure. A high death rate from septic shock would be postulated to occur without early treatment using streptomycin, gentamycin, or members of the tetracycline or fluoroquinolone classes of antibiotics. These drugs could also be used for prophylactic purposes.

Pulmonary Anthrax and *Bacillus anthracis* *B. anthracis* is a gram-positive spore-forming bacillus that infects cattle, sheep, and horses in addition to humans. The bacteria are currently found among both wild and domestic animals in Asia, Africa, South and Central America, eastern and southern Europe, the Caribbean, and the Middle East. The hardy spores resist dehydration and other adverse environmental conditions to persist in the soil of pastures for years (up to 200 years, according to some reports). *B. anthracis* produces the highly pathogenic anthrax toxin, encoded by a plasmid. It is composed of three synergistically acting proteins: edema factor, lethal factor, and protective antigen. *B. anthracis* has been postulated to be a genetic variant of the nonpathogenic *B. cereus* and *B. thuringiensis*, which acquired plasmids that produce the toxin and a protective capsule.

Disease manifestations take three forms: cutaneous, gastrointestinal, and inhalational. **Cutaneous anthrax** is the most common. An ulcerative skin lesion is produced following exposure of the skin to spores. The lesion later transforms into a black scab containing a necrotic core surrounded by blood-stained fluid and edema prior to self-resolution. **Gastrointestinal anthrax** is very rare and is acquired by ingesting undercooked meat contaminated by spores. **Inhalational (pulmonary) anthrax** is the form that bioterrorists seek to induce. This form is acquired by inhaling 8,000 to 50,000 aerosolized spores. After the bacteria are ingested by macrophages in the lungs, they are transported to regional lymph nodes, where they germinate, divide, and begin to produce toxin. Several days of malaise, mild fever, and cough are followed by progressive respiratory distress, cyanosis with massive edema in the neck and chest, and elevated pulse, respiration, and body temperature. Large numbers of bacteria are present in the lungs, blood, and other tissues. Local necrosis and edema may compress respiratory passages, and the toxin may depress the respiratory centers of the brain. This form of disease is rapidly fatal if untreated due to thrombosis of the pulmonary capillaries. The mortality rate is 95% when therapy is initiated longer than 48 hours after the beginning of symptomatic disease. Fortunately, several antibiotics are very effective against all forms of anthrax infection if administered early.

The use of anthrax as a bioweapon began early in the twentieth century as Germany infected livestock during World War I. In 1941, Britain tested the effect of anthrax on sheep on the island of Gruinard in Scotland. Decontamination

FIGURE 30.3   Hemorrhage of the brain due to anthrax

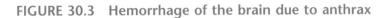

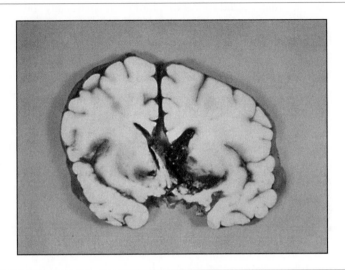

Source: CDC.

proved very difficult, and the island was not considered safe until 1990. During World War II, Unit 731 of the Japanese army stockpiled 400 kilograms of anthrax spores for use in bombs. The United States and the Soviet Union as well as other nations developed anthrax as a bioweapon in the 1950s and 1960s. An accidental release of spores occurred from a Soviet weapons facility in Sverdlovsk in April 1979. During this outbreak of inhalational anthrax, 68 of 79 victims died and animal infections were reported more than 50 kilometers from the facility. The Soviet government at the time claimed that the fatalities resulted from gastrointestinal anthrax contracted by ingestion of infected meat. In 1992, President Yeltsin revealed the involvement of a military facility in this outbreak.

Several attacks with anthrax spores have occurred since 1990. In 1993, the Japanese Aum Shinrikyo terrorist cult released aerosolized spores from the top of a building in Kameido, a city near Tokyo. Fortunately, they used a nonpathogenic strain, Sterne 34F2, which is usually used for vaccination. An unknown group was responsible for a moderately successful series of anthrax attacks in the United States in September and October 2001, not long after the destruction of the World Trade Center in New York City. Five letters were sent containing anthrax spores. The first two were sent to NBC Television in New York and the *New York Post*. These contained only 10% spores but used the Ames strain, one of the most virulent strains of naturally occurring *B. anthracis*. Several people were sickened as a result of exposure. The other three letters were sent to a Florida tabloid newspaper, *The Sun*, and to the offices of U.S. Senators Patrick Leahy and Tom Daschle. These letters were far more sophisticated and contained pure 10-micrometer-sized spores that had been chemically stabilized. Five people died during this attack, and two dozen more were infected, several of these people being exposed at a post office after handling the sealed letters.

One of the difficulties in the weaponization of anthrax is production of the most effective spores. Spores must be of a proper size to stay airborne until inhaled and must be able to pass into the lower reaches of the respiratory tree to inflict the most harm to the greatest number of individuals. Ten micrometers is believed to be the optimal size for deep lung penetration. The anthrax letter attack in the United States may have produced this size of particles by spray-drying. Weaponized *B. anthracis* has often been genetically modified so as to be resistant to many antibiotics.

Tularemia (Rabbit Fever) and *Francisella tularensis* *F. tularensis* is a small, nonmotile, aerobic, gram-negative coccobacillus with a thin lipopolysaccharide-containing envelope. These bacilli are facultative intracellular bacteria that multiply within macrophages, targeting the lymph nodes, lungs, spleen, liver, and kidneys. Hardy and non-spore-forming, these bacteria are able to survive for weeks at low temperatures in water, moist soil, hay, straw, and decaying animal carcasses.

Tularemia is common in humans in parts of Europe, including Sweden, Finland, Spain, and Kosovo. It is also present in North America (1,368 cases were reported in the United States during the 1990s). Two major subspecies (biovars) exist, differing in virulence and epidemiological features. Biovar tularensis (type A) is the most common type in North America and is highly virulent in humans and animals. Biovar palaearctica (holarctic; type B) is most common in Europe and Asia and is relatively avirulent. Bacteria may enter humans through the skin, mucous membranes, gastrointestinal tract, and lungs; following bites by infective arthropods (ticks, deerflies, or mosquitoes); handling infected animal tissues; contact with or ingestion of contaminated water, food, or soil; or inhalation of infective aerosols generated by a lawn mower or brush cutter. Wild animals, including rabbits, squirrels, muskrats, beaver, and deer, may be infected, as may, less commonly, domestic animals such as sheep, cats, and dogs.

Infection with *F. tularensis* may take several forms. **Respiratory tularemia (tularemia pneumonia)** is the form that would follow a biological attack; it results from inhalation of bacteria-laden aerosols. Onset of disease is abrupt and is characterized by fever, headache, chills and rigor, generalized body ache, and sore throat followed by profound sweating, progressive weakness, anorexia, and weight loss, all of which may become incapacitating within a day or two. Symptoms of pulmonary infection include dry cough and substernal pain or tightness in the presence or absence of objective signs of bronchopneumonia, including purulent sputum, difficulty breathing, and rapid breathing rate. Hemorrhagic airway inflammation may occur as alveoli fill with exudates of mononuclear cells, leading to inflammation of the pleural membranes and hilar lymphadenopathy that rapidly progresses to severe pneumonia, respiratory failure, and death. Untreated, symptoms may remain for weeks to months and may be spread via the circulatory system, resulting in secondary pneumonia, sepsis, and occasionally meningitis. **Tularemia sepsis** is severe and may be fatal. It is characterized by fever, abdominal pain, diarrhea, and vomiting early after infection. If not treated promptly, affected persons may present with confusion and coma followed by septic shock, disseminated intravascular coagulation and bleeding, acute respiratory distress syndrome, pericarditis, mild hepatitis, and multiorgan failure.

Other manifestations of *F. tularensis* infection include **ulceroglandular tularaemia** (75% to 85% of naturally occurring cases), acquired from an infected carcass or an arthropod bite. Symptoms are relatively mild and include fever, painful ulcerative skin lesions, and enlarged lymph nodes.

Glandular tularemia is similar but does not produce skin ulcers. The **oculoglandular tularemia** form of disease follows airborne exposure or exposure while cleaning contaminated animal carcasses. This form leads to ulceration of the cornea. **Oropharyngeal tularemia** is acquired by consumption of contaminated water or food, by hand-mouth contact, or by inhalation of infectious droplets. It is characterized by exudative pharyngitis or tonsillitis in the presence or absence of mucosal ulcers. **Typhoidal tularemia** is an acute flulike

FIGURE 30.4   Skin lesion due to *Francisella tularensis* infection

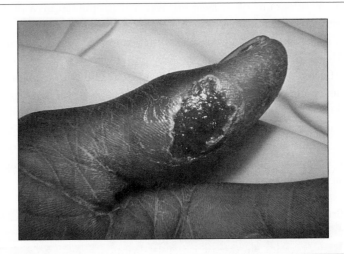

Source: CDC.

illness accompanied by diarrhea, vomiting, headache, chills, muscle and joint pain, prostration, and weight loss. This form of the disease follows ingestion or inhalation of bacteria. Without proper treatment, the mortality rate for type A tularemia is 5% to 15% overall, 4% for ulceroglandular tularemia, and 30% to 50% for typhoidal, septicemic, and respiratory forms. Use of antibiotics lowers the mortality rate to 1%. Type B tularemia is rarely fatal.

F. tularensis was first discovered to be a disease agent during a plaguelike outbreak of rodents in 1911. Its potential to cause human epidemics was seen during the 1930s and 1940s when large waterborne outbreaks occurred in Europe and the Soviet Union. It was one of the agents studied at the Japanese germ warfare research unit in Manchuria from 1932 to 1945 and was developed as a bioweapon by the Soviet Union and the United States. The former head of the Soviet bioweapons development effort, Kanadjan Alibekov, suggested that tularemia outbreaks affecting tens of thousands of Soviet and German soldiers during World War II may have been be due to intentional release. Military strains of *F. tularensis* were engineered for resistance to antibiotics and vaccines.

F. tularensis is a dangerous potential biological weapon due to its extreme infectivity (requiring fewer than ten inhaled bacteria to initiate pulmonary infection), ease of dissemination, and capacity to cause illness and death. Disease is, however, expected to progress more slowly and have a lower fatality rate than inhalational plague or anthrax. The lack of a stable spore phase complicates the bioterrorism application. If a weapon of airborne bacteria were released in a dense population center, however, it would be predicted to result in a large outbreak of pulmonary tularemia within three to five days. An aerosol dispersal of 50 kilograms of *F. tularensis* over a metropolitan area of 5 million inhabitants is projected to result in 250,000 incapacitated persons and 19,000 deaths. Illness may persist for weeks, with relapses potentially occurring for months. Vaccinated individuals may be only partially protected against such an exposure. Affected individuals should be promptly treated with streptomycin, gentamycin, doxycycline, or ciprofloxacin, which may also be useful as prophylactic agents. The Soviet Union immunized tens of millions of persons living in tularemia-endemic areas with a live attenuated vaccine. The United States also uses such a vaccine to protect laboratory workers routinely exposed to this bacterium. It is not known, however, if these vaccines provide protection against weaponized strains of *F. tularemia*.

Brucellosis and *Brucella* Species Brucellosis (also known as Mediterranean fever, Gibraltar fever, Malta fever, Cyprus fever, undulant fever, and typhomalarial fever) is an ancient disease that remains the most commonly occurring zoonotic infection in the world. It is endemic to the Middle East, Central Asia, India, the

Mediterranean regions of Europe and Africa, Central and South America, and Mexico. It is caused by infection with *Brucella* species, several small, highly contagious, gram-negative aerobic coccobacilli. Brucellosis is primarily a zoonotic infection that causes abortions in sheep and goats (*B. melitensis*), cows and bison (*B. abortus*), and pigs (*B. suis*). *B. canis* is pathogenic to dogs. Each of these bacterial species may induce human disease as well, although *B. melitensis* is the most pathogenic species and the one that most commonly infects humans.

Although *Brucella* species do not produce spores and are heat-sensitive, they are able to survive in the environment for several years under the correct conditions and continue to infect both humans and animals of the region during that period. Natural infection occurs primarily through consumption of unpasteurized milk and soft cheese or through areas of abraded skin (especially in slaughterhouse workers). Bacteria may also be acquired via mucous membranes, such as the conjunctiva lining the eyelids, the throat, and the respiratory tract—the route favored by bioterrorists. After entering a person, the bacteria may grow either outside of or within cells, such as macrophages and neutrophils, occupying special acidic compartments where they work to ensure the host cell's continued survival. An unusual lipopolysaccharide in the cell wall inhibits killing of the bacteria by these phagocytic cells. *Brucella* also dampens the production of the cytokine TNF-α by other immune cells.

Symptoms of brucellosis vary, the most common presentation being a flulike illness with protracted fever, muscle and joint pain, fatigue, malodorous perspiration, swollen lymph nodes, and enlarged liver and spleen. Complications are common, including arthritis and inflammation of the vertebrae. Other disease manifestations include formation of abscesses in a variety of sites, inflammation of the male reproduction tract, respiratory dysfunction, mild hepatitis, rash, and buildup of fluid in the abdominal cavity. The most dangerous complications of brucellosis are neurobrucellosis and endocarditis, the major cause of mortality. Chronic infection persists for more than six months and may lead to behavioral changes and other neurological syndromes, weight loss, and fatigue. Chronic brucellosis is similar to the chronic fatigue syndrome reported among U.S. troops serving in the first Gulf War. *Brucella* was endemic to the battlefield regions, and suspicions have been raised as to whether the American forces were deliberately targeted.

Brucella species have been the subject of biological weapons research for many years due to the ease of airborne transmission, the production of chronic debilitating disease that requires treatment using a six-week course of a combination of antibiotics, its abundance throughout the world, and its long incubation period and vague clinical symptoms that impede rapid detection and diagnosis. Its dissemination among enemy forces would incapacitate many troops for extended periods of time and also require the attention of many noncombat personnel. Agricultural communities could be crippled. In 1954, *B. suis* was the first biological agent to be weaponized by the United States. The United Kingdom may also have developed this agent for biological attack purposes. No evidence exists that *Brucella* species were ever deployed as weapons. Currently, the minimal mortality rate associated with infection, the availability of effective treatment options, and the emergence of newer and more virulent biological weapon agents have restricted the value of brucellosis for use by bioterrorist groups.

Q fever and *Coxiella burnetii* *C. burnetii* is one of several rickettsiae that have been explored for use as bioweapons. Rickettsiae are gram-negative, obligate intracellular bacteria. They are found worldwide and pass through zoonotic cycles with occasional epidemic outbreaks into the human population. Rickettsiae have several characteristics that appeal to bioterrorism groups, such as environmental stability, low infectious dose, high morbidity, and a substantial mortality rate. This group of bacteria has several properties that complicate their use as well. They must be propagated in eukaryotic cells and then isolated from the cell components, procedures that require skilled personnel and specialized laboratory equipment. *C. burnetii* and *Rickettsia prowazekii* are highly contagious as well and may easily cause infections of laboratory workers. *C. burnetii* and other rickettsiae are also not directly transmitted between humans, and their use as weapons is dependent on either the presence of the appropriate arthropod vectors or large amounts of aerosolized bacteria. The process of aerosolization requires trained personnel and a well-equipped weaponization facility.

Almost half of all infections with *C. burnetii* are asymptomatic. The acute form of **Q (query) fever** is characterized by abrupt onset of fever, severe sweats, chills, headache, weakness, and fatigue. Approximately 1% of individuals with acute disease progress to chronic illness. The major symptom of chronic disease is endocarditis, often requiring valve replacement operations. Mice infected by inhalation of aerosols of bacteria develop lung, liver, and spleen lesions. Untreated, chronic Q fever is typically fatal. A substantial numbers of persons having acute disease (10% to 30%) later develop a form of chronic fatigue syndrome that persists for over a year after infection. Immunosuppressed persons, especially pregnant women, are more prone to develop serious disease manifestations. Approximately one-third of these women experience spontaneous abortions or neonatal death, and another third give birth prematurely.

C. burnetii produces a sporelike form that is highly stable to heat and drying and is very resistant to many disinfectants. It accumulates in high concentrations in many organs, particularly the placenta, and only a single organism may be needed to infect a human. *C. burnetii* is found in sheep, cattle, goats, cats, dogs, birds, and ticks throughout the world. Populations at risk include farmers, sheep and cattle workers, and veterinarians, as well as workers in rendering and meat processing plants. People are usually infected by inhaling dust containing bacteria from animal placentas or associated fluids after birthing or from animal excreta. Transmission may also occur by direct contact with animals, their wool or bedding materials, or the clothing of infected persons.

If used during a biological attack, bacteria might be disseminated as an aerosol or in food, water, or the mail. One estimate projects that the release of 50 kilograms of aerosolized bacteria upwind of a city of 500,000 would incapacitate 125,000 people, kill 150, and lead to 9,000 cases of chronic Q fever. Other estimates place the numbers of individuals who experience severe disease or death much higher. Effective antibiotics are available to counter the effects of a deliberate release.

Epidemic Typhus and *Rickettsia prowazekii* Epidemic (louseborne) typhus is distributed around the world and is due to infection with *Rickettsia prowazekii*. These rickettsiae are transmitted via the bite of human body lice (*Pediculus humanus corporis*), whose temperature preference leads them to rest in areas of clothing that are not in direct contact with the skin. A rise in body temperature, as occurs during a fever, causes the louse to seek a new host, thus disseminating the bacteria throughout the human population.

Epidemic typhus occurring during and in the aftermath of World War I caused over 30 million infections and approximately 3 million deaths. More recently, a large epidemic of this disease struck the refugee population of Burundi. Human populations in which overcrowding, poverty, and unsanitary conditions encourage louse infestation are at risk for acquiring this disease. Massive population movements, as occur during times of war, civic unrest, and famine, can fuel the spread of disease. Epidemic typhus is currently endemic in the highlands and colder regions of Africa, Asia, South and Central America, and eastern Europe. Zoonotic transmission in wild animal populations occurs in the eastern United States. Symptoms include rash, high fever, stiffness, very painful muscles and joints, and cerebral dysfunction progressing to delirium and stupor. Blood clots may clog small blood vessels in the extremities, leading to gangrene. Epidemic typhus usually has a mortality rate of 20%, but this may reach 40% in extreme cases.

The median infectious dose of *R. prowazekii* is fewer than ten bacteria. Preparative work with this agent should be done in a BSL-3 laboratory due to the hazardous nature of propagating and isolating the bacteria. The WHO estimates that the release of 50 kilograms of aerosolized bacteria would result in 85,000 persons incapacitated and another 19,000 dead. Fortunately, this infection responds well to antibiotic therapy.

Endemic Typhus and *Rickettsia typhi* Endemic (murine) typhus is found throughout the world and results from infection with *Rickettsia typhi* or *R. felis*. The reservoir hosts of *R. typhi* are rats and mice, while those of *R. felis* are cats, opossums, and dogs. These rickettsiae are transmitted to humans via rat or cat flea bites. The course of disease is similar to that of epidemic typhus but milder. The overall mortality rate is 1%, which increases with age.

Rocky Mountain Spotted Fever and *Rickettsia rickettsii* Rickettsia rickettsii is the causative agent of **Rocky Mountain spotted fever** (RMSF; also known as New World spotted fever and São Paulo fever). Small mammals, rabbits, dogs, and birds serve as the reservoir hosts for the bacteria, and humans become infected by the bite of infected ticks. This disease is confined to North and South America. Despite its name, the highest incidence of infection in the United States occurs in North Carolina and Oklahoma. RMSF is characterized by a rash that begins in the extremities, extends to the soles and palms, and then progresses to much of the remaining skin area.

This is followed by abrupt onset of moderate to high fever, deep muscle pain, malaise, chills, and conjunctival infection. In the 1920s, before the beginning of the antibiotic era, the mortality rate for RMSF could reach 66%. More recently, 3% to 5% of infected persons have died in the United States, especially those who delayed treatment or were over the age of 40 years.

FIGURE 30.5   Rash typical of Rocky Mountain spotted fever

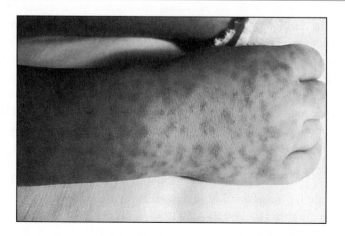

Source: CDC.

FIGURE 30.6 *Burkholderia*, obligate aerobic bacteria

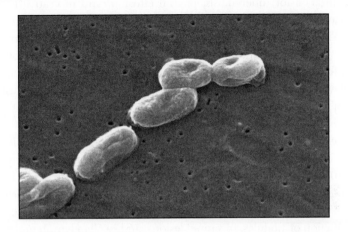

Source: CDC.

Glanders and Melioidosis, *Burkholderia mallei* and *B. pseudomallei* Glanders and melioidosis are similar diseases that result from infection with *Burkholderia mallei* and *B. pseudomallei*, respectively. These bacteria primarily attack animals and may thus be used to either cripple a country's agriculture or target humans. *Burkholderia* species are small, gram-negative, obligate aerobic bacteria (require oxygen for survival) with a bipolar, safety-pin appearance. *B. pseudomallei* have flagella and are motile; *B. mallei* have no flagella and are not motile. Cultures of these bacteria produce a grapelike odor.

Glanders is a disease of horses, donkeys, and mules and can also affect goats, dogs, and cats. Though rare, glanders is endemic in Africa, Asia, the Middle East, and Central and South America. *B. mallei* bacteria have a low rate of transmission to humans but may infect persons in prolonged contact with animals. No epidemics of human glanders have occurred. Melioidosis is endemic in Southeast Asia and northeast Australia, and cases have also occurred in Africa, the South Pacific, India, the Middle East, and Central and South America, where *B. pseudomallei* is common in the soil and water. Humans may become infected through direct contact of damaged skin with contaminated soil or water, through the mucous membranes of the nasal cavity and eyes, or via ingestion of contaminated water or dust.

Glanders and melioidosis may be manifest in several clinical forms: pulmonary, septicemic, localized, and chronic infection. Pulmonary infection follows inhalation or is spread via the blood and may be the primary disease manifestation occurring after a bioterrorist attack. The onset of symptoms is abrupt and includes chest pain, fever, pneumonia, pulmonary abscesses that may be mistaken for tuberculosis, pleural effusion, and ulcerative lesions of the nasal cavity. Inhalational melioidosis may be accompanied by skin abscesses as well. Without specific treatment, disease may progress to bacteremia or septicemia.

The septicemic form of *Burkholderia* infection may follow one to five days after infection by inhalation, skin exposure or ingestion. The initial symptoms of fever, muscle ache, headache, and diarrhea are followed by flushing and cyanosis of the skin, swollen regional lymph nodes, and cellulitis. Infected persons may be light-sensitive and release tears, have slightly enlarged liver or spleen, rapid heart rate, jaundice, and generalized papular or pustular lesions. Multiorgan failure leads to death within seven to ten days, with a mortality rate approaching 50% even after antibiotic therapy (over 90% if untreated). Immunosuppressed patients are particularly vulnerable to this form of melioidosis.

Localized infection follows bacterial penetration of the skin followed by production of nodules, ulcerated lesions, and swollen lymph nodes. The nodules are firm, either gray or white, and are surrounded by a reddened hemorrhagic zone. Infection of mucous membranes leads to increased mucus production. Abscesses may develop in the salivary glands in children with melioidosis. Osteomyelitis, arthritis, and abscesses of the brain or internal organs may also be seen.

Chronic infection results in multiple abscesses of the skin, in the muscles of the arms and legs, or in the spleen and liver. Melioidosis may also be reactivated years after the primary infection.

B. mallei have been used at least twice in biological attacks against animals. During World War I, it infected Russian horses and mules on the Eastern Front, slowing troop movements. During World War II, the Japanese infected animals and people in China. *B. pseudomallei* has not been used as a bioweapon, although such studies have been conducted.

Humans have been infected by aerosolized bacteria in laboratories, with attack rates as high as 46%. A very low number of organisms are required to cause human infection by this route. Human-to-human transmission of glanders is not common, decreasing its utility as a bioweapon.

Both glanders and melioidosis respond to antibiotics. Postexposure prophylaxis with trimethoprim-sulfamethoxazole is recommended following a biological attack. No protective vaccine is currently available for human use.

Viral Diseases

Smallpox and Variola major Smallpox is an ancient disease that was once one of the most dreaded plagues of humankind, causing many deaths and leaving many survivors horribly scarred for life. Many of these scars were on the head and face. Smallpox was usually caused by the highly lethal *Variola major* virus. Its clinical presentation is similar to monkeypox (described in Chapter Twenty-Three), and the vaccinia vaccine used to immunize people against smallpox during the smallpox eradication campaign is cross-protective against monkeypox. During the campaign, which eventually completely eliminated variola from nature and stopped all cases of naturally transmitted smallpox in 1977, massive numbers of people were immunized. All remaining variola virus was kept in storage in two specialized BSL-4 facilities, one in the United States and the other in the Soviet Union. Following the elimination of the disease in nature, immunization with the vaccinia vaccine was stopped due to its high potential to cause pathological reactions, especially in the very young and other immunosuppressed populations. Over the subsequent decades, protective immunity in previously vaccinated individuals declined, leaving them again susceptible to developing disease should variola ever again be released from the laboratories harboring the virus. These persons are, however, likely to retain at least some degree of protection in comparison to younger persons who never received the vaccinia vaccine.

Smallpox is most contagious during its incubation period before the appearance of the characteristic rash, which is not present for at least three days after the beginning of symptoms. The initial signs include headache and myalgia as well as a diffuse maculopapular rash, followed later by the vesicular eruptions on the head and extremities and crusting of the lesions. Smallpox is highly contagious via the airborne route, and containment requires strict isolation. People are no longer contagious after the crusting occurs.

If smallpox were to be identified in a patient, it must be assumed to have originated from a bioterrorism attack, since variola major no longer exists in nature.

Viral Hemorrhagic Fevers **Viral hemorrhagic fevers** (HFs) are illnesses associated with fever and hemorrhagic manifestations caused by viruses belonging to four families: Filoviridae, Arenaviridae, Bunyaviridae, and Flaviviridae. These are all small RNA viruses surrounded by lipid envelopes.

Most HF viruses are transmitted to humans by the bite of an arthropod or contact with excreta or carcasses of a reservoir host. Filoviruses and arenaviruses may be spread between humans, leading to local outbreaks or nosocomial infections. Bunyaviruses and flaviviruses are not transmitted by person-to-person contact.

The viral HFs have an incubation period of 2 to 21 days, followed by nonspecific prodromal symptoms that include high fever, headache, malaise, joint and muscle ache, nausea, abdominal pain, and diarrhea. Early signs of disease

Table 30.2   Agents of viral hemorrhagic fever

Viral Family	Virus	Virus Morphology	Viral Genome
Filoviridae	Ebola virus, Marburg virus	Filamentous	Single-stranded RNA (negative sense)
Arenaviridae	Lassa virus, American hemorrhagic fever viruses	Spherical	Single-stranded RNA (ambisense)
Bunyaviridae	Rift Valley fever virus, Crimean-Congo hemorrhagic fever virus	Spherical	Single-stranded RNA (negative sense)
Flaviviridae	Yellow fever virus, Omsk hemorrhagic fever virus, Kyasanur Forest disease virus	Isometric	Single-stranded RNA (positive sense)

Table 30.3   Distribution of the viruses that cause hemorrhagic fever (HF)

Virus	Disease	Natural Vector	Distribution
Ebola virus	Ebola HF	Unknown (bats?)	Africa
Marburg virus	Marburg HF	Unknown (bats?)	Africa
Lassa virus	Lassa HF	Rodents	West Africa
Junin virus	Argentine HF	Rodents	South America
Guanarito virus	Venezuelan HF	Rodents	South America
Machupo virus	Bolivian HF	Rodents	South America
Sabia virus	Brazilian HF	Rodents	South America
Whitewater Arroyo	Whitewater Arroyo HF	Rodents	North America
Rift Valley fever virus	Rift Valley fever	Mosquito	Africa, Saudi Arabia, Yemen
Crimean-Congo HF virus	Crimean-Congo HF	Tick	Southeastern Europe, southwestern Asia and Russia, tropical Africa
Yellow fever virus	Yellow fever	Mosquito	Africa, tropical Americas
Omsk HF virus	Omsk HF	Tick	Central Asia
Kyasanur Forest virus	Kyasanur Forest disease	Tick	India

include sore throat, conjunctivitis, fever, low blood pressure, slow heart rate, and skin flushing or rash. As the disease progresses, hemorrhagic manifestations occur, including petechiae, mucous membrane and conjunctival hemorrhages, and bloody vomit, followed by disseminated intravascular coagulation and shock.

Blood irregularities include elevated levels of liver enzymes and low numbers of platelets, leukocytes, and erythrocytes, although hemoconcentration may also be found. Coagulation abnormalities include prolonged bleeding time, increased degradation of fibrin products, and decreased levels of fibrinogen. Platelet function is adversely affected during Ebola HF, Lassa fever, and Argentine HF. The loss of coagulation factors may result from liver dysfunction during Rift Valley fever and yellow fever. Ebola and Marburg viruses also damage endothelial cells lining the blood vessels directly or indirectly via pathogenic immune or inflammatory responses. Both protein and blood may be present in the urine. Central nervous system involvement may involve delirium, convulsions, cerebellar dysfunction, and coma. Recovery may be prolonged and accompanied by weakness, fatigue, anorexia, wasting, hair loss, and joint pain. Other conditions resulting from infection include hearing or vision loss, decreased coordination, and inflammation of the salivary glands, eyes, pancreas, testes, and pericardium. The fatality rate ranges from 0.5% (Omsk HF) to 90% (Ebola Zaire), and death is often preceded by hemorrhagic symptoms, shock, and multiorgan system failure.

Filoviruses are cytotoxic and induce necrosis of liver, spleen, and kidney cells either directly or by impairing the organs' microcirculation. The filoviruses that infect humans are Ebola virus and Marburg virus (described in Chapter Twelve). Ebola HF has a fatality rate of 50% to 90% (depending on subtype), while that of Marburg is 23% to 70%. The current treatment for each infection is supportive care. Most filovirus infections result from contact with blood, secretions, or tissues of infected patients or nonhuman primates. Nosocomial infections have played a major role in large outbreaks.

Arenaviruses, unlike other HF viruses, generally do not directly kill cells but produce their pathogenic effects by stimulating the production of inflammatory compounds by macrophages. The arenaviruses that cause hemorrhagic disease in humans are Lassa fever virus (described in Chapter Fourteen) and New World arenaviruses (described in Chapter Thirteen). Hemorrhagic manifestations are less common during Lassa fever, which may, however, lead to some degree of permanent deafness. Complications of the American HFs may include tremors and seizures. The fatality rate for Lassa fever is 15% to 20%, while that of the American HFs is 15% to 30%. Treatment for arenavirus disease is supportive and may also include the use of the antiviral compound ribavirin. Most arenavirus infections result from contacting rodent excreta via inhalation of aerosols of dried urine or feces, ingestion of contaminated food, or direct contact with abraded skin or mucous membranes. Person-to-person transmission may result from contact with infectious blood or bodily fluids, leading to nosocomial outbreaks.

Two bunyaviruses that cause hemorrhagic disease in humans are the Rift Valley fever virus and the Crimean-Congo HF virus. Jaundice due to liver dysfunction is common during Rift Valley fever, but fewer than 1% of infected individuals develop hemorrhagic fever or encephalitis, leading to a very low fatality rate for this disease. Inflammation of the retinas of the eyes does, however, occur in 10% of the infected. As is the case for arenavirus infection, treatment for Rift Valley fever is supportive and may include ribavirin. IFN-α protects against liver damage in rhesus macaques. Humans are infected by the bite of an infected mosquito, contact with infected animal tissues, inhalation of aerosolized virus from animal carcasses, or perhaps ingestion of unpasteurized animal milk. During Crimean-Congo HF, severe pain is present in the limbs and loin areas, and substantial anorexia occurs. The range of this disease includes the steppe regions of southeastern Europe, southwestern Asia and Russia, and tropical Africa. Hares, birds, and ticks are commonly infected, as well as some sheep, goats, and cattle. Humans are usually infected via a tick bite, but nosocomial infections are also common.

The yellow fever, Omsk HF, and Kyasanur Forest disease viruses are flaviviruses known to be pathogenic to humans. Yellow fever virus infects and destroys liver cells, leading to jaundice. Renal failure may also occur. Much less is known about the pathogenesis of Omsk HF and Kyasanur Forest disease viruses, although persons infected by the latter were shown to have degeneration of the liver and spleen and hemorrhagic pneumonia. Central nervous system involvement occurs in both Omsk FH and Kyasanur Forest disease. The fatality rate for yellow fever is 20%, for Omsk HF is 0.5% to 10%, and for Kyasanur Forest disease is 3% to 10%. Supportive care is the recommended treatment for all three flavivirus-associated diseases. Yellow fever virus is transmitted by the bite of infected mosquitoes, while Omsk HF and Kyasanur Forest disease viruses are obtained via tick bite. Person-to-person transmission or nosocomial spread of flaviviruses has not been reported.

Many of the agents of viral HF have been weaponized. The former Soviet Union and Russia produced large amounts of weaponized Marburg, Ebola, Lassa, and American HF viruses until 1992. The U.S. offensive biological weapons program explored the use of yellow fever and Rift Valley fever viruses until its termination in 1969. Yellow fever virus may have been weaponized by North Korea as well. The Japanese Aum Shinrikyo cult attempted to obtain Ebola virus for use in its terrorism program. Weapons disseminating HF viruses are believed to be capable of causing illness 2 to 21 days later. Symptoms could include fever, rash, hemorrhagic manifestations, shock, or other pathological conditions, depending on the agent used. Administration of ribavirin during the early stages of the outbreak may be helpful in the treatment of some, but not all, of these diseases. A live, attenuated virus vaccine has been developed with a high degree of protection against the development of Argentine and Bolivian, but not Venezuelan, HF.

Viral Encephalitis Six families contain at least one species that causes **viral encephalitis**—acute, inflammatory disease of the human brain, spinal cord, or meninges. The encephalitis viruses (EVs) are potential agents for use in bioterrorism attacks. The majority of infections are asymptomatic, and mild cases may produce only headache, fever, or aseptic meningitis. More serious infections range in severity, depending on the virus involved, and may lead to high fever, meningitis, confusion, stupor, coma, tremors, convulsions, and spastic paralysis. Mortality rates vary from 0.3% to 60%, with eastern equine, Murray Valley, Japanese encephalitis, Hendra, and Nipah viruses being among the most pathogenic agents.

Toxins as Biological Weapons

Various toxins have been explored for their potential use in biological attacks. Many of these toxins are of bacterial origin. Other potent toxins are derived from nonmicrobial sources. Two such plant toxins are abrin, derived from *Abrus precatorius,* and ricin, derived from *Ricinus communis.* In January 2003, several Arabs with connections to the terrorist group Al-Qaeda were arrested as they

Table 30.4 Agents of viral encephalitis in humans

Family	Encephalitis Virus (Ev) Species	Means of Transmission
Togaviridae	Eastern equine EV	Mosquito
	Western equine EV	Mosquito
	Venezuelan equine EV	Mosquito
Flaviviridae	Saint Louis EV	Mosquito
	Murray Valley EV	Mosquito
	Kunjin EV	Mosquito
	West Nile virus	Mosquito
	Japanese EV	Mosquito
	Rocio virus	Mosquito
	Dengue virus	Mosquito
	Tickborne complex EV	Tick
	Powassan virus	Tick
	Louping ill virus	Tick
Bunyaviridae	La Crosse virus	Mosquito
	Toscana virus	Sand fly
Arenaviridae	Lymphocytic choriomeningitis virus	Rodent
Paramyxoviridae	Hendra virus	Horse
	Nipah virus	Pig
Herpesviridae	Herpesvirus simiae (B virus)	Monkey

attempted to produce the highly lethal ricin in London. Marine toxins may also used as bioweapons, including tetrodotoxin, produced by pufferfish and certain marine bacteria, and saxitoxin, produced by dinoflagellates.

Clostridium botulinum and Botulinum Neurotoxin A

Clostridium botulinum constitutes four genetically diverse groups of gram-positive, spore-forming, obligate anaerobic bacteria that produce **botulinum toxin**. Strains of *C. baratii* and *C. butyricum* may also produce the toxin. These bacteria occur naturally in the soil. Seven non-cross-neutralizing antigenic types of toxin exist (lettered from A to G). Botulism in humans usually results from exposure to toxins A, B, E, or F (in rare cases). These toxins engage cells in a form of a preformed "A-B" complex.

Botulinum toxin A contains a 100-kilodalton heavy chain joined to a 50-kilodalton light chain (A and B chains). The latter is an endopeptidase enzyme that blocks neural vesicles containing the neurotransmitter acetylcholine from fusing with the membrane of the motor neuron. Because acetylcholine transmits the signals needed to stimulate muscle contraction, botulinum toxin inhibits muscle action, leading to flaccid muscle paralysis. Muscles whose actions are tightly controlled, such as those that move the eyes, are affected first, and in severe cases, any striated muscles may be involved, leading to respiratory failure.

Botulism and botulinum toxin are not contagious, nor are they transmitted by person-to-person contact. A microbe intentionally modified to produce the botulinum toxin might, however, be contagious. Three naturally occurring forms of botulism occur—foodborne, wound, and intestinal. Fewer than 200 cases of botulism occur annually in the United States. Inhalational botulism represents a human-created form of the disease resulting from inhaling aerosolized toxin. It is the form favored by bioterrorists and the intended outcome of at least one country's specially designed missiles and artillery shells. All forms of botulism follow absorption of toxin into the circulatory system after entry through a mucosal surface (gut, lung) or a wound. It does not penetrate intact skin. Once the toxin is absorbed, it is carried to cholinergic synapses of the nervous system, particularly the neuromuscular junction, to which it binds irreversibly. Neurological signs found during naturally occurring foodborne botulism may be preceded by gastrointestinal symptoms such as abdominal cramps, nausea, vomiting, and diarrhea.

The classic triad of botulism symptoms is acute symmetric, descending flaccid paralysis with prominent palsies of the bulbar musculature; absence of fever; and clear sensorium. Symptoms are similar regardless of toxin type, but the extent and pace of paralysis may differ between individuals, depending on the levels of absorbed toxin. Some persons are only mildly affected, whereas others may be paralyzed to the point of appearing comatose and requiring months of ventilatory support. Difficulty seeing, speaking, or swallowing may occur, including drooping eyelids, double or blurred vision, enlarged or sluggishly reactive pupils, dry mouth, and loss of the gag reflex, requiring intubation and mechanical ventilation. These signs are followed by loss of head control and muscle tone, generalized weakness, decreased deep tendon reflexes, and constipation. Untreated, death occurs due to airway obstruction resulting from paralysis of pharyngeal and upper airway muscles and inadequate respiratory tidal volume due to paralysis of the diaphragm and accessory respiratory muscles. Recovery results from production of new axonal "twigs" to reinnervate paralyzed muscle fibers.

Botulinum toxin is a bioweapon threat due to its extreme potency and lethality, ease of production and transport, and the need for prolonged periods of intensive care for affected individuals. It is the most poisonous substance known, 100,000 times more toxic than sarin gas. The lethal dose of crystalline toxin A for a 70-kilogram human is estimated to be 0.09 to 0.15 micrograms via the intravenous or intramuscular route, 0.70 to 0.90 micrograms via inhalation, and 70 micrograms orally. One gram of toxin, evenly dispersed and inhaled, could kill over 1 million people. In stark contrast, it is the first biological toxin licensed for treatment of human disease and is beneficial in the treatment of spastic paralysis, cerebral palsy, focal dystonia, essential tremor, headache, and incontinence as well as cosmetic uses (botox).

Terrorists have regrettably already made several attempts to exploit botulinum toxin as a bioweapon. Between 1990 and 1995, aerosols were dispersed at multiple sites in downtown Tokyo and at U.S. military bases in Japan by the Aum Shinrikyo cult using toxin derived from soil. Previous use of botulinum toxin as a weapon occurred in the 1930s as Japanese Unit 731 fed *C. botulinum* to prisoners. During World War II, the United States also developed the toxin, and Germany was reputed to have done so as well. Botulinum toxin was among the agents tested by the Soviet Union at Vozrozhdeniye Island in the Aral Sea. The Soviets attempted to splice the toxin gene from *C. botulinum* into other bacteria to produce a multifaceted bioweapon. After the dissolution of the Soviet Union, some of its bioweapons scientists have found employment in other countries pursuing their own bioweapons program, including Iran, Iraq, North Korea, and Syria. Following the 1991 Persian Gulf War, Iraq admitted to having produced 19,000 liters of concentrated toxin, enough to kill every human on earth three times. Over half of the botulinum toxin, aflatoxin, and anthrax spores were loaded into more than 150 missiles. Not all of it was ever located.

Several difficulties hamper the use of botulinum toxin as a weapon of mass destruction or its use against a military opponent. It rapidly degrades in the environment, becoming nonlethal within minutes of deployment. Its large size prevents the toxin from penetrating the skin. It is also difficult to concentrate. Nevertheless, the release of spores or toxin could disrupt civilian population targets if dispensed as an aerosol or added to foods or beverages, including milk, fruit juices, or canned tomato products. Following such exposure, symptoms typically begin 12 to 72 hours after ingestion. Treatment consists of supportive care such as mechanical ventilation and early passive immunization with horse antitoxin. Timely administration of horse antitoxin minimizes subsequent nerve damage and decreases disease severity but does not reverse existing paralysis.

Decontamination efforts are simplified by the fact that botulinum toxin is easily destroyed by heating. Fine aerosols dissipate into the atmosphere and decay at a rate of 1% to 4% per minute, leading to substantial inactivation after two days. If exposure is anticipated, covering the mouth and nose with clothing provides some protection, and the toxin does not enter through intact skin. Clothing and skin should be washed afterward with soap and water and other objects and surfaces cleansed with 0.1% bleach solution.

Other Bacterial Binary Toxins

Tetanus neurotoxin, produced by *Clostridium tetani*, is another binary toxin, but unlike botulinum toxin, which leads to flaccid paralysis, tetanus toxin provokes spastic paralysis. Both botulinum and tetanus toxin attack the SNARE complex of the synaptic bulb at the ends of neurons. This complex facilitates the fusion of synaptic vesicles with the cell membrane, allowing release of neurotransmitter and neural signal transmission. Botulinum toxin A attacks the synaptosome-associated protein of 25-kilodalton component of SNARE, while tetanus toxin attacks the synaptobrevin 2 component. Other binary bacterial toxins that bind to target cells as preformed A-B complexes include diphtheria toxin (*Corynebacterium diphtheria*), exotoxin A (*Pseudomonas aeruginosa*), pertussis toxin (*Bordetella Pertussis*), heat-labile enterotoxins (*Escherichia coli*), Shiga toxin (*Shigella dysenteriae*), and cholera toxin (*Vibrio cholerae*).

The Threat of Agroterrorism

In addition to direct effects on human health, terrorist groups may target a nation's agriculture and its economic well-being. The contribution of agriculture to the U.S. economy is enormous, at least $1 trillion per year (one-sixth of the gross domestic product) and employs one of every eight Americans, either in food production, distribution, or sales. In addition to state-sponsored terrorist groups, animal rights and vegetarian-motivated organizations may seek nonlegislative means to end animal agriculture in the United States or other countries. In addition to causing economic instability, such activity may result in widespread hunger or starvation, especially in developing nations with few resources. Recent intelligence has outlined the existence of extensive programs in the Soviet Union that specifically targeted agriculture and may have involved six agricultural research centers and up to 10,000 scientists and technicians. Some of the diseases described in this chapter could be used to attack domestic animals (brucellosis, glanders). In light of such threats to the food supply, several comprehensive food security plans for the United States have been proposed, including the Consolidated American Network for Agriculture Resource Intelligence system.

Preparation for Biological Attacks

Public Health and Governmental Responses

To defend against the threat of biological attack, national public health agencies need to develop rapid response plans for each of the potential agents of concern. These plans should contain methods of detection of an outbreak, means of diagnosis and the mechanisms to differentiate a biological attack from a naturally occurring event, effective therapies and plans for delivery to at-risk populations, and whenever possible, vaccines. Education of the medical community and public health workers is a vital component for protection of the public.

In the aftermath of the terrorist attacks of September 11, 2001, and the subsequent release of anthrax spores, President George W. Bush proposed a program to formerly counter the threat of biological, chemical, radiological, and nuclear attack in his 2003 State of the Union address. The Project BioShield Act was signed into law the following year. This project involves multiple agencies including the U.S. Department of Health and Human Services, the Department of Homeland Security, the CDC, the Food and Drug Administration, and the National Institutes of Health. It draws on the Special Reserve Fund, with $5.6 billion available over ten years, for the advanced development and purchase of medical countermeasures to these threats. Funded projects have included research into development of several anthrax vaccines, several anthrax therapeutics, and mass production of botulinum antitoxin and modified smallpox vaccines.

Detection of a Biological Attack

One of the keys to limiting the extent of human casualties following a biological attack is the ability to rapidly diagnose the associated disease and to determine whether the outbreak resulted from natural transmission or deliberate release of the biological agent. This may be difficult in the case of some organisms, such as *B. anthracis*, which bears many similarities to *B. cereus*, a nonpathogenic bacterium that is common in the environment. Assays have been developed, however, to detect the presence of a capsule, a virulence factor for *B. anthracis*. Portable handheld biosensors have also been developed for routine surveillance of microbes such as *B. anthracis*, *F. tularemia*, and *Y. pestis*. Bacteriophages, viruses that infect bacteria, have also been developed to specifically recognize or kill certain pathogenic bacteria.

Protective Vaccines

The threat of biological attack may be diminished by the presence of adequate stockpiles of effective protective vaccines. Such vaccines are now available for use against some of the agents described in this chapter. There is no vaccine currently available to protect against infection with many of the other agents, such as *Y. pestis* and most of the hemorrhagic fever viruses. Fortunately, many of the agents for which no vaccine is available may be neutralized with antibiotics or antitoxin. This section discusses work on the development of safe, effective vaccines against two biological agents of interest.

A vaccine against tularemia has recently been produced by engineering a recombinant bacterial vaccine designed to prevent infection with *F. tularensis*. This vaccine uses attenuated *Listeria monocytogenes*, which was engineered to express seven *F. tularensis* proteins. *L. monocytogenes* is similar to *F. tularensis* in that both dwell within cells. Mice immunized intradermally (through the skin) were protected against intranasal exposure to *F. tularensis*, which mimics airborne infection, and against aerosols of the highly virulent type A *F. tularensis* SchuS4 strain.

Production of the vaccinia vaccine for the prevention of smallpox was halted in the 1980s after the eradication of the variola virus from nature. Vaccinia vaccine was formerly obtained from the skin of infected animals or from chick embryos. It was administered by scarification of the skin using needles or bifurcated needles, by rotary lancets, or by jet injectors. Successful vaccination was determined by the production of a vesicle or pustule at the vaccination site seven to nine days later. Administration of the smallpox vaccine often resulted in adverse effects, some of which were severe or life-threatening. Up to 40% of the recipients experienced mild symptoms such as fever, muscle aches, malaise, and headache. The rate of development of more serious reactions was 40 to 400 cases per million vaccinations. Such reactions included generalized or progressive vaccinia, eczema vaccinatum, encephalitis or encephalopathy, Bell's palsy, Guillain-Barré syndrome, seizures, or death. These occurred more commonly among young children and individuals who had not previously been vaccinated. In 2002, the United States began development of a new smallpox vaccine known as Dryvax. This vaccine has decreased risk for the reactions previously cited but increased risk for developing cardiac manifestations such as cardiomyopathy, cardiac ischemia (decreased blood supply to heart), or heart attack. Vaccination is not recommended for immunocompromised persons, including pregnant women; individuals with a history of eczema, atopical dermatitis, or similar skin disorders; and those in contact with these individuals. More recent strategies have attempted to simplify vaccine production by growing the viruses in cultured animal cells and to make the vaccine safer for the currently counterindicated populations by weakening the virus or by producing vaccines using viral DNA or viral subunits (selected proteins).

To adequately protect human populations, such vaccine development needs to continue against other potential bioweapon agents. Development of vaccines against agricultural pathogens is also important to protect our food supplies. Such vaccines need to be safe, effective, and available to large enough segments of the population to prevent crippling attacks from persons or groups with ill will for other members of humanity.

Summary

Bacterial Bioweapons

- neumonic plague (*Yersinia pestis*) • pulmonary anthrax (*Bacillus anthracis*)
- tularemia (*Francisella tularensis*) • brucellosis (*Brucella* species) • Q fever (*Coxiella burnetii*) • epidemic typhus (*Rickettsia prowazekii*) • endemic typhus (*R. typhi*) • Rocky Mountain spotted fever (*R. rickettsii*) • glanders (*Burkholderia mallei*) • meliodiosis (*B. pseudomallei*)

Viral Bioweapons

- Smallpox (variola major) • viral hemorrhagic fevers (Ebola HFV, Marburg HFV, Lassa virus, Junin virus, Machupo virus, Guanarito virus, Sabia virus, Whitewater Arroyo virus, Rift Valley fever virus, Crimean-Congo HFV, yellow fever virus, Omsk HFV, and Kyasanur Forest disease virus) • viral encephalitis (Eastern, Western, and Venezuelan equine EV, St. Louis EV,

Murray Valley EV, Kunjin EV, West Nile virus, Japanese EV, Rocio virus, dengue virus, tickborne complex EV, Powassan virus, Louping ill virus, La Crosse virus, Toscana virus, lymphocytic choriomeningitis virus, Hendra virus, Nipah virus, and herpesvirus simiae B virus)

Toxins as Biological Weapons

Botulism neurotoxin A (*Clostridium botulinum*) • tetanus neurotoxin (*C. tetani*) • diphtheria toxin (*Corynebacterium diphtheria*) • exotoxin A (*Pseudomonas aeruginosa*) • pertussis toxin (*Bordetella pertussis*) • heat-labile enterotoxins (*Escherichia coli*) • Shiga toxin (*Shigella dysenteriae*) • cholera toxin (*Vibrio cholerae*)

Key Terms

Botulinum toxin A Toxin produced by *Clostridium botulinum*; inhibits muscle action, resulting in flaccid muscle paralysis, and may lead to respiratory failure and death if untreated

Brucellosis Disease resulting from infection with *Brucella* species; flu-like illness with protracted fever, muscle and joint pain, fatigue, malodorous perspiration, swollen lymph nodes, enlarged liver and spleen, arthritis, inflammation of the vertebrae and male reproductive tract, abscess formation, respiratory dysfunction, mild hepatitis, rash, build-up of fluid in the abdominal cavity, neurobrucellosis, and endocarditis

Buboes Swollen, reddened, extremely tender lymph nodes in the groin, axilla, or cervical regions

Bubonic plague One disease resulting from infection with *Yersinia pestis*; characterized by sudden onset of fever, chills, and weakness and production of buboes

Cutaneous anthrax One disease resulting from infection with *Bacillus anthracis*; characterized by an ulcerative skin lesion which later transforms into a black scab with a necrotic core surrounded by blood-stained fluid and edema prior to self-resolution

Endemic (murine) typhus Disease resulting from infection with *Rickettsia typhi* or *R. felis*; symptoms are similar to those of epidemic typhus, but milder

Epidemic (louseborne) typhus Disease resulting from infection with *Rickettsia prowazekii*; characterized by rash, high fever, stiffness, highly painful muscles and joints, cerebral dysfunction progressing to delirium and stupor, and blood clotting that clogs small blood vessels in the extremities, leading to gangrene

Gastrointestinal anthrax One disease resulting from infection with *Bacillus anthracis*; acquired by ingesting undercooked meat contaminated by spores

Glanders Disease resulting from infection with *Burkholderia mallei*; symptoms of pulmonary infection include chest pain, fever, pneumonia, pulmonary abscesses, pleural effusion, and ulcerative lesions of the nasal cavity; symptoms of septicemic infection include fever, muscle ache, headache, diarrhea, flushing and cyanosis of the skin, swollen regional lymph nodes, cellulitis, rapid heart rate, jaundice, multiorgan failure, and death

Inhalational (pulmonary) anthrax One disease resulting from infection with *Bacillus anthracis*; characterized by progressive respiratory distress, cyanosis with massive edema in the neck and chest, elevated pulse, respiration, and body temperature; rapidly fatal if untreated due to thrombosis of the pulmonary capillaries

Melioidosis Disease resulting from infection with *B. pseudomallei*; symptoms resemble those of glanders

Oculoglandular tularemia One infection resulting from infection with *Francisella tularensis*; characterized by ulceration of the cornea

Oropharyngeal tularemia One infection resulting from infection with *Francisella tularensis*; characterized by exudative pharyngitis or tonsillitis in the presence or absence of mucosal ulcers

Pneumonic plague One disease resulting from infection with *Yersinia pestis*; characterized by severe bronchopneumonia, chest pain, dyspnea, cough, and bloody sputum

Q (query) fever Disease resulting from infection with *Coxiella burnetii*: acute form is characterized by abrupt onset of fever, severe sweats, chills, headache, weakness, fatigue; chronic disease characterized by endocarditis, which is typically fatal if untreated

Respiratory tularemia (tularemia pneumonia) One infection resulting from infection with *Francisella tularensis*; characterized by dry cough, substernal pain or tightness, purulent sputum, difficulty breathing, rapid breathing rate, hemorrhagic airway inflammation, and hilar lymphadenopathy rapidly progressing to severe pneumonia, respiratory failure, and death

Rocky Mountain spotted fever Disease resulting from infection with *Rickettsia rickettsii*; characterized by rash, fever, deep muscle pain, malaise, chills, and conjunctival infection

Septicemic plague One disease resulting from infection with *Yersinia pestis*; characterized by disseminated intravascular coagulation, necrosis of small vessels, purpuric skin lesions, and gangrene in the digits or nose

Smallpox Disease resulting from infection with variola major; characterized by headache, myalgia, and a diffuse maculopapular rash progressing to the formation of vesicular eruptions on the head and extremities prior to their crusting

Tularemia sepsis One infection resulting from infection with *Francisella tularensis*; characterized by fever, abdominal pain, diarrhea, vomiting, confusion, coma septic shock, disseminated intravascular coagulation, acute respiratory distress syndrome, pericarditis, mild hepatitis, and multiorgan failure

Typhoidal tularemia One infection resulting from infection with *Francisella tularensis*; an acute flulike illness accompanied by diarrhea, vomiting, headache, chills, muscle and joint pain, prostration, and weight loss

Ulceroglandular tularaemia One infection resulting from infection with *Francisella tularensis*; characterized by fever, painful ulcerative skin lesions, and enlarged lymph nodes

Viral encephalitis Diseases resulting from members of the Togaviridae, Flaviviridae, Bunyaviridae, Arenaviridae, Paramyxoviridae, and Herpseviridae families of viruses; characterized by high fever, meningitis, confusion, stupor, coma, tremors, convulsions, and spastic paralysis

Viral hemorrhagic fevers Diseases resulting from infection with members of the Filoviridae, Arenaviridae, Bunyaviridae, and Flaviviridae families of viruses; symptoms include hemorrhagic manifestations such as petechiae, mucous membrane and conjunctival hemorrhages, bloody vomit, disseminated intravascular coagulation, and shock and central nervous system involvement such as delirium, convulsions, cerebellar dysfunction, and coma

Review Questions

1. What are the symptoms of pneumonic plague? What bacterium causes this disease and how is this form of infection acquired?
2. What diseases are caused by infection with *Rickettsia*? Name the responsible bacteria and how each is each transmitted.
3. Which viruses cause viral hemorrhagic fever? Name the disease associated with each.
4. Which viruses cause viral encephalitis?
5. What toxins have been considered for use as agents of bioterrorism? What organism produces each?

Topics for Further Discussion

1. In addition to the attacks described in this chapter, research other instances in which biological weapons were suspected to have been employed.
2. Research the plans currently in place for first-responders to rapidly respond to any of the diseases described in this chapter.
3. If you were a terrorist who planned to attack the U.S., the Russian Federation, or a European country, which bioweapon would you choose to use? Explain the reasons for your choice.
4. Discuss how the nations of the world may act in concert to decrease the likelihood of a biological attack.

Resources

Arnon, S. S., and others. "Botulinum Toxin as a Biological Weapon: Medical and Public Health Management." *Journal of the American Medical Association*, 2001, *285*, 1059–1070.

Azad, A. "Pathogenic Rickettsiae as Bioterrorism Agents." *Clinical Infectious Diseases*, 2007, *45*, S52–S55.

Bigalke, H., and Rummel, A. "Medical Aspects of Toxin Weapons." *Toxicology*, 2005, *214*, 210–220.

Borio, L., and others. "Hemorrhagic Fever Viruses as Biological Weapons: Medical and Public Health Management." *Journal of the American Medical Association*, 2002, *287*, 2391–2405.

Bossi, P., and others. "Bichat Guidelines for the Clinical Management of Glanders and Melioidosis and Bioterrorism-Related Glanders and Melioidosis," "Bichat Guidelines for the Clinical Management of Tularaemia and Bioterrorism-Related Tularaemia," and "Bichat Guidelines for the Clinical Management of Brucellosis and Bioterrorism-Related Brucellosis." *Eurosurveillance*, 2004, *9*.

Bossi, P., and others. "Bioterrorism: Management of Major Biological Agents." *Cellular and Molecular Life Science*, 2006, *63*, 2196–2212.

Chin, J. *Control of Communicable Diseases Manual* (17th ed.). Washington, D.C.: American Public Health Association, 2000.

Dennis, D. T., and others. "Tularemia as a Biological Weapon: Medical and Public Health Management." *Journal of the American Medical Association*, 2001, *285*, 2763–2773.

Inglesby, T. V., and others. "Plague as a Biological Weapon: Medical and Public Health Management." *Journal of the American Medical Association*, 2000, *283*, 2281–2290.

Jia, Q., and others. "Recombinant Attenuated *Listeria monocytogenes* Vaccine Expressing *Francisella tularensis* IglC Induces Protection in Mice Against Aerosolized Type A *F. tularensis*." *Vaccine*, 2009, *27*, 1216–1229.

Ligon, B. L. "Plague: A Review of Its History and Potential as a Biological Weapon." *Seminars in Pediatric Infectious Diseases*, 2006, *17*, 161–170.

Norton, R. A. "Agro-Terrorism: Biological Threats and Biosecurity Measures: Food Security Issues—a Potential Comprehensive Plan." *Poultry Science*, 2003, *82*, 958–963.

Pappas, G., Panagopoulou, P., Christou, L., and Akritidis, N. "Brucella as a Biological Weapon." *Cellular and Molecular Life Sciences*, 2006, *63*, 2229–2236.

Pohanka, M., and Skládal, P. "*Bacillus anthracis, Francisella tularensis* and *Yersinia pestis*: The Most Important Bacterial Warfare Agents." *Folia Microbiology*, 2009, *54*, 263–272.

Riedel, S. "Plague: From Natural Disease to Bioterrorism." *Baylor University Medical Center Proceedings*, 2005, *18*, 116–124.

Russell, P. K. "Project BioShield: What It Is, Why It Is Needed, and Its Accomplishments So Far." *Clinical Infectious Diseases*, 2007, *45*, S68–S72.

Stein, A., and others. "Q Fever Pneumonia: Virulence of *Coxiella burnetii* Pathovars in a Murine Model of Aerosol Infection." *Infection and Immunity*, 2005, *73*, 2469–2477.

Wiser, I, Balicer, R. D., and Cohen, D. "An Update on Smallpox Vaccine Candidates and Their Role in Bioterrorism-Related Vaccination Strategies." *Vaccine*, 2007, *25*, 976–984.

Acronyms

Aß amyloid ß

ABV adriamycin, bleomycin, and vincristine

ACE-2 angiotensin-converting enzyme 2

ADE antibody-dependent enhancement

AIDS acquired immunodeficiency syndrome

ALT alanine aminotransferase

APP amyloid precursor protein

Ara-C cytosine-arabinoside

ARC AIDS-related complex

AST aspartate aminotransferase

ATP adenosine triphosphate

AZT zidovudine

BA bacillary angiomatosis

BBB blood-brain barrier

BCG bacillus Calmette-Guérin

Bcl-2 B cell leukemia protein-2

BP bacillary peliosis hepatis

BSE bovine spongiform encephalopathy

BSL biosafety level

CA-MRSA community-associated methicillin-resistant *S. aureus*

CA-MSSA community-associated methicillin-susceptible *S. aureus*

CDK cyclin-dependent kinase

CDP CCAAT displacement protein

C/EBPε CCAAT enhancer binding protein epsilon

CFU colony-forming unit

CIA enhanced chemiluminescence immunoassay

CJD Creutzfeldt-Jakob disease

CMV cytomegalovirus

CNS central nervous system

COPD chronic obstructive pulmonary disease

COX-2 cyclooxygenase-2

CSD cat-scratch disease

CSF cerebrospinal fluid

CTLA-4 cytotoxic T-lymphocyte-associated antigen 4

DC dendritic cells

DC-SIGN dendritic cell-specific ICAM-3-grabbing nonintegrin

DEET N,N-diethyl-m-toluamide

DF dengue fever

DFH dengue hemorrhagic fever

DNA deoxyribonucleic acid

DOTS directly observed therapy, short-course

DRC Democratic Republic of the Congo

DSS dengue shock syndrome

EBV Epstein-Barr virus

ECG, EKG electrocardiograph

EHEC enterohemorrhagic E. coli

EIA enzyme immunoassay

ELISA enzyme-linked immunosorbent assay

EM erythema migrans

EMC essential mixed cryoglobulinemia

EPEC enteropathogenic *E. coli*

Epo erythropoietin

ESBL extended-spectrum ß-lactamase

espP enzyme that cleaves pepsin and human coagulation factor V, inhibiting blood clotting

ETAR 1-ß-d-ribofuranosyl-3-ethynyl-[1,2,4]triazole

EV encephalitis virus

FADD Fas-associated protein with death domain

FFI fatal familial insomnia

FLICE FADD-like interleukin-1 beta-converting enzyme

GAS group A streptococci

G-CSF granulocyte colony-stimulating factor

GERD gastroesophageal reflux disease

GI gastrointestinal

GM-CSF granulocyte-macrophage colony-stimulating factor

GSS Gerstmann-Straussler-Scheinker syndrome

GTP guanosine triphosphate

H hemagglutinin (protein on the surface of the influenza virus)

HAART highly active antiretroviral therapy

HA-MRSA hospital-acquired methicillin-resistant *S. aureus*

hCG human chorionic gonadotropin

HCV hepatitis C virus

HF hemorrhagic fever

HFRS hemorrhagic fever with renal syndrome

HGA human granulocytotropic anaplamosis

HHV-8 human herpesvirus-8; also known as Kaposi's sarcoma–associated herpesvirus

HIV human immunodeficiency virus

HLH hemophagocytic lymphohistiocytosis

HME human monocytotropic ehrlichiosis

HNP-1 human neutrophil peptide 1

HPS hantavirus pulmonary syndrome

HTLV human T lymphotropic virus

HUS hemolytic uremic syndrome

ICT immunochromatographic

IDO indoleamine 2,3-dioxygenase

IFA indirect fluorescent-antibody assay

IFN interferon

Ig immunoglobin

IL interleukin

IMPDH inosine 5'-monophosphage dehydrogenase

IP-10 interferon gamma-induced protein 10 kilodalton

IRF interferon regulatory factor

I-TAC interferon-inducible T cell alpha-chemoattractant

IV intravenous

KS Kaposi's sarcoma

LANA latency-associated nuclear antigen

LAV lymphadenopathy-associated virus

LD$_{50}$ lethal dose$_{50}$, the number of organisms required to kill 50% of a host

LEE locus of enterocyte effacement

LPS lipopolysaccharide

LTR long-terminal repeat

LUAT Lyme urine antigen test

MAC *M. avium* complex

MAPK mitogen-activated protein kinase

MCD multicentric Castleman's disease

M-CSF macrophage colony-stimulating factor

MDA5 melanoma differentiation-associated gene 5

MDM2 murine double minute 2 protein

MDR multidrug-resistant

MDR-TB multidrug-resistant TB

MGMT malachite green microtubule assay

MHC major histocompatibility complex

Mig monokine induced by IFN-gamma

Mip macrophage infectivity potentiator

MIP-1 migration inhibitory protein-1

MRI magnetic resonance imaging

mRNA messenger RNA

MRSA methicillin-resistant *S. aureus*

MS multiple schlerosis

MSM men who have sex with men

MyD88 myeloid differentiation protein 88

N neuraminidase (protein on the surface of the influenza virus)

NCR natural cytotoxicity receptor

NF-κB nuclear factor kappa of B lymphocytes

NK cells natural killer cells

NIH National Institutes of Health

NNRRI non-nucleoside-based RNA replicase inhibitors

NOS nitric oxide synthestase

NRRI nucleoside-based RNA replicase inhibitors

NSP nonstructural proteins

NTU nephrelometry turbidity units

OAS 2-5-oligoadenylate synthase

OspC outer surface protein C of *B. burgdorferi*

PCR polymerase chain reaction

PD-1 programmed death-1

PEL primary effusion lymphoma

PLA$_2$ phospholipase A$_2$

PPD purified protein derivative (in connection with tuberculosis)

PrP normal form of the prion protein

Rb retinoblastoma protein

RIA radioimmunoassay

RIBA recombinant immunoblot assay

RMSF Rocky Mountain spotted fever

RNA ribonucleic acid

RNAi interfering RNA

RNS reactive nitrogen species

ROS reactive oxygen species

RT-PCR reverse transcriptase polymerase chain reaction

SARS severe acute respiratory syndrome

SARS CoV SARS-associated coronavirus

siRNA small interfering RNA

SIV simian immunodeficiency virus

SNP single-nucleotide polymorphism

SNV Sin Nombre virus

ssrDNA sequencing small subunit ribosomal DNA sequencing

STARI southern tick-associated rash illness

STSS streptococcal toxic shock syndrome

Stx Shiga toxins

TB tuberculosis

TGF-ß transforming growth factor-beta

Th1 T helper cell type 1

Th2 T helper cell type 2

Th17 T helper cell type 17

TK thymidine kinase

TLR toll-like receptor

TNF-α tumor necrosis factor-alpha

Tpo thrombopoietin

Treg regulatory T lymphocytes

TREM triggering receptor expressed on myeloid cells

tRNA transfer RNA

TSE transmissible spongiform encephalopathies

TTP thrombotic thrombocytopenic purpura

UK-UPRT bifunctional uridine kinase/uracil phosphoribosyltransferase

UPRT uracil phosphoribosyltransferase

vCJD variant Creutzfeldt-Jakob disease

VEGF vascular endothelial growth factor

VEGFR vascular endothelial growth factor receptor-2

vFLIP v-FLICE inhibitory protein

vGPCR viral G protein-coupled receptor

VISA *S. aureus* strains with intermediate resistance to vancomycin

VRE vancomycin-resistant enterococci

VRSA vancomycin-resistant *S. aureus*

WHO World Health Organization

XDR-TB extensively drug-resistant TB

Medical Terms, Prefixes, and Suffixes

A- without, lacking

Acaricides chemicals that kill ticks and mites

Acidic having a pH less than 7

Actin protein component of the cell's cytoskeleton; also involved in skeletal muscle contraction

Active immunization induction of an immune response against a specific agent by the individual's own immune system

Adaptive immunity highly specific immune response that produces memory cells and takes several weeks or longer to generate; due to the action of T and B lymphocytes

Aerobic respiration a process vital to human life that requires oxygen and produces large amounts of ATP from glucose; occurs within mitochondria

AIDS usually fatal final stage of infection with HIV; may be characterized by low numbers of $CD4^+$ T helper cells, wasting, opportunistic infections, malignancies, and dementia

Alanine aminotransferase (ALT) liver enzyme whose levels are often altered in disease states

Allograft transplant received from a different person

Alpha helical protein structure pattern of protein folding that resembles a helix (spiral staircase)

Alveoli terminal air sacs of the lungs

Amino acids building blocks of proteins

Amyloid plaques deposits of tangled amyloid protein in the brain; occurs in several diseases, including Alzheimer's disease

Anaerobic bacteria bacteria that cannot survive in the presence of oxygen

Anchorage-independent growth ability of cancer cells to grow in the absence of attachment to a stratum

Anemia low levels of red blood cells

Angioblastic involving increased blood supply

Angiogenesis production of new blood vessels

Anorexia decreased appetite and food intake

Antibodies immune proteins that bind to one specific antigen

Antigen material that stimulates an immune response

Aphasia decreased ability to comprehend spoken or written language due to brain damage

Apicomplexa protozoan phylum that includes *Plasmodium, Babesia,* and *Cryptosporidium* species

Apoptosis a process of orderly programmed cell death in which cells actively induce a cascading set of enzymatic reactions due to the caspases that ultimately lead to cell death and division of cellular contents into small membrane-enclosed apoptotic bodies that are removed by phagocytic cells without producing inflammation

Arenal cortex outer portion of the adrenal gland; produces several hormones, including the corticosteroids

Arthralgia painful joints

Ascites accumulation of fluid in the abdominal cavity

-ase degradative enzyme

Ashkenazi Jews Jewish persons of eastern European origin

Asplenic lacking a spleen

Astrocyte one type of glia (support cell) of the central nervous system

Astrocytosis increased numbers of astrocytes

Asymptomatic without symptoms

Ataxia unsteadiness and loss of coordination

ATP (adenosine triphosphate) major energy source for cells; produced by aerobic respiration from glucose

Attenuated vaccine vaccine using live, weakened organisms

Autocrine stimulation cell is stimulated by material that it produced itself

Autoimmune immune system attack on the individual's own body components

Autonomic nervous system the portions of the nervous system controlling involuntary actions; composed of sympathetic, parasympathetic, and enteric branches

Autosomal trait characteristics not encoded by the X or Y chromosome

Axilla armpit region

B7.2 cell surface receptor found on T lymphocytes whose binding is required for proper cellular activation; T lymphocyte stimulation in the absence of the binding of B7.2 to its ligand leads to an inability of the T lymphocyte to mount an immune response

B lymphocytes (B cells) cells of the adaptive immune response that produce antibodies

Bacteremia the growth of bacteria in the blood

Bactericide substance that kills bacteria

Bacteriophage virus that infects bacteria

Basal ganglia areas of gray matter deep within the cerebral hemispheres that produce the neurotransmitter dopamine

Basic having a pH greater than 7

Basophil white blood cell involved in inducing allergic reactions

Bcl-2 protein that inhibits apoptosis

Bell's palsy paralysis affecting half of the face

Beta pleated sheet pattern of protein folding that resembles a flattened accordian

Bilirubin a highly toxic breakdown product of hemoglobin

Binary fision asexual form of reproduction that produces two identical offspring

Biofilms complex microbial communities that have adhered to a substrate

Cachexia wasting

Calcium (Ca⁺) ion critical for nervous signal conduction and muscular activity; also serves as an intracellular signaling molecule necessary for the action of numerous enzymes

Carcinoma tumor of the skin or epithelial lining of internal organs

Carditis inflammation of the heart

Caseous cheese-like material

Caspases series of enzymes that increase mitochondrial membrane permeability and lead to cell death by apoptosis

Category A HIV infection initial stage of infection; either asymptomatic or characterized by lymphadenopathy

Category B HIV infection stage of infection characterized by conditions such as thrush, fever, or diarrhea persisting for greater than a month, and shingles; formerly known as AIDS-related complex

Category C HIV infection full-blown AIDS

CD4⁺ T helper cells subset of T lymphocytes that aid other leukocytes through production of cytokines

CD8⁺ T killer cells subset of T lymphocytes that kill virally infected cells and malignant cells

Cell-mediated immunity major type of the immune response that is due to the action of leukocytes as opposed to humoral immunity that involves the action of antibodies

Cellulitis inflammation of cellular tissue, particularly subcutaneous tissue

Central nervous system brain and spinal cord

Cerebellum region in the posterior, dorsal brain that coordinates balance and posture and regulates fine movements

Cerebrospinal fluid fluid that circulates through the ventricles of the brain and bathes the spinal cord

Cerebrum largest region of the brain; involved in thought, memory, awareness, and perception of sensations

Cervical region neck

Chemokines chemotactic cytokines

Chemotaxis movement toward a chemical attractant

Cholecystitis disorder in which large gallstones block movement of bile from the gallbladder into the duodenum

Chorea involuntary twitching movements

Chromosome linear or circular strands of DNA and histone proteins that serve as genetic material and encode the information necessary to produce RNA

Circadian rhythm wake-sleep cycle

Cirrhosis scarring of the liver

Coagulation clotting of the blood

Colitis inflammation of the large intestine that may lead to abdominal pain and bloating, bloody stools, diarrhea, urge to defecate, increased gas production, dehydration, chills and fever

Collectins defense proteins that bind sugars on microbial surfaces and help the immune system to kill these invaders by the action of phagocytes or the complement system

Columnar epithelium epithelium with rectangular cells

Complement enzymatic cascade that results in lysis of the targeted cell or microorganism

Conjunctivitis inflammation of the mucous membrane lining the underside of the eyelid

Constitutive production continual production of a material

Consumption tuberculosis

Corticosteroids immunosuppressive stress hormones produced from cholesterol in the adrenal cortex

Cryoglobins unusual antibodies that tend to precipitate out of solution at temperatures below that of the human body

Cutaneous associated with the skin

Cyanosis bluish cast to the skin; may result from inadequate amount of blood oxygen

Cyclins and cyclin-dependent kinases (CDKs) proteins that positively regulate passage through the cell cycle, leading to cell division

-cyte cell

Cytokines immune mediator molecules

Cytopathic effect death of cells following formation of syncytia

-cytosis increased levels of a cell type

Cytoskeleton flexible cellular framework composed of microtubules, microfilaments, and intermediate filaments

Definitive host host species in which sexual reproduction occurs

Denaturation in a protein, the process of changing shape; typically results in a loss of protein function

Desiccation state of extreme dryness following excessive water loss

Dihydrofolate reductase enzyme that participates in the production of folate, necessary for nucleic acid production during cell division

Dimorphic fungi fungi that can change from a yeast (unicellular) to mold form

Disseminated infection infection that has spread from its point of origin

Disseminated intravascular coagulopathy disorder in which the blood-clotting process is overly active, leading to the formation of small clots that may clog blood vessels and block the supply of oxygen to organs

DNA (deoxyribonucleic acid) nucleic acid that is the hereditary material for most forms of life; produces RNA

Duodenum first portion of the small intestine

Dysesthesia unpleasant distortion of the sense of touch

Dyspenia difficulty breathing

Dystonia loss of muscle tone

Echocardiograph device that uses the differential transmission and reflection of ultrasonic waves to determine abnormalities of the heart

Electroencephalogram graph of the electrical activity of the brain

-emia presence of material in the blood

Empyema accumulation of pus in a body cavity, especially the pleural cavity containing the lungs

Encephalitis inflammation of the brain

Endemic native to a region

Endocarditis inflammation of the inner membrane surrounding the heart

Endoplasmic reticulum membranous cellular organelle that process nascent proteins

Endothelium simple squamous epithelium lining blood vessels

Enteric involving the gut

Enteric nervous system branch of the autonomic nervous system that innervates the gut

Enterocolitis inflammation of the small intestine and colon

Enzootic present among the animals of a given region

Eosinophilia increased numbers of eosinophils; often associated with allergic reactions or infection by parasites

Epicarditis inflammation of the external covering of the heart

Epidemic large-scale outbreak of infectious disease with high morbidity or mortality rates

Epithelium (epithelial cells) type of a membranous cellular tissue that covers surfaces and lines interior regions of organs and blood vessels

Epitope region of an antigen that reacts with lymphocyte receptors

Erythema marginatum pinkish-red macular lesions with a central area of clearing

Erythema nodosum painful, nodular inflammatory lesions of dermal and subcutaneous tissue

Erythematous rash reddened rash

Erythroblastopenia low numbers of immature red blood cells

Erythrocyte red blood cell

Essential mixed cryoglobulinemia noncancerous lymphoproliferative disease B cells

Estrogens female sex hormones that suppress several parts of the immune response

Exogenous of outside origin; added

Extra- outside of

Extracellular found outside of cells

Extrapulmonary present outside of the lungs

Flagellum (*pl.*, flagella) long, whiplike projection from the plasma membrane that propels cells

Florid plaques brain pathology found in Creutzfeldt-Jakob disease; a central area that stains with the red dye eosin is surrounded by a region of spongiform degeneration

Focal localized

Ganglion (*pl.*, ganglia) swollen area along nerves that contains neuron cell bodies outside of the central nervous system

Gangrene localized area of tissue death due to inadequate blood supply to the area

Gastric referring to the stomach

Gastric mucosa cells composing the inner layer of the stomach; they secrete pepsin, hydrochloric acid, and mucus, this last of which protects the stomach from the acidic conditions

Genesis origin; beginning

Genotype sum total of genes inherited by an offspring from its parent

Glial cells neural support cells

Glomerulonephritis inflammation of the glomeruli in the nephron of the kidneys

Gluconeogenesis generation of glucose from materials that are not carbohydrates (sugars or starches)

Glucose monosaccharide sugar that is vital for human energy production

Glutamine amino acid vital for human life

Granuloma aggregation of macrophages, lymphocytes, or fibroblasts

Helminth worm

Hemangiomatous lesions blood-filled lesions

Hematological malignancies cancers of the white blood cells; leukemias and lymphomas

Hematopoiesis production of erythrocytes, leukocytes, and platelets; usually a function of red bone marrow

Hematuria bloody urine

Hemo- pertaining to blood

Hemoconcentration increased concentration of red blood cells due to water loss from the circulatory system

Hemolymph blood-like fluid in the circulatory system of insects

Hemolysis lysis of red blood cells

Hemolytic anemia low level of red blood cells due to their lysis

Hepatic referring to the liver

Hepatitis inflammation of the liver

Hepatomegaly enlargement of the liver

Hepatosplenomegaly enlargement of the spleen and liver

Heterogeneous consisting of a mixture of differing components

Hippocampus region of brain involved in memory formation

HIV human immunodeficiency virus

Homologous similar

Horizontal transmission transmission of an agent between members of a species that does not involve passage from parent to offspring

Humoral immunity antibody-based immune response

Huntington's disease inherited progressive neurodegenerative disease characterized by involuntary movements and dementia

Hyper- over, greater than

Hyperplasia excessive growth

Hypo- under, less than

Hypogammaglobinemia low levels of gamma globulins, including antibodies

Hypoglycemia low levels of blood sugar

Hyponatremia decreased urine output

Hypotension low blood pressure

Hypothermia low body temperature

Hypoxia low blood oxygen levels

Iatrogenic associated with a medical procedure

ICAM-1 cellular recognition molecule found on cells of the immune system

Ileum third and final section of the small intestine

Immune complexes large complexes of antigens and antibodies that may lodge in areas such as joints and kidney tubules, activating complement and resulting in inflammation

Immunocompetent having a fully functional immune system

Immunocompromised (immunosuppressed) having an immune system that is not fully functional

Inflammation (inflammatory condition) state characterized by redness, swelling, pain, and heat

Inguinal region groin area

Innate immunity inborn, nonspecific, and immediate immune response to pathogenic conditions; does not lead to the production of memory cells

Inter- between

Interferons antiviral cytokines

Interleukins group of cytokines produced by leukocytes

Intestinal villi multiple protrusions from the cells lining the intestine; increase the surface area to allow increased absorption of nutrients

Intra- within

Intracellular found inside cells

Intranasal route entry via the nostrils

Intramuscular route entry via the muscles

Intravenous (IV) route entry via the veins

-itis inflammation

In vitro occurring outside of living organisms or cells ("in glass")

In vivo occurring in a live organism or within cells ("in life")

Jaundice yellowish coloration of the skin and eyes

Keritinization addition of the tough, water-proofing keratin protein to an area

Kinases enzymes that attach phosphate ions onto other molecules, including proteins

Kinins compounds that affect blood flow and blood pressure and aid in tissue repair

Lamina propria connective tissue underlying the lining of organs

Langerhans cells dendriticlike cells of the skin and mucous membranes

Leuko- white

Leukocyte white blood cell

Leukocytosis increased white blood cell count

Leukopenia decreased white blood cell numbers

Lichen planus autoimmune disease with chronic dermal or intraorbital keratinization

Lipid fat or oil

Lipid rafts specialized functional areas of a cell's plasma membrane that contain large amounts of lipid that vary depending on the function of a given raft

Liposomes fat droplets

Lymphadenopathy swollen lymph nodes

Lymphoblasts dividing lymphocytes

Lymphocytes white blood cells that produce adaptive immunity

Lymphocytosis elevated white blood cell numbers

Lymphoma cancer of lymphocytes that forms a solid tumor mass

Lymphopenia low numbers of blood lymphocytes

Lysosome cellular organelle that is filled by digestive enzymes at low pH; aids in degradation of proteins and ingested microbes

Lytic infection viral infection that results in the destruction of the host cell

M cells specialized cells associated with Peyer's patches that take up particulate matter from the intestinal contents, including infectious material

Macular lesions flat lesions

Major histocompatibility class I (MHC I) antigens glycoproteins expressed on the surface of most nucleated cells in the body; required to present antigen to and activate $CD8^+$ T killer cells

Major histocompatibility class II (MHC II) antigens glycoproteins expressed only on the surface of specialized "antigen-presenting cells"; required to present antigen to and activate $CD4^+$ T helper cells

Macrogametocyte cell that gives rise to the "female" macrogamete in the life cycle of *Plasmodium* species

Macrophage mature, tissue form of a monocyte; phagocytic cell that produces several cytokines and aids in the stimulation of $CD4^+$ T helper cells; part of the innate immune system

Malaise generalized feeling of unwellness

Malignancy cancer

Megakaryocyte hematopoietic cell type that produces platelets

Meiosis form of cell division that produces male and female gametes while halving the amount of genetic information per gamete

Meninges three layers of material covering the brain and spinal cord

Meningitis inflammation of the meninges

Merozoite asexual reproduction stage in the lifecycle of Plasmodium and Babesia species; infects erythrocytes

Mesangial cells primitive stem cells

Metabolic acidosis excessive amounts of acid are present in body fluids

Metastasis movement of cancerous cells out of the confines of the original location

Microgametocyte cell that gives rise to the "male" microgamete in the life cycle of *Plasmodium* species

Mitochondria cellular organelles that produce energy in the form of ATP by aerobic respiration

Mitogen-activated protein kinase (MAPK) intracellular signaling pathway involved in the division of many cell types

Mitosis form of cell division in which two identical daughter cells are produced

Molluscum contaginiosum viral infection that results in raised, pearl-like papules or skin nodules

Monoclonal antibodies identical antibodies produced by the descendants of a single B lymphocyte

Monocyte phagocytic immune cell found in the blood; immature macrophage

Morbidity rate proportion of illness in a region or due to a particular disease

Mortality rate proportion of deaths in a region or due to a particular disease

mRNA messenger RNA; used as a template for the production of proteins

Multinucleated giant cells huge, hollow, balloonlike cells resulting from the fusion of many small cells; also known as *syncytia*

Myalgia muscle aches

Myocardial pertaining to the heart muscle

Myonecrosis death of muscle tissue

Myositis inflammation of muscle tissue

Necrotic lesion lesion filled with dead cells

Negative-sense RNA virus virus whose genomic DNA is used to produce mRNA that codes for proteins

Nephritis inflammation of the nephrons of the kidneys

Neuritis inflammation of a nerve

Neuromuscular junction area of contact between the axon of a motor neuron and the muscle that it stimulates

Neuropathy nerve pain

Neuropil interwoven network of extensions from neurons and glial cells in the central nervous system

Neurosyphilis progressive destruction of the brain and spinal cord by *Treponema pallidum*

Neutralizing antibody antibody that blocks entry of microbes or toxins into cells

Neutropenia decreased neutrophil number

Neutrophil phagocytic immune cell found in the blood

NF-κ transcription factor involved in activating transcription of many genes involved in immune responses and in cell growth

Nocturnal primarily active at night

Nosocomial infection infection acquired in a hospital setting

Nucleus region of the cell that contains the majority of DNA in the form of chromosomes

Nymph immature life cycle stage occurring during the incomplete metamorphosis of insects; resembles the adult but lacks wings

Obligate aerobes organisms requiring oxygen for growth

Obligate intracellular parasite organisms that must live within cells of another species

-oma cancer

Oncogenes genes associated with cancer; often related to cellular growth

Oocyst hardy, cystlike life cycle stage found in Apicomplexa protozoa

Ookinete mobile zygote stage of *Plasmodium* species

Opportunistic infection pathogenic infection with an organism that is generally not harmful to immunocompetent individuals

Opsonization process that enhances uptake of bacteria by phagocytic cells

Osteolytic lesion area of bone lysis

Osteomyelitis inflammation of the bone marrow

Otitis media inner ear infection

Outbreak (disease outbreak) greater occurrence of disease than is expected to occur in a particular time and place

p27^{kip} protein that functions as part of the cell's normal feedback mechanism to prevent excessive cell growth; inhibits the action of CDK6 during cell division

Pandemic worldwide epidemic with high morbidity or mortality rates

Papular lesions palpable lesions

Parasitemia presence of parasites dividing in the blood

Parenteral route material enters the body by injection

Passive immunization transference of preformed immune components to an individual

Pasteurization heating of a liquid to 142°F to 145°F for 30 minutes to destroy microbes

PCR very sensitive method of detecting specific DNA regions

-penia decreased levels of a cell type

Pericardial cavity chest cavity surrounding the heart

Pericarditis inflammation of the outer membrane surrounding the heart

Pericrine stimulation cell is stimulated by material produced by surrounding cells

Peritoneal cavity upper abdominal cavity

Peritonitis inflammation of the peritoneal cavity

Petechial rash collection of bright red spots in the skin resulting from leakage of blood from the underlying capillaries

Peyer's patches small areas of lymphatic tissue scattered throughout the gut wall

Phagocytosis ingestion of microbes, cells, or cell debris by neutrophils, monocytes, or macrophages

Phagosome internal vacuole in neutrophils, monocytes, and macrophages produced during phagocytosis

Phosphatidylinositol-glycolipid tail unusual chemical group linked to the end of some proteins which serves as an anchor to the plasma membrane

Piroplasms parasites belonging to the *Babesia* genus

Plasma cells antibody-producing B lymphocytes

Plasma membrane lipid bilayer studded with proteins that encloses cells and selectively allows material to enter or exit

Plasmids circular, extrachromosomal DNA found in some bacteria

Pleural cavity chest cavity surrounding the lungs

Pneumonitis inflammatory lesion of the alveoli of the lungs and interstitial spaces

Point mutation change of one nucleotide in DNA or RNA

Polyprotein fused proteins produced from a single mRNA in some viral species

Porphyria cutanea tarda abnormal sensitivity to sun exposure and liver damage due to excessive iron deposition in the liver

Positive-sense RNA virus virus whose genomic RNA codes for proteins

Postauricular region area behind the ear

Postpartum after birth

Prion small proteinaceous infectious particle that resists inactivation by procedures that modify nucleic acids

Proctitis inflammation of the tissue of the rectum

Prodrome early warning sign or group of signs

Prostaglandins class of small molecules that are released during inflammatory responses and increase sensitivity to pain

Prostration being unable to rise from a position of lying

Protease enzyme that degrades proteins

Protease-resistant proteins that are resistant to degradation by proteases

Protease-sensitive proteins that are susceptible to degradation by proteases

Protein long chain of amino acids produced by translation from an mRNA template

Protein kinase C enzyme that adds the phosphate group onto proteins as a part of intracellular signal transduction

Proteinuria presence of protein in the urine

Protozoa single-celled animals

Provirus latent form of a virus integrated into the host's DNA

Pulmonary edema accumulation of fluid in the lungs

Pulmonary infarction dead area of the lung

Pulvinar sign high intensity signal from the pulvinar region of the thalamus detected by magnetic resonance imaging

Purines nucleic acids guanine and adenine

Pustular lesions lesions containing pus

Pyrimidines nucleic acids cytosine, thymine, and uracil

Pyrogenic inducing fever

Quasispecies closely related species differing by small mutations; often involves viruses with a high mutation rate such as HIV

Rehydration restoring body fluid levels

Renal pertaining to the kidneys

Reticulocytes immature red blood cells

Retinitis inflammation of the retina

Retrograde axonal transmission transmission of material from the axon toward the neuron cell body

Retroorbital behind the eye

Rheumatoid arthritis autoimmune disease in which synovial tissues are damaged

Ribosomes cellular organelles that contain protein and rRNA; site of protein synthesis

RNA (ribonucleic acid) nucleic acid that produces proteins and may serve as the hereditary material for some viruses

RNAi group of small, interfering RNA molecules that inhibit protein synthesis

RNA polymerases enzymes that synthesize RNA

rRNA (ribosomal RNA) RNA found within ribosomes

RT-PCR very sensitive method of detecting the presence of specific mRNA

Saprophyte organism that grows and feeds on dead organic material

Sarcoma tumor of connective tissue

Schizogony form of asexual reproduction in apicomplexan parasites that results in multiple progeny (*merozoites*)

Septic shock syndrome hypotension, respiratory distress syndrome or failure, and abnormal functioning of the central nervous system, liver, kidneys, or muscles

Septicemia blood infection

Seropositive producing antibodies to a given material

Shingles herpes zoster; inflammation due to reactivation of infection with varicella virus, the causative agent of chickenpox

Sjögrens's syndrome autoimmune syndrome in which production of tears and saliva are decreased

Sodium (Na$^+$) ion critical for the conduction of nervous impulses

Spleen immune system organ that houses many antibody-producing B lymphocytes and macrophages

Splenomegaly enlarged spleen

Spongiform degeneration brain pathology due to the presence of many small holes

Sporozoite infective stage in the life cycle of Apicomplexa protozoa, achieved through sexual reproduction

Sputum material, such as mucus mixed with pus and saliva, expectorated from the respiratory passageways

Squamous epithelium epithelium with flattened cells

Strictures narrowed region of an area such as the intestine or esophagus

Subcutaneous under the skin

Submandibular region area under the lower jaw

Substance P neurotransmitter involved in pain perception

Substernal pain pain occurring beneath the sternum (breastbone)

Superantigen antigen that causes large-scale stimulation of the immune response

Sydenham's chorea spasmatic muscular movements and incoordination

Synaptic conduction transmission of a signal between neurons

Syncytia multinucleated giant cells

Systemic occurring throughout the body

T helper cells $CD4^+$ T lymphocytes

T killer cells $CD8^+$ T lymphocytes

T lymphocytes (T cells) immune cells of the adaptive immune system that respond in a highly specific manner

Tachycardia rapid heart rate

Tachypnea rapid breathing

Telomerase enzyme that allows cells to escape the normal capping of cell growth after 40–60 divisions

Th1 immune response immune response produced by a subset of T helper cells; correlates with the production of cell-mediated immunity

Th2 immune response immune response produced by a subset of T helper cells; correlates with the production of humoral immunity

Thalamus region of the midbrain that associates sensations with emotions

ß-thalassemia genetic disorder that leads to abnormally low levels of mutant hemoglobin in red blood cells

Thrombocyte platelet

Thrombocytopenia low platelet numbers

Thrombus blood clot

Thrush infection of the oral cavity with the yeast *Candida*

Thymus immune system organ that is responsible for the selection and maturation of T lymphocytes; active thymic tissue decreases as a function of age

Tinnitus ringing in the ears

Toll-like receptors receptors on cells of the innate immune system that recognize molecules from microorganisms

Toxoids inactivated toxins that may be used for vaccination

Transcription process of forming RNA from a DNA template

Transcription factors molecules that stimulate the transcription of a specific set of genes

Transformation process of producing a malignant cell

Translation process of forming a protein from an mRNA template

Transovarial transmitted from mother to offspring during gestation

Transposon "jumping gene": small region of DNA that may duplicate itself and move to other areas of the same chromosome or to other chromosomes

Transstadial transmission transmission of a microbe from one developmental form of a vector to the next

Treg cells regulatory subset of CD4$^+$ T cells

tRNA (transfer RNA) RNA that transports amino acids to the ribosome to be added to the growing protein chain during translation

Trophozoites feeding form

Tumor suppressor genes genes that protect against the development of cancer either by halting division of cells with damaged DNA in order to repair the damage or by killing cells that are unable to be repaired

Type IV hypersensitivity reaction slow-developing allergic reaction caused by activity of T lymphocytes and macrophages

Tyrosine kinases enzymes that add a phosphate group onto the tyrosine amino acid of proteins, often upregulating or downregulating their activity

Valvulitis inflammation of the valves of the heart

Variolation inoculation with infectious matter derived from persons suffering from mild cases of smallpox in the hopes of preventing the later development of severe smallpox

Vascular endothelial growth factor (VEGF) molecule that encourages formation of new blood vessels by stimulating growth of endothelial cells

Vasculitis inflammation of blood vessels

Vasodilation enlargement in diameter of blood vessels

Vertical transmission transmission of an agent from parent to offspring

Vesicular lesions fluid-filled lesions

Viral vector virus containing regions of foreign DNA or RNA; used to stimulate immune responses to the proteins produced by the foreign DNA or RNA

Viremic having viruses present in the blood

Virulence factor factor that increases pathogenicity of a microbe

Virulent characterized by a rapid, severe, destructive course

Xenotransplants transplants using organs from a different species

Yeast unicellular fungi

Zoonotic infection (zoonosis) infection entering the human population from animals

Zygote cell resulting from the union of two gametes prior to its first division